CURRENT THERAPY IN
INFECTIOUS DISEASE - 3

Medical Titles in the Current Therapy Series

CURRENT THERAPY IN
INFECTIOUS DISEASE - 3

EDWARD H. KASS, PH.D., M.D., SC.D.(HON.), M.A. (HON.)

William Ellery Channing
Professor of Medicine, Emeritus
Channing Laboratory
Harvard Medical School

Senior Physician
Brigham and Women's Hospital
Boston, Massachusetts

RICHARD PLATT, M.D.

Assistant Professor of Medicine
Harvard Medical School

Hospital Epidemiologist
Brigham and Women's Hospital
Boston, Massachusetts

B.C. DECKER INC • Toronto • Philadelphia

Publisher

B.C. Decker Inc
3228 South Service Road
Burlington, Ontario   L7N 3H8

B.C. Decker Inc
320 Walnut Street
Suite 400
Philadelphia, Pennsylvania   19106

Sales and Distribution

United States and Puerto Rico
The C.V. Mosby Company
11830 Westline Industrial Drive
Saint Louis, Missouri   63146

Canada
McAinsh & Co. Ltd.
2760 Old Leslie Street
Willowdale, Ontario   M2K 2X5

Australia
McGraw-Hill Book Company Australia Pty. Ltd.
4 Barcoo Street
Roseville East 2069
New South Wales, Australia

Brazil
Editora McGraw-Hill do Brasil, Ltda.
rua Tabapua, 1.105, Itaim-Bibi
Sao Paulo, S.P. Brasil

Colombia
Interamericana/McGraw-Hill de Colombia, S.A.
Apartado Aereo 81078
Bogota, D.E. Colombia

Europe
McGraw-Hill Book Company GmbH
Lademannbogen 136
D-2000 Hamburg 63
West Germany

France
MEDSI/McGraw-Hill
6, avenue Daniel Lesueur
75007 Paris, France

Hong Kong and China
McGraw-Hill Book Company
Suite 618, Ocean Centre
5 Canton Road
Tsimshatsui, Kowloon
Hong Kong

India
Tata McGraw-Hill Publishing Company, Ltd.
12/4 Asaf Ali Road, 3rd Floor
New Delhi 110002, India

Indonesia
P.O. Box 122/JAT
Jakarta, 1300 Indonesia

Italy
McGraw-Hill Libri Italia, s.r.l.
Piazza Emilia, 5
I-20129 Milano MI
Italy

Japan
Igaku-Shoin Ltd.
Tokyo International P.O. Box 5063
1-28-36 Hongo, Bunkyo-ku,
Tokyo 113, Japan

Korea
C.P.O. Box 10583
Seoul, Korea

Malaysia
No. 8 Jalan SS 7/6B
Kelana Jaya
47301 Petaling Jaya
Selangor, Malaysia

Mexico
Interamericana/McGraw-Hill de Mexico, S.A. de C.V.
Cedro 512, Colonia Atlampa
(Apartado Postal 26370)
06450 Mexico, D.F., Mexico

New Zealand
McGraw-Hill Book Co. New Zealand Ltd.
5 Joval Place, Wiri
Manukau City, New Zealand

Panama
Editorial McGraw-Hill Latinoamericana, S.A.
Apartado Postal 2036
Zona Libre de Colon
Colon, Republica de Panama

Portugal
Editora McGraw-Hill de Portugal, Ltda.
Rua Rosa Damasceno 11A–B
1900 Lisboa, Portugal

South Africa
Libriger Book Distributors
Warehouse Number 8
''Die Ou Looiery''
Tannery Road
Hamilton, Bloemfontein 9300

Southeast Asia
McGraw-Hill Book Co.
348 Jalan Boon Lay
Jurong, Singapore 2261

Spain
McGraw-Hill/Interamericana de Espana, S.A.
Manuel Ferrero, 13
28020 Madrid, Spain

Taiwan
P.O. Box 87–601
Taipei, Taiwan

Thailand
632/5 Phaholyothin Road
Sapan Kwai
Bangkok 10400
Thailand

United Kingdom, Middle East and Africa
McGraw-Hill Book Company (U.K.) Ltd.
Shoppenhangers Road
Maidenhead, Berkshire
SL6 2QL England

Venezuela
McGraw-Hill/Interamericana, C.A.
2da. calle Bello Monte
(entre avenida Casanova y Sabana Grande)
Apartado Aereo 50785
Caracas 1050, Venezuela

NOTICE

The authors and publisher have made every effort to ensure that the patient care recommended herein, including choice of drugs and drug dosages, is in accord with the accepted standards and practice at the time of publication. However, since research and regulation constantly change clinical standards, the reader is urged to check the product information sheet included in the package of each drug, which includes recommended doses, warnings, and contraindications. This is particularly important with new or infrequently used drugs.

Current Therapy in Infectious Disease – 3

ISBN 1-55664-066-8

Library of Congress catalog card number: 86-643210   7/15/91   10 9 8 7 6 5 4 3 2 1

CONTRIBUTORS

DONALD ARMSTRONG, M.D.

Professor of Medicine, Cornell University Medical
College; Chief, Infectious Disease Service, and
Director, Microbiology Laboratory, Memorial Sloan-
Kettering Cancer Center, New York, New York
Antifungal Chemotherapy

MARK D. ARONSON, M.D.

Associate Professor of Medicine, Harvard Medical
School; Physician, Beth Israel Hospital, Boston,
Massachusetts
Pharyngitis

MICHAEL C. BACH, M.D., FRCPC

Clinical Professor of Medicine, University of Vermont
School of Medicine, Burlington, Vermont; Assistant
Chief, Division of Infectious Diseases, Maine Medical
Centre, Portland, Maine
Nocardial Infection

ANN SULLIVAN BAKER, M.D.

Assistant Professor of Medicine, Harvard Medical
School; Chief, Infectious Disease, Massachusetts Eye
and Ear Infirmary; Associate Physician, Infectious
Disease Unit, Massachusetts General Hospital, Boston,
Massachusetts
Endophthalmitis

ROBERT S. BALTIMORE, M.D., F.A.A.P.

Associate Professor of Pediatrics and Epidemiology,
Yale University School of Medicine; Attending
Pediatrician, Yale-New Haven Hospital, New Haven,
Connecticut
Infection in the Newborn

DOUGLAS J. BARRETT, M.D.

Associate Professor and Chief, Division of
Immunology, Department of Pediatrics, University of
Florida College of Medicine, Gainesville, Florida
Immunodeficiency Disorders in Infants and Children

THOMAS R. BEAM Jr., M.D.

Associate Professor of Medicine and Microbiology,
SUNY at Buffalo School of Medicine; Associate Chief
of Staff for Education, Buffalo Veterans
Administration Medical Center, Buffalo, New York
Bacterial Meningitis in Adults

STEVEN L. BERK, M.D.

Professor and Chairman, Department of Medicine,
East Tennessee State University Quillen-Dishner
College of Medicine, Johnson City, Tennessee
Pericarditis

ALAN L. BISNO, M.D.

Professor and Vice-Chairman, Department of
Medicine, University of Miami School of Medicine;
Chief, Medical Service, Veterans Administration
Medical Center, Miami, Florida
*Nonsuppurative Sequelae of Group A Streptococcal
Infection*

DONALD L. BORNSTEIN, M.D.

Associate Professor of Medicine, Infectious Disease
Section, SUNY Health Science Center at Syracuse,
Syracuse, New York
Tetanus

SUSAN E. BORUCHOFF, M.D.

Assistant Professor of Medicine, University of
Massachusetts Medical School, Worcester,
Massachusetts
Antiviral Chemotherapy

JOHN P. BURKE, M.D.

Professor of Medicine, University of Utah School of
Medicine; Chief, Infectious Disease Division, LDS
Hospital, Salt Lake City, Utah
Urinary Catheter–Associated Infection

JANE C. BURNS, M.D.

Assistant Professor, Harvard Medical School;
Associate in Medicine, Children's Hospital, Boston,
Massachusetts
Kawasaki Syndrome

DAVID CHARLES, M.D., F.R.C.O.G., F.A.C.O.G.

Former Professor and Chairman, Department of
Obstetrics and Gynecology, Marshall University
School of Medicine; Former Chief of Obstetrical
Service, St. Mary's Hospital, Huntington, West
Virginia
Infection in Pregnancy

SARAH H. CHEESEMAN, M.D.

Associate Professor of Medicine, Pediatrics, Molecular Genetics, and Microbiology, University of Massachusetts Medical School, Worcester, Massachusetts
Antiviral Chemotherapy

CLARE L. CHERNEY, M.D.

Former Instructor in Medicine, The Medical College of Pennsylvania, Philadelphia, Pennsylvania
Bacteriuria and Pyelonephritis

P. JOAN CHESNEY, M.D., C.M.

Professor of Pediatrics, Division of Pediatric Infectious Diseases, University of Tennessee, Memphis, College of Medicine; Attending Pediatrician, LeBonheur Children's Medical Center, Memphis, Tennessee
Aseptic Meningitis Syndrome

GERALD W. CHODAK, M.D.

Associate Professor, University of Chicago Pritzker School of Medicine, Chicago, Illinois
Prostatitis, Epididymitis, and Balanoposthitis

ANTHONY W. CHOW, M.D., FRCPC, FACP

Professor and Head, Division of Infectious Disease, Department of Medicine, University of British Columbia School of Medicine, Vancouver, British Columbia, Canada
Vulvovaginitis, Cervicitis, and Pelvic Inflammatory Disease

DAVID C. CLASSEN, M.D.

Assistant Professor of Medicine, University of Utah School of Medicine, Salt Lake City, Utah
Urinary Catheter–Associated Infection

JOSEPH A. COOK, M.D.

Director, Program in Tropical Disease Research, The Edna McConnell Clark Foundation, New York, New York
Schistosomiasis

DONALD E. CRAVEN, M.D.

Professor of Medicine and Microbiology, Boston University School of Medicine; Director of AIDS Program, Infectious Disease Section, Boston City Hospital, Boston, Massachusetts
Gram-Negative Rod Bacteremia

BURKE A. CUNHA, M.D.

Associate Professor of Medicine, SUNY at Stony Brook School of Medicine, Stony Brook; Chief, Infectious Disease Division, and Associate Chairman, Department of Medicine, Winthrop-University Hospital, Mineola, New York
Tularemia

HARRY E. DASCOMB, M.D.

Professor of Medicine, University of North Carolina at Chapel Hill School of Medicine, Chapel Hill; Professor, Medicine Teaching Service, Wake County Memorial Hospital Area Health Education Centers Program, Raleigh, North Carolina
Biliary Tract Infection

E. PATCHEN DELLINGER, M.D.

Associate Professor of Surgery, University of Washington School of Medicine, Seattle, Washington
Crepitus and Gangrene

ANASTACIO DE Q SOUSA, M.D.

Assistant Professor of Medicine, Universidade Federal do Ceará, Fortaleza, Ceará, Brazil
Leishmaniasis

JAMES P. DUDLEY, M.D.

Associate Professor of Surgery, Division of Head and Neck Surgery, University of California, Los Angeles, UCLA School of Medicine; Staff, UCLA Medical Center, Los Angeles, California
Infection of the Mouth, Salivary Glands, and Neck Spaces

ASIM K. DUTT, M.D.

Professor of Medicine, Meharry School of Medicine, Nashville; Chief, Medical Service, Alvin C. York Veterans Hospital, Murfreesboro, Tennessee
Tuberculosis

MARK R. ECKMAN, M.D.

Clinical Associate Professor of Microbiology and Clinical Medicine, University of Minnesota–Duluth School of Medicine; Staff, Section of Infectious Diseases, Division of Internal Medicine, The Duluth Clinic, Ltd., Duluth, Minnesota
Babesiosis

THEODORE C. EICKHOFF, M.D.

Professor of Medicine, University of Colorado School of Medicine; Director of Internal Medicine, Presbyterian St. Luke's Medical Center, Denver, Colorado
Adult Immunization

CHARLES ELLENBOGEN, M.D.

Clinical Associate Professor of Medicine and Community Medicine, Duke University School of Medicine, Durham; Director of Internal Medicine, Fayetteville Area Health Education Center, Fayetteville, North Carolina
Animal Bite Infections

THOMAS G. EVANS, M.D.

Assistant Professor of Medicine, University of Utah School of Medicine, Salt Lake City, Utah
Leishmaniasis

PATRICK G. FAIRCHILD, M.D.

Assistant Professor of Medicine, University of Massachusetts Medical School; Director, HIV Clinical Center, University of Massachusetts Medical Center, Worcester, Massachusetts
Sternal Wound Infection and Mediastinitis

BARRY M. FARR, M.D., M.Sc.

Associate Professor, University of Virginia School of Medicine, Charlottesville, Virginia
The Common Cold

GREGORY A. FILICE, M.D.

Associate Professor of Medicine, University of Minnesota; Staff Physician, Veterans Administration Medical Center, Minneapolis, Minnesota
Toxoplasmosis

GERALD W. FISCHER, M.D.

Professor of Pediatrics, and Director, Pediatric Infectious Disease Program, Uniformed Services University of the Health Sciences, Bethesda, Maryland
Epiglottitis (Supraglottitis)

GERALD H. FRIEDLAND, M.D.

Professor of Medicine and Epidemiology and Social Medicine, Albert Einstein College of Medicine; Co-Director, AIDS Center, and Member, Division of Infectious Diseases, Montefiore Medical Center, Bronx, New York
Fever and Lymphadenopathy

NELSON M. GANTZ, M.D., F.A.C.P.

Professor of Medicine and Microbiology and Molecular Genetics, University of Massachusetts Medical School; Clinical Director of Infectious Diseases and Hospital Epidemiologist, University of Massachusetts Medical Center, Worcester, Massachusetts
Sternal Wound Infection and Mediastinitis

GARY E. GARBER, M.D., FRCPC

Assistant Professor of Medicine, Department of Medicine, University of Ottawa School of Medicine; Head, Division of Infectious Disease, Department of Medicine, Ottawa General Hospital, Ottawa, Ontario, Canada
Vulvovaginitis, Cervicitis, and Pelvic Inflammatory Disease

JEFFREY A. GELFAND, M.D.

Associate Professor of Medicine, Tufts University School of Medicine; Lecturer in Surgery, Harvard Medical School; Physician, Infectious Diseases Division, New England Medical Center; Associate Immunologist, Trauma Service, Massachusetts General Hospital, Boston, Massachusetts
Infection Following Burn Injury

ANNE A. GERSHON, M.D.

Professor of Pediatrics, Columbia University College of Physicians and Surgeons; Attending Physician, Babies Hospital, New York, New York
Childhood Exanthems

DAVID J. GOCKE, M.D.

Professor of Medicine and Microbiology, and Chief, Division of Allergy, Immunology, and Infectious Diseases, Robert Wood Johnson Medical School, University of Medicine and Dentistry of New Jersey, New Brunswick, New Jersey
Viral Hepatitis

RONALD GOLD, M.D.

Professor of Pediatrics, University of Toronto Faculty of Medicine; Chief, Division of Infectious Disease, The Hospital for Sick Children, Toronto, Ontario, Canada
Bacterial Meningitis in Children

ELLIOT GOLDSTEIN, M.D.

Professor of Medicine and Microbiology, and Chief, Division of Infectious and Immunologic Diseases, University of California, Davis, School of Medicine, Davis, California
Infection Following Trauma

SHERWOOD L. GORBACH, M.D.

Professor of Medicine and Community Health, Tufts University School of Medicine, Boston, Massachusetts
Medical Advice for Travelers

DAVID W. GREGORY, M.D.

Associate Professor of Medicine, Vanderbilt University School of Medicine, Nashville, Tennessee
Psittacosis

DAVID E. GRIFFITH, M.D., F.C.C.P.

Assistant Professor of Medicine, University of Texas Health Center at Tyler, Tyler, Texas
Nontuberculous (Environmental) Mycobacterial Disease in the Non–HIV-Infected Patient

JACK M. GWALTNEY Jr., M.D.

Professor, University of Virginia School of Medicine, Charlottesville, Virginia
The Common Cold

SCOTT M. HAMMER, M.D.

Assistant Professor of Medicine, Harvard Medical School; Director, Research Virology Laboratory, and Member, Infectious Disease Section, New England Deaconess Hospital, Boston, Massachusetts
Herpes Simplex Virus Infections

MARY ALICE HARBISON, M.D.

Research Fellow in Infectious Diseases, Harvard Medical School; Research Fellow in Infectious Diseases, New England Deaconess Hospital, Boston, Massachusetts
Herpes Simplex Virus Infections

HARLEY A. HAYNES, M.D.

Associate Professor of Dermatology, Harvard Medical School; Director, Dermatology Division, Department of Medicine, Brigham and Women's Hospital, Boston; Chief of Dermatology, Veterans Administration Hospital, West Roxbury, Massachusetts
Ectoparasitic Infection

MARTIN S. HIRSCH, M.D.

Professor of Medicine, Harvard Medical School; Physician, Infectious Disease Unit, Massachusetts General Hospital, Boston, Massachusetts
Viral Encephalitis

JAN V. HIRSCHMANN, M.D.

Associate Professor of Medicine, University of Washington School of Medicine; Assistant Chief, Medical Service, Seattle Veterans Administration Medical Center, Seattle, Washington
Systemic Prophylactic Antibiotics in Surgery

DAVID D. HO, M.D.

Assistant Professor of Medicine, Division of Infectious Diseases, University of California, Los Angeles, UCLA School of Medicine; Associate Physician and Research Scientist, and Director, AIDS Virology Laboratory, Cedar Sinai Medical Center, Los Angeles, California
Viral Encephalitis

CYRUS C. HOPKINS, M.D.

Assistant Professor of Medicine, Harvard Medical School; Hospital Epidemiologist and Physician, Massachusetts General Hospital, Boston, Massachusetts
Intravascular Catheter-Associated Infection

DONALD R. HOPKINS, M.D., MPH, D.Sc.(Hon.)

Senior Consultant, Global 2000, Carter Presidential Center, Chicago, Illinois
Nonvenereal Treponematoses

SUSAN J. JACOBSON, M.D.

Infectious Disease Fellow, Tufts University School of Medicine; Geographic Medicine and Infectious Disease, New England Medical Center, Boston, Massachusetts
Malaria

PETER G. JESSAMINE, M.D., Hons. B. Sc., FRCPC

Fellow, Section of Infectious Diseases and Medical Microbiology, University of Manitoba Faculty of Medicine, Winnipeg, Manitoba, Canada
Chancroid, Lymphogranuloma Venereum, Granuloma Inguinale, and Condyloma Acuminata

CANDICE E. JOHNSON, M.D., Ph.D.

Assistant Professor of Pediatrics, Case Western Reserve University School of Medicine; Attending Pediatrician, Metro Health Medical Center, Cleveland, Ohio
Otitis Media

ROYCE H. JOHNSON, M.D., F.A.C.P.

Adjunct Associate Professor of Medicine, University of California, Los Angeles, UCLA School of Medicine, Los Angeles; Chief, Infectious Disease, Department of Medicine, Kern Medical Center, Bakersfield, California
Plague

EDWARD H. KASS, Ph.D., M.D., Sc.D.(Hon.), M.A.(Hon.)

William Ellery Channing Professor of Medicine, Emeritus, Channing Laboratory, Harvard Medical School; Senior Physician, Brigham and Women's Hospital, Boston, Massachusetts
Book Editor

DONALD KAYE, M.D.

Professor and Chairman, Department of Medicine, The Medical College of Pennsylvania, Philadelphia, Pennsylvania
Bacteriuria and Pyelonephritis

THOMAS M. KERKERING, M.D.

Associate Professor of Medicine, Division of Infectious Diseases, Medical College of Virginia/Virginia Commonwealth University, Richmond, Virginia
Localized Infection of the Central Nervous System

ALBERT S. KLAINER, M.D.

Professor of Clinical Medicine, Columbia University College of Physicians and Surgeons, New York, New York; Chairman, Department of Internal Medicine, Morristown Memorial Hospital, Morristown, New Jersey
Pleural Effusion and Empyema

JEROME O. KLEIN, M.D.

Professor, Boston University School of Medicine; Director, Division of Pediatric Infectious Diseases, Boston City Hospital, Boston, Massachusetts
Childhood Immunization

RONICA M. KLUGE, M.D.

Professor and Vice Chair for Educational Affairs, and Director, General Internal Medicine and Geriatrics, Department of Internal Medicine, University of Texas Medical Branch, Galveston, Texas
Infectious Diarrheas

ANTHONY L. KOMAROFF, M.D.

Associate Professor of Medicine, Harvard Medical School; Chief, Division of General Medicine, Brigham and Women's Hospital, Boston, Massachusetts
Pharyngitis

JOSEPH KOO, M.D.

Fellow in Infectious and Immunologic Diseases, Department of Medicine, University of California, Davis, School of Medicine, Davis, California
Infection Following Trauma

DEBORAH PAVAN LANGSTON, M.D.

Associate Professor of Ophthalmology, Eye Research Institute, Harvard Medical School; Surgeon, Massachusetts Eye and Ear Infirmary, Boston, Massachusetts
Infectious Keratitis

BRYAN LARSEN, Ph.D.

Professor of Obstetrics/Gynecology and Microbiology, Marshall University School of Medicine, Huntington, West Virginia
Infection in Pregnancy

CARL B. LAUTER, M.D., F.A.C.P.

Associate Clinical Professor of Medicine, Wayne State University School of Medicine, Detroit; Chief, Medical Services, Divisions of Infectious Diseases, Allergy and Clinical Immunology, William Beaumont Hospital, Royal Oak, Michigan
Sinusitis

JACK L. LeFROCK, M.D.

Scientific Director, Therapeutic Research Institute, Sarasota, Florida
Bacterial Osteomyelitis

PHILLIP I. LERNER, M.D.

Professor of Medicine, Case Western Reserve University School of Medicine; Chief, Infectious Disease Division, Mount Sinai Medical Center, Cleveland, Ohio
Prosthetic Valve Endocarditis

MYRON M. LEVINE, M.D., D.T.P.H.

Professor and Head, Division of Geographic Medicine; Professor and Head, Division of Infectious Diseases and Tropical Pediatrics; and Professor and Director, Center for Vaccine Development, University of Maryland School of Medicine, Baltimore, Maryland
Typhoid Fever and Enteric Fever

SARAH S. LONG, M.D.

Professor of Pediatrics, Temple University School of Medicine; Chief, Section of Infectious Diseases, St. Christopher's Hospital for Children, Philadelphia, Pennsylvania
Pertussis

JAMES H. MAGUIRE, M.D.

Assistant Professor of Medicine, Harvard Medical School; Assistant Professor of Tropical Public Health, Harvard School of Public Health; Associate in Medicine, Brigham and Women's Hospital, Boston, Massachusetts
Trypanosomiasis: African (Sleeping Sickness) and American (Chagas' Disease)

RICHARD J. MANGI, M.D.

Clinical Associate Professor of Medicine, Yale University Medical School; Chief, Infectious Diseases, Hospital of Saint Raphael, New Haven, Connecticut
Nonbacterial Infectious Arthritides

KENNETH H. MAYER, M.D.

Associate Professor of Medicine and Community Health, Brown University, Providence; Chief, Infectious Disease Division, Memorial Hospital of Rhode Island, Pawtucket, Rhode Island
Antibacterial Chemotherapy

WILLIAM R. McCABE, M.D.

Professor of Medicine and Microbiology, and Director of Infectious Diseases, Boston University School of Medicine; Director, Maxwell Finland Laboratory for Infectious Diseases, Boston City Hospital, Boston, Massachusetts
Gram-Negative Rod Bacteremia

JOHN E. McGOWAN Jr., M.D.

Professor of Pathology and Laboratory Medicine, Emory University School of Medicine; Director, Clinical Microbiology, Grady Memorial Hospital, Atlanta, Georgia
Postoperative Wound Infection

KAREN A. MELLO, M.D.

Clinical Fellow, Geographic Medicine and Infectious Diseases, Tufts University School of Medicine; Clinical Fellow, New England Medical Center, Boston, Massachusetts
Medical Advice for Travelers

BURT R. MEYERS, M.D.

Professor of Medicine, Mount Sinai School of Medicine of the City University of New York; Attending Physician, Division of Infectious Diseases, Mount Sinai Medical Center, New York, New York
Lung Abscess

ABDOLGHADER MOLAVI, M.D.

Associate Professor of Medicine, and Chief, Division of Infectious Disease, Hahnemann University School of Medicine, Philadelphia, Pennsylvania
Bacterial Osteomyelitis

THOMAS R. NAVIN, M.D.

Medical Entomology and Research Training Unit, Guatemala
Leishmaniasis

HARRY C. NOTTEBART JR., M.D., F.A.C.P.

Clinical Associate Professor of Medicine, University of Virginia School of Medicine, Charlottesville; Associate Clinical Professor of Pathology, Medical College of Virginia, Richmond, Virginia
Syphilis

DALE W. OLLER, M.D.

Associate Professor of Surgery, University of North Carolina at Chapel Hill School of Medicine, Chapel Hill; Director of Trauma and Surgery, Wake County Memorial Hospital Area Health Education Centers Program, Raleigh, North Carolina
Biliary Tract Infection

JEFFREY PARSONNET, M.D.

Assistant Professor of Medicine, Harvard Medical School; Associate Physician, Department of Medicine, Channing Laboratory, Brigham and Women's Hospital, Boston, Massachusetts
Toxic Shock Syndrome

RICHARD D. PEARSON, M.D., F.A.C.P.

Associate Professor of Medicine and Pathology, University of Virginia School of Medicine, Charlottesville, Virginia
Leishmaniasis

CLARENCE J. PETERS, M.D.

Associate, Department of Immunology and Infectious Diseases, School of Hygiene and Public Health, The Johns Hopkins University, Baltimore; Chief, Disease Assessment Division, U.S. Army Institute of Infectious Diseases, Fort Detrick, Frederick, Maryland
Viral Hemorrhagic Fever

RICHARD PLATT, M.D.

Assistant Professor of Medicine, Harvard Medical School; Hospital Epidemiologist, Brigham and Women's Hospital, Boston, Massachusetts
Book Editor

PETER E. POCHI

Herbert Mescon Professor of Dermatology, Boston University School of Medicine; Visiting Dermatologist, University Hospital; Visiting Physician, Dermatology, Boston City Hospital, Boston, Massachusetts
Acne Vulgaris

SERGIO RABINOVICH, M.D.

Professor of Internal Medicine, and Chief, Division of Infectious Diseases, Southern Illinois University School of Medicine, Springfield, Illinois
Superficial Fungal Infection

CARLOS H. RAMIREZ-RONDA, M.D., F.A.C.P.

Professor of Medicine, University of Puerto Rico School of Medicine; Director, Division of Infectious Diseases, Veterans Administration Hospital and University Hospital, San Juan, Puerto Rico
Diphtheria

JONATHAN I. RAVDIN, M.D.

Associate Professor of Medicine and Pharmacology, Division of Clinical Pharmacology, Department of Internal Medicine, University of Virginia School of Medicine, Charlottesville, Virginia
Amebiasis and Giardiasis

DAVID G. ROBERTS, M.D.

Instructor in Pediatrics, Case Western Reserve School of Medicine; Attending Pediatrician, Metro Health Medical Center, Cleveland, Ohio
Otitis Media

ALLAN R. RONALD, B.Sc., FRCPC, F.A.C.P.

Professor and Chairman, Department of Internal Medicine, University of Manitoba Faculty of Medicine; Physician-in-Chief, Department of Medicine, Health Sciences Centre, Winnipeg, Manitoba, Canada
Chancroid, Lymphogranuloma Venereum, Granuloma Inguinale, and Condyloma Acuminata

WILLIAM SCHAFFNER, M.D.

Professor and Chairman, Department of Preventive Medicine, and Chief, Division of Infectious Diseases, Department of Medicine, Vanderbilt University School of Medicine, Nashville, Tennessee
Psittacosis

WALTER F. SCHLECH III, M.D., F.A.C.P., FRCPC

Associate Professor of Medicine, Dalhousie University School of Medicine, Halifax, Nova Scotia, Canada
Listeriosis

DAVID SCHLOSSBERG, M.D., F.A.C.P.

Professor of Medicine, Temple University School of Medicine; Director, Department of Medicine, Episcopal Hospital, Philadelphia, Pennsylvania
Cellulitis and Soft Tissue Infection

HEINZ-JOSEF SCHMITT, M.D.

Instructor in Medicine, Cornell University Medical College; Fellow in Training, Infectious Disease Service, Memorial Sloan-Kettering Cancer Center, New York, New York
Antifungal Chemotherapy

JOHN W. SENSAKOVIC, M.D., PH.D.

Associate Professor of Medicine and Infectious Diseases, Seton Hall University School of Graduate Medical Education, South Orange; Adjunct Associate Professor of Microbiology, Robert Wood Johnson Medical School, University of Medicine and Dentistry of New Jersey, New Brunswick; Director of Medical Education, St. Michael's Medical Center, Newark, New Jersey
Fever and Rash

ALEXIS SHELOKOV, M.D.

Adjunct Professor, Department of Epidemiology, School of Hygiene and Public Health, The Johns Hopkins University School of Medicine, Baltimore, Maryland; Director of Vaccine Research, The Salk Institute, Government Services Division, Swiftwater, Pennsylvania
Viral Hemorrhagic Fever

JOHN W. SLEASMAN, M.D.

Assistant Professor, Division of Immunology, Department of Pediatrics, University of Florida College of Medicine, Gainesville, Florida
Immunodeficiency Disorders in Infants and Children

BRUCE R. SMITH, PHARM.D.

Associate Director, Therapeutic Research Institute, Sarasota, Florida
Bacterial Osteomyelitis

LEON G. SMITH, M.D., F.A.C.P.

Chairman of Medicine and Infectious Diseases, Seton Hall University School of Graduate Medical Education, South Orange; Professor of Medicine and Preventive Medicine and Community Health, Robert Wood Johnson Medical School, University of Medicine and Dentistry of New Jersey, New Brunswick; Director of Medicine and Chief of Infectious Diseases, St. Michael's Medical Center, Newark, New Jersey
Fever and Rash

JOHN F. STAMLER, M.D., PH.D.

Fellow, Department of Ophthalmology, Harvard Medical School; Fellow, Cornea Service, Massachusetts Eye and Ear Infirmary, and Eye Research Institute of the Retina Foundation, Boston, Massachusetts
Infectious Keratitis

WALTER E. STAMM, M.D.

Professor of Medicine, University of Washington School of Medicine; Head, Division of Infectious Disease, Harborview Medical Center, Seattle, Washington
Acute Dysuria in Women and Urethritis in Men

WILLIAM W. STEAD, M.D.

Professor of Medicine, University of Arkansas School of Medicine; Director, Tuberculosis Program, Arkansas Department of Health, Little Rock, Arkansas
Tuberculosis

RHOADS E. STEVENS, M.D.

Cornea Specialist, Straub Eye Clinic and Hospital; Medical Director, Hawaii Lions Eye Bank and Maleana Foundation, Honolulu, Hawaii
Infection of the Conjunctiva, Eyelids, and Lacrimal Apparatus

IRA B. TAGER, M.D., M.P.H.

Associate Professor of Medicine and Epidemiology and International Health, University of California, San Francisco, School of Medicine; Veterans Administration Medical Center, San Francisco, California
Chronic Bronchitis

MARTIN G. TÄUBER, M.D.

Visiting Assistant Professor, University of California, San Francisco, School of Medicine; The Medical Service, San Francisco General Hospital, San Francisco, California
Acquired Immunodeficiency Syndrome

JAMES R. TILLOTSON, M.D.

Clinical Professor of Medicine and Adjunct Professor of Microbiology, Albany Medical College; Attending in Infectious Diseases, Albany Medical Center, Child's Hospital, Memorial Hospital, and St. Peter's Hospital, Albany, New York
Pneumonia

RALPH TOMPSETT, M.D.

Professor Emeritus, University of Texas Southwestern Medical School; Chief, Infectious Diseases, Baylor University Medical Center, Dallas, Texas
Bacterial Arthritis

BORIS VELIMIROVIC, M.D., D.T.P.H.

Professor of Social Medicine, University of Graz, Faculty of Medicine; Chief of Communicable Diseases, World Health Organization of Europe; Director, Institute of Social Medicine, Graz, Austria
Anthrax

ABRAHAM VERGHESE, M.D., F.R.C.P.

Associate Professor of Medicine, East Tennessee State University Quillen-Dishner College of Medicine; Chief, Infectious Disease, Veterans Administration Medical Center, Johnson City, Tennessee
Pericarditis

C. FORDHAM von REYN, M.D.

Associate Clinical Professor of Medicine, Dartmouth Medical School; Chief, Infectious Disease Section, Hitchcock Medical Center, Hanover, New Hampshire
Infective Endocarditis and Mycotic Aneurysm

MICHAEL D. WAGONER, M.D.

Assistant Clinical Professor of Ophthalmology, Harvard Medical School; Assistant Surgeon, Massachusetts Eye and Ear Infirmary, Boston, Massachusetts
Infection of the Conjunctiva, Eyelids, and Lacrimal Apparatus

RICHARD J. WALLACE Jr., M.D., B.A.

Professor of Medicine and Microbiology, and Chairman, Department of Microbiology, Baylor College of Medicine, Houston; Professor of Medicine, University of Texas Health Center at Tyler, Tyler, Texas
Nontuberculous (Environmental) Mycobacterial Disease in the Non–HIV-Infected Patient

GEORGE WATT, M.D., DTM & H

Chief, Department of Medicine, Armed Forces Research Institute of Medical Sciences, Bangkok, Thailand
Leptospirosis

J. JOHN WEEMS Jr., M.D.

Clinical Assistant Professor, University of Tennessee, Memphis, College of Medicine; Consulting Hospital Epidemiologist, Baptist Memorial Hospital, Memphis, Tennessee
Actinomycosis

BURTON C. WEST, M.D.

Former Professor of Medicine, Division of Infectious Diseases, Louisiana State University School of Medicine; Former Consultant, Shreveport Veterans Administration Medical Center, Shreveport, Louisiana; Chairman, Department of Medicine, Meridia Huron Hospital, Cleveland, Ohio
Leprosy

M. J. WINSHIP, M.D.

Clinical Associate Professor, Department of Internal Medicine, University of Washington School of Medicine, Seattle, Washington
Human Brucellosis

MARTIN S. WOLFE, M.D.

Clinical Professor of Medicine, George Washington University School of Medicine and Health Sciences; Director, Traveler's Medical Service of Washington, Washington, D.C.
Infection Caused by Intestinal Helminths

THEODORE E. WOODWARD, M.D., M.A.C.P.

Professor Emeritus of Medicine, University of Maryland School of Medicine, Baltimore, Maryland
Rickettsial Infection

GARY P. WORMSER, M.D.

Professor of Medicine and Pharmacology, and Chief Division of Infectious Diseases, New York Medical College; Chief, Section of Infectious Diseases, Westchester County Medical Center, Valhalla, New York
Lyme Disease

DAVID J. WYLER, M.D.

Professor of Medicine, Tufts University School of Medicine; Physician, New England Medical Center, Boston, Massachusetts
Malaria

LOWELL S. YOUNG, M.D.

Clinical Professor of Medicine, University of California, San Francisco, School of Medicine; Director, Kuzell Institute for Arthritis and Infectious Diseases; Chief, Division of Infectious Diseases, Pacific Presbyterian Medical Center, San Francisco, California
Infection Complicating Immunosuppression

DORI F. ZALEZNIK, M.D.

Assistant Professor of Medicine, Harvard Medical School; Hospital Epidemiologist, Beth Israel Hospital, Boston, Massachusetts
Intra-abdominal Abscess

JONATHAN M. ZENILMAN, M.D.

Assistant Professor, Division of Infectious Diseases, Department of Medicine, The Johns Hopkins University School of Medicine; Attending Physician, The Johns Hopkins Hospital, Baltimore, Maryland
Disseminated Gonococcal Infection

MOHSEN ZIAI, M.D.

Chair, Department of Pediatrics, Fairfax Hospital, Falls Church, Virginia
Trachoma

STEPHEN H. ZINNER, M.D.

Professor of Medicine, Brown University; Head, Division of Infectious Diseases, Roger Williams General Hospital and Rhode Island Hospital, Providence, Rhode Island
Antibacterial Chemotherapy

PREFACE

The kind reception accorded to the two previous editions of *Current Therapy in Infectious Disease* prompted the preparation of a third edition. The present edition follows the practice outlined previously; virtually all the chapters are written by authors different from those who had contributed previously, and the relatively few exceptions were carefully reviewed and brought up to date. As we have stressed in previous editions, the decision to ask entirely new contributors to share their knowledge and expertise with our readers was based not on any sense of inadequacy of previous chapters, but rather on a desire to bring to our readers as wide a range of viewpoints as possible on the complexities of managing patients with infectious diseases.

We have continued to maintain the philosophy encased in previous editions: we have insisted, wherever appropriate, that authors not use permissive and occasionally ambiguous recommendations (as often appear in contemporary textbooks), but rather that they tell us *what each expert actually does*, with precise dosages and precise statements of preference in terms of the many therapeutic possibilities that are available in contemporary medicine.

Many, if not most, textbooks and manuals are written by experts who consciously or unconsciously seek the approbation of fellow experts; since some disagreement within a field is inevitable (and generally useful), recommendations for treatment commonly contain permissive terms such as "may sometimes be helpful" or "is often recommended." Dosages of drugs are often given in broad ranges. For the busy clinician, who cannot take time to thread through all the details of current controversy or uncertainty, these broad statements can be perplexing in the least and frustrating in the extreme.

If to this problem is added the contemporary one of new therapeutic agents that appear on the market with staggering frequency and are marketed with forcefulness, difficult problems of decision become common.

It seemed to us reasonable to assemble volumes on management of infectious disease that attempted to cut through the problems of choice and consensus by adhering to two simple principles: first, that experts in the field be asked to state what they actually did when faced with specific therapeutic problems, and second, that recommendations be given in clear and unambiguous terms. If there are acceptable alternatives, these were to be given in the order of preference, *in the opinion of the expert who was writing the specific chapter*. Disagreements could be cited, but the expert involved ultimately had to say, in the most precise terms possible, exactly what he or she does when faced with a patient with the disease in question.

As our experience has grown, it has become evident that some diagnostic information was desirable, and so we have encouraged the presentation of such information and of relevant preventive strategies, but in as succinct a form as possible, using algorithms and diagrams when possible.

Therefore, this is intended as a manual for busy practitioners. We are most appreciative of the many helpful suggestions that have come from our readers and consultants; errors and misinterpretations that have arisen as we have tried to edit the various contributions in accordance with our initial principles are ours, and we shall be ready to edit and amend each presentation in response to our readers.

We are particularly grateful to the experts who have contributed their clinical wisdom to this volume and who have put up with our queries, suggestions, and editorial comments with good humor and constructive purpose. Because most of our contributors are members of the Infectious Diseases Society of America, we have, as in the past, attempted to express our appreciation by contributing a share of the royalties to the Lectureship Fund of the IDSA. However, the Society has no official involvement with this volume, has neither approved nor disapproved of its contents, and is in no way responsible for the opinions and judgments expressed.

Our particular gratitude goes to Joan Daniels for her perceptive contributions to this volume, to Inge Smith for her helpful assistance, and to Mary Mansor and Brian Decker of B.C. Decker for their encouragement and advice.

Edward H. Kass
Richard Platt
August 1989

CONTENTS

INFECTIONS AFFECTING MORE THAN ONE SYSTEM AND CAUSED BY PARASITES OR FUNGI

NOSOCOMIAL INFECTIONS

GENERAL THERAPEUTICS

ANTIVIRAL CHEMOTHERAPY

SUSAN E. BORUCHOFF, M.D.
SARAH H. CHEESEMAN, M.D.

The rapid advances being made in antiviral treatment are reflected in the number of chapters in this volume devoted to therapy of specific viral diseases. This chapter provides an overview of the major antiviral agents available or presently under investigation in the United States today, with emphasis on mode of action and pharmacologic properties relevant to clinical use. More detailed discussion of specific therapeutic recommendations are found in other chapters devoted to the individual infections (*Herpes Simplex Virus Infection, Viral Hemorrhagic Fever, Viral Hepatitis*). Topical agents for treatment of ocular herpes simplex virus infections are considered in the chapter on keratitis. The use of topical agents should be reserved for the experienced ophthalmologist. Zidovudine (AZT) and the many other agents under development for treatment of infections caused by human immunodeficiency virus (HIV) are discussed in the chapter *Acquired Immunodeficiency Syndrome*.

GENERAL PRINCIPLES OF ANTIVIRAL CHEMOTHERAPY

Appropriate and effective use of antiviral agents requires a specific virologic diagnosis, by viral isolation or other laboratory techniques, or at least a strong clinical suspicion based on knowledge of distinctive manifestations of disease. Each available drug has a limited spectrum of activity. The mechanism of action of most antiviral agents involves inhibition of viral replication, either through prevention of uncoating (amantadine/rimantadine) or by interference with nucleic acid replication (acyclovir, ganciclovir, vidarabine, ribavirin, zidovudine). It should be noted that no current therapy can eradicate the latent stage of any viral infection, since the antiviral effects involve interference with active viral multiplication. Another approach to antiviral therapy involves the use of immunomodulatory agents (such as the interferons), which alter the host's immune response to viral infection.

ACYCLOVIR (9-[2-HYDROXYETHOXYMETHYL]GUANINE, ACYCLOGUANOSINE, ZOVIRAX)

Acyclovir is the most important and widely used antiviral agent in clinical practice today. It is a synthetic acyclic analogue of guanosine, with specific activity only against viruses of the herpesvirus family. It has clinical efficacy in the treatment of infections caused by herpes simplex virus (HSV) types 1 and 2 and varicella-zoster virus (VZV). In vitro, the concentrations producing 50 percent inhibition of replication (ID_{50}) of these three viruses are 0.02 to 0.2 μg per milliliter, 0.2 to 0.4 μg per milliliter, and 0.8 to 1.2 μg per milliliter, respectively.

Acyclovir has a unique mechanism of selective action in virus-infected cells. It is phosphorylated by a virus-encoded thymidine kinase (TK) to acyclovir monophosphate. This, in turn, is phosphorylated to the active form of acyclovir triphosphate by cellular enzymes. Acyclovir triphosphate's antiviral effect is twofold: it inhibits viral DNA polymerase through irreversible binding, and it is incorporated into viral DNA where it acts as a chain terminator. Low levels of acyclovir triphosphate can be found in uninfected cells, indicating that cellular TKs are able to phosphorylate acyclovir to some degree. These levels, although 40- to 100-fold lower than in HSV-infected cells, are enough to produce in vitro inhibition of Epstein-Barr virus, which lacks a viral TK but possesses an especially sensitive DNA polymerase. Viral mutants may become resistant to acyclovir in vitro by alterations in either TK or DNA polymerase. There is as yet little clinical evidence to support the notion that TK deficiency leads to poor outcomes in patients treated with acyclovir; indeed, animal studies suggest that TK-deficient strains of HSV may be less virulent.

Pharmacology and Toxicity

Acyclovir is available in topical, intravenous, and oral forms. Topical administration leads to little percutaneous absorption. Infusions of 5 or 10 mg per kilogram every 8 hours in patients with normal renal function produce average peak concentrations of 9.8 μg per milliliter and 20.7 μg per milliliter, respectively, with corresponding trough levels of 0.9 μg per milliliter and 2.3 μg per milliliter. Only 15 to 30 percent of an oral dose of acyclovir is absorbed. Mean steady-state peak and trough plasma concentrations of 0.7 and 0.4 μg per milliliter, respectively, are achieved in adults taking 200 mg orally five times a day. The bioavailability is further reduced with increasing doses, and 800 mg orally five times a day produces peaks of 1.6 μg per milliliter and troughs of 0.8 μg per milliliter. Cerebrospinal fluid (CSF) concentrations are approximately one-half of plasma levels. Acyclovir and its major metabolite are excreted by the kidneys by glomerular filtration and tubular secretion, with an average plasma half-life of 2.9 hours after intravenous administration in adults with normal renal function. Patients with renal insufficiency require adjustments in dosing (Table 1). Peritoneal dialysis is ineffective in removing acyclovir, but in anuric patients receiving hemodialysis, acyclovir should be given after a dialysis session, as up to 60 percent is removed during each 6-hour dialysis.

Acyclovir is relatively nontoxic. Intravenous acyclovir in doses of at least 5 mg per kilogram every 8 hours has been associated with reversible renal dysfunction caused by tubular crystal deposition in 5 percent of patients. Associated risk factors include dehydration, bolus infusion, and preexisting renal insufficiency. Approximately 1 percent of patients develop encephalopathic changes, including lethargy, tremors, confusion, hallucinations, delirium, seizures, and coma. These changes are more common in the presence of renal insufficiency and resolve when therapy is stopped. Rapid infusion of intravenous acyclovir may cause phlebitis, and extravasation causes blistering and burning at the site. Oral acyclovir is benign and is only infrequently associated with headache and nausea. Topical acyclovir may cause transient burning when applied to genital lesions, especially in females. It is not approved for intravaginal use.

Clinical Uses

Acyclovir is most frequently used in treatment of infections caused by herpes simplex viruses, which are the subject of a separate chapter in this volume.

Varicella-Zoster Virus

Acyclovir is the treatment of choice in infections caused by VZV. In immunosuppressed patients with herpes zoster (shingles), treatment with high-dose intravenous acyclovir (500 mg per square meter every 8 hours or 12.4 mg per kilogram every 8 hours) for 7 days significantly reduces the likelihood of cutaneous or visceral dissemination, the duration of viral shedding, the duration of pain, and the time to complete healing of lesions. This is especially true if treatment is begun within 72 hours of onset of lesions. Studies in a similar population of immunosuppressed patients comparing treatment with intravenous acyclovir and intravenous vidarabine found better results in the acyclovir group in all parameters mentioned above. Acyclovir treatment does not seem to decrease the incidence of postherpetic neuralgia. Therefore, although intravenous acyclovir treatment reduces the duration of uncomplicated zoster in adults who are not immunodeficient, its use in this population does not seem

TABLE 1 Dosage Adjustment for Intravenous Acyclovir in Patients With Impaired Renal Function

Creatinine Clearance (ml/min/1.73 m²)	Percentage of Standard Dose	Dosing Interval (hours)
> 50	100	8
25–50	100	12
10–25	100	24
0–10*	50	24

* Administered after hemodialysis.

worth the cost and inconvenience. Trials of oral acyclovir for herpes zoster are underway, and early results show that oral acyclovir may also reduce the duration of lesions and symptoms in uncomplicated zoster. These require the use of much larger doses (800 mg orally five times daily) than are used for HSV. Intravenous acyclovir is also effective in treatment of immunocompromised children with primary varicella (chickenpox). Administration of 500 mg per square meter every 8 hours for 7 days, beginning within 72 hours of onset of skin lesions, reduces the incidence of pneumonitis and other visceral involvement. We infuse each dose over 1 hour and maintain urine output (in milliliters) equal to the number of milligrams of acyclovir in the total daily dose.

Other Herpesviruses

Despite in vitro sensitivity of Epstein-Barr virus (EBV) to acyclovir at clinically achievable levels, the role of acyclovir in treatment of EBV-associated diseases remains limited. Although a rapid decrease in pharyngeal shedding of EBV occurs in patients with severe infectious mononucleosis given high doses of intravenous acyclovir (10 mg per kilogram every 8 hours), treatment does not significantly shorten the clinical course of the disease. Acyclovir has no proven utility in treatment of infections caused by cytomegalovirus; the related compound, ganciclovir, is much more effective and will be discussed below.

GANCICLOVIR (9-[1,3-DIHYDROXY-2-PROPOXYMETHYL]-GUANINE, DHPG, BW759U)

Ganciclovir, like acyclovir, is an acyclic analogue of guanine, but it is active against all human herpesviruses, especially cytomegalovirus (CMV). Like acyclovir, it is selectively phosphorylated in infected cells to the triphosphate form, which inhibits viral DNA polymerase and acts as a DNA chain terminator. It has had extensive investigational use in treatment of serious CMV infections in immunocompromised hosts and has now been licensed by the U.S. Food and Drug Administration (FDA). The ID_{50} of ganciclovir for CMV is in the range of 1 to 4 μM, a level exceeded several-fold by peak plasma levels in patients treated with the usual dose of 5 mg per kilogram. The drug is excreted unchanged in the urine, and patients with renal insufficiency require adjustments in dosage. The major adverse effect of ganciclovir is neutropenia, which is often dose-related and usually resolves when therapy is stopped. This is a frequent limiting factor in patients with underlying immunosuppressive conditions who are receiving other drugs that suppress the bone marrow.

Studies in immunocompromised patients with serious CMV infections (retinitis, pneumonia, hepatitis, and gastrointestinal tract involvement) have shown that ganciclovir treatment at 5 mg per kilogram every 12 hours rapidly clears viremia and viruria in 70 to 80 percent of patients. Stabilization of retinitis and clearing of gastrointestinal symptoms on therapy are frequent, but CMV pneumonia is more refractory to treatment. Clearing of viral shedding does not always correlate with clinical improvement and, unfortunately, most patients relapse when ganciclovir treatment is stopped. This is especially true of patients with the acquired immunodeficiency syndrome (AIDS), who may respond more poorly than transplant recipients to ganciclovir therapy, in part because reversal of immunosuppression in conjunction with the use of ganciclovir is not possible in AIDS patients. Some studies demonstrate prolongation of clinical improvement with maintenance ganciclovir (5 to 6 mg per kilogram once daily) for an indefinite period following initial therapy, although viremia may recur during maintenance therapy.

VIDARABINE
(9-β-D-ARABINOFURANOSYLADENINE, ARA-A, ADENINE ARABINOSIDE, VIRA-A)

Vidarabine was the first drug licensed by the FDA for systemic treatment of life-threatening viral infections. It is active against most herpesviruses, with the exception of CMV, as well as pox viruses and hepatitis B. Multiple clinical studies have documented the efficacy of vidarabine in the treatment of serious infections caused by HSV and VZV. Because of its toxicity, vidarabine has now been replaced by acyclovir as the drug of choice in treatment of infections caused by these viruses.

Vidarabine is an analogue of adenine deoxyriboside, which is phosphorylated in host cells to vidarabine triphosphate. This triphosphate form selectively inhibits viral DNA polymerase and acts as a chain terminator in both viral and cellular DNA. Vidarabine inhibits strains of HSV and VZV that are resistant to acyclovir in vitro.

Pharmacology and Toxicity

Vidarabine is available in intravenous form and as a topical preparation for ophthalmic use. A major problem in the clinical use of intravenous vidarabine is its poor solubility (0.45 mg per milliliter at 25°C). It is administered in a 12-hour continuous infusion of several liters of fluid daily. This fluid load complicates the management of cerebral edema in herpes simplex encephalitis. Infused vidarabine is rapidly deaminated to hypoxanthine arabinoside (ara-Hx), which is much less active than the parent drug. About 50 percent of a daily infusion is excreted in the urine within 24 hours, most in the form of ara-Hx. Excretion is reduced in the presence of renal insufficiency,

and the dose of vidarabine must therefore be reduced. Allopurinol interferes with metabolism of ara-Hx, and its use is contraindicated in patients treated with vidarabine.

At the usual dose range of 10 to 15 mg per kilogram per day, the most common adverse effects involve the gastrointestinal system, including anorexia, nausea, vomiting, diarrhea, and weight loss. These are dose-related and tend to resolve within several days despite continued treatment. Central nervous system toxicity is found in 2 to 10 percent of patients, with manifestations including hallucinations, tremors, ataxia, painful paresthesias, myoclonus, confusion, and coma. These are most common in the presence of renal or hepatic insufficiency and in patients on concurrent interferon therapy. Some of these reactions, especially the pain syndromes, may take several months to resolve. At high doses (20 mg per kilogram per day) vidarabine may cause megaloblastic bone marrow changes and pancytopenia. Rashes, infusion-related thrombophlebitis, and, rarely, syndrome of inappropriate secretion of antidiuretic hormone have also been reported. Vidarabine is teratogenic in some animal systems and is therefore not recommended for use in pregnant women.

Clinical Uses

The use of vidarabine in herpes simplex infections is discussed in a separate chapter. Like acyclovir, vidarabine is effective in limiting the severity of VZV infections in the immunocompromised patient, and it is the only drug that has been shown to reduce the incidence of postherpetic neuralgia. Vidarabine reduces replication of hepatitis B virus; potential applications of vidarabine in treatment of chronic hepatitis B infection is discussed in the chapter *Viral Hepatitis*.

RIBAVIRIN
(1-β-D-RIBOFURANOSYL-1,2,4-TRIAZOLE-3-CARBOXAMIDE, VIRAZOLE)

Ribavirin is a synthetic guanosine analogue with a broad spectrum of in vitro antiviral activity. It appears to have multiple antiviral mechanisms that are not yet well defined. Ribavirin monophosphate, produced via phosphorylation of ribavirin by host cellular enzymes, competitively inhibits guanine nucleotide synthesis. In addition, ribavirin triphosphate inhibits the capping of viral messenger RNA. Ribavirin is generally ineffective against viruses with single-stranded RNA genomes that act directly as messenger RNA, such as the enteroviruses, but has in vitro activity against a range of other RNA and DNA viruses including influenza A and B viruses, respiratory syncytial virus, HSV, Lassa fever virus, and HIV. Resistance to ribavirin is not known to develop as a result of therapy.

Pharmacology and Toxicity

Ribavirin has been studied in intravenous, oral, and aerosolized forms. The pharmacology of the drug is not well understood. Intravenous and oral treatment have been complicated by a mild, dose-related hemolytic anemia due to accumulation of ribavirin within erythrocytes. This is readily reversible upon cessation of therapy. Aerosolized ribavirin reaches high levels in the lungs, with plasma concentrations only 1 percent of those found in respiratory secretions. No hematologic or other systemic effects are associated with the aerosolized form; with the exception of conjunctival irritation, it is extremely well tolerated. Its use is contraindicated in pregnant women, as it has teratogenic effects in animals.

Clinical Uses

Aerosolized ribavirin is approved by the FDA for treatment of infants with lower respiratory tract disease due to respiratory syncytial virus (RSV). RSV infections are implicated in about 100,000 pediatric admissions yearly in the United States. Ribavirin administered in small-particle aerosolized form (20 mg per milliliter at 12 L per minute for 12 to 20 hours daily over 3 to 7 days) has been shown to decrease the severity of fever and systemic symptoms as well as the duration of viral shedding in both normal infants and those with underlying cardiopulmonary disease, although no study has yet shown that these beneficial effects correlate with shorter hospital stays or with less need for oxygen or ventilatory assistance. Aerosolized ribavirin has generally been used in infants who require hospitalization and who have evidence of severe lower respiratory tract disease and RSV on immunofluorescent staining of nasal wash specimens. Treatment of patients on mechanical ventilators requires the use of prefilters in order to prevent precipitation of drug in the tubing. Measurable quantities of drug in the air around the beds of patients receiving ribavirin aerosol have recently raised concerns about exposure of health care workers to this potentially teratogenic agent. This has led to greatly diminished enthusiasm for the use of this therapy.

Studies in small numbers of young adults with naturally occurring influenza A or B have shown modest decreases in duration of clinical illness when they are treated with oral or aerosolized ribavirin, but the results are not striking. Intravenous or oral ribavirin appears quite effective in the treatment of Lassa fever (see the chapter *Viral Hemorrhagic Fever*).

AMANTADINE (1-ADAMANTANAMINE HYDROCHLORIDE, SYMMETREL)

Amantadine is a symmetric tricyclic amine. It is active only against influenza A viruses. The mechanism of action is not entirely clear, but amantadine appears to prevent uncoating of the viral genome following penetration of the virus into the host cell. Most isolates of influenza A are inhibited in vitro at concentrations of 0.2 to 0.6 μg per milliliter. Although strains of influenza A can be made resistant to amantadine by laboratory passage, resistance to amantadine in treated patients is not a clinical problem. There has, however, been a report of isolation of resistant strains from untreated patients during an outbreak in East Germany. Amantadine was the first systemic antiviral drug licensed by the FDA and is indicated for treatment and prophylaxis of influenza A infection.

Pharmacology and Toxicity

Oral amantadine is well absorbed. Steady-state plasma levels in healthy adults taking the usual oral dose of 200 mg daily average 0.7 to 0.8 μg per milliliter, with CSF levels 60 percent of those in plasma. Amantadine also reaches therapeutic concentrations in respiratory secretions. Approximately 90 percent is excreted unchanged in the urine; the mean plasma half-life of 12 to 18 hours in healthy young adults increases to 7.4 days in patients with severely impaired renal function (creatinine clearance less than 10 ml per minute). Hemodialysis removes less than 5 percent of a dose, whereas substantially more is removed by peritoneal dialysis. Dosage adjustment is therefore essential in patients with renal insufficiency.

Oral amantadine is relatively well tolerated. Adverse effects are limited to the gastrointestinal and central nervous systems and appear to correlate with high plasma levels. One to 10 percent of treated patients experience nausea, anorexia, insomnia, difficulty in concentrating, headache, and dizziness, but in several studies the incidence of these complaints was not appreciably different between amantadine and placebo recipients. These minor side effects usually occur within 3 to 4 days of initiation of treatment and may resolve despite continued treatment. Toxic plasma levels (more than 1.0 μg per milliliter) in elderly patients or those with impaired renal function more rarely produce severe central nervous system effects, including delirium, hallucinations, convulsions, and coma. These adverse effects may be related to the dopamine-potentiating effects of amantadine, which are the basis for this drug's other common use, the treatment of Parkinson's disease. Patients with known seizure disorders have an increased risk of seizures with amantadine; this risk may be reduced by decreasing the dose. Oral amantadine is contraindicated in patients with gastric ulceration. High doses of amantadine (50 mg per kilogram daily) are teratogenic in rats; therefore amantadine therapy is not appropriate for pregnant women.

Clinical Uses

Amantadine is useful for treatment and prophylaxis of infections caused by influenza A viruses. When administered prophylactically, amantadine is 50 to 91 percent effective in preventing illness due to influenza A. It is more effective in preventing illness than in preventing infection, as documented by virus isolation or seroconversion. This may in fact be beneficial, as subclinical infection may lead to the development of immune responses that will protect against further exposure to antigenically related strains of influenza A virus. Because flu-like symptoms may be caused by several different infectious agents (only one of which is susceptible to amantadine) and because widespread use of amantadine is quite costly and associated with side effects, amantadine prophylaxis should begin only after there is a documented outbreak of influenza A in the community. The prophylactic efficacies of amantadine and influenza vaccine are roughly equivalent, but amantadine is not a substitute for vaccination as it does not protect against influenza B. In addition, amantadine as sole prophylaxis must be continued for the entire duration of the community outbreak, often 4 to 6 weeks, and the incidence of side effects increases with prolonged use. Thus amantadine prophylaxis should be considered an adjunct to immunization; the combined efficacy of amantadine and vaccine approaches 90 percent.

The target population for prophylaxis includes hospitalized patients; children and adults with chronic cardiovascular, pulmonary, metabolic, or renal disorders; immunodeficient patients; and persons over 65 years of age, especially those in nursing homes. Because of the risk of nosocomial transmission of influenza, vaccination and outbreak-period prophylaxis are recommended for health care workers (both hospital and community based) who have extensive contact with high-risk patients and for the entire staff of chronic care facilities.

High-risk patients who have not been immunized before the beginning of an outbreak of influenza A should begin amantadine as soon as possible and be vaccinated as well. Amantadine should be continued for 2 weeks after vaccination or for the duration of the outbreak if the patient is unable to tolerate vaccination (because of a severe allergy to eggs or a history of severe immediate allergic reaction to a previous dose of vaccine) or is at risk of having a poor antibody response to vaccination (for example, the immunocompromised patient).

Several studies have shown that therapeutic use of amantadine, if begun within 24 to 48 hours of onset of flu-like symptoms, reduces the duration of fever and systemic symptoms by one-third, or 1 to 2 days. It also hastens the resolution of minor small airway abnormalities in patients with uncomplicated influenza A and reduces viral shedding. Its efficacy in the treatment or prevention of primary influenza pneumonia is not clear. Nevertheless, oral amantadine therapy should be considered for high-risk patients with an illness compatible with influenza during a period of known or suspected influenza A activity in the community. Therapy should be initiated within 24 to 48 hours of onset of symptoms and continued for 48 hours after resolution.

The usual dose of oral amantadine for both prophylaxis and therapy in normal adults is 100 mg twice daily. For adults over 65 years of age, the recommended daily dose should not exceed 100 mg. Further dosage reductions are needed for patients with impaired renal function (Table 2) and in patients with known seizure disorders. The approved dosage for children 1 to 9 years of age is 4.4 to 8.8 mg per kilogram per day, up to 150 mg per day. Aerosolized amantadine is also effective in treating uncomplicated influenza A infection, producing therapeutic levels in the lungs with little systemic absorption, but the inconvenience of administration fails to warrant its use, especially in comparison with the equally effective oral form.

TABLE 2 Dosage Adjustment for Oral Amantadine in Patients With Impaired Renal Function

Creatinine Clearance (ml/min/1.73 m^2)	Suggested Oral Maintenance Regimen After 200 mg (100 mg b.i.d.) on the First Day
≥ 80	100 mg b.i.d.
60–80	100 mg b.i.d. alternating with 100 mg daily
40–60	100 mg daily
30–40	200 mg (100 mg b.i.d.) twice weekly
20–30	100 mg 3 times each week
10–20	200 mg (100 mg b.i.d.) alternating with 100 mg q7d
< 10*	100 mg q7d

* Including patients on hemodialysis.
Modified from Horadan et al. Ann Intern Med 1981; 94:454–458.

RIMANTADINE (α-METHYL-1-ADAMANTANEMETHYLAMINE HYDROCHLORIDE)

Rimantadine is a structural analogue of amantadine. It has the same antiviral spectrum and mechanism of action but is somewhat more effective in vitro than amantadine. Rimantadine is less well absorbed and more extensively metabolized, with less than 10 percent excreted unchanged in the urine. When given in equal doses, steady-state plasma levels of rimantadine are 61 to 65 percent of amantadine values, and the plasma half-life is twice as long. Central nervous system adverse effects are less frequent with rimantadine, correlating perhaps with lower plasma concentrations. Indeed, comparable plasma concentrations produce comparable symptoms, and the incidence of gastrointestinal complaints is the same with the two drugs. Rimantadine has been used extensively in the Soviet Union. It has been studied in several controlled trials in the United States and found to be as effective as amantadine in prophylaxis and therapy of infections caused by influenza A but is not yet licensed for clinical use.

OTHER AGENTS

Foscarnet (trisodium phosphonoformate) is a DNA polymerase inhibitor that is virustatic for herpesviruses. It has some efficacy in treatment of herpes simplex virus infections and is undergoing trials for therapy of CMV infections in immunosuppressed patients. It may also have activity against HIV. Its use is limited by the need for continuous intravenous infusion, and the major adverse effect appears to be renal dysfunction.

Human interferons (IFNs) have multiple antiviral effects, both in inhibition of viral replication and in modulation of host immune responses. Trials are underway to investigate the efficacy of the various interferons, either alone or in combination with other antiviral agents, in the therapy of several different viral diseases. Intralesional human IFN-α is efficacious in therapy of genital papillomavirus infections (condyloma acuminata).

SUGGESTED READING

Dolin R, Reichman RC, Madore HP, et al. A controlled trial of amantadine and rimantadine in the prophylaxis of influenza A infection. N Engl J Med 1982; 307:580–584.

Dorsky DI, Crumpacker CS. Drugs five years later: acyclovir. Ann Intern Med 1987; 107:859–874.

Hall CB, McBride JT, Walsh EE, et al. Aerosolized ribavirin treatment of infants with respiratory syncytial viral infection. N Engl J Med 1983; 308:1443–1447.

Shepp DH, Dandliker PS, Meyers JD. Treatment of varicella-zoster virus infection in severely immunocompromised patients. N Engl J Med 1986; 314:208–212.

ANTIBACTERIAL CHEMOTHERAPY

STEPHEN H. ZINNER, M.D.
KENNETH H. MAYER, M.D.

The past half century of antibiotic chemotherapy has provided physicians with many choices to treat bacterial infections. Several new antibiotic classes have been introduced in the past decade, and a consideration of the appropriate use of these drugs is important in the current practice of medicine.

While many of the newer, expensive antimicrobial agents are active against a wide range of bacterial pathogens, the physician should use less expensive drugs whenever possible. Often, antibiotics may be given for inappropriate indications (e.g., viral syndromes). Antibiotic resistance continues to cause treatment failures, and any unnecessary use of antibiotics that alters the bacterial ecology and enhances the development of antibiotic resistance should be avoided.

This chapter considers the use of specific classes of antibiotics, their pharmacology, the use of antibiotic susceptibility testing, and studies of antibiotic activity in vitro and in vivo.

GENERAL PRINCIPLES OF ANTIBIOTIC THERAPY

The appropriate use of antibiotics requires an estimation of the likelihood of the presence of bacterial infection. A careful history and physical examination should be performed. Whenever possible, a sample should be obtained from the affected body site or from blood, urine, or other body fluid for stain and culture before the selection of an appropriate antibiotic.

If an empiric antibiotic choice is necessary, this should be based on an evaluation of the most likely pathogen responsible for infection at a given clinical site. The spectrum of activity of the drug, its pharmacology, cost, and the frequency of adverse toxic or side effects all affect the choice of antibiotic. If drugs are administered orally, efforts should be made to ensure patient compliance. In general, it is preferable to use a narrow-spectrum or specific antibiotic whenever the organism is known. The use of broad-spectrum agents can result in the suppression of endogenous, commensal bacterial flora, with resulting diarrhea and overgrowth of resistant pathogens.

The optimal duration of antibiotic therapy has not been clearly established for most infections. In many acute infections, it is appropriate to administer antibiotics for approximately 3 to 5 days after the patient has defervesced. Serious infections such as osteomyelitis, bacterial endocarditis, and septic arthritis require longer therapy, often intravenously, for 4 to 6 weeks. Other infections such as meningitis and gram-negative rod bacteremia are usually treated for 10 to 14 days.

ANTIBIOTIC PHARMACOLOGY

The physician should select a drug that is active against the infecting organism at the site of infection. Antibiotic pharmacology includes consideration of pharmacodynamics, which describe the effects of the drug on the bacteria, and of pharmacokinetics, which consider the absorption, distribution, metabolism, and excretion of these agents.

Pharmacodynamics

Pharmacodynamic considerations include evaluations of the in vitro susceptibility of the bacteria to the antibiotic. Several methods exist to determine antibiotic susceptibility. The Kirby-Bauer-Turck disk test is still commonly used in many hospital microbiology laboratories. This method requires the seeding of an agar plate with the test organism and the application of small disks that have been impregnated with known concentrations of antibiotics. The plates are incubated overnight and the zone of inhibition of bacterial growth around the disk is measured. This method provides an estimate of antibiotic inhibition of bacterial growth and not its bactericidal activity.

The minimal inhibitory concentration (MIC) and minimal bactericidal concentration (MBC) are laboratory tests to determine concentrations of a drug that will inhibit or kill a standard bacterial inoculum (usually 10^4 cfu per milliliter). Several automated methods have been introduced in laboratory microbiology to supply clinicians with specific MICs and MBCs.

In general, bactericidal activity is required in the treatment of bacterial infections that are deep seated or occur in an area of minimal host defense, such as osteomyelitis and endocarditis, as well as infections the treatment of which requires the rapid elimination of the bacterial load, e.g., meningitis or bacteremia in immunocompromised patients. Bactericidal agents include penicillins, cephalosporins, aminoglycosides, quinolones, vancomycin, metronidazole, rifampin, and trimethoprim-sulfamethoxazole. Tetracycline, chloramphenicol, erythromycin, clindamycin, and sulfona-mides inhibit bacterial growth and are thus bacteriostatic.

More specialized procedures exist to determine anti-biotic pharmacodynamics, such as time-kill curves, in which standard bacterial inocula are exposed to variable concen-trations of drugs, usually as multiples of the MIC. The ef-fect of these drug concentrations over time is determined by counting the remaining viable bacteria, usually over an 8- or 12-hour period. Time-kill curves are time- and labor-intensive, usually requiring specially trained technologists, and are not routinely performed for clinical isolates.

The minimum antibiotic concentration (MAC) describes the smallest amount of antibiotic that has any measurable effect on bacteria, such as reduction in bacterial growth rates, bacterial elongation or filamentation, or changes in the ad-herence of bacteria to various tissues or surfaces. These MACs could result in enhanced phagocytosis at infected tis-sue sites. Some antibiotics exert an effect on bacteria at con-centrations below the MIC. Subinhibitory effects also might enhance local phagocytosis and synergistically abet the activ-ity of other antibiotics when combination chemotherapy is used.

The effect of antibiotics on bacteria can persist after the extracellular drug has been removed. This is known as the postantibiotic effect (PAE) and can be measured in vitro by bacterial exposure to antibiotics, subsequent removal of the drug by washing or enzymatic inactivation, and then comparing the rate of bacterial growth to that of unexposed bacteria. The PAE reflects the difference in time for con-trol and treated bacteria to increase in number by one log. The clinical significance of the PAE is not clearly known, but it may contribute to the clinical activity of aminoglyco-sides and quinolones.

Local conditions at the site of infection may influence the activity of certain antibiotics. For example, the pH of the surrounding tissues can affect antibiotic activity. Aminoglycosides and erythromycin are more active at an alkaline pH. These drugs are less effective within an ab-scess or other infected tissues with low pH. Aminoglyco-sides are not active in an anaerobic environment. Other drugs may be relatively inhibited in the presence of certain uri-nary components. The activity of aminoglycosides and some of the new quinolone antibiotics may be decreased in the presence of high concentrations of calcium, magnesium, or other cations. All antibiotics may reversibly bind to serum albumin, but tightly bound compounds such as certain cephalosporins may not achieve high concentrations of free or active drug in the central nervous system or in other tissues.

Pharmacokinetics

Some new drugs have been developed in order to take advantage of pharmacokinetic properties. In general, the clinical activity of a drug depends upon the ability to achieve peak serum concentrations of free or unbound drug that are well in excess of the MIC for a given bacterial pathogen. Other important considerations include the time above the MIC, the area under the concentration–time curve above the MIC, as well as the ratio of peak serum concentration to the MIC (Fig. 1). The clinical significance of these vari-ables is especially important with agents such as aminoglyco-sides, which demonstrate concentration-dependent bactericidal activity.

The route of administration, bioavailability, volume of distribution, and administered dose independently affect the concentration of antibiotic achieved in serum and tissue. The highest serum concentrations usually follow the intravenous administration of an antibiotic. However, some well-

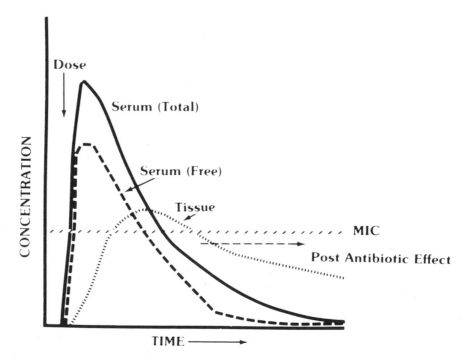

Figure 1 Diagram showing the re-lation between drug concentrations in serum and those in tissues after a sin-gle dose. The postantibiotic effect be-gins when levels in tissues fall below the MIC. (Reprinted with permission from Kunin CM. Dosage schedules of antimicrobial agents: a historical review. Rev Infect Dis 1981; 3:4–11.)

absorbed drugs (e.g., chloramphenicol and the fluoroquinolones) achieve similar concentrations by mouth as well as by intravenous administration, although the time to achieve this concentration after oral dosing is delayed by about 1 hour.

The distribution of antibiotics may also depend on the drug's lipid-partition coefficient. Lipophilic drugs, such as chloramphenicol and rifampin, are more diffusible across cell and tissue membranes. Clinically, this is most important in the treatment of bacterial meningitis where chloramphenicol, rifampin, tetracyclines, sulfonamides, and metronidazole achieve acceptable concentrations even in the absence of inflammation. In the presence of inflamed meninges, adequate therapeutic concentrations are usually achieved with penicillins and most third-generation cephalosporins. Aminoglycosides, clindamycin, erythromycin, and vancomycin cannot reliably achieve therapeutic concentrations in cerebrospinal fluid. Experience with the new quinolones in meningitis is limited.

The absorption of some drugs, notably tetracyclines and the quinolones, may be decreased in the presence of bivalent or trivalent cations. These drugs are less well absorbed following the administration of calcium- or aluminum-containing antacids, respectively.

The volume of distribution of an antimicrobial agent influences the duration of the peak concentration as well as the penetration into tissues. Drugs such as the quinolones, which have a high volume of distribution, have a relatively prompt decrease in their peak concentrations following intravenous administration.

The rate of elimination of an antibiotic is expressed as its elimination half-life (t½). The t½ of antibiotics ranges from less than 1 hour for the penicillins and first-generation cephalosporins to between 3 and 5 hours for some of the new quinolone drugs. In general, the shorter the t½, the more frequently a drug must be administered to achieve an antibacterial effect. Drugs with a very long t½ (e.g., ceftriaxone) may be administered once daily. The dosing of antimicrobial agents that are primarily excreted by the kidney is often reduced in the presence of renal failure. In most cases either each dose is reduced or the interval between doses is prolonged in order to provide appropriate levels and minimize toxicity. Metabolism and excretion of antibiotics are also important factors to consider in determining the ability of active drug to reach the site of infection.

Serum drug concentrations are usually measured for antibiotics having a narrow therapeutic range. Aminoglycosides have variable pharmacokinetics, and their use requires frequent monitoring of serum levels. High trough concentrations of aminoglycosides have been associated with nephrotoxicity.

The serum bactericidal assay utilizes a sample obtained following an antibiotic dose. The ability of successive serum dilutions (e.g., 1:2, 1:4, etc.) to kill a standard inoculum of the patient's infecting organism is determined. The serum bactericidal titer (SBT) is expressed as the highest dilution that kills 99.9 percent of the inoculum. This test describes the relation of achievable drug concentration to the MBC and is useful in the treatment of bacterial endocarditis and osteomyelitis, as well as in bacteremia in the immunocompromised patient. In general, SBTs 1:16 or higher have been associated with good clinical outcome.

ANTIBIOTIC RESISTANCE

Bacteria may become resistant to antibiotics by several mechanisms. Mutations (changes in the bacterial chromosome) may result in antibiotic resistance by alterations in cell wall or membrane components with subsequent drug impermeability. A mutation may result in the alteration of a specific target or binding site of the antibiotic. Mutation in a bacterial regulatory gene may result in overproduction of a substrate or result in the loss of a biochemical intermediate on which the antibiotic acts. Mutations are not readily transferable between species. Although mutated bacteria are resistant to antibiotics, they also have growth disadvantages when compared to their wild-type counterparts. Antibiotic selection pressure clearly may be related to an increase in resistant mutants.

Antibiotic resistance also may be mediated by self-replicating, transferable genetic material called plasmids. These plasmids may contain multiple genes in addition to those mediating antibiotic resistance, and more than one plasmid may exist within a given bacterial cell. In this setting, genetic exchange or recombination can occur, and resistance determinants may move from one plasmid to another or from a plasmid to a chromosome by smaller motile genes called transposons.

Several clinically common mechanisms are responsible for antibiotic resistance in many bacterial species. Enzymes that hydrolyze the β-lactam ring of penicillins and similar compounds render these antibiotics inactive, as they are no longer able to bind specific binding proteins. These β-lactamases may be chromosomally or plasmid-mediated and are common in many species. The ability of bacteria to produce β-lactamases may be constitutive (substrate independent), as in the case of many gram-negative bacilli, or inducible (substrate dependent), as with many gram-positive cocci. The β-lactamases may be excreted extracellularly, as in most gram-positive cocci, or may be retained within the periplasmic space between the inner and outer membranes of gram-negative bacilli.

β-Lactam antibiotics also may be inactive against resistant bacteria by means of changes in porins, which are cell wall proteins responsible for the water-filled channels that limit the permeability of the bacterial cells for specific compounds.

Aminoglycosides are most often inactivated because of the production of aminoglycoside-modifying enzymes. These acetylating, adenylating, or phosphorylating enzymes decrease the ability of the aminoglycosides to bind to their ribosomal targets. Some bacteria resist aminoglycosides by mutations in their oxidative phosphorylation mechanisms, which may affect the uptake of aminoglycosides into the bacterial cell. Bacteria also produce enzymes that inactivate

TABLE 1 Antibiotics in Clinical Use

Category, Agent	Available by Oral Route	Category, Agent	Available by Oral Route
Penicillins		Other β-lactam drugs	
Penicillin	Yes	Aztreonam	
Ampicillin (±βLI)	Yes	Imipenem-cilastatin	
Amoxicillin (±βLI)	Yes		
Oxacillin	Yes	Aminoglycosides	
Methicillin		Gentamicin	
Nafcillin		Tobramycin	
Cloxacillin	Yes	Amikacin	
Dicloxacillin	Yes	Netilmicin	
Azlocillin			
Mezlocillin		Quinolones	
Piperacillin		Nalidixic acid	Yes
Ticarcillin (±βLI)		Cinoxacin	Yes
Carbenicillin		Norfloxacin	Yes
Amdinocillin		Ciprofloxacin	Yes
		Enoxacin (I)	Yes
Cephalosporins and cefamycins		Ofloxacin (I)	Yes
First-generation*		Lomefloxacin (I)	Yes
Cephalothin		Fleroxacin (I)	Yes
Cefazolin		Pefloxacin (I)	Yes
Cephapirin			
Cephalexin	Yes	Other antibacterial drugs	
Cephradine	Yes	Chloramphenicol	Yes
Cefaclor	Yes	Clindamycin	Yes
Cefadroxil		Erythromycin	Yes
Second-generation†		Metronidazole	Yes
Cefamandole		Nitrofurantoin	Yes
Cefuroxime	Yes	Rifampin	Yes
Cefoxitin		Sulfonamides	Yes
Cefotetan		Trimethoprim	Yes
Cefonicid		Tetracycline (minocycline, doxycycline)	Yes
Ceforanide		Vancomycin	
Third-generation‡		Spectinomycin	
Cefotaxime			
Ceftizoxime			
Ceftriaxone			
Cefoperazone (±βLI)			
Ceftazidime			
Moxalactam			
Cefpiramide			
Cefsulodin			
Cefmenoxime			

Note: (±βLI): may be administered in combination with a β-lactamase inhibitor to enhance antibacterial spectrum; (I): investigational drug.
* First-generation drugs are active against gram-positive cocci and some gram-negative rods.
† Second-generation drugs are also active against *Haemophilus* species and some anaerobic organisms.
‡ Third-generation drugs are more active against gram-negative bacilli and less active against gram-positive cocci, and some have activity against *P. aeruginosa*.

chloramphenicol. Resistance to erythromycin is often mediated by ribosomal methylation, which prevents antibiotic binding. Resistance to sulfonamides and trimethoprim may be mediated by plasmid-encoded target enzymes that are not susceptible to these drugs.

ANTIBIOTIC CLASSES

The antibiotics in clinical use are listed in Table 1. Table 2 describes the spectrum of activity of some commonly used antibiotics against prevalent bacterial pathogens.

Penicillins

The penicillins kill bacteria by inhibiting cell wall synthesis. Penicillins bind to specific proteins that prevent peptide cross-linkages, and thus the cell wall becomes osmotically fragile. Some penicillin-binding proteins mediate bacterial lysis, and others, elongation or filament formation. Their spectrum includes the streptococci, clostridia, *Neisseria* species, some anaerobic gram-negative rods, and *Treponema pallidum*. Semisynthetic penicillins, such as nafcillin, oxacillin, methicillin, cloxacillin, and dicloxacillin are

TABLE 2 Spectrum of Activity of Some Commonly Used Antibiotics Against Prevalent Bacterial Pathogens

Antibiotic Class	Organism					
	Nonenterococcal Streptococci	Enterococcus*	S. aureus†	Enterobacteriaceae	P. aeruginosa	Anaerobes‡
Natural penicillin	++++	+++	+/−	−	−	+++/−
Ampicillin	+++	++++	+/−	+	−	+++/−
Gram-positive semisynthetic penicillin	++	++	++++/−	−	−	+/−
Ureidopenicillin	++	++++	+/−	++++	+++	+++/−
First-generation cephalosporin	++	−	+++/−	++++	−	+/−
Second-generation cephalosporin	++	−	+/−	+++	−	+++
Third-generation cephalosporin§	+	−	+/−	++++	++	+++
Monobactam	−	−	−	+++	++	−
Carbapenem	+++	+++	+++/+	++++	++++	+++
Aminoglycoside#	−	+	++	+++	++	−
Fluoroquinolone	+	−	+++	++++	++++	−
Tetracycline	++	−	+	+	−	+/−
Erythromycin	++	−	++	−	−	+/−
Chloramphenicol	+++	−	++	++	−	+++
Vancomycin	++++	++++	++++	−	−	−
Metronidazole	−	−	−	−	−	++++
Clindamycin	++	−	++	−	−	++++

Specific susceptibilities should be performed on any clinical isolate, since the acquisition of chromosomal- or plasmid-mediated resistance may inactivate a generally efficacious antibiotic. The site of an infection may make an antibiotic with excellent in vitro activity less desirable (e.g., vancomycin for a staphylococcal brain abscess). Allergic reactions and common drug toxicities may limit the use of an agent for a specific infection.

− = no activity
+ = some activity
++ = moderate activity
+++ = good activity
++++ = first-line agent
* Systemic enterococcal infection requires therapy with a β-lactam or vancomycin (cell wall active compounds) *plus* an aminoglycoside.
† Methicillin susceptible/methicillin resistant.
‡ Anaerobes above the diaphragm/anaerobes below.
§ Specific agents may differ greatly in their activity against gram-negative aerobes.
# Aminoglycosides are rarely used as monotherapy.

bactericidal for *Staphylococcus aureus* and some strains of *Staphylococcus epidermidis*. The extended-spectrum penicillins such as ampicillin and amoxicillin are not active against penicillinase-producing strains of *S. aureus*, but they are active against some gram-negative enteric bacilli such as *Salmonella*, *Shigella*, and many urinary tract strains of *Escherichia coli*. In addition, these drugs are active against many strains of *Haemophilus influenzae*. The antipseudomonal penicillins are frequently active against Enterobacteriaceae and include carbenicillin, ticarcillin, piperacillin, azlocillin, and mezlocillin, the latter of which is least active against *Pseudomonas aeruginosa*. These penicillins do not resist the activity of β-lactamases, but amoxicillin, ticarcillin, and ampicillin have been combined with β-lactamase inhibitors such as clavulanic acid and sulbactam, with enhanced activity against many β-lactamase-producing strains of gram-negative rods, including some anaerobic organisms.

Cephalosporins

The cephalosporins have a similar mechanism of action to the penicillins and are active against many gram-negative rods as well as methicillin-sensitive staphylococci and streptococci. The first-generation cephalosporins (cephalothin, cefazolin, cefapirin, and others) are primarily active against staphylococci and urinary isolates of *E. coli*. Newer cephalosporins are also active against β-lactamase-producing *H. influenzae*. Cefotetan and cefoxitin are particularly active against anaerobes. The most recently developed cephalosporins have extended spectra that include most aerobic, multiresistant gram-negative rods. Ceftazidime is also active against *P. aeruginosa*.

Other β-lactam agents include aztreonam, a monobactam agent with activity only against gram-negative bacteria, including *P. aeruginosa*. Imipenem is a carbapenem antibiotic with broad-spectrum activity against most aerobic and anaerobic bacteria. Clinically, it is combined with cilastatin, which inhibits its renal degradation.

Aminoglycosides

The aminoglycoside antibiotics are rapidly bactericidal against gram-negative aerobic bacteria including *P. aeruginosa*. These antibiotics also kill *S. aureus* and, in combination with penicillin or ampicillin, are bactericidal for enterococci. They act on ribosomes and their activity requires metabolic uptake across the bacterial membranes. These drugs are administered intravenously or intramuscularly and are often used in combination with β-lactam agents in the treatment of gram-negative rod bacteremia.

Quinolones

The older quinolones, nalidixic acid and cinoxacin, are primarily limited to the treatment of susceptible urinary tract infections. The new fluoroquinolones, norfloxacin and ciprofloxacin, have enhanced activity against most gram-negative rods, including *P. aeruginosa,* and are active against enteric bacterial pathogens. The new quinolones are also active against staphylococci, *Legionella* species, *Chlamydia trachomatis*, and *Ureaplasma urealyticum.* Some quinolones may be active against some mycobacterial species. These drugs have limited activity against streptococci and no activity against anaerobic gram-negative rods. The quinolones are well absorbed orally, have a large volume of distribution, and act intracellularly. Norfloxacin is clinically limited to urinary and some gastrointestinal infections.

Other Antibacterial Drugs

Chloramphenicol is primarily limited to treatment of bacterial meningitis, brain abscess, and typhoid fever. Clindamycin is a useful antibiotic active against anaerobic gram-negative rods and many gram-positive cocci, including *S. aureus*. Erythromycin is the treatment of choice for Legionnaire's disease and is active against many gram-positive cocci.

Metronidazole's activity is limited to anaerobic organisms, and it is frequently used in the treatment of intra-abdominal infections. Nitrofurantoin is limited to the treatment of urinary tract infections due to susceptible aerobic gram-negative rods. Rifampin is an agent that is usually limited for use in the treatment of tuberculosis but also has activity against gram-positive cocci and many gram-negative rods. It is never used alone because mutational resistance develops rapidly. Its use should be limited to special clinical situations and should be in combination with other antibiotics.

The sulfonamides are primarily used in the treatment of urinary tract infections and in infections caused by *Nocardia asteroides*. They are frequently combined with trimethoprim to enhance activity and bactericidal effects. Tetracyclines are broad-spectrum antimicrobial agents active against a number of intracellular organisms including rickettsiae, mycoplasmas, chlamydiae, and some parasitic infections, as well as some bacteria. Vancomycin is active against most gram-positive organisms, including methicillin-resistant staphylococci. Oral vancomycin may also be used to treat *Clostridium difficile*-related colitis. Spectinomycin is primarily used in the treatment of gonococcal infections.

ANTIBIOTIC COMBINATIONS

Antibiotic synergism occurs with antibiotic combinations in a few clinical circumstances, notably bacteremia in neutropenic patients and enterococcal endocarditis and in-

fections caused by *P. aeruginosa*. Antibiotics may be combined in mixed infections and possibly to limit the emergence of antibiotic-resistant bacteria. Unnecessary antibiotic combinations needlessly contribute to increased costs and could result in drug antagonism.

ANTIBIOTIC PROPHYLAXIS

It is impossible to prevent all infections with antibiotic prophylaxis. However, the preventive use of these agents is clearly valuable in some surgical operations, notably, foreign-body implants, cardiovascular surgery, operations on an infected biliary tract, contaminated intra-abdominal procedures, vaginal and abdominal hysterectomy, and trauma associated with ruptured abdominal viscera or compound fractures. Antibiotic prophylaxis should be started just before surgery and should be stopped within 24 hours after surgery. Two doses of most agents, or one dose of a long-acting agent, are usually sufficient. Longer courses may lead to superinfections and obviously increase costs without benefit to patients.

Prophylactic antibiotics are also used to prevent bacterial endocarditis following instrumentation, surgery, or dental treatment. Prophylaxis is also useful in the prevention of secondary cases of rheumatic fever and following exposure to meningitis caused by *N. meningitidis* and *H. influenzae*. These issues are addressed more fully in other chapters.

CONCLUSIONS

Judicious use of antimicrobial agents requires consideration of the spectrum, pharmacodynamics, and pharmacokinetics, as well as the cost of these frequently expensive drugs. The current trend appears to favor the use of single or twice daily doses of intravenous drugs for serious infections. The use of oral agents with excellent pharmacokinetic properties may minimize hospitalization-associated costs. The utilization of intravenous antibiotics at home is becoming more common, and physicians should closely supervise and monitor the patient's care. Potential adverse effects and pharmacologic interactions of antibiotics should always be considered so that the physician can choose the least expensive and least toxic but most specific and efficacious antibiotic for any given infection.

SUGGESTED READING

Handbook of antimicrobial therapy. New Rochelle, NY: The Medical Letter, 1986.
Kucers A, Bennett N. The use of antibiotics: a comprehensive review with clinical emphasis. Philadelphia: JB Lippincott, 1987.
Neu H. Chemotherapy of infection. In: Braunwald E, ed. Harrison's principles of internal medicine. 12th ed. New York: McGraw-Hill, 1987:485–502.
Sande MA, Mandell GL. Chemotherapy of microbial diseases. In: Goodman and Gilman's the pharmacological basis of therapeutics. 7th ed. New York: Macmillan Publishing, 1980:1066–1198.
Young LS. Antimicrobial therapy. In: Wyngaarden JB, Smith LH, eds. Cecil textbook of medicine 18th ed. Philadelphia: WB Saunders, 1988:112–125.

ANTIFUNGAL CHEMOTHERAPY

HEINZ-JOSEF SCHMITT, M.D.
DONALD ARMSTRONG, M.D.

This chapter reviews antifungal agents that can be used for the treatment of systemic fungal infections. Table 1 shows agents currently available or in various states of clinical evaluation. Ever since its introduction in the 1950s, amphotericin B has been the "gold standard" of treatment of most invasive fungal diseases, despite its considerable toxicity. New agents are on the horizon. The evaluation of their efficacy in human disease, however, as compared with the evaluation of antibacterial agents, is difficult for several reasons:

1. In vitro tests are not standardized, and determination of minimal inhibitory concentrations (MICs) often differs more than 1,000–fold among different laboratories.

2. Animal models more reliably reveal antifungal activity. However, data are sometimes conflicting, and the disease produced may not reflect the counterpart seen in humans (e.g., injection of aspergillus spores intravenously does not produce pulmonary aspergillosis).

3. Clinical trials are difficult to perform because (1) the diagnosis of many systemic fungal infections is difficult to prove without invasive techniques (exception, cryptococcal meningitis); (2) some fungal diseases are rare, and it may take years to complete clinical trials; and (3) in some cases fungal infections heal spontaneously, e.g., when the immune system of a patient recovers or when immunosuppressive therapy is stopped.

These limitations should always be kept in mind when in vitro test results or cases of "successful treatment" of a fungal disease with a new agent are reported. For many diseases the optimal duration of treatment is not known. As a rule of thumb, immunocompromised patients require longer, and sometimes indefinite, treatment.

POLYENES

Polyenes, of which amphotericin B is an example, share a similar structure, mechanism of action, pharmacology, and toxicity. There is practically complete cross-resistance. They are all poorly absorbed from the gastrointestinal tract and remarkably toxic when given parenterally. The common mechanism of action is binding of the lipophilic polyene component to the ergosterol in fungal cytoplasmic membranes, thus causing the membrane to become porous.

Modification of membrane sterols leading to a less efficient binding with amphotericin B and a decrease in membrane ergosterol are mechanisms for resistance. With rare exceptions, however, emergence of resistance is not of major clinical concern. However, a lack of bioavailability of amphotericin B probably contributes to therapeutic failures, especially in immunocompromised patients: Patients dying of invasive aspergillosis and candidiasis had

TABLE 1 Antifungal Agents for Treatment of Systemic Mycoses

Polyenes
Amphotericin B
Nystatin*
5-Fluorocytosine
Azoles
Clotrimazole*
Miconazole
Ketoconazole
Fluconazole[†]
Itraconazole[†]
Allylamines
Naftifine*[†]
Terbinafine[†]
Lipopeptides
Cilofungin[†]

* Topical use only.
† Investigational antifungal agents.

amphotericin B concentrations in infected organs that exceeded their MIC by 100-fold, as determined from isolates cultured from the autopsy specimens.

Filipin, trichomycin, candidin, and other compounds of the polyene group have no advantage over amphotericin B, nystatin, and natamycin (pimaricin only as 5 percent ophthalmic suspension), which are the only polyenes marketed in the United States. Nystatin and natamycin are only used topically. None of the others has any proven advantage in terms of clinical efficacy.

Amphotericin B

Amphotericin B is produced by *Streptomyces nodosus*. It is given intravenously in 250 (lower doses) to 1,000 ml of 5 percent dextrose in water (D5W; the recommended final concentration is 0.1 mg per milliliter) over 4 to 6 hours. When it is freshly prepared, protection of amphotericin B from light is not necessary. Addition of electrolytes, sodium, or potassium salts causes aggregation of the amphotericin B suspension and results in decreased effectiveness.

In serum, amphotericin B is separated from the desoxycholate with which it is packaged and binds to β-lipoproteins (probably cholesterol). It leaves the bloodstream rapidly and accumulates in the liver, spleen, and kidneys. The highest amphotericin B concentrations are found in these organs, and lung concentrations are about one-fifth to one-tenth of those found in the liver. Amphotericin B does not penetrate inflamed or normal meninges very well; drug concentrations in inflamed peritoneum, pleura, joints, and vitreous and aqueous humor are about 50 percent of serum concentrations or higher. Serum levels are not helpful in predicting outcome, efficacy, or side effects. Only a small amount of amphotericin B is excreted via the urine. The exact mode of excretion is unknown, although in dogs and rats biliary excretion accounts for some elimination.

No dose-adjustment is necessary in patients with renal failure, except for the purpose of decreasing renal toxicity. Hemodialysis does not change blood levels unless a patient is lipemic and loses amphotericin B because it binds to the dialysis membrane.

Dosage and duration of therapy depend on the type and severity of infection, the underlying disease, the patient's general condition and tolerance, and side effects. Candidal esophagitis usually responds to doses as small as 0.2 to 0.3 mg per kilogram given intravenously for 5 to 7 days. We treat life-threatening fungal infections in immunocompromised patients with 1 mg per kilogram per day, usually for a total dose of 1.0 to 2.5 g. First, a 1-mg test dose is given over 4 hours, and vital signs are monitored at least every 30 minutes. If the dose is tolerated, immediately thereafter 5 mg, followed by 10 mg, 20 mg, and 40 mg, are administered every 4 to 6 hours. Thus, the total dose given on day 1 of amphotericin B treatment is about 1 mg per kilogram, which is the usual dose on the following days.

About 50 percent of all patients receiving amphotericin B experience acute reactions (fevers, chills, malaise), which usually last for a few hours and become less severe with continued therapy. These seem to be due to release of interleukin 1 and tumor necrosis factor and can be ameliorated, if necessary, by premedication with acetaminophen (700 mg orally) and meperidine (50 mg intravenously). Hydrocortisone (50 mg intravenously) can be given if reactions are extreme, but this must be weighed against the possible immunosuppressive effects of glucocorticoids. It is not helpful in patients already receiving steroids for other reasons.

An increase in creatinine level occurs in virtually every patient on amphotericin B. The amount of permanent reduction in the glomerular filtration rate is related to the total dose given. Salt supplementation administered by antibiotic solutions containing large amounts of sodium (e.g., ticarcillin) or by sodium chloride solution (e.g., 1 L of 0.9 percent sodium chloride per day) may minimize amphotericin B–induced nephrotoxicity.

Since only a small amount of amphotericin B is excreted via the kidneys, no dosage adjustment is necessary for patients with a rising creatinine level. For a serum creatinine concentration between 3.0 and 3.5 mg per milliliter, however, a dose reduction may become necessary in order to prevent dehydration and cachexia secondary to nausea and vomiting. In this situation, amphotericin B is often given in a somewhat higher single dose (1.25 mg per kilogram) every other day if the patient is stable and clearly responding. Kidney toxicity is only prevented if the dose given every other day is not doubled.

Electrolytes in serum should be monitored carefully. Hypokalemia and hypomagnesemia occur regularly. Other adverse effects of amphotericin B include anemia, weight loss, headache, phlebitis, renal tubular acidosis, and, in rare cases, thrombocytopenia, leukopenia, burning sensation on the soles of the feet, hypotension, and anaphylaxis. In one report, aggregation of leukocytes by amphotericin B given directly after a white blood cell transfusion was believed to be the cause of acute pulmonary deterioration.

With the first dose, the patient's blood pressure should be checked at least every half hour. Further monitoring should include at least a thrice-weekly determination of the complete blood count, K^+, Na^+, Mg^{++}, and urinalysis. Since amphotericin B is eliminated slowly, its side effects may persist for months after completion of therapy.

Diseases that usually respond to intravenous therapy with amphotericin B include aspergillosis, blastomycosis, candidiasis, coccidioidomycosis, cryptococcosis, histoplasmosis, mucormycosis, paracoccidioidomycosis, and extracutaneous sporotrichosis. In patients with prolonged fever and neutropenia some investigators recommend amphotericin B empirically from day 5 to 7 on, even without documenting a fungal infection. The diagnosis of invasive fungal disease is missed in many of these patients, even when optimal diagnostic approaches are used, and early treatment improves outcome of opportunistic fungal infections.

In order to improve efficacy (bioavailability) or to decrease the amount of adverse effects, local therapy with amphotericin B is used in some instances. Intracisternal or intraventricular amphotericin B is essential for treating meningitis due to *Coccidioides immitis*. In a series from our institution, intraventricular amphotericin B given through an Ommaya reservoir was correlated with improved survival among cancer patients with cryptococcal meningitis. After test doses of 0.05 and 0.1 mg per day on days 1 and 2, a total of 0.2 to 0.5 mg amphotericin B is given once daily to three times a week. More frequent administration is given for more severe disease along with the higher doses. There is no evidence that intrathecal injection in the lumbar area is beneficial. If lumbar injections are used, 10 percent glucose may be preferred for dilution of the stock solution in order to facilitate hyperbaric flow to the brain. Additional intrathecal injection of 5 to 15 mg of hydrocortisone may decrease fever, headache, and nausea. In cystitis due to *Candida*, bladder irrigations with amphotericin B (0.05 mg per milliliter in distilled water) have been suggested. Joint mycosis due to *Sporothrix schenckii* or *C. immitis* may respond favorably to intra-articular injection of amphotericin B (5 to 15 mg). For keratomycoses, corneal baths with amphotericin B (1 mg per milliliter) are used.

New Methods of Delivering Amphotericin B

First reports indicate that amphotericin B encapsulated in liposomes is much better tolerated than amphotericin B desoxycholate. There appears to be virtually no acute toxicity, and adverse reactions occur in only about 3 percent of all patients. The incidence of nephrotoxicity is also decreased. One study group, however, reported somnolence in some patients. The mode of preparation and composition of liposomes may be crucial. The main advantage of liposomal amphotericin B appears to be the increased therapeutic index: much higher doses can be given with fewer adverse effects. Controlled clinical trials will have to show whether there will also be an increased therapeutic efficacy.

Nasal amphotericin B (10 mg per day in three divided doses) given with a sterile atomizer is currently under investigation for prophylaxis of pulmonary aspergillosis in patients with neutropenia and fever. Since the pathogenesis of pulmonary aspergillosis involves direct inhalation of *Aspergillus* spores into distal airways as well as colonization of the upper nasopharynx, we believe that additional measures should be taken. Aerosol amphotericin B has been effective in both preventing and treating pulmonary aspergillosis in our rat model of this disease, and clinical trials are underway.

Amphotericin B in Combination With Other Agents

The rationale in combining amphotericin B with other agents is to increase its efficacy and/or to reduce its toxicity. Many combinations have been shown to act synergistically with amphotericin B in vitro or even in animal models. To date, the only generally accepted indication is cryptococcal meningitis, for which amphotericin B is combined with 5-fluorocytosine (5-FC). Prospective, randomized controlled clinical trials have documented this indication.

Systemic candidiasis due to *Candida tropicalis* we believe to be another indication for the combined use of amphotericin B and 5-FC as suggested from one retrospective study.

In vitro, there is a two- to fourfold reduction in MICs against *Aspergillus, Candida, Cryptococcus, Histoplasma*, and *Mucor* when amphotericin B is combined with rifampin. In our animal model of systemic candidiasis, rifampin acts "synergistically" with amphotericin B, at least in part by increasing about twofold peak serum concentrations of amphotericin B (unpublished data). Clinical studies are needed to further investigate the role of amphotericin B plus rifampin in the treatment of fungal infections.

In various animal models, the combination of ketoconazole and amphotericin B was no better than amphotericin B alone. Some studies even suggested antagonism. Theoretically, antagonism may result when azoles block the synthesis of ergosterol, thus leaving amphotericin B without a target.

Nystatin

Nystatin is available in the United States for topical and oral administration, and it can be used to treat candidal infections of the skin and mucous membranes. Ringworm and subcutaneous fungal infections do not respond. There is no systemic absorption.

Indications for its use are oropharyngeal and esophageal candidiasis (5 ml of the 100,000 U per milliliter suspension four times daily swished in the oral cavity and swallowed thereafter) and vaginal candidiasis (1 tablet with 100,000 U inserted once or twice a day with an applicator high into the vagina for 14 days). For this indication, however, miconazole or clotrimazole cream given for 1 week only might have a lower failure rate. The one-week regimen with clotrimazole or miconazole is more convenient.

Whether nystatin given orally reduces the risk of recurrence of vaginal candidiasis by preventing fecal-vaginal recolonization is less clear. It has been used in doses of up to 30 million U per day in immunocompromised patients in protected environments, and, again, the benefit of this kind of prophylaxis is controversial. We do not use it. The only major side effect, however, is the bad taste of nystatin.

FLUCYTOSINE

5-Fluorocytosine (5-FC) was initially developed to be used as an anticancer agent. Although it was ineffective for this indication, it was found to be effective in experimental fungal infections.

After uptake into a fungal cell by a cytosine permease, 5-FC is deaminated by a cytosine deaminase to 5-fluorouracil (5-FU) and converted to 5-fluorodeoxyuridylic acid monophosphate. The latter is a noncompetitive inhibitor of thymidylate synthetase, interfering with DNA synthesis. Another mechanism of action is replacement of uracil by 5-FU in fungal RNA, leading to a disturbance in protein synthesis.

The two prerequisites for the antifungal activity of 5-FC are enzymatic uptake into the fungal cell and enzymatic conversion to the finally active inhibitor. A decreased permeability (loss of activity of cytosine permease) and a loss of activity of cytosine deaminase as well as other enzymes may lead to resistance to 5-FC. An increase in the amount of de novo synthetized pyrimidines is another mechanism of resistance.

5-FC is marketed in the United States as 250-mg and 500-mg capsules. An intravenous solution is available in other countries, but may only be obtained in the United States for compassionate use from the producer.

5-FC is readily and completely absorbed from the gastrointestinal tract. There is virtually no protein binding, and about 90 percent is excreted unchanged into the urine. In the cerebrospinal fluid (CSF) more than 70 percent of the serum concentration can be achieved. Hemodialysis and peritoneal dialysis remove the medication from the body. In patients with normal renal function, the half-life of 5-FC is about 4 hours, but it is remarkably prolonged in patients with azotemia.

The usual dose is 150 mg per kilogram per day in four divided doses (orally or intravenously). We recommend starting with a daily dose of 100 mg per kilogram per day of 5-FC in order to take into account renal function in older people or those on renally toxic antibiotics, such as aminoglycosides and amphotericin B. Blood levels (see below) should be monitored. It has been suggested to calculate the dose of 5-FC to be given by dividing the usual dose (150 mg per kilogram per day) by the serum creatinine. Patients on hemodialysis should receive a single dose of 37.5 mg per kilogram after each dialysis.

In any case, subsequent doses in all patients should be adjusted according to serum levels obtained before and

2 hours after the administration of 5-FC. A bioassay as well as chemical method give reliable results. Recommended optimal values should range between 50 and 100 μg per milliliter of serum. Levels above 100 μg per milliliter have been associated with severe and even fatal adverse effects. MICs of either *C. neoformans* and *Candida* species are usually in the range of 1 μg per milliliter, so a 5-FC level of 25 to 50 μg per milliliter would be ample.

In patients with normal renal function, adverse effects are rare. Nausea and vomiting (common with the 150 mg per kilogram regimen), rash, diarrhea, and hepatic dysfunction are seen. More severe and even fatal effects may occur in patients with impaired renal function. Thrombocytopenia is often the first sign of bone marrow toxicity, soon followed by neutropenia. Enterocolitis should be suspected in any patient receiving 5-FC and complaining of abdominal pain. If any of these symptoms occur, therapy should be stopped—even if serum levels of 5-FC are within normal limits. These patients usually tolerate lower doses of 5-FC, and it can be restarted after the side effects disappear. Rare cases of permanent marrow aplasia have been reported. It has been assumed that secretion of 5-FC into the gastrointestinal tract, followed by subsequent conversion to 5-FU by intestinal bacteria and reabsorption are the cause of bone marrow and abdominal adverse effects.

Except in treating chromomycosis, 5-FC should never be given as a single agent. It is usually less clinically effective than amphotericin B, and secondary resistance is common. 5-FC in combination with amphotericin B is the treatment of choice for cryptococcal meningitis. Recommended dosages are amphotericin B 0.3 mg per kilogram per day intravenously plus 5-FC 150 mg per kilogram per day by mouth for 4 to 6 weeks. We start out with higher doses of amphotericin B (0.6 to 1 mg per kilogram per day) and lower doses of 5-FC (75 to 100 mg per kilogram per day). We also may treat for longer than 6 weeks if the clinical situation warrants it, which it may in both normal and immunocompromised hosts. Spinal fluid cell counts and sugar and protein levels should be normal, and cryptococcal antigen levels should be absent or should be low (less than 1:16) and stable.

In patients with human immunodeficiency virus infection and cryptococcal meningitis, the antigen levels are much higher and remain higher. Once the patient is stable both clinically and in terms of CSF and serum antigen levels, he is given a maintenance dose of amphotericin B (1 mg per kilogram per week). Relapse rates of 50 percent to 90 percent were evident when this was not done. Many investigators do not use 5-FC in patients with acquired immunodeficiency syndrome (AIDS) because of their poor marrow reserve and because early experience in patients with AIDS suggested that it was not necessary in acute cryptococcosis. Maintenance therapy with ketoconazole and fluconazole have been under study and are discussed below.

Studies in animal models as well as uncontrolled clinical trials suggest that systemic candidiasis may also be an indication for the combination of 5-FC and amphotericin B. We do not use the combination in any other fungal infection except cryptococcosis or candidiasis due to *C. tropicalis*, and especially not in pulmonary aspergillosis, where 5-FC only adds to toxicity without any evidence of benefit for the patient.

AZOLE ANTIFUNGAL AGENTS

The severity and frequency of adverse effects encountered with amphotericin B have stimulated the search for new antifungal agents. Although the antifungal properties of the imidazole benzimidazole have been known since 1944, more extensive research was not done until the 1970s. The common structure of all azole compounds is a five-membered azole ring, which is bound by a carbon nitrogen to other aromatic rings. Triazoles contain a third nitrogen atom in the azole ring as compared with the two nitrogen atoms in imidazoles.

In vitro test results with azoles depend largely upon many factors like culture medium, pH, and inoculum size and may not be helpful in comparing the different compounds. As for other antifungal agents, animal models more reliably allow assessment of the activity of the different agents. The spectrum of activity of azoles is broad, including most clinically relevant species of dermatophytes, yeasts, and dimorphic fungi. Azoles exhibit their antifungal properties by binding to cytochrome P-450, resulting in an inhibition of cytochrome activation and enzyme function. This results in an inhibition of ergosterol synthesis by inhibition of the demethylation of lanosterol. Additional mechanisms of action have been reported. Decreased uptake at the cytoplasmic membrane is a possible mechanism of resistance; however, currently this appears not to be clinically relevant.

Many agents are available or in various stages of laboratory or clinical evaluation. Some are available for topical use only and are not discussed here.

Clotrimazole

Clotrimazole was the first available azole that was shown to be active in fungal infections in experimental animals and in humans. It induces microsomal enzymes in the liver, resulting in increased drug metabolism and decreased antifungal activity. It is used as a 1-percent solution for the treatment of cutaneous fungal infections (candidiasis, ringworm, pityriasis versicolor), as a 1-percent vaginal cream or as 100-mg tablets for vaginal candidiasis, and as 10-mg oral lozenges for oropharyngeal candidiasis.

Miconazole

Miconazole as topical cream or lotion or as a 2-percent vaginal cream can be used interchangeably with clotrimazole for the indications mentioned for clotrimazole. Since ketoconazole has become available, intravenous miconazole is indicated only for severely ill patients with an infection due to *Pseudoallescheria boydii*. There is no rapid metabolism when miconazole is given systemically (an intravenous form is available). However, there are multiple toxic effects such as nausea, vomiting, anaphylactoid reactions, central nervous system reactions (including seizures), pruritus, and cardiorespiratory arrest. The latter may be related to the rate and duration of drug administration, and it is recommended that miconazole be given in at least 200 ml of diluent over a minimum of 2 hours. Some of the adverse effects mentioned have been attributed to the vehicle Cremophor El, which is required for colloidal stabilization.

Ketoconazole

Ketoconazole was the first azole that could be used in a variety of superficial and systemic fungal infections. It is available in 200-mg tablets. Peak serum concentrations of about 2 to 4 μg per milliliter can be observed 2 to 3 hours after oral intake of one tablet. Absorption is markedly decreased in patients with achlorhydria. Only a minimal amount of the drug appears in the CSF. The serum half-life is about 90 minutes (for a 200-mg dose). Ketoconazole is metabolized in the liver and excreted into the bile. Only a small amount appears unchanged in the urine. Serum protein binding is more than 90 percent. Altered liver or kidney function does not result in a change in plasma drug levels. Hemodialysis and peritoneal dialysis do not remove ketoconazole from the body.

Simultaneous therapy with ketoconazole and rifampin leads to decreased plasma levels of both medications; failures of both compounds have been reported. Coadministration of ketoconazole and cyclosporin A prolongs the half-life of the latter, and coadministration with H_2 blockers, such as cimetidine, or with antacids leads to an impaired absorption of ketoconazole.

In contrast to miconazole intravenously administered, oral ketoconazole is well tolerated. Dose-related nausea and vomiting are the most commonly observed side effects. Increases in liver function test values can be seen in up to 2 to 5 percent of patients and usually disappear spontaneously. Progressive hepatotoxicity that is not dose dependent occurs in about 0.01 percent of patients. It may be fatal if the drug is not discontinued. Interference with steroidal hormone production may lead to a dose-related inhibition of testosterone synthesis (resulting in gynecomastia, menstrual irregularity, sexual impotence, oligospermia) and a decreased ACTH-cortisol response.

Ketoconazole, like other azoles, has a broad spectrum of activity. It is not active, however, against molds such as *Aspergillus* species. Response to treatment is usually slow, and therefore ketoconazole should never be used in the initial treatment of systemic fungal infections in critically ill patients, cancer patients, transplant recipients, or patients with AIDS. It should not be used in any form of fungal meningitis because it crosses the blood-brain barrier poorly.

With these limitations in mind, ketoconazole (400 to 800 mg per day for 6 to 12 months) is effective in the treatment of nonmeningeal blastomycosis and pulmonary and disseminated histoplasmosis. If the 400 mg per day dose is not effective, increasing the dose to 600 mg per day or even 800 mg per day may be. Duration of therapy depends on severity of disease and clinical response. Coccidioidomycosis of the skin, soft tissue, bone, and joints and noncavitary lung infection also respond to 400 to 800 mg per day. Patients with paracoccidioidomycosis have responded to daily doses of 200 to 400 mg. Other indications may include griseofulvin-resistant ringworm, onychomycosis, and tinea versicolor. Chronic mucocutaneous candidiasis requires prolonged administration of 3 to 5 mg of ketoconazole per kilogram per day. Oropharyngeal and esophageal candidiasis may not respond better to ketoconazole than to nystatin. We would, however, always try ketoconazole before resorting to amphotericin B. Candidal vaginitis can be treated with 400 mg per day for 5 days, although hepatotoxicity and the possibility for teratogenicity in pregnant women are major concerns.

We do not recommend the use of ketoconazole in patients with prolonged neutropenia and fever, since important fungi like *Aspergillus* species and *Candida glabrata* would not be treated adequately. There is no good evidence that ketoconazole is effective against invasive candidiasis with dissemination. In one animal model, ketoconazole given prophylactically diminished the protective effect of amphotericin B against *Aspergillus fumigatus*.

Azoles Currently Under Clinical Investigation

Itraconazole

Itraconazole is lipophilic, and more than 99 percent is bound to serum proteins. It is well absorbed after oral ingestion, with improved absorption when taken after a meal. It is metabolized, and the (inactive) metabolites are excreted in bile and urine. The area under the curve (AUC) as well as the peak serum concentration increases remarkably with multiple dosages. A steady state is reached after about 2 weeks. Itraconazole is widely distributed throughout the body, with concentrations in lungs, kidneys, and brain being up to five-fold higher than in plasma. Low concentrations are found in saliva and bronchial secretions, and itraconazole does not penetrate into the CSF.

Adverse effects reported so far are rare and not severe. Nausea and vomiting are observed in 1 to 20 percent of patients and elevation of liver enzymes is seen in less than 5 percent. Hypokalemia and pedal edema were noted in some patients. There seems to be no interference with the production of testicular or adrenal steroidal hormones.

First clinical studies suggest that itraconazole may be used for the same indications as ketoconazole. In addition, it may be active in sporotrichosis and aspergillosis. Its activity against aspergilli in vitro is noteworthy, although carefully designed controlled clinical studies will be needed to substantiate the in vitro promise.

Itraconazole is experimental and can only be used in clinical trials or by compassionate-use approval.

Fluconazole

In contrast to other azoles, fluconazole is water soluble and only weakly protein bound. It is well absorbed and undergoes little metabolism, and more than 90 percent of the drug appears unchanged in urine and feces. Two pharmacokinetic properties are of high clinical interest: fluconazole penetrates well into CSF (60 percent and 80 percent of corresponding serum levels are found in uninflamed and inflamed meninges, respectively), and more than 60 percent of the drug can be recovered from urine. The β half-life is 22 hours. There is a slight accumulation with administration over time, and a dosage reduction is necessary in patients with renal impairment.

Fluconazole appears to be well tolerated. Less than 5 percent of patients develop minor side effects such as gastrointestinal symptoms or elevations in liver function tests.

First clinical studies indicate that fluconazole may be used in fungal infections of the skin and in vaginal candidiasis. Its possible use in systemic mycoses is less clear. It appears, however, to be a promising agent for cryptococcal meningitis, and it is currently under evaluation in a randomized trial with once weekly amphotericin B as standard treatment for prevention of relapse of cryptococcal meningitis in patients with AIDS. It is also under prospective, randomized controlled trials in comparison with amphotericin B as initial treatment of cryptococcal meningitis in patients with and without AIDS.

Fluconazole is experimental and can only be used in clinical trials or by compassionate-use approval.

ALLYLAMINES

Naftifine and terbinafine are members of a new group of antifungal agents, the allylamines. They are synthetic naphthalenemethanamines and act as antifungal agents by inhibiting squalene epoxidase, a key enzyme in ergosterol biosynthesis. Their mode of action is highly specific, i.e., they are much more inhibitory to fungal than to mammalian sterol biosynthesis. Lack of bioavailability after systemic administration may be a mechanism of resistance. Naftifine and terbinafine are experimental agents and can only be used in clinical trials or by compassionate-use approval.

Naftifine

The first compound of this group to be discovered was naftifine. It is active in vitro against a wide variety of fungi and can be used for the topical treatment of infections due to dermatophytes and *Candida*. Activity was not seen after oral administration, even with high doses.

Terbinafine

In vitro, terbinafine is even more active than naftifine against a wide variety of fungi. Of high clinical interest is the fact that it showed in vitro activity against *A. fumigatus*, *Aspergillus flavus*, and *Aspergillus niger* that was comparable to or even better than the activity of amphotericin B. In our animal model of pulmonary aspergillosis, however, we could not detect any activity against *A. fumigatus* despite adequate tissue concentrations. Lack of bioavailability may be the explanation for this in vivo resistance. Terbinafine is currently under clinical investigation as topical and oral medication.

CILOFUNGIN (LY121019)

Cilofungin (LY121019), an analogue of echinocandin B, is a novel semisynthetic lipopeptide. Its mode of action is to inhibit the synthesis of the β-(1,3)-glucan cell-wall component of sensitive fungi.

In vitro it is more active than amphotericin B against *C. albicans* and *C. tropicalis* but less active against other *Candida* species. First animal data indicate that intravenous cilofungin is less toxic than intravenous amphotericin B, and it showed efficacy in the treatment of local and systemic infections due to *C. albicans*.

SUGGESTED READING

Heel RC, Brogden RN, Carmine A, et al. Ketoconazole: a review of its therapeutic efficacy in superficial and systemic fungal infections. Drugs 1982; 23:1–36.
Iwatak K, Vanden Bossche H, eds. In vitro and in vivo evaluation of antifungal agents. New York: Elsevier, 1986.
Rev Infect Dis, January/February 1987, Supplement 1. (The whole issue is devoted to itraconazole.)
Rippon JW. Medical mycology. Philadelphia: WB Saunders, 1988.
Schmitt HJ, Bernard EM, Andrade J, et al. MIC and fungicidal activity of terbinafine against clinical isolates of *Aspergillus* spp. Antimicrob Agents Chemother 1988; 32:780–781.
Speller DCE, ed. Antifungal chemotherapy. New York: Wiley, 1980.
Warnock DW, Richardson MD, eds. Fungal infections in the compromised patient. New York: Wiley, 1982.

MEDICAL ADVICE FOR TRAVELERS

KAREN A. MELLO, M.D.
SHERWOOD L. GORBACH, M.D.

Increasing international travel has prompted the growth of travel clinics and the medical specialty of emporiatics (from Greek *emporus*, traveler). Travelers to developing countries are exposed to societies with different standards of sanitation, and these conditions impart increased risk of certain bacterial, viral, and parasitic diseases not seen with frequency in the United States. In addition, travelers must cope physiologically with changes in time zones, climate, and geography. This chapter reviews the main health risks associated with travel to developing countries and their treatment and prevention.

TABLE 1 Suggested Items for a Medical Kit

First-Aid Materials	Nonprescription Items	Prescription Items
Band-Aids, sterile gauze tape, scissors, knife*	Aspirin, acetaminophen, ibuprofen	Epinephrine kit
Bactericidal soap solution	Hydrocortisone cream 0.5%	Scopolamine transdermal patches
Alcohol wipes	Antihistamine/decongestant tablets or capsules	Compazine 25 mg tablets
Thermometer	Dimenhydrinate HCl (Dramamine) liquid or tablets	Triazolam 0.25 mg tablets
Snake bite kit	Diphenhydramine HCl (Benadryl) elixir, tablets or capsules	Chloroquine 500 mg tablets
Sunscreen (containing PABA)	Glucose-electrolyte mixture† (e.g., Infalyte)	Fansidar 3 tablets/person
Repellant lotion and spray (both containing diethyltoluamide)	Bismuth subsalicylate (Pepto-Bismol) tablets or liquid	Diphenoxylate HCl 2.5 mg tablets or Loperamide HCl 2.0 mg capsules or liquid
Iodine-release tablets	Mild oral laxative	TMP/SMZ 160 mg/800 mg tablets
		Doxycycline 100 mg tablets

* Swiss army–type combination knife with a straight blade, scissors, and tweezer recommended
† Recommended if traveling with infants or small children

PREPARATION

A traveler with a planned itinerary should be encouraged to contact his or her physician or a local hospital-associated travel clinic 6 months before departure in order to plan the necessary immunizations. If a low-risk trip (defined in this setting as a stay of less than 3 months with activities not involving health care or animals) is planned, 4 to 6 weeks in advance is adequate. The traveler should provide information on the itinerary, particularly on travel outside urban areas, the season of travel, duration of stay, and planned activities. A medical history and immunization record are also necessary.

A medical supply kit should be prepared (Table 1). For established health problems, a traveler should be given a medical problem summary and a list of medications and doses to carry on his or her person, along with the name of the personal physician. An adequate amount of medications and medical supplies should be taken for the duration of travel because of unknown availability and quality of supplies abroad. An extra pair of prescription eyeglasses, and the prescription itself, should be carried. Travelers should learn whether their health insurance covers emergency medical visits or evacuation costs if these are necessary outside the United States. If these are not covered, it might be advisable to obtain additional insurance.

GENERAL PRECAUTIONS WHILE ABROAD

Because of the high transmission rate of food and water-borne illnesses in developing countries, especially outside the higher-class hotels and restaurants, the traveler should be instructed to pay careful attention to avoidance of contaminated food and water. (This is discussed further in the section on diarrheal illness.)

Disequilibrium problems often precede the arrival of the traveler on land. Motion sickness can occur during all modes of transportation, but especially aboard ship. The symptoms include nausea, vomiting, malaise, fatigue, headache, and dizziness. Prophylactic use of anticholinergic agents, such as transdermal scopolamine patches, is effective when the patches are applied at least 4 hours before departure, and protection lasts up to 3 days. This drug should not be used in children, in patients with known hypersensitivity to scopolamine or to any components of the adhesive matrix, or in patients with glaucoma. The most common adverse effect from transdermal scopolamine is dryness of the mouth, occurring in about two-thirds of people. Other effects include drowsiness, blurred vision, and dilated pupils. Severe rare adverse effects include hallucinations, disorientation, precipitation of acute angle-closure glaucoma, and urinary retention. Elderly persons are more susceptible to these reactions, and the patch should be immediately removed upon suspicion of an untoward effect.

Other useful agents for motion sickness include antihistamines such as diphenhydramine (Benadryl), dimenhydrinate (Dramamine), and meclizine (Antivert). These agents should be taken ½ to 1 hour before departure. A typical regimen for Dramamine is one or two 50-mg tablets every 4 to 6 hours, depending on travel conditions. Pregnant women should refrain from taking these products, and they should not be used during breast feeding. Both diphenhydramine and dimenhydrinate are available in liquid formulations and can be used in children. A typical pediatric dose of diphenhydramine would be 12.5 to 25 mg three to four times daily in children over 20 pounds. These agents should not be used concurrently with alcohol. Caution should be taken in prescribing antihistamines in patients with angle-closure glaucoma, symptomatic prostatic hypertrophy, bronchial asthma, hyperthyroidism, cardiovascular disease, and hypertension.

Jet lag refers to the sensation of disequilibrium and fatigue experienced by travelers after time-zone changes. Eating well and obtaining adequate sleep prior to departure may be helpful in lessening jet lag. In studies of military personnel, the use of caffeine products, adherence to local wake-sleep cycles, and social interaction were shown to decrease symptoms and adjustment time. Triazolam (Halcion), a benzodiazepine, has also been shown to improve wake-sleep cycles in travelers. Triazolam can be recommended to travelers who spend at least 6 continuous hours in flight, require a high level of mental alertness upon arrival (e.g., business meetings), and have no contraindications to benzodiazepines. A dose of 0.25 mg taken at the start of the new sleep cycle for one or two nights should be adequate. A lower dose of 0.125 mg is recommended for use in the elderly. Alcohol should not be taken concurrently because of reports of retrograde amnesia. There are also reports of occasional idiosyncratic disorientation occurring after triazolam exposure.

Acute mountain sickness (AMS) can occur when travelers rapidly ascend to altitudes of more than 9,000 to 12,000 feet during trekking expeditions in mountainous regions. The syndrome is characterized by headache, nausea, vomiting, insomnia, and lassitude. The most severe complications are high-altitude pulmonary edema and cerebral edema, both of which are associated with high mortality. Prevention involves acclimatization, a process of spending a few days at an intermediate altitude of 5,000 to 7,000 feet, with subsequent gradual ascent to higher elevations. Acetazolamide, a carbonic anhydrase inhibitor, hastens acclimatization in climbers starting out at higher elevations. However, it cannot be depended upon to prevent AMS. Doses of 250 mg two or three times daily taken 24 to 48 hours before and a few days during the ascent have been used. Adverse effects include increased urination and circumoral and peripheral paresthesia. Acetazolamide is contraindicated in sulfa-allergic individuals. If AMS develops, travelers should descend and not attempt treatment with acetazolamide.

Travelers should be aware of the local weather conditions in the season of the countries being visited. Packing appropriate clothing for outdoor exposure is important, e.g., raingear for monsoon season, or lightweight long-sleeved garments for the tropics.

Tropical climates put the unprotected traveler at risk for arthropod-borne diseases such as malaria, yellow fever, dengue, and trypanosomiasis. Personal protection measures for insect control include (1) protective clothing with long-sleeved garments; (2) avoidance of outdoor exposure before dawn and after dusk; (3) use of insect-repellent lotion containing a high concentration of *N,N*-diethylmetatoluamide (DEET) on skin; (4) use of insect-repellent spray containing pyrethrins in living and sleeping areas; and (5) mosquito netting, especially for infants and young children. Mosquito netting headgear is also available for heavy exposure.

Travelers should avoid excessive sun exposure to prevent heat exhaustion, heat stroke, sunburn, and photosensitivity reactions if taking predisposing medication (e.g., tetracyclines). Sunscreens with high sun protection factor numbers that contain para-aminobenzoic acid (PABA) offer the best protection, especially for the fair-skinned traveler. Shoes and sandals should be worn at all times to prevent nematode penetration, which can occur at the beach. Dermatophytid infections, such as tinea versicolor, may worsen in warm, humid conditions. The skin should be kept as clean and dry as possible, and topical antifungal agents should be carried for early treatment of exacerbations.

Swimming in nonchlorinated fresh water should be avoided in certain areas because of the potential risk of schistosomiasis ("swimmer's itch"). Areas of risk for systemic schistosomal infections include the Middle East, Africa, South America, the Caribbean, Japan, China, and the Phillipines. Saltwater swimming is safe from most parasites, but swimmers should be on guard for jellyfish stings. Snorkelers and divers should use caution in approaching abrasive coral, and they need to be aware of locally dangerous fish and eels.

In general, domestic and wild animals in developing countries should be avoided because of the potential for animal bites and the transmission of rabies. In some areas merchandise made from animal products has been known to transmit infections such as anthrax, and shoppers need to be made aware of this risk.

Travelers should be advised of the worldwide risk of sexually transmitted diseases (STDs). Many STDs in the developing world are relatively rare in the United States; these include chancroid, lymphogranuloma venereum, and granuloma inguinale. However, gonorrhea, syphilis, and genital herpes are common and the usual risk factors apply. The heterosexual transmission rate of human immunodeficiency virus (HIV) is significantly higher in the developing world, especially in central and East Africa. Because of the high seroprevalence of HIV antibody in prostitutes from this region (in some areas greater than 50 percent), avoidance of sexual activity with residents is recommended. Condoms manufactured abroad may not confer protection against HIV transmission. Any genital lesion present should be an absolute contraindication to sexual contact, even with condom use, because of the higher potential for contracting HIV. Some countries have begun to require a negative HIV test in certain travelers before permitting entrance. An up-to-date list of these countries should become available through the Centers for Disease Control (CDC) (see Appendix).

If medical care is needed abroad, a reputable physician or medical clinic should be sought, preferably one recommended by a U.S. physician or health care agency. The local U.S. embassy or consulate usually maintains a list of recommended English-speaking physicians. In general, blood products and injectables should be avoided because of the unstandardized procedures for blood screening, care of hypodermic needles, and sterility practices in many developing countries. The transmission of HIV, hepatitis B, hepatitis non-A, non-B, and other bloodborne pathogens is possible in this setting. If blood products are absolutely indicated, available family members, fellow travelers, or local expatriates who have tested negative for hepatitis B and HIV or have no risk factors for either disease should be blood donors if blood types are compatible.

IMMUNIZATIONS

Depending on the areas of travel and anticipated exposures (e.g., a business trip limited to major urban areas or visits or work in rural or agricultural areas, game preserves, ruins), recommended immunobiologics will vary. In certain circumstances, vaccination schedules should begin

6 months before departure in order to gain maximal antibody response before exposure. In most instances, however, a period of 4 to 6 weeks before departure is adequate time to schedule vaccinations, some of which require two or more injections for minimal antibody response. Shorter pretravel periods for vaccinations are possible, albeit with a higher probability of minor side effects when more than one vaccine is given per session.

Routine Immunizations

Both adults and children should have completed a primary series with DPT or DT; they should receive a booster injection of DT if more than 10 years have elapsed since the last booster. MMR (measles-mumps-rubella) immunization is given only once in infancy. Individuals born before 1965 with a history of natural disease should be immune for life. However, those who received measles vaccine between 1963 and 1967 should be revaccinated with the new vaccine because of inadequate response to the earlier vaccine. If time permits, the immunologic status for each of these diseases can be determined and monovalent vaccines can be given if there are inadequate serum antibody levels ($<1:8$). Rubella vaccine should be avoided 3 months before and during pregnancy. MMR is an attenuated live virus and is contraindicated in individuals with a history of egg allergy (anaphylactic), altered immunologic status (malignancies, treatment with immunosuppressive agents, hypogammaglobulinemia, immunodeficiency syndromes[1]), pregnancy, and age less than 6 months.

Polio Vaccine

Poliomyelitis regularly occurs in developing countries but can occur in unexpected areas, as evidenced by an outbreak in Israel in 1988. Because of the devastating illness, especially in older individuals, and the excellent protection provided by the vaccine, travelers should be encouraged to be adequately vaccinated. Polio vaccination is currently administered in oral form (OPV) during childhood, and a booster injection is given in adolescence. OPV is an attenuated live virus that is shed in the feces of recipients for up to 30 days. Because there have been rare cases of vaccine viruses causing paralytic polio in nonimmune recipients as well as in close contacts of OPV recipients, such as household members, careful consideration must be given to its use. Health practitioners should know the immunologic status of the potential vaccine recipient and their contacts before giving OPV.[1] This vaccine is not recommended for people over the age of 17 years unless previously immunized with OPV, and a booster is needed prior to travel. One booster is probably adequate for lifetime protection.

Inactivated polio vaccine (IPV) is given by injection. A primary series consists of four injections in adults, the first three injections given 4 to 6 weeks apart and a fourth injection given 1 year after the third. If insufficient time remains before departure, the first two or three injections can be given on the 4- to 6-weekly schedule, with the final injection given after the return home. If the person has been previously immunized with OPV or IPV, a single dose of IPV to boost immunity is recommended at least 2 months before departure. Protection is estimated to persist for 5 years.

Since 1978, an enhanced potency IPV (e-IPV) has been available and is currently recommended for unvaccinated adults. The schedule consists of two doses, 1 to 2 months apart, with a third dose 6 to 12 months later. If less time is available, two doses can be given 1 month apart or one dose of e-IPV or OPV can be given, although there are risks associated with the latter. Adults incompletely immunized with OPV or IPV should receive doses to complete the series regardless of the interval since last dose or type of vaccine received.

International Certificate of Health

International health regulations regarding vaccinations are adopted and revised by the World Health Organization (WHO) in order to control the international spread of diseases. A proof of vaccination in the form of a yellow International Certificate of Health may be required at the time of visa application or upon entry into a country. In recent years, required vaccination for smallpox has been dropped in all countries and for cholera in most countries because of worldwide eradication of the former and inadequacy of the vaccine in preventing spread of the latter. Cholera is both endemic and epidemic in southern and Southeast Asia, the Middle East, and Africa and occurs infrequently in certain European countries. There are also endemic foci of cholera in certain U.S. states on the Gulf of Mexico. The following countries require a vaccination certificate for cholera for travelers coming from an endemic area: Albania, Madagascar, Malta, Pakistan, Pitcairn, Somalia, and Sudan. Some countries change their requirements at short notice, causing considerable inconvenience for travelers without proof of vaccination. The International Certificate is valid for 6 months after vaccination or revaccination. A booster for cholera is required every 6 months. Because the killed vaccine demonstrated only 50 percent efficacy in field trials, most health authorities do not recommend its use even in high-risk areas and would allow a single-dose injection for certificate purposes. A completed series involves two doses subcutaneously 1 week apart. There is no information on safety in pregnancy. Adverse effects consist of pain, redness and induration at the injection site, as well as fever, malaise, and headache.

Yellow Fever

Yellow fever is an acute disease caused by an arthropod-borne flavivirus that induces fever, chills, headache, gastrointestinal bleeding, liver failure, bradycardia, and albuminuria. It is endemic in certain areas of tropical America and

---

[1]The Immunization Practices Advisory Committee (ACIP) of the CDC recommends routine DTP, IPV, and MMR vaccinations and boosters, when necessary, in both asymptomatic and symptomatic HIV-infected children and adults; however, OPV is not recommended in these individuals.

Africa. Although epidemics of the disease can be confined to small areas, many countries require vaccination of travelers coming from an endemic zone. An updated list of countries requiring yellow fever vaccination certification can be obtained from the CDC publication *Health Information for International Travel.* Anyone traveling to an endemic zone should receive prior vaccination. Because yellow fever vaccine is a live virus formulation, the contraindications to its use are those previously outlined for the MMR vaccine. The most common adverse effect is pain at the injection site. Yellow fever and cholera vaccines can be given on the same day without loss of individual vaccine potency. The yellow fever vaccine must be WHO approved and administered at a designated yellow fever vaccination center. The location of these centers is available from the local department of health.

Other Vaccines

Typhoid Vaccine

Typhoid fever is a severe illness with fever, headache, and abdominal pain in its early phase and rash, prostration, and delirium during the second and third weeks of illness. In the fourth week, defervescence and recovery occurs. More than 50 percent of cases reported in the United States are acquired during travel or residence outside the country. Infection occurs via ingestion of food or water contaminated with *Salmonella typhi,* which invades the gastrointestinal tract and gains access to the lymphatics and blood. The organisms multiply in phagocytic cells and reenter the blood, causing recurring waves of bacteremia. Typhoid is common in most developing countries. Because of limited efficacy and a high incidence of uncomfortable side effects, the current typhoid vaccine is not recommended for most conventional trips, even to developing countries. The vaccine can be offered to travelers who anticipate long exposures to potentially contaminated food and water in smaller cities and villages or rural areas. Typhoid vaccine is a killed bacterial formulation given in two injectable doses at least 1 month apart. For individuals previously immunized, a single booster is necessary if more than 3 years have elapsed since primary immunization. If insufficient time exists, the unvaccinated traveler can receive three injections, each 1 week apart; however, this schedule may not confer as much protection as the standard series. Other typhoid-like enteric fevers caused by *Salmonella paratyphi* A or B or various *Salmonella* serotypes are not prevented by standard typhoid vaccine.

Meningococcal Vaccine

Meningococcal vaccine is a polysaccharide vaccine recommended to travelers to areas in which outbreaks of meningococcal disease are being reported. A single dose of vaccine confers long-lasting protection against the serotypes in the vaccine (A,C,Y,W-135). Serotype B, an important cause of meningitis in some outbreaks, is not prevented by this vaccine. The vaccine should be administered 10 days prior to departure. If travelers are exposed during an epidemic, rifam-

pin prophylaxis should be given when exposure is less than 7 days after leaving the epidemic area. In recent years, outbreaks have been reported in Saudi Arabia, Nepal, sub-Saharan Africa, and New Delhi. Information regarding recent epidemics can be obtained from the CDC, although there is often a delay in reporting.

Plague Vaccine

Plague is a killed bacterial vaccine recommended for travelers who anticipate direct contact with wild rodents in areas enzootic for plague.

Rabies Vaccine

Prophylaxis for rabies includes preexposure vaccination for individuals with a high probability of exposure and postexposure vaccination for actual blood or mucous membrane contact with a high-risk animal. Preexposure immunization is recommended for missionary families, Peace Corps workers, field biologists, agricultural consultants, spelunkers, and others who will work or travel in an endemic area for prolonged periods. Domestic as well as wild animals can transmit the disease through unprovoked attacks. Children are more vulnerable than adults. The preexposure regimen consists of three injections given on days 1, 7, and 30, and 90 percent protective antibody levels can be expected. A booster is needed every 2 years. Six percent of recipients have a hypersensitivity reaction after the booster dose. Booster dosing is unnecessary if an adequate rabies antibody titer can be demonstrated.

When a traveler is attacked by an animal, immediate medical attention should be sought. If possible, the animal should be captured and, depending on the circumstances, either observed for a 10-day period for signs of rabies or sacrificed for postmortem examination. The wound should be immediately cleaned with soap and water and any mucous membrane contact irrigated. Postexposure vaccination should proceed with one dose of rabies immune globulin (RIG) given immediately and injections of human diploid cell vaccine (HDCV) administered on days 0, 3, 7, 14, and 28 if the individual has not been previously immunized. In the setting of previous immunization (preexposure or postexposure regimens), HDCV is given on days 0, 3, and 7 without RIG. If RIG or HDCV is not available locally, the CDC or local U.S. embassy should be contacted for advice.

Japanese B Encephalitis Vaccine

Japanese B encephalitis is a mosquito-borne flavivirus-induced encephalitis that occurs in many areas of the Indian subcontinent and Asia. In China, endemic areas include all but the two most western provinces, with over 10,000 cases reported annually. From June to September, Korea, the lowlands of Nepal, Burma, northern India, Thailand, and eastern USSR are high-risk areas. The tropical zones of southern India and Thailand, Indonesia, Malaysia, and Singapore are high-risk areas throughout the entire year.

Travelers to the Far East have rarely contracted Japanese B encephalitis. Despite its low incidence in travelers, the disease carries significant morbidity and mortality, and there is no effective therapy. Two inactivated vaccines have been available in countries other than the United States. A recent placebo-controlled vaccine trial utilizing inactivated purified virus in either univalent or bivalent formulations in Thai children yielded a 91 percent efficacy rate. In addition, a significant reduction in the severity of cases of dengue, caused by a closely related flavivirus, was noted. Although these data cannot necessarily be extrapolated to nonindigenous people, travelers to rural Asia in the epidemic season may be candidates for immunization, especially if a prolonged stay (longer than 3 weeks) is planned. Travelers to rural areas having anticipated exposure to rice and pig farming during the summer months or those planning prolonged residencies in endemic areas should be immunized. No Japanese B encephalitis vaccine is currently available commercially in the United States; however, up-to-date information regarding the vaccine for at-risk travelers can be obtained from the CDC.

Hepatitis Vaccine

Hepatitis B is transmitted via inoculation with blood or body fluid secretions from infected individuals and through sexual contact. Most developing countries report a high prevalence of this disease. Travelers at risk include health care workers, missionaries, Peace Corps workers, and others who anticipate residence and work in areas where hepatitis B is prevalent. In these circumstances, hepatitis B vaccine, a killed-virus vaccine, is recommended for adults and children. The vaccine is given in three injections, the first two given 1 month apart and the third given 6 to 12 months after the first. The injections should be administered in the deltoid muscle for adequate absorption.

Hepatitis A is transmitted through ingestion of food and water contaminated with human excrement. Hepatitis non-A, non-B can also be transmitted in this manner. The risk of infection with both groups of viruses is highest in rural areas with inadequate sewage disposal. Outbreaks of enterically transmitted non-A, non-B hepatitis have been reported in the Soviet Union, central Asia, Nepal, Burma, India, and Pakistan and in Ethiopian refugee camps in Somalia and Sudan. No vaccine for hepatitis A or non-A, non-B hepatitis is currently available.

Immune serum globulin (ISG) will prevent hepatitis A for a 3- to 6-month period, depending on the dose received. Despite initial concerns that pooled serum for ISG preparations might transmit viral infections, especially HIV, no reported cases have been associated with ISG use in the USA. The risk of hepatitis A in persons not protected by ISG varies from one to 10 cases per 1,000 travelers during a 2- to 3-month stay in developing countries. The prevalence of protective antibody levels is high in adults over the age of 40 years (78 percent in a 1985 Glasgow study), and antibody prevalence increases steadily with age; however, because ISG is safe and inexpensive, it is recommended for all persons over the age of 12 years traveling to endemic areas. Controversy exists over the use of ISG in younger chil-

dren and infants because of the milder course of the disease in these age groups. Immune globulin preparations are probably not effective against non-A, non-B hepatitis in developing countries. ISG preparations should be given at least 2 weeks before departure, and protection lasts for a 3-month period. The dose recommended for travel of less than 2 months is 0.02 ml per kilogram (or 2 ml for most adults). For long-term travel or residence, a dose of 5 ml every 4 to 6 months is recommended. Local discomfort at the injection site may occur, and rare hypersensitivity reactions have been reported. If possible, ISG should not be given for 3 months before or at least 2 weeks after a live virus vaccine because of abatement of an adequate immunologic response. However, studies have demonstrated that ISG does not interfere with the immunologic response to yellow fever or OPV vaccines. ISG is safe for use in pregnant women.

Influenza and Pneumococcal Vaccines

The indications for use of these vaccines in travelers are the same as those for nontravelers. Recent influenza outbreaks have occurred among travelers aboard cruise ships in the Pacific Basin. Because different virus strains were probably involved in these cases, individuals vaccinated in their home countries were not necessarily protected.

DIARRHEA

Probably the most common socially debilitating affliction of the international traveler is infectious diarrhea. With the booming number of international travelers to developing countries and the popularity of itineraries that take adventurous travelers off the beaten path, it is not surprising that diarrhea is such a common problem. It often occurs despite the most careful preventive measures, attacking 30 to 60 percent of visitors to developing countries.

Most acute diarrheal syndromes occur during the first week following arrival. Symptoms consist of frequent unformed stools, abdominal cramps, nausea, bloating, urgency, and malaise. Diarrheal pathogens isolated from cases of travel-related diarrhea are listed in Table 2. In this setting, enterotoxigenic *Escherichia coli* accounts for approximately 40 percent of diarrhea associated with travel.

High-risk areas for travelers' diarrhea include Central and South America, the Middle East, and Asia. Intermediate-risk areas are the Mediterranean countries, including southern Europe, and a few Caribbean islands.

Diarrheal pathogens are acquired by ingesting fecally contaminated food or water. Both cooked and uncooked foods may be implicated if handled improperly. Risky foods include raw vegetables; raw or undercooked meats, seafood, and fish; unpeeled fruit; tap water and ice; and unpasteurized milk and dairy products. Dairy products are also potential carriers of organisms that cause nondiarrheal diseases, such as tuberculosis and brucellosis. Safe beverages include bottled carbonated liquids, beer, wine, hot black coffee or tea, and water boiled or treated with iodine or chlorine.

The clinical course of noninvasive infectious diarrhea is usually 4 days. More than one episode can occur per trip.

TABLE 2 Pathogens in Travelers' Diarrhea

Noninvasive	*Invasive*
Bacteria	
Enterotoxigenic *E. coli* (ETEC)	*Shigella*
Enteropathogenic *E. coli* (EPEC)	*Salmonella*
Vibrios (*V. cholerae*, non-01vibrios)	*Campylobacter jejuni*
Clostridium perfringens	*Aeromonas*
Staphylococcus aureus	*Yersinia enterocolitica*
Bacillus cereus	*Vibrio vulnificus*
	Vibrio parahaemolyticus (invasive strains)
	Clostridium difficile
Parasites	
Giardia lamblia	Enterohemorrhagic *E. coli* (0157:H7)
	Entamoeba histolytica
	Balantidium coli
	Cryptosporidium
Viruses	
Rotavirus	
Norwalk virus	

Invasive diarrhea is characterized by fevers, usually over 102°F, and bloody mucoid stools.

Prevention

Most of these organisms are transmitted directly via the fecal-oral route. In areas where hygiene and sanitation are inadequate or questionable, the following precautions are recommended:

1. Assume tap water is contaminated unless one is in a major hotel or restaurant where the water is filtered or chlorinated. However, chlorination does not kill some enteric viruses, *Giardia lamblia*, or amebae.
2. Bottled water is usually available and is usually safe.
3. Avoid brushing teeth or bathing in contaminated water.
4. Use safe water or liquids to take medication.
5. If no source of safe drinking water can be obtained, hot tap water in a clean container can be used.
6. Water can be "disinfected" by boiling or chemical means. Boiling is the most effective method. Water is heated above 65°C for more than 3 minutes at sea level (longer at higher elevations and with cloudy water). Chemical disinfection with tincture of iodine or chlorine will kill giardial cysts in most circumstances. Chemical kits with instruction are available for both agents. Iodine is available in both liquid and tablet form but should be avoided in pregnant women and in travelers with thyroid disorders.
7. Avoid prepared salads and ice cubes in drinks.
8. Eat only cooked food that is still hot and has not been reheated. Avoid fresh fruit or vegetables that have not been peeled by the traveler. Avoid food from street vendors. Undercooked or raw meat, fish, and shellfish carry various intestinal parasites, and some species of fish and shellfish contain biotoxins even when well cooked.

For the traveler who ventures off the usual tourist routes or into rural areas, safe water should be carried or carefully collected. Vessels should be washed with hot soap and water and drinking directly from the container after wiping the contact surface is advised.

The use of bismuth subsalicylate (Pepto-Bismol) has been demonstrated to decrease the incidence of diarrhea significantly when a dose of 60 ml four times a day is taken every day of travel. The chewable tablet form has also been effective in doses of two tablets taken every 6 to 8 hours. Although the exact mechanism of action is unknown, it may relate to the antiprostaglandin effect of salicylate, with reduction of toxin-associated fluid secretion. The bismuth moiety also has antibacterial properties. Caution must be taken in recommending Pepto-Bismol to travelers with salicylate sensitivity, bleeding disorders, impaired renal function, or concomitant salicylate or anticoagulant therapy. This drug may cause toxicity if used for prolonged periods (longer than 2 months) or in higher than recommended doses. As with all salicylate compounds, bismuth subsalicylate should be used only sparingly in young children.

Prophylactic antibiotic regimens have been demonstrated to be effective in preventing travel-related diarrhea for periods of up to 3 weeks. Trimethoprim-sulfamethoxazole (TMP/SMZ), doxycycline, norfloxacin, and ciprofloxacin have been effective. However, the "Traveler's Diarrhea Consensus Development Conference Panel" convened by the National Institutes of Health in 1985 recommended that travelers be advised to carry effective antibiotics for presumptive treatment and not for prophylactic use against diarrhea. Potential problems with prophylactic antibiotic usage in this setting include:

1. Increased susceptibility to infections with antibiotic-resistant pathogenic organisms due to alteration of bowel flora;
2. Risk of severe sulfonamide reactions, including Stevens-Johnson syndrome and erythema multiforme;
3. Other adverse medication effects (see Table 3);
4. Bacterial resistance to tetracyclines may exist in the area of travel, e.g., high incidence of resistant ETEC in the

TABLE 3 Antibiotics for Treatment of Diarrhea

Antibiotic	Adult Dose	Adverse Effects	Contraindications
TMP/SMZ	160 mg TMP/800 mg SMZ* b.i.d.	Gastrointestinal, rash, urticaria; rarely Stevens-Johnson syndrome, toxic epidermal necrolysis, hepatic necrosis	Previous hypersensitivity to TMP or sulfonamides, folate deficiency, pregnancy at term, breast feeding, infants <2 mo
TMP	100 mg b.i.d.	*See* TMP/SMZ	Previous hypersensitivity
Tetracycline	250 mg q.i.d. or 2.5 g single dose	Gastrointestinal, rash, photosensitivity, candidal vaginitis	Previous hypersensitivity, age <12 yr, pregnancy
Doxycycline	100 mg b.i.d.	*See* Tetracycline	*See* Tetracycline
Norfloxacin	400 mg b.i.d.	Gastrointestinal, headache, dizziness, CNS stimulation, crystalluria[†]	Previous hypersensitivity to quinolones, children, pregnancy
Ciprofloxacin[‡]	500 mg b.i.d.	*See* Norfloxacin	*See* Norfloxacin

Note: Ciprofloxacin and norfloxacin—oral fluorinated carboxyquinolones—are highly effective against most enteric pathogens including *E. coli, Salmonella, Shigella, Yersinia enterocolitica, Campylobacter jejuni,* and *Vibrio* species.
* Pediatric dose: 8 mg TMP/40 mg SMZ in two divided doses.
† Patients should be well hydrated and an alkaline urine avoided.
‡ Ciprofloxacin prolongs the elimination of theophylline, thereby increasing its serum level.

Philippines, Korea, Indonesia, and Mexico;
5. Antibiotic-associated colitis with *Clostridium difficile.*

Oral Rehydration

In most cases, fluid and electrolyte balance can be maintained by potable fruit juices, caffeine-free soft drinks, and salted crackers. Safe liquids can be prepared from commercially available powdered forms of balanced electrolyte solutions, especially those high in glucose, NaCl, NaHCO$_3$ and KCl. The WHO oral rehydration formula is well known and described elsewhere (see Appendix). Solid food and milk products should be avoided until diarrhea abates. Infants should receive commercially available oral rehydration solutions given in small sips with continued regular feedings. Immediate medical attention is needed for adults and infants with signs of moderate to severe dehydration, bloody diarrhea, or fever higher than 103°F. Travelers taking diuretics should discontinue them if they develop febrile diarrhea.

Symptomatic Treatment

Relief of abdominal cramps and diarrhea can be obtained with bismuth subsalicylate in doses of 60 ml or two tablets four times a day. The narcotic analogues such as loperamide (Imodium) and diphenoxylate and atropine (Lomotil) relieve symptoms by decreasing intestinal motility. Loperamide in a 2-mg dose can be taken as two capsules initially followed by one capsule after each loose stool, not to exceed eight capsules per day. The antimotility drugs should not be used for bloody diarrhea or dysentery. Over-the-counter antidiarrheal agents with unfamiliar names in other countries should be avoided.

Antibiotics

Empiric antibiotic use is recommended when diarrhea exceeds three or more loose stools in a 8-hour period or is associated with severe abdominal cramps, bloody stools, or fever. Appropriate regimens are described in Table 3. Three days of treatment is recommended, although fewer days may be sufficient. Loperamide can be used concurrently with antibiotics, except in the setting of bloody diarrhea or dysentery.

Because of the emergence of tetracycline and TMP/SMZ resistance in *E. coli* reported in recent years in developing countries, ciprofloxacin or norfloxacin may soon become the antibiotics of choice for travel-related diarrhea. The use of ciprofloxacin or norfloxacin is recommended in areas endemic for *Campylobacter jejuni* because of its resistance to TMP/SMZ. These drugs are also recommended for use in adults with sulfonamide allergy or TMP or TMP/SMZ intolerance, and in areas of the world where TMP/SMZ and/or tetracycline resistance is common.

In conclusion, travelers should be cautious in their selection of food and drink and should carry a supply of bismuth subsalicylate, antimotility agents, and a 3-day treatment course of TMP/SMZ, doxycycline, ciprofloxacin, or norfloxacin.

MALARIA

Malaria is a protozoan infection spread via bites of infected female *Anopheles* mosquitos in endemic areas. The disease can be severe and even fatal in its malignant form (*Plasmodium falciparum*). It afflicts 100 to 200 million people annually worldwide and approximately 1,000 persons each year in the United States. Thus, prevention and treatment of malaria are vital to travelers in endemic areas.

Four species of malarial parasite cause disease in humans. *Plasmodium vivax* and *P. falciparum* occur worldwide, but disease caused by the latter, when untreated, can rapidly progress to severe illness and death in nonimmune individuals. *Plasmodium ovale* infection is acquired in western Africa and is relatively uncommon. *Plasmodium malariae* occurs worldwide, and an asymptomatic, low-level erythrocytic infection can persist for years. Areas of risk for malaria are shown in Table 4. Malaria due to chloroquine-resistant strains of *P. falciparum* (CRPF) occur in tropical zones of both hemispheres. Because malarial risk and chloroquine-resistance patterns can change, it is important to contact the local health department, travel clinic, or the Malaria Branch of the CDC (see Appendix) for the most updated information.

Chemoprophylaxis

In addition to fever, malaria often presents with nonspecific symptoms such as malaise, headache, myalgia, fatigue, chest pain, and arthralgias. Because of the severity of illness when it occurs, and the potential for late diagnosis, chemoprophylaxis is recommended for all travelers to moderate- and high-risk areas. The choice of prophylactic drugs is becoming increasingly difficult due to the emergence and spread of drug-resistant strains of *P. falciparum*.

Chloroquine phosphate (chloroquine) is the primary suppressive agent used against *P. vivax*, *P. malariae*, *P. ovale*, and susceptible strains of *P. falciparum*. It is a 4-aminoquinoline compound that is highly effective against erythrocytic forms of malarial species, including most strains of *P. falciparum*, but will not kill the gametocyte forms of the latter or prevent relapses in patients with *P. vivax* or *P. malariae* infection when administered as a prophylactic. It will suppress the infection in patients with *P. vivax* and *P. malariae* infection and lengthen the interval between treatment and relapse. Chloroquine can be used to treat susceptible *P. falciparum* infections.

Prophylaxis is begun 1 to 2 weeks before travel and is continued every week for at least 4 weeks after leaving the endemic area.

The exact duration of posttravel malaria prophylaxis is debated by malaria experts, but the range is 4 to 8 weeks. (The reader is referred to the chapter on malaria for specific medication dosage regimens, contraindications, and adverse effects.) Because of recent reports of accidental chloroquine ingestion by children, the drug should be kept out of reach of children and disposed of after completion of prophylaxis.

Few alternatives to chloroquine for routine prophylaxis are available. When there is intolerance to the minor side effects of chloroquine, such as headache, pruritus, or gastrointestinal symptoms, the dose can be divided and taken twice weekly with food. Hydroxychloroquine sulfate (Plaquenil) can be substituted in a dose of 400 mg (155 mg of base) given in the same manner as chloroquine and may be better tolerated. Proquanil (Paludrine), a dihydrofolate reductase inhibitor, is effective against most malarial species but is not commercially available in the United States. Proquanil-resistant strains of *P. falciparum* have been reported in Southeast Asia where resistance to Fansidar exists (see the chapter *Malaria*). The prophylactic regimen consists of one 100-mg tablet taken daily beginning 1 week before travel and continuing for 6 weeks after return. A dose of 200 mg per

TABLE 4 Guidelines for Malaria Chemoprophylaxis

	Malaria Endemic	Low-Risk CRPF*	High-Risk CRPF	Multiply Drug-Resistant CRPF
Drug of choice Alternatives	Chloroquine Proguanil‡ (100 mg)	Chloroquine Proguanil (100 mg)	Doxycycline† (qd) Chloroquine† *plus* Fansidar (g wk§) *or* Proguanil (qd) (200 mg)	Doxycycline (qd) Proguanil *plus* Chloroquine *or* Mefloquine# (g wk)
Regions/countries	S. Africa, Mexico (rural and Yucatan Peninsula), Central America, Middle East, People's Rep. of China, Singapore, S. America (except for areas in other categories), Sri Lanka	W. Africa, S. America, (Brazil, Bolivia, Colombia, Ecuador, Venezuela, northern Peru, Surinam), Philippines, Indian subcontinent, People's Rep. of China (Hainan Island, southern provinces)	W. Africa (Gambia), E. Africa, S. America (Amazon basin), S.E. Asia (rural areas of Thailand, Kampuchea, Laos, Malaysia, Vietnam), S. Pacific (Irian Java, Papua New Guinea, Solomon Islands, Vanuatu)	S.E. Asia (esp. forested areas of Thailand, Burma, Kampuchea)

Note: See the chapter *Malaria* for specific dose regimens in adults and children.

* CRPF = chloroquine-resistant *Plasmodium falciparum*.

† Recommended for short-term (<3 wk) travel periods only in both high-risk and multiply drug-resistant CRPF categories.

‡ Not available in the U.S. Indicated only in cases of severe intolerance or contraindications to 4-aminoquinolone agents.

§ Fansidar (pyrimethamine 25 mg + sulfadoxine 500 mg) recommended only in areas with prolonged (>3 wk) exposures in highly endemic areas where medical care is not readily available (see text).

Not available in the U.S. Ineffective in preventing infection in Thailand and Papua New Guinea; may be effective in Kenya.

day is recommended for prophylaxis in Africa and certain CRPF areas. Proquanil is recommended only in cases of severe chloroquine intolerance or hypersensitivity. Its current availability may be determined by contacting the Malaria Branch of the CDC (see Appendix).

Prevention of Relapsing Malaria

Primaquine phosphate (Primaquine) is used to prevent relapsing forms of malaria. This is referred to as terminal prophylaxis or "radical cure." Primaquine is an 8-aminoquinoline compound highly active against the exoerythrocytic stages of *P. vivax* and *P. ovale*. It is used to prevent delayed attacks or later relapses after chloroquine is discontinued in areas of high endemicity. It is indicated for use in individuals returning home after prolonged periods of heavy exposure in areas with *P. vivax* or *P. ovale* or less-extensive periods in areas of intense exposure. These areas would include India, Pakistan, Bangladesh, Sri Lanka, Central America, and Africa.

If primaquine use is anticipated, the traveler should have a glucose-6-phosphate dehydrogenase (G6PD) blood level determined in order to avoid a potential hemolytic reaction upon exposure to primaquine. Because the fetus cannot be tested for G6PD deficiency, primaquine is contraindicated in pregnancy. Exposed pregnant women should continue chloroquine throughout pregnancy and begin the usual 2-week course of daily primaquine after delivery. Primaquine should not be used during breast feeding unless the infant is determined to have a normal G6PD level. Those at highest risk of G6PD deficiency include travelers of African, Asian, or Mediterranean descent. Primaquine is to be used cautiously with laboratory testing in patients with systemic diseases that are associated with a tendency to leukopenia (e.g., rheumatoid arthritis) or in those receiving concurrent bone marrow suppressive agents. The concurrent use of quinacrine (e.g., for treatment of giardiasis) enhances the toxicity of primaquine.

Chloroquine-Resistant *P. falciparum*

Because of the coexistence of chloroquine-susceptible strains with chloroquine-resistant strains of the same parasite in areas with chloroquine-resistant *P. falciparum*, chloroquine remains the agent of choice in these regions. Fansidar (pyrimethamine 25 mg and sulfadoxine 500 mg) is used to treat CRPF in areas where concomitant Fansidar resistance does not exist. For travel to low-risk CRPF areas (see Table 4), a single-treatment dose of Fansidar should be carried and taken at the first sign of possible acute malaria. Symptoms include a flu-like syndrome with headaches, chills, myalgias, and erratic fever. Medical attention should be sought concurrently with presumptive treatment because of the possibility of other infectious diseases that present similarly. Contraindications to Fansidar use include severe renal insufficiency, liver damage, blood dyscrasias, allergy to sulfonamides or pyrimethamine, megaloblastic anemia, age less than 2 months, and pregnancy at term or breast-feeding. Major adverse effects, including severe cutaneous reactions (erythema multiforme, Stevens-Johnson syndrome, and toxic epidermal necrolysis) have been reported among travelers using Fansidar prophylaxis. Because of these occasionally fatal reactions, prophylactic Fansidar use has limited indications. It is recommended on a weekly basis with chloroquine for travel involving prolonged exposure in highly endemic areas with CRPF. At the first sign of skin rash, mucous membrane symptoms, fever, arthralgia, pallor, or jaundice, Fansidar should be discontinued and medical attention sought.

Alternatives to Fansidar prophylaxis for CRPF exist. Doxycycline has been shown to be an effective prophylactic agent against sensitive CRPF strains. It is taken 1 to 2 days before travel to malarious areas and then every day until 4 weeks after departure from these areas. Doxycycline is recommended for the short-term traveler to areas of Thailand, Burma, and Kampuchea. It is also appropriate for chemoprophylaxis in individuals with sulfonamide allergies or intolerance. Adverse effects and contraindications are outlined in Table 3.

Proguanil, as previously mentioned, is also effective against sensitive CRPF. Amodiaquine, a 4-aminoquinoline like chloroquine, has been used in other countries for CRPF prophylaxis, but is not recommended because of reports of agranulocytosis in European travelers. The CDC recommends the use of proguanil over amodiaquine in select circumstances. Proguanil is widely available in other countries and has been effective in preventing infection with CRPF in Thailand and Papua New Guinea.

Mefloquine is an aminoalcohol currently under study for prophylaxis and treatment of multidrug resistant *P. falciparum*. It is available in France and Switzerland and in Thailand in a fixed-dose combination with Fansidar. When approved in the United States, mefloquine will probably be an alternative to doxycycline for CRPF prophylaxis.

Multiply drug-resistant *P. falciparum* has been a problem in rural Thailand in recent years. Travelers to this area are advised to seek up-to-date information from local health experts regarding resistant malaria upon arrival.

Travelers should be advised that prevention of malaria is not complete with chemoprophylaxis because of continuing spread of drug-resistant strains, and prompt medical attention is necessary when symptoms develop during travel or upon return home. The specific regimens used to treat malarial syndromes are outlined in the chapter on malaria.

APPENDIX

1. Centers for Disease Control (CDC), Atlanta, Georgia 30333
   Telephone numbers:
main switchboard	(404) 639–3311 (working hours),
	(404) 639–3670 (other times),
	(404) 639–2888 (emergency),
Malaria Branch	(404) 452–4046,
Rabies Branch	(404) 329–3095.

2. Centers for Disease Control. Health Information for international travel—1988. USDHHS, USPHS. Order from: Superintendent of Documents, U.S. Government Printing Office, Washington, D.C. 20402. Ref. Stock #88–8280.

3. U.S. State Department, Overseas Citizens Emergency Center, Washington, D.C., (202) 632–5225.
4. World Health Organization. Vaccination certificate requirements and health advice for international travel. Geneva: WHO, 1988.

SUGGESTED READING

Centers for Disease Control. Recommendations for the prevention of malaria in travelers. MMWR 1988; 37:no.17.

Hill DR, Pearson RD. Health advice for international travel. Ann Intern Med 1988; 108:839–852.
Hoke CH, Nisalek A, Sangawhipa N, et al. Protection against Japanese encephalitis by inactivated vaccines. N Engl J Med 1988; 319:608–614.
Jong EC. The travel and tropical medicine manual. Philadelphia: WB Saunders, 1987.
Krogstad DJ, Herwaldt BL. Chemoprophylaxis and treatment of malaria [editorial]. N Engl J Med 1988; 319:1538–1540.
Traveler's Diarrhea: National Institutes of Health Consensus Development Conference. Rev Infect Dis 1986; 8(Suppl 2).

CHILDHOOD IMMUNIZATION

JEROME O. KLEIN, M.D.

Immunization for children can be divided according to products recommended for all children and products recommended for special children or special situations. Eight products are considered routine immunization; these include diphtheria and tetanus toxoids and pertussis whole cell vaccine; measles, mumps, and rubella live vaccines; oral poliovirus vaccine; and *Haemophilus influenzae* type b conjugate polysaccharide vaccine. Special products include influenza virus vaccine, pneumococcal, and meningococcal polysaccharide vaccines, bacille Calmette-Guerin (BCG), hepatitis B vaccine, and live rabies vaccine. Immune globulins are available for prevention and treatment of measles, hepatitis A and B, varicella-zoster, rabies, and tetanus.

Recommendations for immunization in the United States are provided by the Committee on Infectious Diseases of the American Academy of Pediatrics (AAP) and published in the Report of the Committee (revised every 3 to 4 years) and the Advisory Committee on Immunization Practices (ACIP) of the United States Public Health Service, published in the *Morbidity and Mortality Weekly Report* (MMWR). In most circumstances the recommendations of the two groups coincide. Current recommendations for immunization of adults (18 years of age and older) are provided in an MMWR supplement (September 28, 1984; vol. 33, no. 1S).

RECOMMENDATIONS FOR IMMUNIZATION OF NORMAL INFANTS AND CHILDREN

The schedule recommended by the AAP and ACIP for active immunization of normal infants and children is provided in Table 1.

Diphtheria and Tetanus Toxoids and Pertussis Vaccine (DTP)

The primary series of DTP is given at 2, 4, 6, and 18 months, with a booster administered between 4 and 6 years. The primary series of DTP is carried out up to the seventh birthday. After the seventh birthday primary immunization should consist of adult-type tetanus toxoid and reduced dose of diphtheria toxoid (Td). A lapse in the schedule does not require restarting the schedule; subsequent doses are given at the recommended time intervals. Although the optimal age for beginning immunization in infants who are born prematurely is unknown, available data suggest that DTP can be administered at the same chronologic age to premature as to term infants.

The preferred site of administration for DTP and other products administered by the intramuscular route is the anterolateral aspect of the upper thigh (preferred in infants because it is the largest muscle mass) and the deltoid muscle of the upper arm (appropriate for most older children). For routine usage, the buttocks should be avoided as a site for injection. Large volumes may require use of the buttocks; the site should be the upper outer mass of the gluteus maximus to avoid injury to the sciatic nerve.

Approximately one-half of children who receive DTP vaccine have local (tenderness, pain) and systemic (fever, irritability) adverse effects; seizures occur, with or without fever, in approximately one in 2,000 children who receive

TABLE 1 Recommended Schedule for Active Immunization of Normal Infants and Children

Recommended Age	Vaccine	Comments
2 months	DTP; OPV	Can be initiated earlier in areas of high endemicity
4 months	DTP; OPV	
6 months	DTP; (OPV)	OPV optional for areas where polio may be imported
15 months	MMR	
18 months	DTP; OPV; PRP-D	
4–6 years	DTP; OPV	Up to the 7th birthday
14–16 years	Td	Adult tetanus toxoid (full dose); diphtheria toxoid (reduced dose); repeat every 10 years

Abbreviations: DTP = diphtheria, tetanus, pertussis; OPV = oral poliovirus vaccine; MMR = measles, mumps, rubella; Td = tetanus, diphtheria; PRP-D = *Haemophilus* b–diphtheria toxoid conjugate vaccine.

DTP, and brain damage has been identified 1 year later at a frequency of one in 310,000 doses. These effects are associated with the whole-cell pertussis component of the vaccine. Most public health experts agree that, on balance, the benefits of pertussis vaccine far outweigh the risks and it should be administered as part of the routine schedule. However, concern about toxicity of whole-cell pertussis vaccine has led to reconsideration of contraindications of its use in children. Deferral of DTP is recommended for children who have previously had convulsions (febrile or nonfebrile) until it can be determined whether an evolving neurologic disorder is present. If an evolving disorder is identified, infants or children should be given DT rather than DTP. Pertussis vaccine is also contraindicated if the child has a history of severe reaction following a prior dose (usually within 48 hours). Severe reactions include shock, collapse, persistent screaming episodes, temperature of 40.5 °C (105 °F) or greater, alterations of consciousness, generalized or local neurologic signs, or systemic allergic reactions,

Measles, Mumps, and Rubella Live Vaccines (MMR)

Live attenuated vaccines for measles, mumps, and rubella are administered in a combined vaccine. Single vaccines are also available for special use. A single dose of MMR provides durable protection with minimal side effects when administered at 15 months of age. Reimmunization is not recommended except for children who received immunization at earlier age (under 12 months for measles vaccine), with other products (killed measles vaccine), or in modified dosage or form (administered with gamma globulin).

Rubella vaccine results in viremia and infection of the placenta and fetus, but available data indicate vaccine virus is not a teratogen. Use of rubella vaccine is encouraged for susceptible nonpregnant women in the childbearing age group.

Immunization after exposure to disease may be of value for measles, but not for mumps or rubella. Measles virus vaccine administered as late as 5 days after exposure is protective in a majority of individuals. Administration of immune globulin is preferred for infants 12 months of age and younger who are exposed to measles because of the chance of vaccine failure in this age group.

Oral Poliovirus Vaccine (OPV) and Inactivated Poliovirus Vaccine (IPV)

OPV is administered at ages 2, 4, 18 months, and 4 and 6 years of age. In areas where exposure to wild virus is possible (some of the states in the Southwest), an additional dose at 6 months is recommended.

Paralytic poliomyelitis has resulted from administration of live vaccine to children with immune defects. Live virus vaccines, including OPV, should not be administered to children with known or suspected immunodeficiency. Because the vaccine virus is excreted by the vaccinee and may infect contacts, the live vaccine should not be used in families with a member who is immunodeficient. Inactivated poliovirus vaccine (IPV) should be used in children with immune defects and members of their households.

Routine immunization against poliovirus is not recommended for susceptible adults. For parents or travelers who may be exposed to wild or vaccine virus, IPV should be administered. The primary series of IPV consists of four doses; the first three may be given at the same time as DTP (in a separate syringe); the fourth dose is given 6 to 12 months after the third or on entry to school for children.

Haemophilus influenzae Type b Vaccines

Haemophilus influenzae polysaccharide vaccine (PRP) was introduced in the United States in April 1985 and recommended for administration to children 24 months of age or older. Conjugate vaccines consist of PRP covalently linked to a carrier protein directly or by a spacer. Examples of protein carriers include diphtheria toxoid, tetanus toxoid, a toxic mutant of diphtheria toxin, and an outer membrane protein of *Neisseria meningitidis* group b. The conjugate vaccines are consistently more immunogenic than the polysaccharide vaccines. A diphtheria toxoid conjugate vaccine (PRP-D) was licensed in 1987 and is now recommended for administration to all children at 18 months of age. Trials of PRP-D and other conjugate vaccines are in progress in younger infants; initial results of a study in Finland indicate protective efficacy of PRP-D against invasive *H. influenzae* type b disease in infants immunized at ages 3, 4, and 6 months.

VACCINES FOR SPECIAL CHILDREN OR SPECIAL CIRCUMSTANCES

Hepatitis B Vaccine for Prevention of Perinatal Infection

Mothers who are hepatitis B antigen (HBsAg)-positive may infect their newborn infant. The initial infection is usually asymptomatic, but about 25 percent of infant carriers may ultimately develop chronic active hepatitis, cirrhosis, and, possibly, primary hepatocellular carcinoma. The severity and chronicity of the disease warrant protection of any infant born to a mother who is hepatitis B antigen-positive. The recommended schedule combines hepatitis B immune globulin (HBIg) and hepatitis B vaccine. HBIg, 0.5 ml intramuscularly, is administered as soon after birth as possible. The vaccine, 0.5 ml intramuscularly, is given before the infant leaves the hospital or within 1 week after birth and at 1 and 6 months of age. The first dose of vaccine may be given at the same time as HBIg at a separate site.

Pneumococcal Vaccine

A 23-valent polysaccharide vaccine against disease due to *Streptococcus pneumoniae* was licensed in the United States in 1983, replacing the 14-valent vaccine introduced in 1977. Although the vaccine contains serotypes responsible for most pneumococcal disease in children, the immune response to most types for children under 2 years of age is limited. Because of the lack of immunogenicity, the vaccine is not recommended for infants. The vaccine should be used for children 2 years of age and older who are at increased risk for pneumococcal disease; these include children with anatomic or functional asplenia, those with sickle cell disease, and children with nephrotic syndrome, cerebrospinal fluid leaks, and conditions associated with immunosuppression. The vaccine may have some value in prevention of recurrent episodes of otitis media in the older children. Duration of immunity is uncertain; until data are available, reimmunization is not recommended.

Meningococcal Vaccine

A polysaccharide vaccine for groups A, C, Y, and W-135 is now available as a quadrivalent product. Group A vaccine produces satisfactory immune response in infants as young as 5 months, but the other group polysaccharides are poor immunogens for infants younger than 18 months of age. Immunity is group-specific, and protective levels of antibody are achieved in 1 week. The duration of immunity is uncertain, but is estimated to be 1 to 3 years. Group B meningococcus is the most prevalent group in the United States today; the polysaccharide is a poor immunogen and does not elicit protective antibody. Current indications in children older than 18 months of age (or younger if disease due to group A is to be prevented) include control of epidemic disease, use for travelers to endemic or epidemic areas, and prolonged prophylaxis for household contacts (because half of the secondary family cases occur more than 5 days after the primary case).

Influenza Vaccine

Influenza is a mild illness in most children, and, therefore, there is no basis for routine immunization. Annual immunization with current influenza vaccines is recommended for children with chronic disorders of the cardiovascular or pulmonary systems that are severe enough to have required regular follow-ups or hospitalization during previous years. If the physician believes the child would be harmed if infected, influenza vaccine should be used. Current influenza vaccines are prepared in eggs and contain trace amounts of egg antigens. Children known to be allergic to eggs should not receive influenza vaccine.

Bacille Calmette-Guerin (BCG)

Selective usage of BCG vaccine may be of value in infants and children: those in a household with repeated exposure to patients with infectious tuberculosis; and those in groups with excessive rates of new infection and for whom usual medical care is not feasible. BCG should not be given during isoniazid administration since multiplication of the bacillus is inhibited by the drug. Skin test with purified protein derivative is done 2 months after vaccination; if skin test is negative, BCG is repeated.

Rabies Vaccine

Human diploid cell vaccine (HDCV) and human rabies immune globulin (HRIg) are recommended following bite by a wild animal of a species known to carry the virus (skunk, fox, coyote, raccoon, bat, and other carnivores)

TABLE 2   Dosage Schedules for Immune Globulins for Prevention and Treatment of Disease

Agent	Condition	Preparation	Dose
Measles	Normal children	Ig	0.25 ml/kg
	Immunodeficient children	Ig	0.5 ml/kg
Hepatitis A	Household contacts	Ig	0.02 ml/kg
	Day care contacts	Ig	0.02 ml/kg
Hepatitis B	Newborn infants	HBIg	0.5 ml
	Exposure to infected blood	HBIg	0.06 ml/kg
Varicella	Immunodeficient children	VZIg	125 units/10 kg
	Newborn infants	VZIg	125 units
Rabies	Postexposure	HRIg	20 IU/kg; $^1/_2$ dose IM $^1/_2$ dose at wound
Tetanus	Postexposure	HTIg	250–500 units IM

Abbreviations: Ig = immune globulin; HBIg = hepatitis B immune globulin; VZIg = varicella-zoster immune globulin; HRIg = human rabies hyperimmune globulin; HTIg = human tetanus immune globulin.

unless the animal is proved to be virus-negative by laboratory test. HDCV and HRIg are also recommended if a domestic animal (dog or cat) is known or suspected to be rabid. If the animal's health is unknown or the animal has escaped, consultation with a local public health official is important to provide information on the risk of rabies in the area (see the chapter *Animal Bite Infection*).

Human Immune Globulin

Immune globulin (Ig) is prepared from pooled serum of adults. Ig is of value for prophylaxis against hepatitis A and measles. Special preparations of high-titer immune globulin are available for prevention or treatment of disease due to varicella, hepatitis B, rabies, and tetanus. Dosage schedules for immune and hyperimmune globulins are given in Table 2. Immune globulins are administered intramuscularly; 1 to 5 ml is administered at one site, depending on the size of the muscle mass.

Ig can be administered to susceptible children who are exposed to measles and is effective for prevention or modification of disease. Ig should be administered to children during the first year of life, to older children who have been exposed for more than 5 days (too late for use of vaccine), and to immunocompromised children. Vaccine should be given 3 or more months after administration of Ig to immunocompetent children.

Ig is recommended for prevention of hepatitis A in households and day care centers. Ig should be administered to all household contacts of a clinical case. If a case of hepatitis A occurs in a child or member of the staff of a day care center or in the households of two or more attendees, Ig should be given to children and staff of the center. Exposure in schools is not a reason for administration of Ig.

Hepatitis B immune globulin is administered to infants of mothers who are HBsAG-positive and to children or adults who are exposed to infected blood.

Varicella-zoster immune globulin should be used for immunocompromised children, for newborns of mothers with peripartum varicella (within 5 days before and 48 hours after delivery) and for premature infants with significant post-natal exposure.

Human rabies hyperimmune globulin should be administered with rabies vaccine (except for those who have been previously immunized). It provides antibody until the initial doses of vaccine have stimulated an immune response. Vaccine and human rabies hyperimmune globulin are administered via the intramuscular route in different sites. If feasible, one-half the dose of human rabies hyperimmune globulin is infiltrated in the area of the wound and one-half, intramuscularly.

Human tetanus immune globulin is indicated for patients whose tetanus toxoid immunization is unknown, those who have received an incomplete series of toxoid immunizations, and those whose wound is older than 24 hours.

SUGGESTED READING

Klein JO, ed. Current status of *Haemophilus influenzae* type b conjugate vaccines. Pediatrics (Suppl). In Press.

Peter G, ed. Report of the Committee on Infectious Diseases. 21st ed. Elk Grove Village, IL: American Academy of Pediatrics, 1988.

Plotkin SA, Mortimer EA Jr. Vaccines. Philadelphia: WB Saunders, 1988.

ADULT IMMUNIZATION

THEODORE C. EICKHOFF, M.D.

Renewed interest in immunization of adults in the United States began in the early 1980s. Despite the successes of pediatric immunization programs, the utilization of some vaccines recommended primarily for use in adults, such as the vaccines against influenza, pneumococcal infection, and hepatitis B, was poor. The latter two products, introduced in the last decade, were targeted primarily for adult populations and did not receive as much acceptance as was hoped.

Several sources give current information on vaccines for adults. The Advisory Committee on Immunization Practices of the Centers for Disease Control publishes periodic recommendations for the use of vaccines in *Morbidity and Mortality Weekly Report*. Recommendations from MMWR are reprinted regularly in JAMA, and are available as well from other journals. In addition, the American College of Physicians publishes a guide for adult immunization that is available from the American College of Physicians, P.O. Box 7777-R0325, Philadelphia, Pennsylvania 19175. A second edition is planned for release in 1989.

Tables 1 and 2 summarize the vaccines generally recommended for adult use, as well as vaccines recommended in the context of certain occupations or travel. Most of these vaccines are discussed in the chapters in this book that address the specific diseases that may be prevented by the vaccines.

TETANUS AND DIPHTHERIA

Tetanus and diphtheria toxoid (Td) consists of formalinized toxoids, derived from tetanus and diphtheria toxins. It is indicated for use in all adults. Individuals who are primarily immunized as children or earlier in adult life need receive only booster doses at 10-year intervals in order to maintain adequate immunity. Because pediatric immunization schedules generally end with a preschool booster dose of these antigens, the mid-decade birthday (e.g., 15 years, 25, 35) is a convenient recall date to provide the recommended booster dose.

Adults who are not known to have completed a three-dose primary immunization series in childhood should be given three 0.5-ml doses of Td. The second dose should be given 4 weeks after the first, and the third dose given 6 to 12 months after the second.

For wound management, an additional dose of Td is recommended only when there have been major or contaminated wounds and then only if more than 5 years have elapsed since the last dose. Td is preferred to T alone.

MEASLES, MUMPS, RUBELLA

These three vaccines are considered together, inasmuch as the immunizing agents are all attenuated live viruses and are frequently given together. They are available singly as well as in the combination product, MMR vaccine.

All adults should be immune to measles, mumps, and rubella. For measles, a physician-documented diagnosis or

TABLE 1 Summary of Vaccines Recommended for Adult Use

Age (yr)	Vaccine					
	Td	MMR	Polio	Influenza	Pneumococcal	Hepatitis B
18–24	+	1	2			3
25–64	+	1	2			3
≥65	+			+	+	

1. Check for documentation of rubella vaccine or serologic test. See text for measles and mumps. MMR vaccine is contraindicated in pregnancy.
2. Inactivated poliovirus vaccine should be used for nonimmune parents of children to be given live oral poliovirus vaccine.
3. Target populations: homosexual or bisexual males, intravenous drug abusers, health care workers at risk of contact with blood or body fluids, and travelers to endemic areas.

TABLE 2 Additional Considerations for Certain Occupations and Travel

Indication	Vaccine
Occupation	
Hospital, laboratory, and other health care personnel	Hepatitis B Measles Rubella Influenza Polio
Staff of institutions for the mentally retarded	Hepatitis B
Veterinarians and animal handlers	Rabies
Selected field workers	Plague
International travel, consider:	Polio, yellow fever, hepatitis B, rabies, meningococcal polysaccharide, typhoid, cholera, plague, immune globulin

laboratory evidence of immunity is acceptable. Individuals vaccinated against measles between 1963 and 1967 may have received inactivated vaccine or vaccine of unknown type and should be reimmunized with live measles vaccine to prevent severe atypical measles, a disease that has occurred among young adults such as college students and military recruits. Adults over the age of 35 years may generally be considered immune to measles and mumps, but younger adults should be investigated more thoroughly.

Since the clinical diagnosis of rubella is too uncertain to be dependable, laboratory evidence of immunity should generally be required unless a record of immunization with rubella vaccine is present. The risks of rubella vaccine during pregnancy are known to be low; nonetheless, women should be counseled not to become pregnant within 3 months after immunization. Transient arthralgias and arthritis after rubella vaccine have been reported in susceptible recipients of rubella vaccine and are believed to be manifestations of the mild vaccine-induced infection.

Most adults are immune to mumps virus; however, a surprising proportion of adults are still susceptible. Since a safe and effective vaccine is available, adults who are not known to be mumps-immune should be immunized.

The combined measles-mumps-rubella (MMR) vaccine is the immunizing agent of choice if the recipient is likely to be susceptible to more than one of the three diseases. There are no adverse effects of giving any of these three components of this vaccine to individuals already immune to one or more of the components.

Since these vaccines are grown in eggs, anaphylactic hypersensitivity to eggs represents a contraindication. Other contraindications include immunoincompetence, pregnancy, and the administration of immune globulin within the preceding 3 months. Commercially available immune globulin provides enough passive antibody directed at measles, mumps, and rubella to inhibit replication of the vaccine virus, thus preventing effective immunization.

POLIOMYELITIS

Two types of poliovirus vaccines are currently available in the United States: live oral poliovirus vaccine (OPV) and inactivated poliovirus vaccine (IPV). An IPV of enhanced potency was introduced in the United States in 1987 and is expected to become the only inactivated poliovaccine available. OPV has been by far the most widely used vaccine in this country. A primary vaccination series with either vaccine produces immunity to all three poliovirus types in over 95 percent of recipients.

Routine polio vaccination of adults living in the United States who have not been primarily immunized is no longer necessary because of the very low risk of poliomyelitis in the United States. When susceptible adults have children, however, they should be immunized against polio at the same time, or preferably before their children are immunized. Since the risk of OPV-associated paralysis is slightly higher in adults than in children, IPV is preferred for susceptible adults who have not received a primary series of polio vaccine in childhood. Similarly, for adults who may be at increased risk of exposure to polioviruses because of international travel or health care occupation, IPV is the preferred product for immunization.

INFLUENZA

Influenza vaccine consists of inactivated influenza virus, either as whole virus or viral subunits. Influenza vaccine differs from other products routinely recommended for use in adults in that its composition is likely to be changed each year, depending on the specific immunologic characteristics of circulating influenza viruses and the fact that the vaccine must be given annually because of the relatively short-lived immunity conferred by the vaccine. The vaccine is recommended for annual use in adults of any age with high-risk conditions such as chronic pulmonary, cardiac, renal, or metabolic diseases, and for all adults over 65 years of age.

Influenza outbreaks in the United States are regularly associated with increased mortality, and the impact of influenza is most severe among elderly persons, who account for 60 to 80 percent of all influenza-associated deaths. Approximately 90 percent of these deaths occur in persons with recognized underlying diseases, but deaths may also occur among apparently healthy elderly adults. For this reason, the annual use of influenza vaccine is strongly recommended to prevent or reduce the excess mortality associated with influenza.

PNEUMOCOCCAL VACCINE

The currently available pneumococcal vaccine consists of 25 μg of each pneumococcal polysaccharide from the 23 pneumococcal capsular types that account for the majority of bacteremic pneumococcal infections in this country. Indications for this vaccine include splenic dysfunction or anatomic asplenia, chronic diseases associated with increased risk of pneumococcal disease, such as chronic cardiopulmonary disease, and all adults over 65 years of age. The indications for pneumococcal vaccine in adults are similar to those for influenza vaccine, but in contrast to influenza vaccine, which is recommended for annual use, pneumococcal vaccine need be given only once. Influenza and pneumococcal vaccines may be given safely and effectively at the same time but in separate sites.

The need for reimmunization of patients at high risk of pneumococcal infection is not clearly defined, but consideration should be given to reimmunizing adults at highest risk who were immunized 6 or more years ago or patients known to have a rapid decline in pneumococcal antibody levels, such as patients with the nephrotic syndrome, renal failure, or organ transplants. It would be prudent to immunize adults at an earlier age, for example, at 55 years, before the age-related increase in frequency of underlying disease occurs, and at a time when a brisk immunologic response might be expected.

HEPATITIS B

The first vaccine directed against hepatitis B consisted of purified, inactivated hepatitis B surface antigen (HBsAg), derived from plasma obtained from chronic HBsAg carriers. A more recently introduced hepatitis B vaccine is derived from yeast cells into which the gene coding for the production of hepatitis B surface antigen has been inserted. This product will eventually fully replace the plasma-derived hepatitis B vaccine.

The vaccine should be administered intramuscularly in the deltoid region in three doses, the second dose 1 month after the first and the third dose 6 months later. The need for booster doses of hepatitis B vaccine after the primary immunizing series is not yet fully clarified. Major target populations for whom the vaccine is recommended include homosexual males, intravenous drug abusers, certain institutionalized populations, household and sexual contacts of chronic carriers of HBsAg, health care personnel who have occupational exposure to blood or blood-contaminated body fluids, and travelers to areas with high endemicity for hepatitis B.

Table 2 should be consulted for additional recommendations relating to certain occupational groups as well as international travel.

SUGGESTED READING

Guide for adult immunization. 2nd ed. Philadelphia: American College of Physicians, 1989.

Morbidity and mortality weekly report. Recommendations of the advisory committee on immunization practices. Atlanta: Centers for Disease Control.

Plotkin, SA, Mortimer EA, eds. Vaccines. Philadelphia: WB Saunders, 1988.

SYSTEMIC INFECTIONS

FEVER AND RASH

JOHN W. SENSAKOVIC, M.D., Ph.D.
LEON G. SMITH, M.D., F.A.C.P.

Fever and rash contribute one of the most challenging clinical syndromes in infectious disease. Many infectious and noninfectious conditions can present in this fashion; many of these are benign and diagnostically elusive. More important, when faced with the patient with fever and rash, the physician must be acutely aware of those several very serious infections that are commonly fulminant and can be rapidly fatal. Thus, the physician must quickly address a series of important issues (Table 1). These include the question of contagious potential to the medical staff, the need for rapid resuscitation in those patients who present in shock, the rapid recognition of and therapeutic intervention for those infections that tend to be fulminant, and the need for a thorough evaluation and work-up for the extensive list of diagnostic possibilities that can present with fever and rash.

URGENT CONDITIONS PRESENTING WITH FEVER AND RASH

Rapid recognition and therapeutic intervention are essential in certain diseases presenting with fever and rash in order to minimize the associated morbidity and mortality. The major conditions include meningococcemia, Rocky Mountain spotted fever, staphylococcal toxic shock syndrome, bacteremia with septic emboli, and the rapidly spreading cellulitides (Tables 2 and 3). All of these conditions can present with fever and rash in a fulminant, rapidly progressive form, requiring urgent therapeutic intervention, often on an empiric basis, prior to confirmation of the diagnosis if the associated mortality rates are to be minimized.

Meningococcemia

Of all the diseases presenting with fever and rash, meningococcemia is the most likely to be rapidly fatal if it is not recognized and treated promptly. Purpura in an acutely ill, febrile patient characteristically suggests this disease, unfortunately too often at a late stage of the illness. Other features that may be helpful in earlier diagnosis include more vague complaints, such as muscle tenderness, sore throat, fever, and headache. The illness tends to occur in late winter and early spring, and is well known to occur under crowded living conditions.

TABLE 1   Major Issues in Patients With Fever and Rash

Contagious potential
Resuscitation
Rapid therapy
Diagnostic evaluation

The initial rash may be maculopapular, with the earliest petechial lesions occurring over pressure points, such as the small of the back, and can easily be overlooked. The rash can progress rapidly over a few hours to the more classic, petechial form with peripheral acrocyanosis.

Management requires immediate recognition, vigorous fluid replacement, rapid therapy with aqueous penicillin, 24 million units intravenously daily. Patients presenting with signs of adrenal insufficiency also require steroid replacement. More controversial therapeutic approaches include the additional use of intravenous gamma globulin, which might benefit certain individuals, and the use of steroids for shock, which are probably not beneficial. Rifampin, 600 mg orally every 12 hours for 2 days, should be given to those patients who survive, to eradicate a possible nasopharyngeal carrier state. Rifampin is also indicated for immediate household contacts and for medical personnel with significant respiratory exposure, such as might occur during a difficult intubation without a protective mask. Rifampin prophylaxis is at best about 70 percent effective, so exposed individuals should also be informed of the signs and symptoms of infection. An alternative to penicillin for penicillin-allergic patients is chloramphenicol at a dose of 100 mg per kilogram per day intravenously up to 4 g daily. Because of its high serum levels and good cerebrospinal fluid penetration as well as its excellent bactericidal activity against *Neisseria*, many experts consider ceftriaxone, 50 mg per kilogram per day intravenously every 12 hours, to be a superior agent.

Rocky Mountain Spotted Fever

Rocky Mountain spotted fever can also present with fever and petechial rash in an acutely ill patient, yet is characteristically different from meningococcemia in several respects. The illness begins with fever and severe headache and occurs between May and September in temperate-zone states, and there is a history of tick bite in 75 percent of the cases. The rash appears after several days of illness, begins as a maculopapular rash on wrists and ankles, and progresses to a petechial form, spreading to palms, soles, and trunk.

TABLE 2 Approach to Seriously Ill Patients With Fever and Rash

Disease	Clues	Diagnosis	Therapy
Meningococcemia	Multiple purpuric lesions, earliest on small of back; rapid progression over hours	Gram stain of lesions; blood cultures	Aqueous penicillin 300,000 U/kg/day up to 24 × 10⁶ U × 5–7 day IV; vigorous fluid support; steroids, controversial; IV gamma globulin, controversial
Rocky Mountain spotted fever	Tick exposure; headache, fever, rash 2–6th day on wrists, ankles, progressing to palms, soles, trunk	Immunofluorescence staining of skin biopsy; serology (CF)	Tetracycline 25 mg/kg/day × 7 days PO; vigorous fluid support
Toxic shock syndrome	Fever, rash, hypotension in menstruating female using tampons; surgical wound or skin infection	Isolation of staphylococci, absence of antibody	Vigorous fluid replacement; remove tampon; drain focus; nafcillin 2 g IV q4h × 10 days
Bacteremia with septic emboli	Elderly or immunocompromised patient; several lesions, macular to necrotic pustules	Gram stain of lesions; blood cultures; Gram stain of buffy coat	Nafcillin IV 2 g q4h and gentamicin IV 5 mg/kg/day × 14 days (longer if endocarditis)
Rapidly spreading cellulitis	Painful spreading lesions; local trauma	See Table 3	

Leukocytosis with thrombocytopenia is frequently present. Therapy is tetracycline, 500 mg every 6 hours, and must be instituted early on a presumptive basis, prior to serologic confirmation, if mortality is to be significantly reduced. Alternative therapy is chloramphenicol, 50 mg per kilogram per day intravenously. In those institutions where available, immunofluorescence staining of a skin biopsy specimen of the rash can yield a rapid diagnosis.

Toxic Shock Syndrome

Toxic shock syndrome due to an exotoxin of *Staphylococcus aureus* characteristically presents in a young menstruating female using a tampon. The tampons that have been epidemiologically most often associated with the disease have been withdrawn from the market. Cases have also occurred, however, that are due to nonvaginal foci of staphylococcal infection, including surgical wound infections and infectious endocarditis. The rash tends to be diffuse and scarlatiniform in character, with associated conjunctival hyperemia and a "strawberry tongue." The rash is associated with fever, hypotension, and evidence of multisystem derangement and is followed during the second week by desquamation. Therapy is vigorous fluid replacement, removal of the tampon, or drainage of any identified infected focus, and administration of nafcillin or oxacillin, 12 g daily. Some experts also recommend vaginal lavage with a Betadine-containing solution as a local antibacterial agent as well as to remove any nonabsorbed exotoxin.

Septic Emboli

The diagnosis of septic emboli associated with bacteremia or fungemia must be considered in any seriously ill patient presenting with fever and rash. Such infections

TABLE 3 Approach to Seriously Ill Patients With Rapidly Spreading Cellulitis

Disease	Clues	Diagnosis	Therapy
Streptococcal or staphylococcal	Minor trauma; insect bite; chronic stasis; lymphangitis; "brawny" edema; serous drainage post-bypass	Culture of drainage; streptozyme titer	Nafcillin 2 g IV q6h × 10 days
Clostridial gas gangrene	Peripheral vascular disease; traumatic wound with deep muscle involvement; leukemia; paucity of WBCs; "rotten apple" odor	Gram stain; anaerobic culture	Aqueous penicillin 4 × 10⁶ U/day IV q4h × 14 days; debridement
Synergistic gangrene	Diabetic; peripheral vascular disease; local trauma; necrotic tissue; fetid odor	Gram stain; aerobic/anaerobic cultures	Clindamycin 600 mg IV q6h and gentamicin 5 mg/kg/day; or ticarcillin/clavulanate 3.1 g IV q6h; debridement; vascular reconstruction
Necrotizing fasciitis	Diabetic; obesity; IVDA; "brawny" edema; toxic patient; subcutaneous gas	Gram stain; aerobic/anaerobic cultures	Clindamycin 600 mg IV q6h and gentamicin 5 mg/kg/day; extensive surgical debridement
Vibrio cellulitis	Saltwater wound; rapidly advancing cellulitis; toxic patient; bullae formation	Gram stain; culture on NaCl enrichment media	Tetracycline 500 mg q6h × 10 days; gentamicin 5 mg/kg/day; local debridement

most commonly present in elderly or immunocompromised patients. Solitary or widely scattered purplish lesions, non-blanching, and often with necrotic centers suggest the diagnosis. The lesions frequently involve the digits. Ecthyma gangrenosum is one such lesion, seen with *Pseudomonas aeruginosa* bacteremia. Such lesions are also seen most often in *Staphylococcus aureus* bacteremia, *Candida albicans* fungemia, and infectious endocarditis. Gram stain of aspirates from the skin lesions and Gram stain of the buffy coat of the blood can be rapidly diagnostic; blood cultures are confirmatory. Presumptive therapy should be with nafcillin and gentamicin pending cultural confirmation. In those institutions in which methicillin-resistant *Staphylococcus aureus* is a problem, vancomycin (1 g intravenously every 12 hours) and ceftazidime (1 g intravenously every 8 hours) are recommended.

Rapidly Spreading Cellulitis

Rapidly spreading cellulitis is not difficult to recognize in most instances, because of the presence of the painful, spreading, inflammatory lesion on the skin. The diagnostic difficulty involves differentiating the various types of rapidly spreading cellulitis based on probable causative organism or organisms and determining whether infection is confined to the surface or extends to deeper structures, including fascia and muscle, in which case adequate surgical debridement is essential, along with appropriate antibiotic therapy (see Table 3).

OTHER CONDITIONS WITH FEVER AND RASH

Most diseases associated with fever and rash are not as rapidly progressive as those previously discussed. They mainly include viral exanthems, drug eruptions, and vasculitis. Several characteristics of the rash suggest the more serious conditions (Table 4). Viral exanthems are most often maculopapular and blanch with pressure. The patients appear less toxic, the complete blood count and the erythrocyte sedimentation rate often suggest a nonbacterial etiology, and oral lesions (enanthema) are common.

TABLE 4 Characteristics of Serious Rashes

Onset with or after fever
Petechial lesions
Rapid spread
Purpuric lesions
Palmar/plantar involvement

Drug eruptions range from maculopapular to petechial to vesiculo-bullous, and can have mucous membrane involvement, as in the Stevens-Johnson syndrome. A history of drug exposure is important. Patients frequently are not toxic in proportion to the fever, there is often a pulse-temperature discrepancy, and associated eosinophilia, increase of hepatic transaminase concentration, or nephritis can sometimes be found. Vasculitis of the skin is often the cause of a nonblanching, petechial rash with associated findings of multisystem involvement, but the diagnosis usually requires skin biopsy along with serologic diagnostic testing.

Several other specific entities are commonly seen with fever and rash. Erythema nodosum lesions are painful, tender, reddish-brown nodules, mainly on the shins. They occur in a variety of infectious diseases (tuberculosis, histoplasmosis, coccidioidomycosis, and infection due to *Yersinia* and β-hemolytic streptococci) and may be drug induced (sulfonamides, penicillins, oral contraceptives). Erythema multiforme characteristically presents as target lesions, often on the palms, but which can become vesiculo-bullous. They are seen in a variety of infections (herpes, *Mycoplasma*) and drug reactions (penicillin, sulfonamides, dilantin).

Although a wide variety of diagnostic tests and procedures can be helpful in the work-up of the patient presenting with fever and rash, none of these is as important as a careful history and physical examination.

SUGGESTED READING

Kingston M, Mackey D. Skin clues in the diagnosis of life-threatening infections. Rev Infect Dis 1986; 8:1–11.
Oblinger M, Sande M. Fever and rash. In: Internal medicine. Stein JH, ed. Boston: Little, Brown & Co, 1983.

FEVER AND LYMPHADENOPATHY

GERALD H. FRIEDLAND, M.D.

The logical evaluation of a patient with fever and lymphadenopathy requires that four questions be answered:

1. Is the adenopathy local or generalized?
2. Is the process acute or chronic?
3. Is the etiology infectious or noninfectious?
4. Is there a primary peripheral lesion?

To answer the first question a thorough physical examination of all accessible major lymph-node-bearing areas should be performed. These include the nodes of the head and neck and the axillary, epitrochlear, and inguinal nodes. Radiologic studies are necessary to define the two other clinically important major node-bearing areas: the mediastinum and hilum of the lung and the retroperitoneum. The somewhat arbitrary period of 1 month separates acute and chronic lymphadenopathy in adults. In children, a period of 2 or 3 months is more reasonable. Although they are less common, noninfectious causes should be considered in puzzling cases, and in localized lymphadenopathy, a primary lesion should always be sought. See Figure 1 for an overview of guidelines to the differential diagnosis of fever and lymphadenopathy.

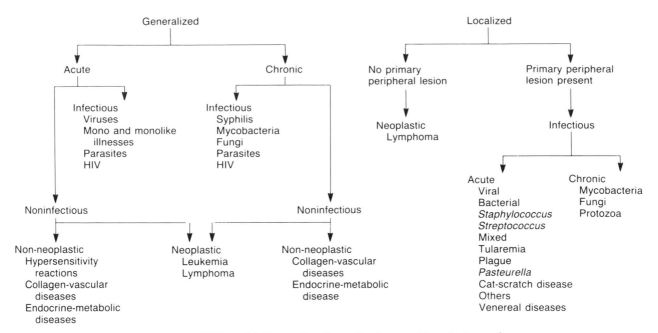

Figure 1 Differential diagnostic scheme for fever and lymphadenopathy.

GENERALIZED LYMPHADENOPATHY

Generalized lymphadenopathy is present if nodes in two or more noncontiguous major lymph-node-bearing areas are enlarged.

Acute generalized infectious lymphadenopathy is most commonly viral and rarely bacterial in origin. Generalized lymph node enlargement is a constant feature of many of the common viral infections of childhood, including rubella, measles, and varicella. It may be present during the prodromal period in hepatitis A and B and is a common feature of infectious mononucleosis, cytomegalovirus mononucleosis, toxoplasmosis, and enteroviral infections as well. Acute generalized lymphadenopathy is a feature of acute human immunodeficiency virus (HIV) infection, occurring 1 to 3 months after infection. In all of these infections the nodes are typically tender, discrete, firm to touch, and without fluctuance. The tenderness and enlargement as well as the fever gradually subside over a period of days to a few weeks without specific therapy.

Acute generalized noninfectious lymphadenopathy is frequently due to hypersensitivity reactions, most commonly drug-induced. Among those agents known to cause fever and lymphadenopathy are the sulfonamides, hydralazine, and phenytoin. The syndrome rapidly disappears with the withdrawal of the drug. Collagen-vascular diseases, including rheumatoid arthritis and systemic lupus erythematosus, may be causes of acute generalized lymphadenopathy and fever. The mucocutaneous lymph node syndrome (Kawasaki's disease), a disease of uncertain origin, must be considered in children with lymphadenopathy, fever, mucosal inflammation, and peripheral rash with desquamation.

Chronic generalized infectious lymphadenopathy is much less commonly encountered but raises more serious diagnostic possibilities. If the fever and lymphadenopathy have been present for 1 month or longer in adults and 3

months in children, viral etiologic agents become unlikely. An exception to this rule is the persistent generalized lymphadenopathy seen in HIV infection. Disseminated bacterial and fungal diseases must also be considered, including tuberculosis, syphilis, histoplasmosis, cryptococcosis, and coccidioidomycosis. The lymph nodes are firmer than those in cases of acute infection and there may be fusion and matting of adjacent nodes. Infection with HIV is associated with chronic generalized lymphadenopathy. When present in association with characteristic immunologic abnormalities, the term *AIDS-related complex* or ARC is used.

Chronic generalized noninfectious lymphadenopathy is most often neoplastic in origin. Lymphoreticular neoplasms (Hodgkin's disease, lymphosarcoma, chronic lymphatic leukemia) predominate. In patients with neoplastic generalized lymphadenopathy, fever may be due either to the underlying malignant process or to secondary infection. This is always a difficult clinical situation, made increasingly so by the frequency with which such patients' host defenses are altered by chemotherapy, radiotherapy, or immunosuppressive agents. Infrequently, hyperthyroidism may present with generalized lymphadenopathy and signs and symptoms suggesting infection.

AIDS

The recently described acquired immunodeficiency syndrome must be considered in patients with chronic weight loss, malaise, fever, generalized lymphadenopathy, and lymphopenia. Such patients typically are homosexual men, intravenous drug abusers, recipients of multiple transfusions or clotting factors, or heterosexual partners of individuals in the above groups. Oral candidiasis is often encountered. An immunopathy consisting of depressed T helper-inducer cells, cutaneous anergy, and hypergammaglobulinemia is found. By definition, these patients have life-threatening opportunistic infections and/or Kaposi's sarcoma (see AIDS chapter).

Lastly, hyperthyroidism may present with generalized lymphadenopathy and signs and symptoms suggesting infection.

LOCALIZED LYMPHADENOPATHY

Localized lymphadenopathy is present if not more than two contiguous lymph-node-bearing areas are involved. Anatomically and clinically the local node-bearing areas are divided into five major groups: the nodes of the head and neck, the axilla, the inguinal area, the mediastinal-hilar areas, and the retroperitoneal para-aortic nodes. The physician again must consider both infectious and noninfectious etiologic agents. A further question will help distinguish between these categories: Is there a primary peripheral lesion?

Noninfectious local adenopathy is not associated with a primary peripheral lesion. The most likely cause is lymphoproliferative neoplasm, particularly if the lymphadenopathy is chronic.

Infectious local adenopathy is usually associated with a primary peripheral lesion and requires an appreciation of the anatomic areas which each nodal area drains. The evaluation of localized lymphadenopathy should always include a thorough examination of these areas. In the following sections each nodal area is discussed separately, with particular reference to those infections that are most characteristic in each area. This is a convenient separation but is somewhat artificial, since many of the infections discussed may present in any of the anatomic sites. Any regional group of nodes may be involved in a disease producing generalized lymphadenopathy, and it is worth stressing again that careful examination of other areas is always indicated.

The *lymph nodes of the head and neck* can be further divided into several more local anatomic and clinical areas.

The *occipital* and *posterior auricular* nodes drain large areas of the scalp and face, and drain in turn into the posterior and inferior cervical nodes. Careful examination of the scalp is essential when these nodes are enlarged. A small primary lesion may be overlooked when the hair is thick. In children, secondarily infected insect, tick, or spider bites and ringworm are common causes. Posterior auricular and occipital adenopathy is a feature of many acute viral illnesses.

The *anterior auricular* nodes drain the eyelids, the palpebral conjunctivae, the external auditory meatus, and the pinna. Primary infections in these sites must be sought in patients with involvement of these nodes. A large number of organisms have been reported to produce the "oculoglandular syndrome" (conjunctivitis and anterior auricular adenopathy) by direct inoculation of the conjunctiva, including *Neisseria gonorrhoeae, Francisella tularensis*, the presumed agent of cat-scratch fever, and epidemic keratoconjunctivitis.

The *"tonsillar," submaxillary, and submental* nodes drain the tonsils and other structures of the pharynx and mouth and as such are of great clinical significance. Involvement of these nodes requires careful inspection and often palpation of the mouth, teeth, and pharynx. The "tonsillar" nodes belong to the superior deep cervical node group and lie below the angle of the mandible. They drain the posterior and

lateral pharynx, including the tonsils, and are thus most frequently enlarged in bacterial and viral infections of the tonsils. The submaxillary nodes lie within the submaxillary fascial compartment, surrounded by the deep cervical fascia. Some of the nodes are imbedded within the submaxillary gland and are often indistinct on palpation even in acute infections. This important group of nodes drains the lateral margins of the tongue, the gums, the angle of the mouth and cheek, the lateral part of the lower lip and the entire upper lip, and the medial aspect of the conjunctiva. They are commonly involved in dental infections, and they, in turn, drain into the deep cervical nodes. The submental nodes drain the floor of the mouth, the tip of the tongue, the central part of the lower lip, and the skin of the chin. They drain into the submaxillary nodes and are also commonly involved in dental infections.

The *posterior cervical* nodes are located in the occipital triangle of the neck above the inferior belly of the omohyoid muscle and posterior to the sternomastoid. They are commonly involved in scalp infections and are often prominently involved in the generalized lymphadenopathy of infectious mononucleosis and monolike syndromes. Involvement of these nodes is highly unlikely in localized infections of the mouth and pharynx.

The *inferior deep cervical nodes* lie below the level of the inferior belly of the omohyoid muscle and both posterior (the supraclavicular nodes) and anterior (the scalene modes) to the sternomastoid muscle. Those nodes receive drainage from the scalp, the superior deep cervical nodes, the axillary nodes, and also the nodes of the hilum of the lung, mediastinum, and abdominal viscera. Their enlargement may signify primary disease at any of these distant sites. Adenopathy in this area not readily palpable may be detected by performance of the Valsalva maneuver.

Acute cervical adenopathy is most likely to be of pyogenic bacterial or viral origin. Staphylococci and streptococci predominate among bacterial etiologic agents, the former from primary skin sites and the latter from oral and dental infections. Infections of the tonsils, pharynx, and skin are the most frequent primary sites in children, whereas dental infections more commonly result in cervical adenopathy in adults. Appreciation of the primary site of infection, as well as aspiration, Gram stain, and culture of fluctuant or grossly enlarged and tender nodes are of therapeutic as well as diagnostic importance. Penicillin is prescribed in those infections of oral and dental origin. A semisynthetic penicillinase-resistant penicillin is used when the primary site of infection is in the skin. Rupture of cervical nodes into their fascial spaces may additionally require surgical drainage if there is fluctuance, impingement on vital structures, or both.

Chronic cervical adenopathy raises the possibility of granulomatous infections, particularly *Mycobacterium tuberculosis* and nontuberculous mycobacterial infection. Toxoplasmosis may cause chronic cervical lymphadenopathy, particularly involving the posterior cervical nodes.

The importance of histologic as well as microbiologic diagnosis in all chronic infections, and the need to exclude lymphoproliferative neoplasm, require that surgical excision of an entire intact node be carried out in cases of chronic cervical lymphadenopathy. More specific indications for surgical excision will be discussed later in this chapter.

The *mediastinal and hilar nodes* are rarely involved in acute suppurative disease. The structures drained include the lungs, pleura, and mediastinal contents. Of particular importance diagnostically is the continuity of these nodes with the inferior deep cervical nodes (supraclavicular and scalene groups) and axillary nodes, since these represent an accessible area for both examination and biopsy. Biopsy at this site in the presence of intrathoracic disease may yield a diagnosis in from 30 percent to 80 percent of selected cases. Anatomically, the drainage remains on the homolateral side except for the left lower lobe, where drainage is to both lateral nodal areas via the interbronchial nodes. Since the nodes within the thorax and their drainage areas are not readily accessible to direct examination, more indirect methods must be used to elicit a diagnosis. In addition to the history and general physical examination, the radiologic characteristics or absence of coexistent pulmonary lesions and examination of sputum are of obvious importance. The differential diagnosis of hilar and mediastinal adenopathy most frequently includes granulomatous disease of both infectious and uncertain origin (sarcoidosis) and lymphoproliferative disorders. In the former, *M. tuberculosis* and fungal disease predominate. In these infections, adenopathy is almost always unilateral—a useful differential diagnostic point. Bilateral hilar adenopathy is present in approximately three-fourths of patients with sarcoidosis and in 10 percent of cases of lymphoma. Looked at from another perspective, 90 percent of patients presenting with bilateral hilar adenopathy have sarcoidosis and only 10 percent have neoplastic disease. Additionally, in the absence of constitutional symptoms or peripheral adenopathy, bilateral hilar adenopathy is almost always caused by sarcoid. Transbronchial lung biopsy, inferior cervical node biopsy, or both are indicated in most patients with hilar adenopathy. Mycobacterial skin tests, sputum examination, cultures, and sputum cytology are also indicated.

Finally, it is worth noting that systemic lupus erythematosus and other collagen-vascular diseases may present with hilar adenopathy.

The *axillary nodes* drain the entire upper extremity as well as the lateral parts of the chest wall, back, and the breast. This cluster of nodes is most frequently involved in acute pyogenic infections of these drainage areas. Careful examination of the readily accessible and often obvious primary site is essential. By far the most common organisms involved are the staphylococcus and streptococcus, often associated with primary areas of cellulitis, lymphangitis, or furunculosis. The upper extremity and axillary nodes may be involved by many additional infecting organisms.

Several zoonoses (discussed in detail in other chapters) should be considered in the appropriate epidemiologic setting. Tularemia, transmitted by bite or skin contact with wild rodents, is seen most frequently in hunters and butchers. Aspiration of nodes and serologic testing will confirm the diagnosis. Agents of choice include tetracycline, chloramphenicol, and streptomycin. Plague must be considered in the southwestern United States where transmission still occurs. Aspiration of nodes should be carried out. Giemsa stain of aspirated material demonstrates the characteristic safety pin appearance of plump rodlike organisms. The organism can be cultured from buboes and blood on routine culture media. Treatment with streptomycin, tetracycline or chloramphenicol should be instituted upon suspicion of the disease.

Pasteurella multocida infections are common following cat and dog bites and scratches. The infection presents with a lesion at the primary site, lymphatitis and/or cellulitis, and tender regional adenopathy. Gram stain of the primary lesion of draining aspirated nodes reveals characteristic gram-negative coccobacillary organisms that are easily cultured. Penicillin is the drug of choice.

Cat-scratch disease may present as lymphadenopathy and fever. The diagnosis is made on the basis of history of cat contact; a papule at the inoculation site; tender regional lymphadenopathy that is often fluctuant and draining, and shows granulomatous inflammation on biopsy; and the exclusion of other definable etiologic agents. There is no specific treatment.

Inguinal lymphadenopathy is commonly encountered clinically. The inguinal nodes drain not only the lower extremities, but the lower abdominal wall, the genitalia, perineum, and perianal area as well. Careful examination of all these drainage areas is an essential part of a thorough evaluation of inguinal adenopathy, including a careful pelvic and rectal examination if other areas of primary infection are not apparent. Acute pyogenic bacterial infection is most common, usually caused by the same organisms enumerated in the discussion of axillary adenopathy. The drainage of the perineum and perianal area suggests the possibility that enteric aerobic gram-negative organisms and gram-positive and gram-negative anaerobic organisms may be present. Because of the drainage of the genitalia, sexually transmitted infections often involve the inguinal nodes. Those likely to present with prominent inguinal adenopathy are syphilis, lymphogranuloma venereum, chancroid, and herpes progenitalis. The appearance of the primary lesion is useful in distinguishing among these entities.

The *abdominal and retroperitoneal nodes* drain the abdominal viscera and retroperitoneal and pelvic organs and may receive drainage from the inguinal nodes as well. Neither the nodes nor the primary site of infection are directly clinically accessible, making assessment difficult. Radiologic procedures must be employed for evaluation, including the intravenous pyelogram, lymphangiogram, and computed tomographic scan. Although the nodes are involved in acute intra-abdominal systemic infections, the possibility of chronic infections, particularly tuberculosis, and of lymphoproliferative disorders involving them is the usual reason for using these diagnostic tools.

GENERAL DIAGNOSTIC APPROACHES

Indirect

In most cases of infectious and non-neoplastic lymphadenopathy with fever, the diagnosis is apparent on the basis of the history and the extranodal features of the illness on examination. This is particularly true of lymphadenopathy of less than 1 month's duration. Other clinical and laboratory findings short of biopsy often suggest the etiologic agent in the enlarged nodes. Some of these findings are:

1. Primary site of infection—clinically apparent and characteristic; streptococcal cellulitis, staphylococcal furuncle, syphilitic chancre, and so on.
2. Characteristic rash—rubella, rubeola, varicella-zoster, secondary syphilis, drug eruption, oral candidiasis.
3. Typical hematologic findings—atypical lymphocytes in mononucleosis and monolike illnesses, eosinophilia in drug hypersensitivity reactions.
4. Skin tests—tuberculosis, lymphogranuloma venereum, tularemia.
5. Serologic tests—infectious mononucleosis and monolike illnesses (cytomegalovirus and toxoplasmosis), HIV infection, hepatitis, syphilis, tularemia, fungal infections.
6. Stains and culture of material from peripheral primary lesions and pulmonary lesions—acute pyogenic infections, including staphylococci, streptococci, tularemia, plague, *P. multocida*, herpes simplex, chancroid, mycobacteria, fungi.
7. Radiologic appearance of primary sites, particularly the character of pulmonary infiltrate.

Direct

Although the diagnosis is often apparent by the methods noted above, careful evaluation of enlarged nodes is always indicated.

The physical characteristics of nodes often reveal important information: discrete, tender, firm nodes that are acutely enlarged suggest acute bacterial or viral infections. Chronic firm and rubbery nodes are characteristic of lymphoproliferative diseases and granulomatous infections. Matted, fluctuant nodes suggest the presence of pyogenic organisms. Hard, fixed nodes are characteristic of carcinoma.

Aspiration of fluctuant but nondraining nodes in palpable areas is a simple and valuable diagnostic technique that is not carried out as frequently as it is indicated. Aspirated material should be stained (Gram, Giemsa, acid-fast) and cultured for all suspected pathogens.

Excision of a lymph node or lymph node biopsy is usually carried out to distinguish between chronic infection and neoplasm. The indications for lymph node biopsy are often vague. The following general guidelines are intended to suggest to the clinician circumstances in which biopsy is appropriate.

Indications for Lymph Node Biopsy

1. Undiagnosed chronic lymphadenopathy (of more than 1 month's duration in adults, 3 months' in children).
2. Localized lymphadenopathy without an accessible or apparent peripheral lesion.
3. Enlarging, undiagnosed lymphadenopathy, after 2 weeks of observation.
4. Nontender, matted to hard lymphadenopathy.
5. Systemic signs and symptoms suggesting granulomatous or lymphoproliferative disease (prolonged fever, sweats, weight loss, fatigue).
6. Radiologic findings suggesting granulomatous disease.
7. Positive tuberculin test.

8. New adenopathy in immunocompromised patients including those with AIDS.
9. Lymphadenopathy in the setting of fever of undetermined etiology.

Technique of Lymph Node Biopsy

Approximately half of lymph node biopsies lead to a specific diagnosis. All too frequently, excision of abnormal lymph nodes does not reveal the diagnosis because of technical errors. Careful attention to several rules maximizes the usefulness of this invasive diagnostic procedure.

1. Consider all of the diagnostic possibilities before performing surgery and make appropriate arrangements for the handling of the excised tissue.
2. Select the best site. Lymph nodes that are frequently involved in common minor inflammatory processes should be avoided, as they may show only nonspecific chronic inflammatory changes or fibrosis. In the presence of generalized lymphadenopathy the inferior or posterior cervical nodes are preferred. The submandibular nodes should be avoided. The axillary nodes are the next best and the inguinal nodes, except in the presence of localized adenopathy in this area, are least likely to provide a diagnosis.
3. Select the best node—the most superficial and accessible node is not necessarily the most desirable or diagnostic node. The biopsy area should be carefully explored and the largest node in a cluster of enlarged nodes should be removed.
4. Remove the node or several nodes in their entirety with their capsules intact. Bisect the nodes, sending half of the specimen to the pathology laboratory and the other half to the bacteriology laboratory for stains and culturing of common pathogens, *M. tuberculosis*, fungi, viruses, and other suspected organisms.
5. Request that the pathologist make additional sections of the tissue excised if the node is abnormal but not diagnostic.
6. Consider a repeat biopsy and the excision of more tissue if the node is abnormal but not diagnostic and the clinical picture is unclear.

Interpretation of Lymph Node Biopsy

The interested reader will find detailed histologic descriptions elsewhere. Entities discussed in this chapter for which a characteristic histologic pattern exists and for which a specific or strongly suggestive diagnosis can be made histologically are lymphoma and other neoplasms, tuberculosis, fungal diseases, sarcoidosis, toxoplasmosis, HIV infection, and cat-scratch disease. Most noninfectious, non-neoplastic disorders show nonspecific lymphadenitis or hyperplasia only, as do most acute viral infections. However, it is important to note that a significant number of patients with initially nondiagnostic lymph node biopsies and persistent lymphadenopathy will ultimately prove to have a serious underlying disease. If the biopsy is not initially diagnostic it is essential to follow the patient carefully and to consider repeat biopsy if adenopathy persists.

SUGGESTED READING

Abrams DI, Lewis BJ, Beckstead JH, et al. Persistent diffuse lymphadenopathy in homosexual men: endpoint or prodrome? Ann Intern Med 1984; 100:801.

Byrnes RK, Chain WC, Spira TJ, et al. Value of lymph node biopsy in unexplained lymphadenopathy in homosexual men. JAMA 1983; 250:1313.

Greenfield S, Jordan MC. The clinical investigation of lymphadenopathy in primary care practice. JAMA 1978; 240:1388.

Ioachim HL. Lymph node biopsy. Philadelphia: JB Lippincott, 1982.

Solnitsky O, Jeghers H. Lymphadenopathy and disorders of the lymphatic system. In: McBryde CM, Blacklow LS, eds. Signs and symptoms. 5th ed. Philadelphia: JB Lippincott, 1970.

INFECTION IN PREGNANCY

DAVID CHARLES, M.D.
BRYAN LARSEN, Ph.D.

In this survey of the infectious diseases that affect the gravid host, emphasis will be placed on systemic infections that present unique problems because of the pregnancy. It is probable that the gravid patient is susceptible to any infectious disease, but some of these complicate the pregnancy by threatening the baby in utero (often without the mother becoming seriously ill). Moreover, some infectious processes, although not posing a direct threat to the baby, are associated with premature delivery. Table 1 contains a summary of these infections.

A further topic addressed in this chapter is antimicrobial therapy inasmuch as the pregnant patient is characterized by pharmacodynamic and pharmacokinetic differences from the nonpregnant individual. The potential toxicity of chemotherapeutic agents to the fetus is of concern to the physician who must prescribe them during pregnancy.

VIRAL INFECTIONS DURING PREGNANCY

The deleterious potential of viral infections for the conceptus has been a major stimulus to research and has resulted in the incorporation of a series of immunologic tests into the routine assessment of the mother prior to pregnancy. Assessment of the pregnant patient for susceptibility to rubella is now standard. Other viral infections may be similarly evaluated in the gravid patient in the future. The possibility that specific viral infections may be more severe in pregnant women than among those who are not pregnant, coupled with the fact that the unborn child may be especially liable to damage by infectious agents that cross the placenta, emphasizes the importance of detecting viral infections encountered during the gravid state.

Infections responsible for perinatal mortality and morbidity may be acquired by the embryo without eliciting symptoms in the mother, but the conceptus may experience significant damage. Many viral diseases have been associated with spontaneous abortion. It should be noted that spontaneous abortion may result from the fever associated with such infections.

Approximately 20 percent of perinatal deaths are ascribed to congenital malformations; however, the identification of viral teratogens is not simple since retrospective studies may be unable to establish that infection definitely did occur, especially if the infection was sub-

TABLE 1 Infectious Complications of Pregnancy That Have Fetal Sequelae

Infection	Maternal Consequences	Fetal Consequence
Viral		
Influenza	Moderate to severe respiratory infection	Prematurity (?)
Hepatitis	Possibly more severe than in nonpregnant patient	Prematurity (?)
Cytomegalovirus	Mild febrile illness or no symptoms	Congenital infection
Rubella	Mild illness with rash	Congenital rubella syndrome with multisystem damage
Genital herpes	Genital lesions	Neonatal infection may be severe or fatal
Bacterial		
Syphilis	Primary or secondary lesions or no symptoms	Possibly abortion if acquired early or stigmata of congenital disease if acquired late
Listeriosis	Mild febrile illness associated with bacteremia	Abortion or stillbirth
Group B Streptococcus	Intrapartum vaginal colonization, postpartum endometritis	Congenital infection, lung, CSF infection
Gonorrhea	Endocervical infection, possibly disseminated gonococcal infection	Possibly premature delivery; neonatal opthalmia
Normal vaginal flora	No untoward maternal intrapartum effect, postpartum	Chorioamnionitis; neonatal septicemia, pneumonia
Pneumonia	More severe in gravid than nongravid patient	May prevent carriage to term

clinical. Prospective studies demand a great number of cases to provide consequential data. Congenital anomalies can, however, be correlated with the stage of gestation at which the infection was acquired.

Many prenatally acquired maternal viral infections appear to have no deleterious effect on the mother or fetus. Viral agents for which a teratogenic role is established include rubella virus, herpesvirus group, mumps virus, influenza viruses, coxsackievirus, cytomegalovirus, and Venezuelan equine encephalitis virus. Not every encounter with one of these viral agents during pregnancy results in fetal infection. Other viruses are of interest, but, as yet, they have not been assigned any embryopathic role.

Possible long-term effects of intrauterine viral infection not apparent at birth are now beginning to be documented. The congenital rubella syndrome may not manifest itself until late childhood when the child develops diabetes and has abnormal dermatoglyphics. Congenital cytomegaloviral infection may be responsible for hearing defects—originally ascribed to hypoxia—as well as some cases of mental retardation discernible only when the children enter school.

Rubella is one of the few congenital infections for which an estimate of the relative risk for congenital damage has been assigned following exposure to the virus at a given gestational age. Generally, the earlier in pregnancy the infection occurs, the greater the risk of detrimental effects to the fetus. In contrast, infection with herpesvirus hominis is likely to cause greater damage, particularly to the central nervous system, when it is acquired late in pregnancy or during parturition. Since no antiviral agent is approved for use during pregnancy, the prevention of rubella by testing for susceptibility and protecting the susceptible host by vaccination, where feasible, should be undertaken before pregnancy.

Attenuated viral vaccines are potentially harmful for the fetus, despite the lack of any adverse effects upon the mother. For this reason, pregnancy is a contraindication to rubella vaccination. Rubella vaccine is unusual among immunogenic agents in that the major purpose for its introduction was for the protection of a future conceptus. The live-attenuated virus can be transferred across the placenta, but its effects on the fetus have not been determined. The duration of protection from rubella vaccination has not been established, and consequently all patients who have not been recently vaccinated should be tested for susceptibility at their initial prenatal visit.

Additional live viral vaccines that are contraindicated in pregnancy are trivalent oral poliomyelitis, mumps, rubella, yellow fever, and vaccinia. There is no indication at present for smallpox immunization.

Adverse effects ascribed to other live viral vaccines may be unpredictable and idiosyncratic. Such a reaction is illustrated by the recipients of swine influenza vaccine who developed the Guillain-Barré syndrome. This complication may be associated with vaccines other than the swine influenza preparation. Currently, vaccines are not available for varicella-zoster, herpesvirus hominis, or cytomegalovirus. The over-riding concern centers on the neurotropic nature of these agents and their possible association with carcinogenesis.

Influenza vaccination should be offered to the gravid patient if the pregnancy includes a period of high influenza activity. The gravid patient may experience more severe symptoms of influenza than the nonpregnant individual. Moreover, the influenza virus may exert adverse effects on the fetus as a result of transplacental infection. Vaccination of pregnant women is desirable, but only an inactivated vaccine should be used.

PROTOZOAL INFECTIONS

The incidence of protozoal infections during pregnancy and the relative importance of these infections as causes of fetal loss and perinatal disease remain to be determined. The risk of such pregnancy complications is dependent on geographic location and the population group being considered. Maternal infection with any species causing human malaria may result in congenital malaria.

Another common protozoal infection capable of causing congenital infection is toxoplasmosis. The reader is referred to the chapter *Toxoplasmosis* for additional information. Congenital infection has also been reported from Chagas' disease because of the transplacental transmission of *Trypanosoma cruzi*. This organism may produce hepatosplenomegaly, fetal hydrops, jaundice, seizure disorders, and cataracts. The frequency of such complications is unknown. Other protozoal infections in pregnancy may also have a deleterious effect on the fetus.

BACTERIAL INFECTIONS

It is difficult to define the incidence of bacterial infections in pregnancy, but they are a major cause of morbidity and severe illness in the gravid patient. Although the fetal risk of transplacental bacterial infection is not known, serious perinatal bacterial illnesses can result from ascending infections. Comprehensive studies of stillbirths and early neonatal deaths have shown that about one-third are associated with chorioamnionitis, and it is recognized that many bacteria encountered by the fetus during the second stage of labor—during its passage through the birth canal—can cause serious disease. Maternal genitourinary bacterial infections are recognized as a major danger to the preterm infant and contribute in large measure to neonatal morbidity and mortality.

Among the most significant systemic infections that threaten the well-being of mother and fetus during pregnancy are syphilis and listeriosis. Although these are encountered relatively infrequently in the United States, they pose a serious threat to the fetus, and prenatal care should include consideration of these diseases. Serologic testing for syphilis is a mandatory part of prenatal care, and satisfactory outcome is possible only if adequate treatment of the disease is prescribed.

Listeriosis represents a challenging problem during pregnancy primarily because the disease is usually a mild, albeit bacteremic, illness in the mother that usually does not generate concern. The physician must therefore be responsible for suspecting listeriosis, especially if the patient has an influenza-like syndrome and provides a history of contact with animals or animal products. In addition it should be noted that *Borrelia* and *Leptospira* may cause febrile illness and fetal infection, although these infections are rarely encountered in gravid patients.

An emerging problem is that of campylobacteriosis. Awareness of this disease process is beginning to develop, and, as a result, complications of pregnancy are now being recognized. A recent case, which consisted of maternal fever and chills accompanied by diarrhea, resulted in the delivery of a 900-g infant 2 weeks after the initial maternal symptoms. The mother had not consumed unpasteurized milk products but did have a positive vaginal culture for the organism. Obstetricians and pediatricians will need to be aware that more cases of campylobacteriosis in pregnancy are likely to emerge.

URINARY TRACT INFECTION AND PYELONEPHRITIS

Urinary tract infections are among the commonest complications of pregnancy, and in former years, fulminant upper urinary tract infections were frequently associated with endotoxic shock. Since antimicrobial agents were introduced, however, this complication is infrequently encountered. Much interest has been generated in the relationship of bacteriuria to obstetric complications. The realization that significant bacteriuria can occur in the absence of symptoms or signs of urinary tract infection and is encountered in at least 5 percent of all gravid patients has resulted in a better understanding of urinary tract infections associated with the gravid state.

The occurrence of asymptomatic bacteriuria in pregnancy is now recognized as a condition requiring therapy because in the absence of appropriate therapy, one-third of such patients will develop overt pyelonephritis. In many instances the bacteriuria antedates the gestation and, in fact, is probably no more frequent in the gravid than in the nongravid state. Furthermore, the vast majority of gravid women with asymptomatic bacteriuria can be identified by routine use of urine culture at the initial prenatal visit. Screening of prenatal patients has been facilitated by the availability of relatively inexpensive methods for the detection of significant bacterial growth. The finding of more than 100,000 organisms per milliliter in a clean voided specimen of urine represents significant bacteriuria and, thereby, identifies individuals who require treatment.

Asymptomatic bacteriuria is observed in at least 2 percent of women. This fact justifies the routine prenatal screening of all patients and treatment of bacteriurics if clinically overt pyelonephritis is to be effectively prevented. This strategy may be important in the prevention of preterm birth. Most urinary tract infections during pregnancy are caused by *Escherichia coli*. The majority of strains of this organism are cured by a short-acting sulfonamide. Such a drug is ideal for the initial therapy of asymptomatic bacteriuria. An alternative therapeutic agent is ampicillin, although treatment should always be based on the antimicrobial susceptibility of the isolated organism.

Single-dose therapy has been studied, but one-third or more patients fail treatment on such a regimen. The majority of patients appear to be cured by a 14-day course of the agents mentioned. Urine culture should be repeated during, and again 1 week after, completion of therapy. If asymptomatic bacteriuria persists after treatment, further therapy is indicated, and the agent prescribed will depend on the in vitro susceptibility of the organism. A combination of trimethoprim-sulfamethoxazole should be avoided in the first trimester because of potential teratogenicity and, likewise, in the last trimester of pregnancy because of the small risk of kernicterus in the neonate.

The presence of underlying renal disease should always be suspected when such organisms as *Proteus, Pseudomonas,* or *Klebsiella* are isolated. Women with urinary tract infection due to these organisms should be thoroughly evaluated after the pregnancy. Approximately one-third of women with recurrent or refractory asymptomatic bacteriuria during pregnancy have some urinary tract abnormality demonstrable by excretion urography.

Acute pyelonephritis in pregnancy remains a serious complication and can result in growth retardation of the fetus, preterm birth, or intrauterine fetal death. Such infections frequently occur at the end of the first half of pregnancy. The major clinical features are high fever, chills, and flank pain. The patient may be acutely ill and may complain of headache, malaise, anorexia, vomiting, and colicky abdominal pain. Acute pyelitis almost invariably involves the right kidney and marked tenderness is elicited in the right costovertebral angle and along the course of the right ureter. The clinical manifestations may simulate acute appendicitis, but the diagnosis is readily established by urine culture.

In severe infections, aggressive treatment with parenteral antibiotics and intravenous fluids are of prime importance. The initial antibiotic therapy should consist of ampicillin, 2 g every 6 hours, until the result of the antimicrobial susceptibility testing of the organism is available. Ampicillin is usually ineffective for therapy of resistant organisms. Bacteria, such as strains of *Klebsiella* and indole-negative *Proteus* species, are susceptible to high concentrations of cephalosporins, which are readily attainable in the urine. The newer cephalosporins are highly effective and are preferred to the aminocyclitols in these individuals because of the latter's potential for nephrotoxicity and VIIIth cranial nerve involvement. Compared with the penicillins and cephalosporins, the margin between toxic and therapeutic doses of the aminocyclitols is narrow. It is especially narrow for gentamicin and tobramycin because of vestibular nerve damage and nephrotoxicity.

Although most patients with urinary tract infections respond rapidly to appropriate therapy, they are, however, liable to have further exacerbations of infection—if they have had a previous upper tract infection—unless therapy is prolonged for at least 3 weeks. Intravenous antimicrobial therapy should be continued for 5 days in patients with pyelonephritis or pyelonephritis associated with bacteremia, but before any form of oral antimicrobial therapy is substituted, urine cultures and susceptibility patterns should be repeated. In less severe cases of acute pyelitis of pregnancy, oral medication can be instituted as soon as the patient has been afebrile for 48 hours. The

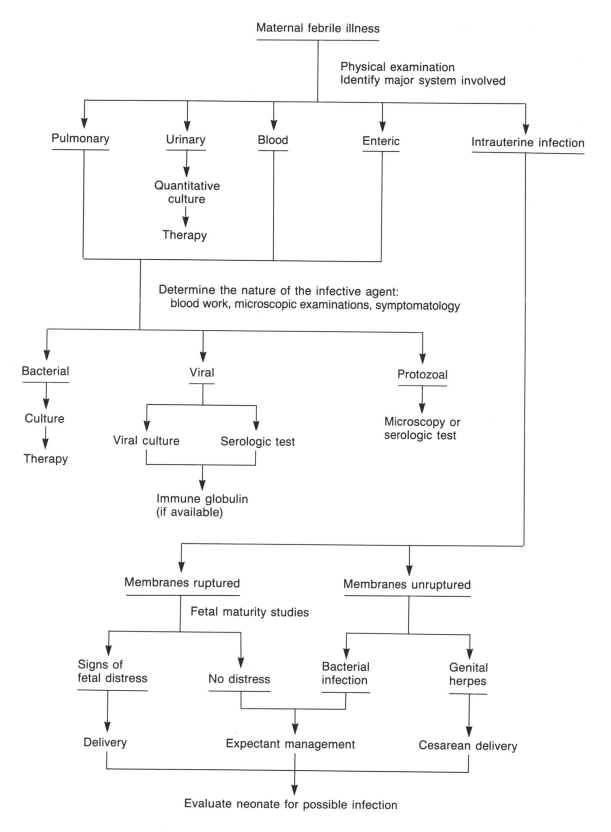

Figure 1 Identifying systemic infections during pregnancy.

patient's recovery is expedited by instructing her to maintain a liberal fluid intake and to lie in the lateral recumbent position. After completion of appropriate therapy, the patient's urine should be screened at each subsequent prenatal visit for the remainder of the pregnancy.

CHORIOAMNIONITIS

Inflammation of the fetal membranes results from an ascending infection from the cervical-vaginal ecosystem. Once the bacterial colonization is established in the lower female genital tract, the periodic fluctuations in physiologic conditions— including hormonal changes, mucus secretion, menstruation, and pregnancy—influence the quantitative composition of the flora. The composition of the cervical-vaginal flora is of importance in the decisions involving therapy for neonatal sepsis following chorioamniotic infection or maternal therapy for endomyometritis, which is a sequel of chorioamnionitis. The presence of mixed aerobic and anaerobic organisms helps to guide therapy before specific microorganisms are identified. Routinely, cultures are not performed in cases of chorioamnionitis; amniotic fluid may be cultured, if available, but the results are not at hand soon enough to influence therapy. The fetus cannot be adequately treated in utero by administering parenteral antibiotics to the mother, and if chorioamnionitis threatens the fetus, expeditious delivery should be performed. Therapy of mother and fetus is instituted independently. Culture of the corporeal endometrium can be performed but is problematic because of contamination with cervical flora, even with the most exacting sampling techniques. Therefore, therapy is usually empiric and based on the normal composition of cervical-vaginal flora. There is even some interest in obtaining prenatal cultures for organisms, such as the group B *Streptococcus*, associated with particularly serious consequences for the baby. Culture for group B *Streptococcus* should be obtained in women who have previously lost an infant to group B *Streptococcus*, but is not generally advocated in routine clinical practice.

Currently, it is not possible to predict which patients will develop chorioamnionitis, although premature rupture of the fetal membranes and lower socioeconomic circumstances are obvious risk factors. Moreover, early and accurate diagnosis of impending chorioamnionitis is not presently available. Thus, diagnosis is usually made relatively late in the course of ascending intrauterine bacterial infections, and the nature of the infectious agents and subsequent therapy is based on the predicted composition of the genital microflora.

When intrauterine infection of the fetus occurs, parenteral antibiotics administered to the mother are generally ineffective for the fetus. The fetus is usually infected by aspiration of the contaminated amniotic fluid, but perfusion of the fetal lung is poor until after birth. For this reason, successful therapy cannot be assured for the intrauterine patient. In the face of serious intra-amniotic infection, it is usually preferable to deliver the fetus, provided that it can be cared for in a neonatal intensive care unit. Figure 1 contains a summary of the best approaches to identifying systemic infections during pregnancy.

PREMATURITY

The problem of prematurity and preterm labor remains the single largest cause of perinatal morbidity and mortality. Among the contributing factors are economic deprivation, poor maternal nutrition, medical illness and obstetric complications, but none of these emerges as the dominant etiologic factor. The recent recognition that bacteria may produce mediators that initiate the production of prostaglandins and, hence, labor, provides an explanation for an apparent association between infections and prematurity. There is a growing consensus that subclinical chorioamnionitis is responsible for many cases of premature birth. The microorganisms usually involved are members of the microbial flora of the lower female genital tract and may include aerobic and anaerobic species that do not possess potent virulence factors causing fulminant disease. Among the organisms implicated in initiating premature labor are mycoplasmas. Finally, an association has been recorded between untreated asymptomatic urinary tract infection and low birth weight. The mediators involved in untimely delivery of infants from mothers with urinary tract infection have not been identified, but it is clear that this represents an additional area in which therapeutic intervention may improve the outcome of pregnancy.

ANTIMICROBIAL THERAPY DURING PREGNANCY

A dual danger exists in inappropriate antibiotic use in pregnancy: the fetus may be damaged by uncontrolled infection, or injury to the fetus may occur as a result of drug toxicity.

Almost all available pharmacokinetic information has been derived from nongravid patients. These data are inadequate for pregnant women because several physiologic changes take place during pregnancy that substantially alter the way in which drugs are handled. The fetal-placental unit comprises a separate compartment into which antibiotics may be transported or diffused or from which they may be excluded. The tissues of the fetus are, in some cases, more sensitive to the toxic effects of certain drugs. As noted before, perfusion of the fetal lung is poor. Other factors affecting pharmacokinetics during pregnancy are expansion of maternal plasma volume, increased glomerular filtration rate, and altered gastrointestinal motility and absorption. Blood flow to the skin, skeletal muscles, kidneys, and uterus is increased, and serum proteins are decreased. The alteration of plasma protein levels—particularly albumin, which provides most of the drug binding sites—may have a significant effect on drugs that are highly bound to plasma protein. Bound drugs are generally considered to be incapable of passage through the capillary walls into tissues. Thus, the effectiveness of a standard dose of a drug may be modified in the pregnant patient.

The absolute amount of a therapeutic agent transferred to the fetus is proportional to the amplitude and duration of the maternal plasma concentration and the rate constant for placental transfer. Low-molecular-weight drugs, such as antibiotics, are considered to be transported

TABLE 2 **Therapeutic Recommendations for Infections in the Pregnant or Parturient Patient**

Infection	Causative Organism	First Choice for Therapy	Alternate Therapy
Asymptomatic bacteriuria	E. coli	Sulfonamides 0.5 g PO q6h	Ampicillin 500 mg q6h
Acute cystitis	E. coli Group B Streptococcus, Klebsiella	Ampicillin 500 mg PO q6h	Trimethoprim 160 mg + sulfamethoxazole 800 mg q12h × 12–14 days
	P. aeruginosa	Amikacin 15 mg/kg/day in 2–3 divided doses IV *plus* Ticarcillin 1 g IV q6h	—
Acute pyelonephritis	E coli	Ampicillin 500 mg IV q6h	Cefotaxime 1.0 g IV q6h
Mastitis	S. aureus	Penicillinase-resistant synthetic penicillin, e.g., methicillin 1.0 g IM q4h	Cloxacillin 0.5 g PO q6h
Pneumonia	S. pneumoniae	Penicillin G 600,000 units IM q6h	Erythromycin stearate 500 mg PO q6h
	H. influenzae	Ampicillin 2.0 g PO q6h	Cefuroxime 500 mg IV q6h Cefotaxime 500 mg IV q6h
	M. pneumoniae	Erythromycin stearate 500 mg PO q6h	—
Tuberculosis	M. tuberculosis	Isoniazid 5 mg/kg/day PO *plus* Ethambutol 25 mg/kg/day × 2 months. then 15 mg/kg/day PO	If triple therapy add rifampin 9 mg/kg/day
Gonorrhea	N. gonorrhoeae	Procaine penicillin 4.8 million units IM *plus* Probenecid 1.0 g orally; for patients with penicillin allergy, erythromycin stearate 1.5 g PO followed by 0.75 g PO q6h for 5 days	Spectinomycin 2.0 g IM *or* Cefotaxime 2.0 g IM and probenecid 1.0 g PO
Syphilis	T. pallidum	Benzathine penicillin G 1.4 million units IM weekly × 3 weeks	For patients with penicillin allergy, erythromycin stearate 0.75 g PO q6h × 15 days; repeat course after an interval of 6 weeks
Listeriosis	L. monocytogenes	Ampicillin 1.0 g PO q6h	Erythromycin 750 mg PO q6h
Campylobacteriosis	Campylobacter fetus ssp. jejuni	Erythromycin 500 mg PO q6h	Clindamycin 600 mg followed by 300 mg PO q6h
Postpartum endomyometritis or septic abortion	Enterobacteriaceae Bacteroides bivius Bacteroides disiens	Cefoxitin 1.0 g IV q6h	Clindamycin 600 mg IV q6h *plus* Cefotaxime 1.0 g IV q6h
	Bacteroides fragilis	Clindamycin 600 mg IV q6h	Metronidazole* 0.5 g IV qh6 *plus* Cefotaxime 1.0 g IV q6h
	Peptostreptococci	Piperacillin 1.0 g IV q6h	Cefotaxime 1.0 g IV q6h

Table continues on following page

TABLE 2 *(continued)*

Infection	Causative Organism	First Choice for Therapy	Alternate Therapy
Puerperal septicemia	Enterobacteriaceae *Bacteroides* species *Peptostreptococcus* *Streptococcus*	Cefotaxime 1.0 g IV q6h *plus* Clindamycin 600 mg IV q6h	Cefotaxime 1.0 g IV q6h *plus* Metronidazole* 500 mg IV q6h

*In the absence of lactation.

through the placenta by diffusion. Pathologic changes in the placenta associated with maternal hypertension and diabetes can alter placental permeability. Placental transmission of a drug may be modified by such abnormalities of the umbilical cord as velamentous insertion of the vessels or absence of one umbilical artery.

Fetal hemodynamics also affect drug distribution in the fetal compartment and characteristics of the fetal circulation whereby much of the umbilical venous blood bypasses the liver via the ductus venosus and the lungs by the ductus arteriosus and results in elevated drug concentrations in the fetal heart and central nervous system.

We are relatively ignorant of the effect and toxicity of these drugs on the intrauterine patient. The majority of antibiotics cross the placenta and attain therapeutic levels in the fetus. Some agents, however, should never be administered to the pregnant patient because of toxicity; these are exemplified by tetracycline, which may cause hypoplasia of fetal bone and discoloration of the primary and secondary dentition. The primary reason for concern about antimicrobial agents administered to the pregnant host is not the known deleterious effects, but the lack of information about the safety of these agents.

Ampicillin achieves plasma levels in pregnant women that are approximately 50 percent of levels attained in nongravid patients. This effect persists until the third postpartum day. Despite this, the levels in urine are similar in the two groups. An increased dose of ampicillin is not particularly hazardous, and if the identical ratio between the plasma levels of ampicillin and the mean inhibitory concentration for the infective organism is to be attained in pregnant women, the dose should be twice that used in nongravid patients. The same applies to other antibiotics, although the actual adjustment required must be based on the measurement of serum levels and these data are as yet not available for all compounds. Although drug dosage in pregnancy probably needs to be increased for a variety of antimicrobial compounds, such adjustments need to be guided by determinations of plasma levels and consideration of potential toxic reactions associated with increased drug dosage. In some situations, such as impaired hepatic or renal function, one must be especially careful about the precise drug concentrations.

It is important for the physician managing individuals with postpartum endometritis to recognize that the hemodynamic changes and altered pharmacokinetics of pregnancy do not immediately return to normal at parturition. In the majority of instances, therefore, patients who become infected after cesarean section require 50 percent more antibiotic for the first 3 days of therapy than is recommended for the nongravid patient. Failure to observe this fact may result in prolonged morbidity.

Table 2 has been provided as a guideline for antibiotic therapy and an overall concept of the agents available that can be prescribed to the pregnant patient. The physicians who have an adequate understanding of the mechanisms of action of currently available therapeutic agents and the rationale for their use will be able to use current and future agents to the maximum advantage of their gravid patients. Finally, the effectiveness of these agents must not be viewed as license to neglect the general management of obstetric patients with infections.

INFECTION IN THE NEWBORN

ROBERT S. BALTIMORE, M.D.

Therapy of infection in the newborn is a specialized area of clinical infectious diseases because of the host's relative immunosuppression and the facts that signs of infection are generally subtle and therapeutic agents available for use in other age groups may have altered toxicities, altered pharmacology, or less well-proven benefit. In common with the principles of treatment of immunosuppressed patients beyond the neonatal period, one must frequently institute treatment when infection is suspected but not proven, and empiric treatment must be appropriate for multiple possible pathogens until specific therapy can be given for a diagnosed pathogen. Thus, the prevalence of antimicrobial use is extremely high in neonatal intensive care units, and these units may have a high incidence of nosocomial infections and colonization with antimicrobial-resistant microorganisms. In order to initiate therapy in a timely and appropriate fashion it is important to recognize the epidemiologic risk factors and microbiology of neonatal infections.

BACTERIAL INFECTIONS

Epidemiology of Neonatal Bacterial Infections

For the purpose of epidemiology, neonatal infections are usually classified according to time and mode of onset into three categories: (*1*) infection with prenatal onset; (*2*) infection acquired in the perinatal period—shortly before or during the process of birth (early-onset neonatal infections); and (*3*) infection acquired in the nursery environment (late-onset neonatal infections). The division in time between early- and late-onset infections is usually 4 to 7 days of age. Infections that have an onset within the first month of life are considered to be neonatal infections, but intensive care units for sick neonates now frequently provide continuing care for infants several months of age with complex problems that are the result of neonatal complications.

Bacterial infections due to the rapidly dividing high-grade pathogens that have an onset substantially before birth usually result in a stillbirth and are not dealt with here. Generally, it is not possible to distinguish between infections acquired shortly prior to birth and those acquired as a result of contact with maternal flora during the process of delivery.

Several risk factors have a strong influence on postnatal neonatal infection rates. Full-term infants born without incident actually have a low incidence of infection, lower than any other population of hospitalized patients. Infants susceptible to early-onset postnatal infections are primarily those born to mothers with an infection or to mothers who have had stress due to a complication of the pregnancy or the delivery. Table 1 lists the well-recognized risk factors for early- and late-onset postnatal infections. Prematurity is the most important risk factor for early-onset infections. This is because the premature infant has relatively poor immune protective mechanisms, with disability roughly proportional to the degree of prematurity. In profoundly premature infants extra vigilance is required for early recognition and treatment of infection. Infants born to mothers whose membranes have been ruptured for longer than 6 hours are also at increased risk of infection, with risk increasing with a greater duration of rupture. Prematurely born infants are much more likely to develop sepsis as a consequence of the amnionitis caused by ascending infection from premature rupture of the membranes than are full-term infants. Similarly, premature infants are at a greater risk of developing an invasive infection if born to a mother with peripartum infection.

Nosocomial infection in the nursery is an important and growing problem. As the technology for treating very premature and very sick infants increases, there is a commensurate increase in the population of surviving immunocompromised infants who require life support equipment, such as respirators, intravascular catheters, total parenteral nutrition, and surgical drains, each of which carries a substantial risk of infection (Table 1). Finally, the liberal use of broad-spectrum antibiotics increases the risk of acquisition of pathogens by interfering with the development of normal flora. In contrast, the risk of acquiring nosocomial viral infections appears to depend mostly on the chances of contact with the virus. Therefore, community activity of respiratory and gastrointestinal viruses and the absence of barriers to prevent spread within the unit appear to be the most important risk factors. Studies of nosocomial infections in intensive care nurseries demonstrate overall infection rates similar to other intensive care units, approximately 20 cases per 100 discharges (20 percent).

Microbiology of Infection

Table 2 lists the major bacterial organisms responsible for early- and late-onset postnatal sepsis and neonatal meningitis. *Escherichia coli* and group B *Streptococcus* currently account for about 80 percent of these infections when there is an early onset. There has been some recent change in the microbiology of late-onset sepsis, with an increase of coagulase-negative *Staphylococcus* and *Candida* species. This change appears to be due to the increased survival of extremely premature infants and the use of parenteral alimentation and broad-spectrum antibiotics. Empiric therapy is guided by this historical information on the microbiology of neonatal infections. The organisms associated with late-onset sepsis listed here are meant to be a guide but may vary from institution to institution. There is a tendency for certain species to be introduced into a nursery and cause an increased proportion of infections for a limited time. Thus, it is necessary to have continuous surveillance of the microbiology and antimicrobial susceptibility of organisms in any institution caring for sick newborns.

TABLE 1   Risk Factors for Neonatal Bacterial Infections

Early-Onset Infections	*Late-Onset Infections*
Prematurity	Contact with hands of
Prolonged premature rupture	colonized personnel
of membranes	Contact with aerosols
Septic or traumatic delivery	of bacteria
Maternal infection:	Contaminated equipment
especially urogenital	Isolettes
Fetal anoxia	Humidifiers
Male sex	Ventilators
Other maternal factors	Bathing fluids
Poverty	Intravascular cannulas
Pre-eclampsia	Adhesive electrodes
Cardiac disease	Debilitating illness
Diabetes mellitus	Congenital anomalies
	Surgery
	Treatment for early-
	onset infection

TABLE 2 Microbiology of Neonatal Bacterial Sepsis: The Most Common Etiologic Agents

Early-Onset Sepsis	Late-Onset Sepsis
Escherichia coli	Those causing early-onset
Group B *Streptococcus*	infections
Klebsiella species	*Staphylococcus aureus*
Enterococcus species	*Staphylococcus epidermidis*
Listeria monocytogenes	*Pseudomonas aeruginosa*
	Other Enterobacteriacae
	(Proteus, Citrobacter, Enterobacter)

Antimicrobial Therapy

Empiric Therapy for Early-Onset Sepsis

Antibiotics for early-onset infections are generally commenced before the identification of the infecting organism. Neonates, especially those who are premature, typically fail to exhibit classic signs and symptoms of infection. Thus, many schemes have been developed for empiric antibiotic treatment of infants with multiple epidemiologic risks alone or nonspecific signs and laboratory test abnormalities plus epidemiologic risk factors. These schemes recognize the risk factors listed in Table 1 and also the possibility that severe infection may present as temperature instability or other changes in vital signs, unexplained hyperbilirubinemia, vomiting, or changes in feeding, and they recognize that a very short delay in treatment may result in overwhelming sepsis and death. Such schemes vary from hospital to hospital depending upon the population served, the type of hospital, and the resources for screening.

Empiric therapy is designed to provide activity against the organisms listed in Table 2. Often the focus of infection is unknown, but therapy is directed against bacteremia and meningitis because these are the most likely foci. Physical examination, chest roentgenogram, and urinalysis will demonstrate pneumonia or urinary tract infection. Empiric treatment generally consists of a combination of a broad-spectrum penicillin and an aminoglycoside antibiotic or a broad-spectrum penicillin and an extended-spectrum (third-generation) cephalosporin. This author and a majority of pediatric infectious diseases practitioners continue to use the combination of an extended-spectrum penicillin, usually ampicillin, with an aminoglycoside, usually gentamicin. The advantages of this combination are low cost, considerable experience, and known low toxicity. The advantages of the extended-spectrum cephalosporin are greater potency against many of the pathogens and excellent central nervous system (CNS) penetration in the presence of inflammation. If there is gram-negative bacillary meningitis on the basis of examination of the cerebrospinal fluid (CSF), it is reasonable to use the combination of ampicillin and an extended-spectrum cephalosporin as a first choice, although it has not yet been proved that this combination results in an outcome superior to that of ampicillin and gentamicin.

Sometimes the aminoglycoside antibiotic of choice should be an agent other than gentamicin. If, for some reason, *Pseudomonas aeruginosa* is a likely agent, tobramycin would be a better choice since it has greater activity against this species. If it is known that there have been gentamicin-resistant gram-negative bacillary infections in the community or in the nursery unit, amikacin would be a better choice. Amikacin is more expensive than gentamicin and has no better activity against gentamicin-susceptible organisms, but it is resistant to most of the aminoglycoside-inactivating enzymes produced by gram-negative bacilli.

Empiric Therapy for Late-Onset Sepsis

As shown in Table 1, infants likely to have late-onset infections are most likely to be ill residents of an intensive care nursery. Empiric antibiotic therapy should take into consideration the resident flora of the nursery, especially isolates from previously infected neonates, and the particular risk factors of the patient. If intravascular cannulae have not been used, if the infant has not been treated for a previous infection, and if there have not been isolates of gentamicin-resistant gram-negative aerobic bacilli, it is appropriate to use the same empiric treatment as for early-onset sepsis.

In fact, this is usually not the case, and another regimen is often more appropriate. Ill infants frequently have intravascular catheter(s) in place, and these may be the focus of infection. The most common causes of catheter-associated infections are *Staphylococcus aureus* and *Staphylococcus epidermidis*. Although penicillinase-resistant semisynthetic penicillins (oxacillin, nafcillin, methicillin) are usually the agents of choice against staphylococci, resistance to this class (commonly referred to as methicillin resistance) is occurring more commonly in many institutions. In addition, *S. epidermidis* appears to have a higher incidence in very low birthweight infants, and this species is more likely to show methicillin resistance. Therefore, in institutions with substantial methicillin resistance of staphylococci, it is reasonable to use vancomycin for empiric treatment of late-onset, possibly catheter-associated infections. Generally an aminoglycoside is added. We usually add gentamicin, but if an infant develops new symptoms of infection while receiving gentamicin, either amikacin or a third-generation cephalosporin is substituted.

Blanket use of vancomycin for all late-onset sepsis is generally not warranted as this agent is very expensive, is toxic compared with the penicillins, and has activity only against aerobic gram-positive bacteria. Likewise, antibiotics active against gentamicin-resistant bacteria should be used in situations only where there is a high risk for resistant pathogens, since frequent use of such agents in an enclosed nursery population will encourage the emergence and persistence of even more-resistant strains of bacteria.

Adjunctive Therapy for Sepsis

In addition to antibiotic therapy, infants with sepsis require intensive care for physiologic support. Intravenous fluid management and treatment for shock and respiratory failure are of paramount importance and should be carried out in facilities designed for the treatment of critically ill newborns. Use of agents to support or enhance the immune system is more controversial. At this time there is evidence from a number of small studies that exchange transfusion, transfusion of concentrated white blood cells (when there is severe neutropenia and bone marrow failure), specific immune serum globulin preparations, and commercial intravenous gamma globulins are effective in the reduction of mortality. Because this is a new investigative area in which key studies are currently undergoing analysis and because the various modalities have not been compared or combined, it is impossible to recommend one as the most effective. In most hospitals, in the treatment of overwhelming sepsis, that adjunctive agent with which the facility has the most experience may be the best, since complications are known to occur with each agent.

Therapy and Management for Other Focal Infections

Often when a focal infection is apparent in the newborn, one cannot rule out the possibility of associated sepsis or meningitis; the recommendations listed above for sepsis and the doses listed in Table 3 may be the most appropriate starting points.

Meningitis. As shown in Table 3, the doses of some antibiotics are increased when treating meningitis. This allows for the lower antibiotic concentrations in CNS tissue and CSF compared with blood. Local instillation of antibiotics is generally not effective. The use of intrathecal or intraventricular administration of antibiotics has not been associated with improvement in outcome. Intraventricular instillation may occasionally be warranted when treating resistant organisms that have not been eradicated using conventional antibiotic dosing. Intraventricular administration should not be used routinely and, in general, not when using antibiotics that diffuse into the CNS relatively well, such as the penicillins, third-generation cephalosporins, or chloramphenicol. Improvement in the prognosis of neonatal meningitis appears to be unrelated to the availability of newer antibiotics. Respirators, aggressive treatment of shock, acidosis, inappropriate antidiuretic hormone secretion, and seizures are most important after antibiotic therapy has commenced. Every infant with bacterial meningitis or severe sepsis should, if possible, receive care at a treatment facility capable of close monitoring and intervention for any of these problems.

Complications and delayed sterilization are more common with gram-negative bacillary meningitis in the newborn than with childhood meningitis beyond the neonatal period. When treating this type infection, I generally

TABLE 3 Appropriate Parenteral Antibiotics, Doses, and Dose Schedules for the Treatment of Infections in Newborns

Antibiotic Agent	Dose/kg/24 h			
	Age <7 days (No. of doses/day)		Age >7 days (No. of doses/day)	
Penicillins				
Penicillin G	50,000–100,000 units	(2)	100,000–200,000 units*	(3)
Penicillinase-resistant penicillins				
(oxacillin, methicillin, nafcillin)	50–100 mg	(2)	100–200 mg	(3–4)
Ampicillin	50–150 mg	(2)	100–200 mg	(3)
Carbenicillin	200–300 mg	(2–3)†	400 mg	(4)
Ticarcillin	150–225 mg	(2–3)	225–300 mg	(3–4)
Mezlocillin	150 mg	(2–3)	225–300 mg	(3–4)
Aminoglycosides				
Amikacin‡	15–20 mg	(2)	22.5–30 mg	(3)
Gentamicin‡	5–6 mg	(2)	7.5 mg	(3)
Tobramycin‡	4–5 mg	(2)	6 mg	(3)
Cephalosporins				
Moxalactam	100 mg	(2)	150 mg	(3)
Cefotaxime	100 mg	(2)	150 mg	(3)
Ceftazidime	60 mg	(2)	90 mg	(3)
Miscellaneous				
Clindamycin	10–15 mg	(2–3)	15–20 mg	(3–4)
Vancomycin	20–30 mg	(2)	30–45 mg	(3)
Chloramphenicol‡	25 mg	(1–2)	25–50 mg	(1–2)
Adenine arabinoside				
(vidarabine)	15 mg	(1)	15 mg	(1)
Acyclovir	30 mg	(3)	30 mg	(3)
Ribavirin (by aerosol)	6,000 mg	(1)	6,000 mg	(1)
Amphotericin B	0.25–1.0 mg	(1)	0.25–1.0 mg	(1)

* Where a dose range with a single suggestion for the number of doses per day is indicated, the higher dose is used for the treatment of neonates with meningitis. In non-meningitic infections the higher end of the dose range is used for more severe infection or when serum antibiotic concentrations are lower than the therapeutic range.

† Where a range of number of doses per day is indicated, those neonates with a birth weight >2,000 g should receive the larger number of doses per day and the higher daily dose, and neonates with a birth weight <2,000 g should receive the lower number of doses per day and the lower daily dose.

‡ Dosing should be guided by laboratory determination of serum antibiotic concentrations.

repeat the lumbar puncture every 48 hours until the CSF is sterile and at the end of therapy to monitor antibiotic efficacy. Assuming no complications, antibiotics are usually continued for 3 weeks. For group B streptococcal meningitis, repeat lumbar puncture has little value if there is a good clinical response and no late complications. Length of treatment is 2 to 3 weeks. Hydrocephalus is an unfortunately common complication of neonatal meningitis, and it is important to monitor the head circumference. Ventricular size may be monitored with ultrasound examinations. Infants who develop an increase in ventricular size should be evaluated by a neurosurgeon for the possible placement of a CSF shunt.

If meningitis develops in an infant with a CSF shunt in place, the most likely microorganisms are normal skin flora (*S. epidermidis, S. aureus,* and diphtheroids) and occasionally gram-negative aerobes. Empiric treatment is generally vancomycin or a penicillinase-resistant penicillin plus an aminoglycoside.

Pneumonia. Neonatal pneumonia can occur in association with early-onset sepsis, as a complication of a noninfectious respiratory condition (e.g., respiratory distress syndrome, meconium aspiration), or as a nosocomial pneumonia. In general, the bacterial agents are the same as for early- and late-onset sepsis, and antimicrobial treatment suggestions are the same. When clusters of staphylococcal infections are seen in hospital nurseries, staphylococcal pneumonia, a severe and necrotizing infection, should be suspected.

Urinary Tract Infection. Cultures of urine as part of a complete work-up for neonatal sepsis have a low rate of significant bacterial growth. Percutaneous bladder puncture is the best method of obtaining uncontaminated specimens for culture. If the same organism is recovered from the urine and the blood, it may not be clear whether the urinary tract was the initial focus of infection or secondarily seeded from blood unless there is an obvious urinary tract anatomic abnormality. Urinary tract infections may occur as a late-onset infection, either associated with a congenital malformation or urinary tract instrumentation, or spontaneously with no discoverable underlying cause.

Antibiotic treatment should be one of the agents listed in Table 3, guided by the results of susceptibility testing of the isolate. Treatment for 10 days with an agent that has renal concentration and excretion is conventional; however, the neonate, like older individuals, may have a poor response or relapse in the presence of obstruction, a foreign body, or incomplete voiding. Thus, there should be a search for an underlying focus, usually with a renal ultrasound examination. Consultation with a urologist should be obtained in order to correct the problem. The urinary tract should be sterilized before any elective genitourinary procedure. If the abnormality is initially uncorrectable, antibiotic suppression should be considered. The suppressive agent chosen should be active against *E. coli*, and oral amoxicillin or trimethoprim/sulfamethoxazole is generally used.

Skeletal Infections. Septic arthritis and osteomyelitis in the neonate are generally secondary to bacteremia.

In the infant who develops such an infection with no predisposing surgery or intravascular appliance in place, *S. aureus* is by far the most common etiologic agent. In addition, group B *Streptococcus* and gram-negative aerobes (especially *E. coli*) may be the cause. *S. aureus* skeletal infections in the neonate are often severely destructive, are associated with later disabilities, and have a tendency to be associated with multiple foci and rupture through the incompletely formed epiphyseal plate in the neonate.

Even when there is only a single symptomatic focus, I generally use nuclear imaging scans in search of other foci. Surgical drainage or aspiration should be performed. Length of treatment is generally at least 3 weeks for septic arthritis and at least 4 weeks for osteomyelitis. A longer course may be necessary if there is delayed sterilization, late appearance of a second focus, or other complications. The use of an oral agent after the patient has had an initial favorable response to intravenous antibiotic treatment may be considered. Experience in neonates is limited, and oral treatment should only be considered if the isolate is susceptible to low concentrations of an acceptable antibiotic, high blood levels are achievable, and compliance is assured.

VIRAL INFECTIONS

Herpes Simplex Infections. Herpes infections of the newborn are transmitted from the mother to the infant, generally at the time of delivery, and the incubation period before symptoms is from 3 or 4 days to a month. Most neonatal herpes infections are due to herpes simplex type 2. Mothers with primary infection appear most likely to transmit infection to offspring. The presentation of these infections varies and includes cutaneous manifestations (vesicles) alone, isolated CNS infection, disseminated visceral infection, and combinations of the three. Severity and prognosis are worst for disseminated visceral disease and best for cutaneous disease.

Treatment with antiviral agents adenine arabinoside (Ara-A, Vidarabine) and acyclovir appears to be equally efficacious. Moderately ill infants who are treated early appear to benefit the most from treatment.

Cytomegalovirus. Cytomegalovirus (CMV) infections are generally transmitted to the infant during gestation, but infection can be transmitted during delivery or after delivery via blood transfusion. Congenital infection is associated with characteristic signs (e.g., low birth weight, hepatosplenomegaly, jaundice, petechiae, microcephaly, occasionally pneumonia, retinopathy), while postgestational infection is more likely characterized by fever, pneumonitis, and mononucleosis. No agent has proved effective for treatment of gestational or neonatal CMV infection.

Hepatitis. At this time the only form of neonatal hepatitis for which treatment is recommended is for the offspring of mothers who are carriers of hepatitis B antigen in the blood, and this treatment is essentially prophylactic. Children of mothers who have hepatitis B antigenemia are likely to acquire infection. Manifestations may show up in weeks or not for decades, as there is an association between hepatic carcinoma and early hepatitis B infection. Currently it is recommended that infants of antigenemic mothers receive 0.5 ml of hepatitis B immune globulin (HBIG) at birth as well as 0.5 ml (10 µg) of hepatitis B vaccine intramuscularly at birth and at 1 and 6 months of age. The HBIG should be given as soon after birth as possible and certainly within 48 hours.

Varicella-Zoster Virus. Infants born of mothers who have active varicella are in danger of developing an aggressive, overwhelming varicella-zoster virus (VZV) infection if the mother's lesions appear from 5 days *before* to 2 days *after* delivery. The rationale is that infants exposed during this period may have received a large viremic dose of VZV transplacentally, and yet not have received any maternal antibody. Infants exposed earlier in utero receive antibody transplacentally from the mother and generally develop a mild infection. Infants exposed after birth also develop mild chickenpox. If an infant is exposed to VZV during the critical perinatal period described above, treatment of the infant with varicella-zoster immune globulin (VZIG) is indicated. The dose is 125 U (one vial of 1.25 ml), given as soon after delivery or after exposure as possible. The other neonatal use of this agent is for premature infants who have had postnatal exposure to chickenpox and whose gestation was too short (less than 28 weeks) to have acquired transplacental antibody. For severe disseminated VZV infection, infants should be treated with acyclovir or vidarabine (ARA-A). I generally prefer acyclovir for its easier administration and lower toxicity.

Viral Pneumonia. In addition to bacteria, nonbacterial agents are also important causes of nosocomial pneumonia. Respiratory syncytial virus, parainfluenza viruses, and adenoviruses can cause severe respiratory disease in neonates. In general, antimicrobial treatment is not available. Ribavirin by aerosol, which appears to be effective in shortening the course of respiratory syncytial virus–associated bronchiolitis in infants, may be used, but there is little information concerning efficacy in neonates. The dose is one 6,000-mg vial per day independent of age. Special expertise is required for use with intubated patients on assisted ventilation.

SUGGESTED READING

Baltimore RS, Andiman WA. Infectious diseases of the newborn. In: Warshaw JB, Hobbins JC, eds. Principles and practice of perinatal medicine. Maternal-fetal and newborn care. Menlo Park, CA: Addison-Wesley, 1983:309.

Committee on Infectious Diseases, American Academy of Pediatrics. Report of the committee in infectious diseases (the red book). 21st ed. Elk Grove Village, IL: American Academy of Pediatrics, 1988.

Feigin RD, Cherry JD. Textbook of pediatric infectious diseases. 2nd ed. Philadelphia: WB Saunders, 1987.

Koren G, Prober CG, Gold R. Antimicrobial therapy in infants and children. New York: Marcel Dekker, 1988.

McCracken GH Jr, Nelson JD. Antimicrobial therapy for newborns. New York: Grune & Stratton, 1983.

IMMUNODEFICIENCY DISORDERS IN INFANTS AND CHILDREN

DOUGLAS J. BARRETT, M.D.
JOHN W. SLEASMAN, M.D.

The normal immune system includes four major components, antibody-mediated immunity (B cell), cell-mediated immunity (T cell), the phagocytic cell system, and the serum complement system.

Cells involved in the immune system are derived from a primitive pleuripotential stem cell capable of differentiating along several pathways (Table 1). Lymphoid stem cell progeny may migrate to the thymus gland, where they differentiate into immunologically competent thymus-derived T cells capable of cell-mediated immune reactions. These include delayed-type hypersensitivity, lymphokine secretion, lymphocytotoxicity, helper T cell function, and suppressor T cell function. Alternatively, some of the stem cell lymphoid progeny populate the fetal liver and later the bone marrow, where they differentiate along a separate lineage to become immunocompetent B cells capable of secreting antibodies. Separate stem cell differentiation pathways lead to development of phagocytic cells, including granulocytes and monocyte/macrophages. The complement system is a series of serum proteins that interact in cascade fashion to produce active complement fragments, which are necessary for bacterial lysis, viral neutralization, opsonization of particles, neutrophil chemotaxis, and mediation of the inflammatory response.

Congenital or acquired defects in any of the four major components of immunity will lead to one of the specific immunodeficiency states listed in Table 2. This is a comprehensive listing of the primary immunodeficiency diseases recognized and classified by the World Health Organization. Given the number and complexity of immunodeficiency diseases, it is obvious that the practitioner must have a logical and organized approach to the diagnosis and treatment of suspected immunodeficiency.

DIAGNOSIS OF IMMUNODEFICIENCY DISEASES

General Approach

A careful medical history and a detailed physical examination often lead to the suspicion of a defect in immunity. Most patients present with increased susceptibility

TABLE 1 Components of the Immune System: Functional Role and Clinical Manifestations of Deficiency

Component of the Immune System	Primary Immunologic Function	Clinical Symptoms Suggestive of Immunodeficiency
T cells	Delayed type hypersensitivity Lymphokine elaboration Cytotoxic killer cell function Induction of B cell immuno- globulin synthesis Immunoregulation	Recurrent infections with viral, fungal, or protozoal pathogens Graft-vs.-host disease B cell or T cell–derived malignancies Autoimmune disease Failure to thrive
B cells	Antibody synthesis Antigen presentation	Recurrent bacterial sinopulmonary infection Chronic gastroenteritis
Phagocytes	Phagocytosis Bacterial killing Antigen presentation to T cells and B cells	Soft tissue abscesses Recurrent infections with catalase- positive organisms Lymphadenitis
Complement system	Microbial lysis Opsonization Neutrophil chemotaxis Inflammatory mediators	Severe recurrent pyogenic infections Recurrent neisserial infections Angioedema Autoimmune disease

to infection: either recurrent infection with common organisms or infection with opportunistic pathogens. The clinical manifestations will generally be related to the degree of deficiency and to the particular component of the immune system that is deficient, as outlined in Table 1. For example, patients with defective antibody-mediated immunity have frequent sinopulmonary infections with common pyogenic bacteria, whereas patients with defective cell-mediated immunity often present with persistent or recurrent fungal, viral, or protozoal diseases. Patients with phagocytic cell defects may have recurrent soft tissue abscesses or systemic infection with uncommon bacteria or fungi of low virulence. Patients with complement defects often present with severe recurrent pyogenic infections, recurrent neisserial infections, or conditions resembling systemic lupus erythematosus.

Physical examination should include attention to those features listed in Table 3. Many findings on physical examination are nonspecific and only indicate evidence of recurrent infection (e.g., lymphadenopathy, hepatosplenomegaly, or chronic pulmonary changes). However, a few findings are peculiar to a specific immunodeficiency.

Since most of the clinical findings in immunodeficiency are not sufficiently distinctive, a definitive diagnosis must include appropriate laboratory testing. Initially, the laboratory investigation should include certain nonspecific laboratory tests, including complete blood cell count with differential and an evaluation of cellular morphology on peripheral smear, erythrocyte sedimentation rate, platelet count, and chest roentgenogram. Before proceeding with a detailed immunologic evaluation, one should exclude nonimmunologic causes of recurrent infection, including cystic fibrosis, allergy, and ciliary dyskinesia syndromes.

Having eliminated nonimmunologic causes of recurrent infection, a detailed immunologic evaluation should assess each of the four components of immunity that are implicated by findings in the history and physical examination. Each of these components can be tested by use of simple and generally available screening studies. If the screening tests are all normal, immunodeficiency is usually excluded and the patient can be assured that gamma globulin therapy or other immunotherapy is not indicated. If the screening tests are abnormal, or if the history is unusually suspicious, it is then appropriate to proceed to more definitive and sophisticated diagnostic tests, some of which are available only in referral medical centers or specialized laboratories. For both screening and diagnostic studies, it is imperative to test both quantitative and qualitative (or functional) aspects of each component of immunity.

Evaluation of Antibody-Mediated Immunity

Screening tests for defects in antibody-mediated (B cell) immunity are listed in Table 4. Quantitation of specific levels of serum immunoglobulins (IgG, IgM, IgA, IgE) should be performed rather than serum protein electrophoresis, since exact quantitative information can be obtained about each immunoglobulin isotype. Results of immunoglobulin quantitation must be carefully interpreted with age-matched controls because of the marked changes that occur with increasing age during childhood. Determination of serum IgG subclass levels is indicated in patients with a history that is suggestive of antibody deficiency, such as severe recurrent purulent sinusitis, recurrent pneumonia, and bronchiectasis. IgG subclass deficiency should be suspected especially when screening total IgG values are low or low normal in patients with this history. The relative contribution of each IgG subclass to the total IgG level is as follows: IgG1 60 to 70 percent, IgG2 14 to 20 percent, IgG3 4 to 8 percent, and IgG4 2 to 6 percent. At present, IgG subclass levels are measured by several different techniques, and, therefore, care must be taken to compare results with age-matched controls run in the same laboratory using the same methodology.

TABLE 2 Classification of Primary Immunodeficiency Diseases

Predominant antibody defects
  X-linked agammaglobulinemia
  Common variable immunodeficiency
    With B cell defect
    With regulatory T cell abnormality
  Immunoglobulin deficiency with increased IgM
  X-linked immunodeficiency with growth hormone deficiency
  Autosomal recessive agammaglobulinemia
  Selective IgA deficiency
  Selective deficiency of other immunoglobulin isotypes
  Kappa chain deficiency
  Antibody deficiency with normal or hypergammaglobulinemia
  Immunodeficiency with thymoma
  Transcobalamin 2 deficiency
  Transient hypogammaglobulinemia of infancy

Predominant defects of cell-mediated immunity
  Combined immunodeficiency with predominant T cell defect
  DiGeorge syndrome
  Purine nucleoside phosphorylase deficiency

Combined antibody and cellular immunodeficiencies
  Severe combined immunodeficiency
    Reticular dysgenesis
    Low T and B cell numbers
    Low T cells and normal B cells (Swiss-type lymphopenic agammaglobulinemia)
    ‘‘Bare-lymphocyte’’ syndrome
  Immunodeficiency with adenosine deaminase deficiency
  Cellular immunodeficiency with abnormal immunoglobulin synthesis (Nezelof's syndrome)
  Ataxia-telangiectasia
  Acquired immunodeficiency syndrome (AIDS)

Phagocytic dysfunction
  Chronic granulomatous disease
  Glucose-6-phosphate dehydrogenase deficiency
  Myeloperoxidase deficiency
  Chediak-Higashi syndrome
  Job's syndrome
  Hyper-IgE syndrome
  Leukocyte adhesion deficiency (iC3b receptor deficiency)

Complement deficiency
  Cl inactivator deficiency (hereditary angioedema)
  Inherited deficiency of complement classical pathway component: Clq, Clr, Cls, C4, C2, C3, C5, C6, C7, C8, C9
  Inherited deficiency of complement alternative pathway component: factor I (C3b inactivator) deficiency; factor P, factor D

After WHO Scientific Group. Clin Immunol Immunopathol 1983; 28:450–475.

Studies to screen for functional defects in B cell immunity include measurement of isoagglutinin titers (for IgM antibody to red blood cell antigens of blood groups A and B) and, if the patient has received diphtheria toxoid immunization, performance of a Schick test (available from the Massachusetts Public Health Biologic Laboratories, Boston, Massachusetts 02130).

If the above screening tests suggest an abnormality, it is then necessary to perform further diagnostic studies for quantitation and functional analysis of B cell immunity to identify the specific defect. These diagnostic studies are listed in Table 4. B cells can be enumerated by immunofluorescence for the CD19 determinant or for surface membrane immunoglobulin. Normally, B cells

constitute approximately 5 to 12 percent of the peripheral blood lymphocytes. Secretory IgA can be measured in tears or saliva.

Diagnostic studies of B cell function include measurement of specific antibody response in serum before and after immunization with inert antigens (or before and after known infection). Antibody responses to both protein antigens (e.g., tetanus toxoid, diphtheria toxoid, streptolysin O) and polysaccharide antigens (e.g., pneumococcal polysaccharide, streptococcal group A carbohydrate, *Haemophilus influenzae* polyribose phosphate) should be tested. It should be emphasized that immunization with live virus vaccines should be avoided in patients with potential or suspected T cell immunodeficiency. The functional capacity of patients' B cells to secrete immunoglobulin and the T cell regulation of immunoglobulin synthesis should be tested in patients with hypogammaglobulinemia. This is determined by pokeweed mitogen stimulation of T cell–B cell cocultures to assess in vitro immunoglobulin secretion.

Evaluation of Cell-Mediated Immunity

Initial screening studies for defects in cell-mediated (T cell) immunity are listed in Table 5. Since T cells comprise the majority of peripheral blood lymphocytes, a total lymphocyte count derived from the white blood cell count multiplied by the percentage of lymphocytes may disclose lymphopenia (<1,000 per cubic millimeter) in

TABLE 3 Features Suggestive of Immunodeficiency on Physical Examination

Abnormality	Associated Immunodeficiency
General: growth failure, short stature, dwarfism	Agammaglobulinemia, T cell deficiencies
Skin	
Eczema	Wiskott-Aldrich syndrome; T cell deficiencies
Candidiasis	T cell deficiency
Telangiectasia	Ataxia-telangiectasia
Petechiae	Wiskott-Aldrich syndrome
Ears/mouth	
Otitis media	Antibody deficiencies
Oral ulcerations	T cell deficiency; granulocyte defects
Lymphatic	
Lymphadenopathy	Some antibody, T cell, or granulocyte defects
Absent tonsils/nodes	Agammaglobulinemia; severe CID
Integument	
Sparse hair	Cartilage-hair hypoplasia syndrome
Albinism	Chediak-Higashi syndrome
Chest: chronic lung disease/ bronchiectasis	Antibody, T cell, or granulocyte defects
Heart: congenital heart defects	DiGeorge syndrome
Abdomen: hepatosplenomegaly	Antibody, T cell, granulocyte defects
Neurologic: ataxia	Ataxia-telangiectasia
Extremities: short limbs	T cell deficiency

TABLE 4 Tests for Defects in Antibody-Mediated Immunity

Screening evaluation
  Quantitative tests
    Serum quantitative immunoglobulins: IgG, IgM, IgA, and IgE
    IgG subclass quantitation
  Functional tests
    Isohemagglutinin titers: anti-A, anti-B
    Schick test
Diagnostic evaluation
  Quantitative tests
    B cell enumeration: CD19 (B1), surface Ig
    Secretory IgA quantitation; IgA1/IgA2 levels
  Functional tests
    Pre- and postimmunization serum antibody levels: tetanus and diphtheria toxoids, KLH, pneumococcal and *Haemophilus* polysaccharides
    Postinfection antibody levels: streptococcal ASO and group A carbohydrate
    In vitro immunoglobulin secretion: pokeweed mitogen induced lymphocyte culture

TABLE 5 Tests for Defects in Cell-Mediated Immunity

Screening evaluation
  Quantitative tests: total lymphocyte count (WBCs × % lymphocytes)
  Functional tests: delayed hypersensitivity skin tests (see Table 6)
Diagnostic evaluation
  Quantitative tests: T cell enumeration (immunofluorescent staining with monoclonal antibodies to T cell subsets [see Table 7])
  Functional tests
    Lymphocyte blastogenesis to mitogens and soluble antigens
    Mixed lymphocyte culture
    Lymphokine secretion: IL-1, IL-2, IL-3, IL-4, IL-5, IL-6, IL-7, interferon-gamma, tumor necrosis factor

should be performed. Further functional studies for T cell lymphokine generation (e.g., interleukin-2, IL-2), interferon gamma, and the B cell growth and differentiation factors (e.g., IL-4, IL-5, IL-6) can be assessed in specialized reference laboratories.

Evaluation of the Phagocytic System

As listed in Table 8, granulocytes and monocytes can be quantitated and assessed morphologically using the white blood cell count and differential smear. Granulocytopenia, defined as less than 1,500 cells per cubic millimeter, is associated with an increased risk of infection; patients with counts below 500 cells per cubic millimeter are unusually susceptible to infection with gram-positive and gram-negative bacteria as well as with fungi such as *Candida albicans* and *Aspergillus* species. The finding of giant granules in neutrophils may suggest a diagnosis of the Chediak-Higashi syndrome. The simplest screening test for metabolic defects of phagocytes leading to recurrent infection is the qualitative histochemical slide test for nitroblue tetrazolium (NBT) dye reduction. Patients with chronic granulomatous disease have less than 1 percent NBT-positive cells, whereas normal individuals generally have more than 10 percent.

Diagnostic studies for granulocyte dysfunction are listed in Table 8. The presence of granulocyte and monocyte

states of severe T cell deficiency. T cell function is best screened by use of delayed hypersensitivity skin tests to evaluate preexisting cell-mediated immunity to microbial agents or immunization. Antigens that are most useful are listed in Table 6. Delayed hypersensitivity skin tests are not generally reliable during the first year of life. False-negative results may also be due to expired lots of antigen or failure to achieve intradermal rather than subcutaneous injection.

Diagnostic testing for definitive characterization of T cell defects should be performed in individuals who have abnormalities in the above screening tests or in whom the diagnosis is highly suspected at an early age (Table 5). The percentage and absolute numbers of T cells can be quantified by immunofluorescent staining using monoclonal antibodies to T cell surface antigens. The T cell specific monoclonal antibodies listed in Table 7 can be used to differentiate functionally distinct T cell subsets. Some patients may be severely deficient in all T cells suggesting a prethymic defect. Others may have a deficiency of mature T cells (CD3+, CD4+, CD8+), with increased numbers of immature cells bearing pre-T or thymocyte markers (CD6+, CD10+), while others may manifest alterations in T helper to T suppressor ratio (normal CD4+:CD8+ = 1.8–2.2).

Diagnostic testing for T cell function involves in vitro lymphocyte activation or transformation (blastogenesis) in response to nonspecific mitogens (e.g., phytohemagglutinin, concanavalin A, pokeweed mitogen, anti-CD2) or to stimulation of the T cell–antigen receptor by soluble antigens (e.g., candidal, tetanus toxoid), by cell surface alloantigens (i.e., mixed lymphocyte culture), or by anti-CD3 antibody. Lymphocyte transformation assays measure the functional capability of T cells (or T and B cells) to become activated and to proliferate. Since the ability to respond to a specific antigen is detectable only with prior host sensitization to that antigen, a complete evaluation with mitogens, soluble recall antigens, and allogenic cells

TABLE 6 Delayed Hypersensitivity Skin Tests

Antigen	Dilution*
Candidal (dermatophyton)	1:100; if negative, use 1:10
Mumps	1 mg/mL undiluted
Trichophyton	1:30
PPD	10 IF; if negative, use 50 IU
Streptokinase/ streptodornase	Under age 10 yr: 40 units→100 units Over age 10 yr: 4 units→40 units
Tetanus toxoid	1:100; if negative, use 1:10
Diphtheria toxoid	1:100; if negative use 1:10

* Each antigen is used in a dose of 0.1 mL of the dilution listed.

TABLE 7 T Cell Surface Determinants

Phenotype	Function
CD2	Pan-T cell marker; alternative pathway of T cell activation
CD3	T cell receptor component; mature T cell marker
CD4	Identifies helper/inducer T cells; interacts with MHC class II
CD6	Common thymocyte marker
CD8	Identifies suppressor/cytotoxic T cells; interacts with MHC class I
CD10	Pre–T cell marker

enzymes, such as alkaline phosphatase, peroxidase, and esterase, can be assessed by histochemical staining. Absence of these enzymes on the qualitative stain should be confirmed by specific quantitative assay. Deficiency of the leukocyte adhesion molecules can be detected using monoclonal antibodies to LFA-1 (CD11a), Mol/CR3 (CD11b), and p150 (CD11c). Fc and C3b receptors can be quantitated by specific monoclonal antibodies to these determinants or by rosettes by use of IgG-coated (EA) or complement-coated (EAC) erythrocytes, respectively. Functional defects in granulocytes include abnormalities of movement, particle ingestion, and intracellular microbicidal systems. Defects in movement, including random migration of neutrophils as well as chemotaxis toward a specific soluble attractant (e.g., C5a, f-met-leu-phe), can be detected by use of the modified Boyden chamber.

Defects in particle ingestion and microbicidal activity are assayed by chemiluminescence, superoxide generation, and neutrophil bacterial killing assays. Recognition, attachment, and ingestion of opsonized particles (such as zymosan) by neutrophils leads to a respiratory burst, with generation of superoxide ion and related toxic oxygen metabolites. As these high-energy oxygen radicals relax

TABLE 8   Tests for Defects in Phagocytic System

Screening evaluation
  Quantitative tests
    Absolute granulocyte count and morphology
    Absolute monocyte count

Diagnostic evaluation
  Quantitative tests
    Bone marrow aspiration to assess granulocyte precursors
    Histochemical staining for alkaline phosphatase, peroxidase, and esterase
    Immunofluorescent staining for leukocyte adhesion molecules with monoclonal antibodies to LFA-1 (CD11a), Mo-1 (CD11b), and p150 (CD11c)
    C3b receptor enumeration
    Fc receptor enumeration
  Functional tests
    Random migration and chemotaxis
    Chemiluminescence of stimulated neutrophils
    Superoxide generation by stimulated neutrophils
    Granulocyte microbicidal assay
    Spectrophotometric analysis of granulocyte membrane cytochrome-b$_{558}$

to ground state, a small amount of electromagnetic energy in the form of light is emitted, a process termed chemiluminescence. This chemiluminescence correlates closely with microbicidal activity. Generation of superoxide can also be directly quantitated by cytochrome reduction assay. Granulocyte bacterial killing can be detected in a kinetic assay in which the test strain is incubated with neutrophils and opsonins from fresh serum. The number of viable intracellular organisms remaining after various times of incubation is then quantitated by culture of neutrophil lysates. Phagocyte membrane-associated cytochrome b$_{558}$, which is absent in X-linked chronic granulomatous disease, can be detected by spectrophotometric analysis.

Evaluation of the Complement System

The complement system is a major effector mechanism involved in clearance of immune complexes, cytolysis, opsonization, chemotaxis, and nonspecific inflammation. Deficiencies of complement should be suspected in patients with recurrent pyogenic infections (especially *Streptococcus pneumoniae* and *Neisseria* species) or conditions resembling systemic lupus erythematosus.

Screening assays for the complement system are listed in Table 9. Serum levels of three basic components can be measured by immunoassay (radial immunodiffusion) to implicate activation or utilization of either the classical or alternative pathway activation. The serum C4 level is depressed with classical pathway activation, serum factor B is depressed with alternative pathway activation, and the serum C3 level is depressed when either pathway is activated leading to initiation of the effector phase of the complement cascade (C5 through C9).

An excellent screening test for functional integrity of the entire complement system is the measurement of total hemolytic complement in the serum, expressed as 50 percent hemolytic units, or CH$_{50}$. While mild decreases in individual components may not be detected as a depression in CH$_{50}$, a low or absent CH$_{50}$ implies a significant defect in one or more components of the classical cascade and requires further diagnostic evaluation. When there is evidence that a complement level or function is abnormal on screening assays, a definitive diagnosis of a depression or deficiency in one or more complement components or regulatory proteins can be made by quantitating the concentration of individual components by immunoassay and by measuring functional activity of individual components independently by hemolytic assay (Table 9). These more sophisticated diagnostic assays are generally available in specialized reference or research laboratories.

Prenatal Diagnosis of Immunodeficiency

With the expansion in knowledge regarding specific cellular, enzymatic, and genetic defects leading to immunodeficiency diseases, prenatal diagnosis of some immunodeficiency diseases has been possible. Enzymatic analysis on cultured fibroblasts obtained at amniocentesis, or fetal blood sampling before 20 weeks' gestation, has been used successfully for the diagnosis of congenital

TABLE 9 Tests for Defects in the Complement System

Screening evaluation
  Quantitative tests
    Serum C3, C4, factor B levels
  Functional tests
    Total hemolytic complement (CH_{50})

Diagnostic evaluation
  Quantitative tests
    Measurement of specific component levels by
      immunoassay: Clq, Clr, Cls, C4, C2, C3, C5, C6, C7,
      C8, C9, factor P, factor D, factor I, factor H
  Functional tests
    Assay of specific component function by factor-limited
      hemolytic assay

immune deficiencies. Many congenital immunodeficiencies are the result of a single, inherited genetic defect. The recent progress in molecular genetics has made carrier detection and in utero diagnosis possible in a number of congenital immunodeficiencies with techniques such as linkage analysis and restriction fragment length polymorphism analysis of DNA (Table 10). Although currently in use at only a few medical centers, these techniques should become more widely available in the near future.

THERAPY FOR IMMUNODEFICIENCY

General Approach

Early diagnosis and rapid institution of specific therapy in patients with immunodeficiency disorders is imperative to prevent mortality and the morbidity of complications from recurrent infections. Early diagnosis is possible using an aggressive and organized approach that includes both screening and diagnostic procedures, as outlined above. Identified infections should be treated with specific antibiotics, the choice being made on the basis of microbial sensitivity patterns. When the infecting agent is unknown, broad-spectrum antibiotic coverage to treat the most likely possibilities is indicated. Prophylactic antibiotics are generally not recommended because of the development of resistant bacteria or fungal superinfection. There are three exceptions to this general rule. These include penicillin prophylaxis for postsplenectomy *S. pneumoniae* infections, trimethoprim-sulfamethoxazole (TMP-SMZ) prophylaxis for *Pneumocystis carinii* pneumonia in patients with deficient cell-mediated immunity, and TMP-SMZ or dicloxacillin prophylaxis for patients with chronic granulomatous disease. These specific indications are discussed in more detail below.

Immunization of patients with suspected immunodeficiency should be performed with great caution. In many instances, immunization will be fruitless because the underlying immunodeficiency results in a poor antibody response. In this situation other forms of protection must be utilized, such as passive immunization with immunoglobulin therapy. In individuals with deficiencies in cell-mediated immunity, live virus immunization (e.g., oral polio, measles, mumps, rubella, smallpox, and influenza) is specifically contraindicated since it may lead to

severe or life-threatening disease in the immunodeficient host.

Blood transfusion should be administered only for clear indications. Whole blood, packed red blood cells, unprocessed plasma, and platelets each contain viable lymphocytes and are capable of producing graft-versus-host disease (GVHD) in susceptible individuals with defects in cell-mediated immunity. Blood products for patients with cell-mediated immune defects should be irradiated with 3,000 R to eliminate viable lymphocytes, which may engraft in the immunodeficient patient and lead to GVHD that may be fatal. The potential of GVHD can also be markedly reduced when blood products are processed by freezing and centrifugation. Cytomegalovirus (CMV) can be transmitted by blood products, and therefore patients with defective cell-mediated immunity should receive CMV-negative transfusions.

Restoration and maintenance of adequate nutritional status is fundamental to the care of patients with immunodeficiency. At the time of diagnosis, many patients are significantly malnourished due to secondary intercurrent gastrointestinal disease, including *Giardia lamblia* infestation and bacterial and fungal overgrowth of the intestinal tract. Malnutrition may contribute to and complicate the immunodeficiency state, further compromising the patient. When enteral feeding is not successful, then parenteral feeding is indicated as long as appropriate precautions to guard against infection are taken.

Therapy for Antibody-Deficiency Syndromes

Since Colonel Ogdon Bruton's description in 1952 of agammaglobulinemia and its subsequent treatment with immunoglobulin, replacement therapy has been the mainstay of treatment for antibody-deficiency syndromes. Currently there are two forms of immunoglobulin for passive administration: modified/stabilized immunoglobulin preparations for intravenous administration and standard immune serum globulin for intramuscular injection. The former has certain advantages over the latter, including less pain on administration (particularly important in patients who require large doses for replacement), ease of achieving physiologic levels of IgG, lower risk of infection and bleeding, rapid acquisition of peak serum levels, and no impediment to frequent administration if required. These advantages must be balanced by the increased cost of intravenous IgG replacement therapy when compared

TABLE 10 Immunodeficiency Diseases in Which Prenatal Diagnosis or Carrier Detection Are Potentially Available

Adenosine deaminase deficiency
X-linked agammaglobulinemia
Chronic granulomatous disease
X-linked lymphoproliferative disease
G6PD deficiency
Purine nucleotide phosphorylase deficiency
Wiskott-Aldrich syndrome
Myeloperoxidase deficiency
Ataxia-telangiectasia
X-linked severe combined immunodeficiency

with the cost of intramuscular standard immune serum globulin.

In patients with clearly defined antibody-deficiency syndromes, intravenous gamma globulin should be begun at a dose of 200 mg per kilogram per dose given every 3 to 4 weeks. Several clinical studies have documented a reduced incidence of infection and fewer missed days of school or work in patients receiving intravenous gamma globulin compared with those receiving standard immune serum globulin intramuscularly. Depending on the patient's clinical response and trough serum IgG levels, the dose may be increased to 400 mg per kilogram per dose. Serum IgG levels can be monitored to achieve optimal therapy. We attempt to maintain a preinfusion trough IgG level in the range of 400 to 500 mg per deciliter or near the lower limit of normal for age.

Adverse effects of both intramuscular and intravenous immunoglobulin replacement therapy include systemic anaphylactoid reactions. These appear to be due to aggregates of IgG injected intravenously and are characterized by rise in body temperature, flushing of the face, tightness in the chest, chills, dizziness, nausea, diaphoresis, and hyper- or hypotension. These reactions may not be true anaphylactic reactions (i.e., not IgE-mediated), since most patients receiving this form of therapy are deficient in their ability to make antibody of the IgE class. In some patients, however, IgG and IgE antibodies against IgA are formed. These patients are at increased risk for anaphylactic reactions to gamma globulin preparations (or other blood products) containing even small amounts of IgA.

As an alternative to intravenous gamma globulin therapy, standard immune serum globulin can be administered in a dose of 0.2 to 0.4 ml per kilogram per dose. It is frequently beneficial to divide the dose into three or four separate injections to minimize the pain associated with administration of large volumes. The subsequent doses of standard immune serum globulin should be adjusted on the basis of the clinical response of the patient, since trough levels of total serum IgG are rarely normalized with intramuscular therapy. In patients who do not tolerate even maximal doses given every 3 to 4 weeks, a more frequent injection schedule using a smaller volume may be better tolerated.

In contrast to most patients with IgG antibody deficiency syndromes, patients with selective IgA deficiency should not be treated with gamma globulin preparation or plasma since these patients are fully capable of forming normal antibodies of other immunoglobulin classes. Consequently, they may recognize traces of IgA contained in gamma globulin or serum as a foreign protein. The use of gamma globulin or plasma may sensitize these patients to make anti-IgA antibodies, which may lead to subsequent anaphylactic transfusion reactions. An exception to this rule is in patients with combined IgA/IgG2 or IgA/IgG2/IgG4 subclass deficiency. These patients may benefit from intravenous immunoglobulin replacement given cautiously in a controlled setting. In this setting it is helpful to measure serum anti-IgA antibodies periodically to avoid potentially serious reactions.

Therapy for Defects in Cell-Mediated Immunity

The correction or therapy of cell-mediated immune deficiency is much more difficult and complex than is the therapy of antibody-deficiency syndromes. Patients with defects of cell-mediated immunity who also show defective antibody synthesis will benefit from immunoglobulin replacement therapy, as outlined above. Most patients with significant impairment of cell-mediated immunity will be susceptible to *P. carinii* pneumonia. When diagnosed, this infection can be treated with TMP-SMZ in a dose of 20 mg per kilogram per day of TMP plus 100 mg per kilogram per day of SMZ in four divided doses for 14 days. If not successful or not tolerated, pentamidine isethionate, 4 mg per kilogram per day intramuscularly in a single daily dose for 14 days, can be utilized. Prophylaxis against *P. carinii* should be instituted in all patients with significant cell-mediated immune deficiency with TMP-SMZ in a dose of 5 mg per kilogram per day of TMP and 25 mg per kilogram per day of SMZ.

Patients with T cell deficiency who require blood transfusion should receive CMV-negative and irradiated blood products to prevent CMV infection and GVHD, respectively (see general measures outline above).

Severe defects in cell-mediated immunity are most effectively treated by transplantation of HLA-genotypically identical bone marrow. Complete immunologic reconstitution with this form of therapy has been documented in more than 150 patients with severe combined immunodeficiency. When an HLA-matched donor is not available for transplant, an alternative for T cell reconstitution is transplant of T cell–depleted haplotype-mismatched parental bone marrow. In this procedure, potential GVHD-producing T lymphocytes are eliminated from the parental marrow before transplantation by differential agglutination by use of soybean lectin or by monoclonal antibodies to human T cells. With this approach, approximately 180 severely T cell deficient patients have received transplants. Nearly 60 percent have achieved engraftment of parental marrow, with subsequent immunologic reconstitution and a state of stable split chimerism.

Bone marrow transplantation is also the treatment of choice in patients with severe T cell immunodeficiency associated with deficiency of enzymes in the purine salvage pathway; however, biochemical therapy is sometimes successful. In patients with adenosine deaminase deficiency, transfusion of frozen irradiated packed red blood cells to replace the deficient enzyme has occasionally been successful in reversing the biochemical abnormalities and partially reversing T cell immunodeficiency. Promising results have recently been obtained with enzyme replacement therapy with polyethylene glycol–conjugated bovine adenosine deaminase.

Some patients with congenital deficiency of cell-mediated immunity appear to have defects in development or function of thymic microenvironment (DiGeorge syndrome, combined immunodeficiency with B cells). Natural and synthetic thymic humoral factors have been prepared and tested for therapy in these patients. Encouraging preliminary results using thymosin fraction V, thymosin alpha-1, or thymic pentapeptide (TP 5) have been obtained in patients with DiGeorge syndrome and in some patients with combined immunodeficiency with B cells. Replacement of lymphokines such as IL-2 or interferon (produced by recombinant DNA technology) has been utilized only in experimental situations.

Therapy for Phagocytic Disorders

At present there is no specific therapy to increase the defective granulocyte microbicidal activity present in chronic granulomatous disease. Management includes antibiotic prophylaxis along with aggressive diagnosis of and specific antimicrobial therapy for infective episodes.

Continuous prophylactic antibiotic therapy with low-dose TMP-SMZ or dicloxacillin is effective in decreasing the incidence of bacterial infections in patients with chronic granulomatous disease. White blood cell transfusions have also been utilized as adjunctive therapies during acute life-threatening infections in patients with chronic granulomatous disease, although experience with this form of therapy is extremely limited. A small number of patients have been successfully reconstituted by HLA-matched bone marrow transplantation.

Therapy for Complement Defects

Defects have been described for all 11 of the complement pathway components in the classical pathway, for factor D in the alternative pathway, and for the complement regulatory proteins C1 inhibitor, factor I (C3b inactivator), factor H, and properdin. There is no satisfactory replacement therapy for most of these deficiencies since the catabolic rates of the proteins are high. Impeded androgens (e.g., danazol) may decrease the frequency of attacks in some patients with hereditary angioedema, presumably by increasing concentrations of C1 inactivator and C4. Therapy with fresh-frozen plasma, 10 mg per kilogram per day, may be used to temporarily restore normal complement function in patients with C3 deficiency (either primary or secondary factor I deficiency) during episodes of severe acute pyogenic infection.

Some patients with deficiencies of terminal complement components such as C5, C6, C7, C8, and C9 have recurrent neisserial infections and require antibiotic prophylaxis with oral penicillin.

SPECIFIC IMMUNODEFICIENCIES

Immunodeficiencies Due to Antibody Defects

Antibody immunodeficiency was the first to be recognized and it represents the most common form of primary immunodeficiency. Deficiencies of all classes and subclasses of immunoglobulins have now been described. The disorders reflect marked decrease or total absence of one or more of the immunoglobulin isotypes, generally due to a defect in B cell maturation or T cell regulation of B cell function. The defect may be congenital or acquired, permanent or transient. In the congenital agammaglobulinemias, symptoms appear during first year of life, fol-

lowing loss of transplacentally acquired maternal immunoglobulins. In the acquired antibody deficiencies, the severity of symptoms varies with the degree of immunoglobulin deficiency. The hallmark of the symptoms of hypogammaglobulinemia is recurrent severe infection by pyogenic organisms. Diagnosis is established readily by quantitation of immunoglobulin isotypes in the serum. Examination of the number and function of B cell and T cell subpopulations helps in identifying the specific nature of the underlying disorder.

X-Linked Agammaglobulinemia (Bruton's Agammaglobulinemia, Congenital or Infantile Agammaglobulinemia)

In this X-linked inherited deficiency, the levels of all classes of immunoglobulins are profoundly decreased. Total absence of immunoglobulins is rare; small amounts of immunoglobulins can usually be detected.

Pathophysiology

The B cell defect appears to be due to a primary block in the maturation or differentiation of pre-B cells to mature B cells. Pre-B cells in bone marrow are usually normal in number, but circulating B cells are greatly diminished (i.e., less than 0.5 percent) and plasma cells can rarely be found. T cells and T cell subsets are usually normal in number and function.

Clinical Manifestations

The defect occurs only in boys. Children rarely manifest clinical evidence of the disease before the age of 6 to 9 months, presumably due to protection from transplacentally acquired maternal antibodies. Thereafter, recurrent sinopulmonary infections or acute, severe, invasive, life-threatening bacterial infections occur. Repeated bacterial infections localized to the upper and lower respiratory tract are usually due to pyogenic organisms, including the pneumococcus, *H. influenzae*, and streptococcus. Septicemia with these organisms or with *Pseudomonas aeruginosa* may occur. Chronic sinopulmonary infections are the major cause of long-term morbidity in patients with agammaglobulinemia. Because of the inability of the patient to produce functional antibody during an active infection, there is a failure to clear antigen. Thus, viral and parasitic infections in patients with X-linked agammaglobulinemia tend to persist.

Vaccine-associated poliomyelitis, persistent enteroviral encephalitis, and gastroenteritis due to rotavirus or *G. lamblia* occur with unusual frequency in these patients. *P. carinii* infections may also be the presenting infection. Rheumatoid arthritis and lymphoreticular malignancies also occur with increased frequency in patients with X-linked agammaglobulinemia.

Diagnosis

All immunoglobulin isotypes are profoundly decreased. Mature immunoglobulin-bearing B cells in peripheral blood are markedly low (i.e., less than 0.5 percent) or absent. The patients are unable to make specific antibody in response to antigenic challenge. T cells are normal in numbers and function. Normal numbers of pre-B cells are present in the bone marrow. Lymph nodes show virtual absence of plasma cells and absence or poor development of germinal centers. Thymic tissue is normal.

Treatment

Replacement therapy with human gamma globulin is effective in reducing morbidity and mortality in patients with agammaglobulinemia. Intravenous immunoglobulin, vigorous and early antibiotic therapy, and supportive care should be provided as outlined above.

Common Variable Immunodeficiency (Late-Onset Hypogammaglobulinemia)

This deficiency is also characterized by abnormally low levels or absence of IgG and other immunoglobulin classes. As implied by the term *hypogammaglobulinemia,* levels of IgG are often somewhat higher in common variable immunodeficiency than in X-linked agammaglobulinemia. This condition includes a heterogenous group of patients with variable age at onset and variable severity of infection.

Pathophysiology

Studies of the number and function of T and B cells in patients with common variable immunodeficiency suggest that there are many causes of this disease. Hypogammaglobulinemia due to an acquired B cell abnormality may occur (1) following Epstein-Barr virus infection (in the X-linked lymphoproliferative syndrome), (2) in association with a failure of B cells to proliferate in response to mitogens or to glycosylate immunoglobulin molecules, or (3) as an idiopathic condition associated with low levels of or absent B cells. Other patients with common variable immunodeficiency may have hypogammaglobulinemia due to defects in regulatory T cells. These include an excess of CD8+ suppressor T cells, or more rarely, a deficiency of CD4+ helper T cells, T cell abnormalities associated with thymoma, or defective cell-mediated immunity associated with autoimmune disease or sarcoidosis. In a few patients, autoantibodies to T or B lymphocytes have been found. The presence of abnormal immunoglobulin levels in family members of patients with this deficiency, as well as a high incidence of autoimmunity (i.e., systemic lupus erythematosus, idiopathic thrombocytopenia, and hemolytic anemia) in first-degree relatives, suggests a hereditary influence on immunoregulation in this condition.

Clinical Manifestation

The hypogammaglobulinemia may occur at any age. Both sexes are equally affected. Patients develop recurrent pyogenic infections. Chronic pulmonary infection with progressive bronchiectasis is a common presentation. A high incidence of gastrointestinal symptoms, often due to *G. lamblia,* and of lymphoreticular malignancy is seen in patients with this form of hypogammaglobulinemia. Pernicious anemia and other autoimmune diseases occur in 30 percent of patients. Noncaseating granulomata of various organs and hepatosplenomegaly occur in hypogammaglobulinemia associated with sarcoidosis.

Diagnosis

Patients may have low or high numbers of circulating immunoglobulin-bearing B lymphocytes. However, these cells usually do not differentiate normally into plasma cells or produce immunoglobulins in vitro, even after polyclonal stimulation. The total number of mature T lymphocytes in the blood is normal, but there may be reversal of the CD4 to CD8 subset ratio. Functional studies may demonstrate diminished helper or increased suppressor T cell activity. Lymphocyte responses to phytohemagglutinin, concanavalin A, and pokeweed mitogen are significantly diminished in some patients.

Treatment

Therapy for patients with common variable immunodeficiency with intravenous immunoglobulin and supportive care is the same as that described above for patients with X-linked gammaglobulinemia.

Transient Hypogammaglobulinemia of Infancy

This uncommon immunodeficiency is characterized by recurrent infection with immunoglobulin levels that are below the lower normal limits for age but not absent. Hypogammaglobulinemia may persist through the first 2 years of life, followed by spontaneous resolution and a rise of immunoglobulin levels to normal.

Pathophysiology

This deficiency may represent a delay in the normal maturation sequence of the humoral immune response. In normal newborns, physiologic hypogammaglobulinemia occurs at 3 to 6 months of age, when loss of maternal immunoglobulins exceeds the infant's ability to synthesize antibodies to environmental antigens. This period may persist longer in premature infants. In patients with transient hypogammaglobulinemia of infancy, the period of hypogammaglobulinemia may extend from 20 to 30 months of age. Despite the low level of serum immunoglobulins, patients respond normally to immunization by forming specific antibodies. This is an important distinction between patients with transient hypogammaglobulinemia of infancy and those with X-linked agammaglobulinemia or common variable immunodeficiency. Circulating B cells are normal in number and function. A numerical and functional deficiency in helper CD4 T lymphocytes has been described in some of these patients. This deficiency resolves spontaneously.

Clinical Manifestations

Two clinical patterns are recognized. The first occurs in a group of patients with relatively mild symptoms who are discovered because they have relatives with immunodeficiencies (especially severe combined immunodeficiency). Infections are mild and immunoglobulin levels return to normal by 2 to 3 years of age. The second pattern occurs in a group with significant recurrent infections beginning in early infancy. These patients have no immunodeficient relatives. Hypogammaglobulinemia usually resolves by 2 years of age, but rarely one or more of the immunoglobulin isotypes may remain below normal levels.

Diagnosis

This deficiency should be considered in a male or female infant with persistent hypogammaglobulinemia but with normal antibody response to antigenic challenge. Hypogammaglobulinemia involves primarily the IgG isotype. The numbers of circulating B and T lymphocytes are normal. T cell subset enumeration may reveal a decrease in the number of CD4+ lymphocytes.

Treatment

The condition is self-limited; hypogammaglobulinemia generally resolves by 2 years of age. Immunoglobulin administration is rarely required except in those few children with marked hypogammaglobulinemia and severe recurrent infections.

X-Linked Hypogammaglobulinemia With Growth Hormone Deficiency

This immunodeficiency has been described in two children and two maternal uncles of one family. It was associated with panhypogammaglobulinemia in three of the four members affected. All had isolated growth hormone deficiency. The patients had short stature, small phallus, delayed onset of puberty, and retarded bone age. Treatment of the antibody deficiency with intravenous immunoglobulin is the same as for X-linked congenital agammaglobulinemia. Growth hormone replacement therapy is now available.

Autosomal Recessive Agammaglobulinemia

A rare form of congenital agammaglobulinemia has been reported in two female siblings. The manifestations of the deficiency are similar to those of X-linked agammaglobulinemia. A defect in B cell differentiation is postulated as being responsible for this disease. The diagnostic criteria used for X-linked agammaglobulinemia apply to the autosomal recessive form. Treatment is also the same.

Selective IgA Deficiency

Selective IgA deficiency is the most common of the primary immunodeficiencies, with a prevalence estimated at one case per 700 general population. This defect is characterized by absent serum or secretory IgA or serum levels below 10 mg per deciliter.

Pathophysiology

Selective IgA deficiency may result from a maturation arrest of IgA-bearing B cells, from inefficient or inaccurate genetic isotype switch mechanisms at the heavy chain constant region alpha-1 or alpha-2 exons on chromosome 14, and in rare cases, from lack of production of secretory component. Acquired IgA deficiency may follow intake of certain drugs such as phenytoin, penicillamine, and sulfasalazine, which may be due to induction of suppressor T cells that depress B cell maturation to IgA synthesis. IgA deficiency has also been described in association with partial deletions of chromosome 18 (18q−) or with ring chromosome 18.

Clinical Manifestations

Individuals with selective IgA deficiency may be relatively healthy. However, many patients with IgA deficiency present with recurrent and severe infections of the respiratory and gastrointestinal tracts. The same encapsulated pyogenic bacterial agents are involved in these infections as in other forms of agammaglobulinemia. Other patients may present with severe atopic disease or autoimmune diseases (e.g., idiopathic thrombocytopenia purpura, rheumatoid arthritis, or lupus).

Diagnosis

The findings of serum IgA levels lower than 10 mg per deciliter on two successive determinations—after the age of 6 to 12 months—establishes the diagnosis of IgA deficiency. IgA deficiency may be associated with deficiency of other classes of immunoglobulins, such as IgE or IgG2 and IgG4 subclasses. Antibody responses to pneumococcal and meningococcal vaccines may be abnormal. A rare deficiency in production of secretory component has been described and is associated with low levels of IgA in saliva and intestinal fluids. Familial IgA2 deficiency has been reported.

Treatment

Therapy should be directed toward the specific disease associated with IgA deficiency (i.e., allergy, autoimmune disease). At present, there is no replacement therapy for IgA deficiency. The propensity of patients to form antibodies to IgA when infused with immunoglobulin preparations or other blood products is a point of serious clinical concern. Near-fatal anaphylactic reactions have followed systemic administration of IgA-containing human blood products to these patients. Up to half of the patients have antibodies to IgA in their serum. Systemic administration of human immunoglobulin to patients with selective IgA deficiency who have anti-IgA antibodies is generally contraindicated. Blood products (red blood cells) should be washed at least five times before administration to remove contaminating IgA and to avoid anaphylactic reactions.

In individuals with drug-induced deficiency, the serum IgA level usually returns to normal upon discontinuation of the offending medication. Although rare, a few patients with primary IgA deficiency have had a spontaneous remission of the deficiency.

Selective IgM Deficiency

This is an extremely rare condition characterized by a selective deficiency in the level of serum IgM, with normal IgG and IgA.

Pathophysiology

Normal or slightly decreased numbers of circulating IgM-bearing B cells are seen. The underlying defect may lie in the differentiation of B cells to IgM-secreting plasma cells. Acquired IgM deficiency has been described in patients with gluten enteropathy, which is reversed following treatment with a gluten-free diet.

Clinical Manifestations

The most common infection associated with IgM deficiency is meningococcemia. Recurrent infection with other bacteria is also seen.

Diagnosis

Levels of serum IgM are subnormal but total absence of IgM is rare.

Treatment

There is no specific therapy. Antibiotics and plasma or immunoglobulin infusions may be beneficial in the patient with serious infections.

Immunoglobulin Deficiency Associated With Elevated IgM (and IgD)

Initially thought to be X-linked, this syndrome has now been observed in females and also as an acquired disease.

Pathophysiology

Increased numbers of IgM-synthesizing plasmacytoid cells are present in the blood and secrete large amounts of IgM on stimulation in vitro. In contrast, the B cells from these patients do not synthesize or secrete IgG or IgA. Likewise, surface IgG- and IgA-bearing B cells are absent. It is hypothesized that these patients have a defect in the normal heavy chain switch from IgM to IgG during B cell differentiation. Several patients have been shown to lack a T cell population of "switch T cells" capable of inducing IgM to IgG and IgA isotype switching. Some patients have developed this form of immunodeficiency as a complication of congenital rubella infection.

Clinical Manifestations

Patients with this form of dysgammaglobulinemia have recurrent pyogenic respiratory infections and autoimmune diseases, such as hemolytic anemia, thrombocytopenia, cyclic neutropenia, or lymphoproliferative disease.

Treatment

Therapy of the antibody deficiency consists of IgG replacement. This may be accompanied by normalization of the IgM levels and regression of lymphoid hyperplasia in some patients.

Deficiency of IgG Subclasses

Patients with absence or selective deficiency of one or more IgG subclasses have been reported. There is often an associated relative or absolute IgA deficiency. In these patients, the total serum IgG level may be normal or below the lower normal range. Patients with IgG subclass deficiency have severe and recurrent sinopulmonary infections often with associated bronchiectasis. Measurement of IgG subclass levels leads to the diagnosis. Many patients respond to a regimen of low-dose antibiotic prophylaxis. IgG replacement should be given to those patients with isolated IgG subclass deficiency who have severe symptoms and who continue to have active infection despite antibiotic prophylaxis. Similar to patients with IgA deficiency, some of these patients may be at higher risk for reactions to intravenous immunoglobulin.

Antibody Deficiency With Normal Immunoglobulin Levels

Rare patients have been described with recurrent infections and normal immunoglobulins, but with inability to form specific antibodies following immunization or in response to antigens of infecting organisms. Some of these patients may have had IgG-subclass deficiency. An imbalance of helper–suppressor T cell function has been considered to be one of the underlying defects. Because of the former association, IgG subclass levels should be determined. Some of these patients will do well on prophylactic antibiotics. Immunoglobulin replacement therapy should be given when a global defect in antibody synthesis is documented with or without IgG-subclass deficiency and the patient continues to have severe infection despite antibiotic prophylaxis.

Hyperimmunoglobulinemia E Syndrome

Children with this syndrome have recurrent staphylococcal infections and very high serum IgE levels (5,000 to 40,000 IU per deciliter). All patients have recurrent skin furunculosis and many have recurrent cellulitis. Lung involvement with pneumonitis is also a universal finding and many patients have persistent pneumatoceles that require surgical resection. While infection of the skin and lungs is most common, involvement of the middle ear, sinuses, eyes, joints, blood, and viscera is reported. Other clinical features include a lichenified dermatitis, growth retardation, and coarse facies. Infection due to *Staphylococcus aureus* is a uniform finding, but many patients also have problems with *Candida albicans, H. influenzae,* pneumococci, group A streptococci, and gram-negative bacteria. Eosinophilia of blood and sputum is virtually always present.

In addition to IgE levels which are three to 80 times the normal level, the patients manifest depressed anamnestic antibody responses. Most have immediate hypersensitivity to inhalant and food allergens and some microbial antigens. Serum levels of other immunoglobulin isotypes are usually normal. T cell number is usually normal. T cell function studies reveal normal mitogen response but depressed responses to candida and tetanus toxoid. Abnormal neutrophil chemotaxis is present in some but not all patients. No definitive therapy is available. Lifelong antibiotic prophylaxis with antistaphylococcal antibiotics may prevent the most frequent clinical problems.

DEFECTS PREDOMINANTLY AFFECTING CELL-MEDIATED IMMUNITY

DiGeorge Syndrome (Third and Fourth Pharyngeal Pouch Syndrome)

This congenital immunodeficiency is characterized clinically by congenital heart disease, abnormal facies, hypocalcemia with tetany, and increased susceptibility to infections. The syndrome results from abnormal embryologic development of the pharyngeal pouches. Dysembryogenesis of neural crest cells participating in the development of these structures results in a syndrome of anomalies of these glands as well as complex cardiac malformations (primarily interrupted aortic arch type B and truncus arteriosis). The clinical and pathologic spectrum of this syndrome ranges from a lethal complete form, with absence of the affected glands, to less severe or partial forms with glandular hypoplasia with or without congenital heart disease.

The clinical manifestations may include all or some of the following features:

1. Abnormal facies with small, low-set, posteriorly rotated, dysmorphic ears with notched pinnae; micrognathia with "fish-mouth," a small mandible, and a short philtrum; hypertelorism and antimongoloid slant of the eyes.
2. Congenital heart defects, especially interrupted aortic arch or truncus arteriosus, but also a variety of severe to mild heart defects have been reported, including septal defects, patent ductus arteriosus, aberrant left subclavian artery, right-sided aortic arch, and tetralogy of Fallot.
3. Hypoparathyroidism presenting as neonatal tetany within the first 24 to 48 hours of life with low serum calcium level, elevated phosphorus level, and absent parathyroid hormone.
4. Cellular immunodeficiency varying from a profound deficiency of T cells to only mild decreases in T cell number with relatively normal T cell function. B cell numbers are generally normal.

The pattern of inheritance of the DiGeorge syndrome is not clearly established. There are reports of families, siblings, and twins with the disorder, as well as selected kindred that show an autosomal dominant mode of inheritance. Clinical features similar to DiGeorge syndrome have been associated with maternal use of alcohol and isotretinoin, a finding suggesting that teratogens may affect embryogenesis. In addition, DiGeorge syndrome has been associated with deletions in chromosome 22.

Persistent hypocalcemia in a child with congenital heart disease is generally the first laboratory abnormality detected in DiGeorge syndrome. The spectrum of T cell defects is considerable. The percentage of peripheral blood T lymphocytes is generally reduced but may be normal. A similar finding is seen with delayed-type hypersensitivity skin testing. Impaired suppressor T cell activity with low CD8 T cell number has been reported in the partial form of the syndrome. In the complete form, the T cell–proliferative response to mitogens is low. In general, B cell number is normal, but hypogammaglobulinemia and dysgammaglobulinemia can occur.

The clinical prognosis is primarily determined by the degree of hypocalcemia and extent of aortocardiac malformation. The acute care of a child with DiGeorge syndrome should include control of hypocalcemia with calcium gluconate infusion, vitamin D supplements, and parathyroid hormone replacement when necessary. The immunodeficiency that results from thymic hypoplasia is lethal in only a minority of cases. The majority of patients with DiGeorge syndrome exhibit steady improvement in their T cell function with time. Some patients have been successfully treated with fetal thymus gland transplantation or thymosin fraction V. Fatal graft-versus-host disease has occurred in patients with DiGeorge syndrome following blood transfusion. Therefore, irradiation of cellular blood products is prudent in the management of DiGeorge syndrome until the T cell defect is corrected. One patient with DiGeorge syndrome and absent T cell function and number has been successfully reconstituted by bone marrow transplantation. Additional management should include prophylaxis against *P. carinii* and avoidance of live virus vaccines.

Combined Immunodeficiency

These disorders consist of a variety of immunodeficiency states involving both cellular and humoral immunity. In general, there is a profound defect in T cell function with variable B cell function. Numerous forms of combined immunodeficiency (CID) are recognized, including reticular dysgenesis, low B and T cell number (classical severe combined immunodeficiency), low T cell numbers with normal B cells (Swiss type lymphopenic agammaglobulinemia, CD4 T lymphocyte deficiency), combined immunodeficiency due to enzyme defects (adenosine deaminase deficiency and purine nucleotide phosphorylase deficiency), combined immunodeficiency with normal immunoglobulins (Nezelof's syndrome), and the "bare lymphocyte syndrome."

Clinical Manifestations

Patients with CID generally have recurrent fungal, viral, protozoal, and bacterial infections beginning before

6 months of age and leading to failure to thrive, chronic lung disease, and death during the first year of life. Clinical findings include persistent oral and gastrointestinal candidiasis, intractable diarrhea, recurrent bacterial sepsis, and interstitial pneumonitis due to *P. carinii* or CMV. Many patients have developed B cell and T cell malignancies in early infancy. With the complete lack of T cell immunity, patients are susceptible to GVHD resulting from maternal T cell engraftment in utero during birth, or following transfusion of unirradiated blood products.

Treatment

General therapy of the T cell–deficient patient is outlined above. Aggressive therapy of defined infections with specific antimicrobial drugs given parenterally is indicated. Gamma globulin replacement should be used in those patients who fail to produce antibody. Immunizations with live virus is contraindicated. Blood products should be irradiated with 3,000 R to prevent GVHD.

Complete immunologic reconstitution can be achieved with HLA-matched bone marrow transplantation. In cases of severe T cell immunodeficiency with no evidence of maternal engraftment, this procedure can be performed without prior bone marrow ablation by radiation or chemotherapy. When engraftment is achieved, the overall survival rate is more than 70 percent. For patients who lack histocompatible donors for bone marrow transplant, the use of T cell–depleted, haplotype-mismatched, parental bone marrow transplantation has been successful in CID.

Diagnosis

Laboratory findings vary from severe lymphopenia, eosinophilia, and absent T cells and B cells (classical severe CID) to some forms that have normal total lymphocyte and T cell numbers. There may be an increase in lymphocytes expressing early thymic T cell markers (CD6 and CD10) and absence of cells with mature T cell markers (CD3, CD4, and CD8). Diminished T cell function can be demonstrated by low lymphocyte blastogenesis after stimulation with mitogens, soluble antigens, and alloantigen. Antibody-dependent cellular cytotoxicity and natural killer cell activity may be increased or absent. Immunoglobulin concentrations are generally low but may be normal or increased. Similarly, B cell number may be low or normal. Immunoglobulin deficiency may be difficult to diagnose in the first few months of life because of transplacentally derived maternal IgG. However most patients with CID will lack serum IgA and IgM. Despite the presence of B cells and relatively normal immunoglobulin levels in some patients with CID, there is no specific antibody formed following antigenic challenge.

CID With Predominant T Cell Defects

Prior to the recent advances in the understanding of T cell biology, this subgroup of CIDs was difficult to define. They have been associated with such diverse etiologies as a failure of stem cell development (classical severe CID), defects in cytokine synthesis or cytokine receptor elaboration, the absence of the CD4 inducer T cell subpopulations, intrathymic maturation arrest (Swiss type lymphopenic agammaglobulinemia), or defects in T cell intracellular signal transduction. All are congenital, with some forms exhibiting an autosomal or X-linked inheritance. In aggregate they comprise 60 percent of all forms of CID.

As in other forms of CID, these patients are susceptible to recurrent viral, fungal, protozoal, and bacterial illnesses. Physical findings vary, but patients with lymphadenopathy and hepatosplenomegaly need to be distinguished from patients with human immunodeficiency virus infection. The common defect in cell-mediated immunity is probably a result of aberrant T cell development within the thymus or a blockade of T cell activation. As a result, even though humoral immunity may be present, it lacks the necessary signals provided by collaborating T cells.

CID Due to Enzyme Defects

The most common enzyme deficiencies associated with CID are adenosine deaminae (ADA) deficiency and purine nucleotide phosphorylase (PNP) deficiency. ADA deficiency results in marked impairment of both B cell and T cell immunity, and PNP deficiency primarily affects T cell immunity. Both enzymes are involved in the purine salvage pathway, necessary for the metabolism of purines to uric acid.

Purine Nucleoside Phosphorylase Deficiency

PNP deficiency leads to an accumulation of inosine, guanosine, deoxyguanosine, and deoxyGTP. These products accumulate, and the defect is manifested in the patients as hypouricemia. Accumulation of purine metabolites results in an inhibition of ribonucleotide reductase activity, with subsequent depletion of deoxyribonucleotide triose phosphate and, ultimately, inhibition of cellular division and absent T cell immunity. In patients with PNP deficiency the toxic nucleotides appear as deoxyguanosine. Humoral immunity is generally normal, but autoantibody formation and recurrent infections are common. Death from overwhelming viral infections, particularly varicella, occurs in many cases. Prenatal diagnosis is available by enzyme analysis of cultured fetal fibroblasts or by restriction fragment length polymorphism analysis of DNA.

Adenosine Deaminase Deficiency

ADA is another enzyme of the purine salvage pathway that catalyzes the conversion of adenosine and deoxyadenosine to inosine and deoxyinosine. Deficiency of ADA leads to accumulation of purine nucleosides, deoxynucleosides, and deoxyATP, resulting in inhibition of ribonucleotide reductase and inhibition of cell division.

In both ADA and PNP deficiency, progressive immunologic attrition is observed. Clinical features are the same as those found in other forms of CID. Approximately one-half of ADA-deficient patients exhibit a characteristic cupping and flaring of the end of the ribs. Diagnosis is established by low or absent ADA levels in the patient's erythrocytes. Optimal treatment is HLA-matched bone marrow transplantation, but replacement treatment with bovine intestinal ADA conjugated to polyethylene glycol has recently been promising.

Other forms of CID that are suspected to be due to an underlying enzyme defect include short-limbed dwarfism with immunodeficiency, cartilage-hair hypoplasia, and multiple carboxylase deficiency.

Bare Lymphocyte Syndrome (MHC Class I or Class II Deficiency)

Patients with the bare lymphocyte syndrome have a form of combined immunodeficiency with deficient or diminished expression of HLA (MHC) cell surface determinants. Clinical manifestations are similar to the other forms of CID with recurrent and opportunistic infections and failure to thrive due to malabsorption. In contrast to many of the other forms of CID, these patients often have easily palpable lymphoid tissue.

Pathophysiology

The basis for the failure to express MHC determinants on the cell surface is not known. DNA analysis by Southern blotting has ruled out a large structural gene loss. Under appropriate conditions MHC antigens can be induced on transformed cell lines from these patients, thus suggesting a regulatory gene abnormality.

Diagnosis

Despite variation in the severity of the defect in HLA expression, all patients have a combined immunodeficiency. In the more-complete forms, T lymphocyte numbers and functions are all depressed. In the less-complete forms, T cells can develop and acquire some normal functions, such as proliferative responses to mitogens and alloantigens, but they do not respond to soluble recall antigens, and they do not provide helper function for B cell differentiation. The diagnosis is made by demonstrating absence or reduced expression of HLA class I (or less commonly, class II) antigen expression on lymphocytes and platelets.

Treatment

Correction of the immunodeficiency can be accomplished by bone marrow transplantation, as described above for the other forms of CID. In the patient with severely deficient expression of the HLA antigens, genotyping can be performed using restriction fragment length polymorphisms to select an appropriately matched marrow donor.

Wiskott-Aldrich Syndrome

Wiskott-Aldrich syndrome is characterized by severe eczema; thrombocytopenia with small, poorly functional platelets; and susceptibility to bacterial, viral, and opportunistic infections. This disorder is inherited in an X-linked recessive fashion although a female variant has been described. Thrombocytopenia leads to petechiae and severe bleeding episodes, usually within the first 6 months of life. Less common clinical manifestations include central nervous system hemorrhage, autoimmune hemolytic anemia or vasculitis, reticuloendotheliosis, or lymphoid malignancy.

Pathophysiology

The pathogenesis of this disorder is uncertain, although recent studies suggest that there may be an alteration in sialophorin, a 115,000-dalton cell surface glycoprotein on T cells and platelets. Monoclonal antibodies to sialophorin are capable of stimulating the proliferation of T cells, a fact indicating that sialophorin may have a role in T cell activation. Patients with Wiskott-Aldrich syndrome either lack sialophorin or express an abnormal form of sialophorin on their T cells and platelets.

Diagnosis

Patients with Wiskott-Aldrich syndrome have a defect in both B and T cells. Serum from affected males shows normal levels of IgG, increased levels of IgA and IgE, and low levels of IgM. An unusual antibody response to antigenic challenge is a consistent characteristic of this immunodeficiency. There is a normal response to protein antigens but a poor response to carbohydrate or polysaccharide antigens. Thus, the serum of these patients lacks isohemagglutinins. Autoantibodies are frequently found in patients with Wiskott-Aldrich syndrome. With age, there is a progressive attrition of T cell number and T cell function. The proliferative responses to the mixed lymphocyte reaction and to soluble recall antigen is often more adversely affected than the proliferative responses to nonspecific mitogens. Platelets of affected males are approximately one-half the normal volume and show abnormal aggregation.

Treatment

The T cell, B cell, and platelet defects in Wiskott-Aldrich syndrome can be corrected by HLA-matched bone marrow transplantation. Although originally thought to be contraindicated in patients with Wiskott-Aldrich syndrome, splenectomy has proved useful in managing severe and life-threatening thrombocytopenia, provided that appropriate precautions are taken to avoid postsplenectomy sepsis. Steroids are generally contraindicated unless required to control autoimmune hemolytic anemia or vasculitis.

For patients with severe recurrent bacterial infections unresponsive to antibiotic prophylaxis, therapy with intravenous gamma globulin may be instituted. Intramuscular gamma globulin therapy is contraindicated because of the risk of bleeding.

Ataxia-Telangiectasia

Ataxia-telangiectasia is an autosomal recessive disorder that consists of progressive cerebellar ataxia, mental retardation, cutaneous and conjunctival telangiectasia, recurrent sinopulmonary infections with bronchiectasis, and a combined immunodeficiency, usually manifested by selective IgA deficiency and partial T cell immunodeficiency. Lymphoreticular malignancies occur with an increased frequency in patients with ataxia-telangiectasia.

Pathophysiology

The pathogenesis of this condition is unknown but may involve a basic defect leading to chromosomal instability and defective cellular DNA repair. Patients demonstrate undue susceptibility to radiation induced cytotoxicity with an increased incidence of chromosomal breaks, translocations, and rearrangements, often involving chromosomes 7 and 14.

Diagnosis

Laboratory investigation reveals lymphopenia, eosinophilia, and selective IgA deficiency in about 70 percent of patients with ataxia-telangiectasia. Other immunoglobulins may be normal or decreased in amount. A subset of patients has combined IgA–IgG2-subclass deficiency, with an increased risk of sinopulmonary infections. Antibody responses to bacterial and viral antigens may be deficient. T cell numbers are frequently, but not always, depressed, as are lymphocyte responses to mitogens and antigens. CD4+ T helper cells appear to be more affected than do CD8+ T suppressor cells.

Treatment

Aggressive supportive therapy may prolong survival; however at present, there is no cure. Gamma globulin may be beneficial in patients with IgA–IgG2 deficiency and severe sinopulmonary infections, although the risks must be weighed carefully. Attempts to reconstitute deficient cell-mediated immunity with thymic factors or fetal thymus gland transplants have been too limited to draw conclusions. Marrow transplantation has not been attempted. No therapy is effective in halting the central nervous system degeneration. Irradiation, including the use of standard x-rays, should be minimized as much as possible to avoid chromosomal damage and the potential for inducing a malignancy.

Natural Killer Cell Deficiency

Natural killer cells are a population of T cell receptor-negative (CD3−) lymphocytes that are capable of spontaneously killing sensitive target cells such as some tumor cells and virus-infected cells. In 1989 a patient who was completely deficient in natural killer cells was described, and we have recently discovered a second case. These patients have recurrent sinopulmonary infections beginning in infancy. Later in childhood, severe herpesvirus infections develop, including overwhelming varicella with pneumonitis, severe cutaneous herpes simplex virus infections, and generalized CMV infection. In addition, polymicrobial septicemia with both bacterial and fungal organisms occurs.

Pathogenesis

It is not yet clear whether the deficiency of natural killer cells in these patients is inherited or acquired, although family members have normal natural killer cell numbers and function. It is likely that there is a defect in natural killer cell precursors, since incubation of the patients' lymphocytes with IL-2 demonstrates a failure of the normal enhancement in natural killer cell number or function.

Diagnosis

Intermittent leukopenia is noted. Lymphocytes bearing natural killer cell surface determinants (NKH-1, CD16) and mediating natural killer function are absent. T cell and B cell numbers and functions are normal.

Treatment

Intravenous gamma globulin is given to enhance the function of cells mediating antibody dependent cellular cytotoxicity (which include natural killer cells, macrophages, and granulocytes). Replacement of natural killer cells with irradiated allogeneic mononuclear cells was not beneficial in one patient. Bone marrow transplantation may reconstitute this defect, although it has not yet been attempted.

IMMUNODEFICIENCY DUE TO PHAGOCYTIC CELL DEFECTS

Phagocytosis of bacteria is a primary function of polymorphonuclear leukocytes and monocytes. Defects in phagocytosis may be due to abnormalities in the number of circulating (or tissue-associated) phagocytes or to an inability of the phagocytic cells to ingest and kill bacteria. Defects in the ingestion of bacteria are usually due to the lack of opsonins (antibody or complement) or to the lack of receptors on phagocytic cells. Such receptors include the immunoglobulin Fc domain and the low-molecular-weight complement-cleavage products C3b and iC3b. Killing of bacteria following phagocytosis depends on fusion of specific granules with the phagosome, and the subsequent burst in the production of superoxide anion, hydrogen peroxide (H_2O_2), hydroxyl radical, and singlet oxygen. The rapid generation of these high-energy oxygen metabolites is due to the activation of a membrane-bound NADPH-oxidase system that utilizes as an electron carrier a b-type cytochrome unique to phagocytes. In the presence of myeloperoxidase and chloride ion, superoxide and H_2O_2 can damage bacteria by the incorporation of the halide ion into the bacterial cell wall. A defect anywhere along this pathway results in lack of microbicidal activity of the phagocytic cell, with intracellular survival of bacteria and persistent tissue infection.

The majority of primary phagocytic cell functional defects are congenital in nature. Acquired defects such as the neutropenias may be due to decreased bone-marrow cell production (i.e., in bacterial sepsis or by antibodies to neutrophils) or due to increased sequestration of these cells in the spleen (Felty's syndrome).

Quantitative Granulocyte Defects

Neutropenia is defined as an absolute granulocyte count of less than 1,500 per cubic millimeter. Increased susceptibility to infection occurs when the count falls below 1,000 per cubic millimeter. At this level, stomatitis, mucositis, and skin infection are the predominant manifestations. As the absolute granulocyte count falls below 500, patients begin to experience pneumonia, cellulitis, and sepsis due to bacteria and fungi.

Congenital granulocytopenia or agranulocytosis (familial, e.g., Kostman's syndrome, versus sporadic), cyclic neutropenia, and neutropenia associated with phenotypic abnormalities (Schwachman syndrome; Fanconi syndrome) account for the majority of the primary neutropenias. Clinical manifestations may vary from total lack of symptoms to recurrent fever and mucous membrane ulcers, mild infection of the skin, recurrent pulmonary infection, or overwhelming systemic infections. In cyclic neutropenia, these symptoms correspond to the nadir of the peripheral granulocyte count, which occurs at 14- to 35-day intervals. The diagnosis of cyclic neutropenia is established by performing serial white blood cell and differential counts, twice weekly, for 4 to 6 weeks. Bone marrow cytology may help differentiate various forms of granulocytopenias associated with aplasia or maturation arrest. Suspected acute bacterial infection in the neutropenic host should be promptly and aggressively treated with bactericidal antibiotics.

Qualitative Granulocyte Defects

Chronic Granulomatous Disease

This is an uncommon inherited disorder in which phagocytic cells fail to produce antimicrobial oxidants. Both X-linked and autosomal recessive inheritance patterns occur. Clinical manifestations of classical chronic granulomatous disease (CGD) appear in infancy and include recurrent infections such as otitis, draining lym-

phadenitis, hepatosplenomegaly, pneumonia, abscess formation, and osteomyelitis due to catalase-positive bacteria and fungi. Variant forms of the disease with a milder clinical course and presentation at a later age have been described.

Pathophysiology. The defect in activation of the PMN oxidase system in the majority of patients with CGD is associated with a complete deficiency of spectrally detected neutrophil cytochrome b. Between different kindreds the specific genetic defects are heterogeneous. Variant X-linked CGD patients have been described who have low but detectable levels of superoxide generation and low levels of mRNA encoding the 90-kDa subunit of the cytochrome b. Variants of CGD and the putative genetic defect are listed in Table 11.

Each of these defects ultimately leads to a deficiency in the neutrophil's ability to generate superoxide, H_2O_2, singlet oxygen, and other high-energy oxygen species. Thus bacteria ingested by phagocytic cells are not killed because of the lack of the superoxide and H_2O_2 needed for the formation of the bactericidal complex. This may explain why the majority of infections in patients with CGD are due to catalase-producing bacteria such as *S. aureus* and *S. epidermidis*, *Serratia marcescens*, *Escherichia coli*, *Pseudomonas* species, *Candida* species, and *Aspergillus* species. These organisms are usually not pathogenic to normal individuals. In contrast, bacteria that are catalase-negative, such as the pneumococcus and streptococcus, only rarely cause infections in patients with CGD, probably because they cannot metabolize their own endogenously produced H_2O_2 and are therefore killed within the phagosome of CGD patients.

Clinical Manifestations. Onset of recurrent and chronic infections in affected children usually starts before the age of 2 years; however, delayed onset of infections is described in variant forms of CGD. Pneumonia and/or lung abscess is present at some time in nearly all patients. Chronic skin infections and persistent, draining adenitis are also common. Generalized lymph node enlargement is seen, together with hepatosplenomegaly and hepatic abscesses. Infections of the lung and bone can be acute or chronic. Abscesses and granulomata may be seen in virtually any organ. Serious infections are often associated with only mild systemic symptoms. Skin infections and subcutaneous abscesses may have minimal erythema and induration. Chronic otitis media and otitis

TABLE 11 Variants of Chronic Granulomatous Disease

CGD Subtype	Cytochrome b	Putative Gene Defect
X−	Absent; very low	Heterogeneous, some RNA defects
X+	Normal or low	90-kDa subunit; missense
A−	Absent or very low	22-kDa cytochrome b subunit; heterogeneous
A+	Normal	Possible cytostolic factor defect
CGD with McLeod or DMD	Absent	Deletion of 90-kDa cytochrome b subunit gene

externa, stomatitis, and perianal abscesses are also encountered.

Diagnosis. A simple screening test is the determination of nitroblue tetrazolium (NBT) dye reduction by polymorphonuclear leukocytes. If NBT reduction is decreased or absent, the diagnosis should be confirmed by a more specific assay of superoxide production.

Treatment. Antibiotic prophylaxis using TMP-SMZ or dicloxacillin has been shown to decrease markedly the incidence of life-threatening bacterial infection in patients with CGD. Acute infections should be treated promptly with broad-spectrum, bactericidal antibiotics given systemically and usually parenterally. A semisynthetic penicillin and aminoglycoside are started empirically. Antibiotics are selectively adjusted when an organism is isolated and its sensitivity is determined. Chloramphenicol and rifampin have been favored by some as empiric initial antibiotics because of their capacity to achieve high intracellular concentrations. Amphotericin should be administered when fungal infections are encountered; if *Aspergillus* is isolated in patients with chronic lung disease, amphotericin plus rifampin is recommended. Prolonged therapy (4 to 6 weeks) is advisable for bacterial and fungal infections in these patients.

Recently, it has been shown that interferon-gamma augments the superoxide production of phagocytic cells. Preliminary in vitro studies in patients with variant X-linked CGD have shown a dramatic partial correction of the defect in superoxide generation. Thus, interferon-gamma is promising as a potential therapy in selected patients with CGD.

Granulocyte Deficiency of Other Metabolic Enzymes

Patients with granulocyte dysfunction due to deficiency of other metabolic enzymes have been described. These include deficiency of glucose-6-phosphate dehydrogenase (G6PD), myeloperoxidase, glutathione reductase, alpha-mannosidase, and leukocyte alkaline phosphatase. The bactericidal activity of the leukocytes of these patients may be only slightly decreased or totally absent, such as with G6PD . The latter defect, which is inherited as an X-linked deficiency, produces clinical manifestations similar to chronic granulomatous disease.

Chediak-Higashi Syndrome

This rare syndrome is characterized by the presence of giant cytoplasmic granules in white blood cells, red blood cells, fibroblasts, and platelets. It is inherited in an autosomal recessive manner. The clinical manifestations consist of recurrent bacterial infections, partial albinism, photophobia, nystagmus, hepatosplenomegaly, neurologic changes, anemia and leukopenia, along with a high incidence of lymphoreticular malignancies. There is defective chemotaxis and delayed but not absent intracellular killing of all bacteria by phagocytes. Hexose monophosphate shunt activity and H_2O_2 production is normal. Granulocyte lysosomal enzyme levels are abnormal, and degranulation is very abnormal with failure of the giant lysosomes to rupture into phagocytic vacuoles. Some patients may benefit from ascorbate therapy.

TABLE 12 Complement Deficiencies

Deficiency	Clinical Findings
C1q	SLE; urticaria; vasculitis; X-linked agammaglobulinemia; and severe CID
C1r	SLE syndrome; glomerulonephritis
C1s	SLE
C1 inhibitor	Hereditary angioedema; SLE
C4	SLE syndrome; IgA nephropathy; Henoch-Schoenlein purpura
C2	SLE syndrome; glomerulonephritis; vasculitis, dermatomyositis, Henoch-Schoenlein purpura; recurrent pneumococcal infection
C3	Pyogenic infections
Factor I (C3b Inactivator)	Pyogenic infections
Factor P	Pyogenic infections
Factor D	Pyogenic infections
C5	Neisserial infections; SLE syndrome
C6	Neisserial infections; Raynaud's phenomenon; sclerodactyly; ankylosing spondylitis; vasculitis; glomerulonephritis
C7	Neisserial infections; SLE; scleroderma, spondylitis
C8	Neisserial infections; SLE syndrome
C9	Usually normal; some neisserial infections

SLE = systemic lupus erythematosus

Disorders in Leukocyte Adherence and Mobility

Patients with leukocyte adhesion deficiency, or iC3b receptor deficiency, have defective leukocyte adherence, migration, and chemotaxis. The leukocytes of these patients lack both the alpha and beta subunits of the iC3b receptor, although the fundamental defect in many of these patients (those with LFA-1, Mac-1, and p150,95 deficiency) appears to involve defective synthesis of a common beta chain. The clinical manifestations include delayed separation of the umbilical cord, recurrent bacterial and fungal infections, poor wound healing, and marked periodontitis, with inability to form pus. Therapy with prophylactic antibiotics is indicated. Bone marrow transplantation can be curative.

Patients with congenital deficiency of neutrophil specific granules all have recurrent bacterial infections, including recurrent skin abscesses and progressive pulmonary disease. Azurophilic granules are present and PMN nuclei are bilobed. Specific granule products, such as cytochrome b, lactoferrin, and vitamin B_{12} binding protein, are absent. Chemotaxis is markedly impaired, and PMN respiratory burst is abnormal to certain stimuli.

COMPLEMENT DEFICIENCIES

Deficiencies for most of the human complement proteins have now been described. A summary of the inherited complement deficiencies is presented in Table 12. Deficiency of the early complement components is frequently associated with recurrent pyogenic infections or rheumatologic disorders, whereas deficiency of late components (C5 to C9) is associated with recurrent (neisserial) infections.

Deficiency of C1 inhibitor, the regulatory protein for C1 activation, leads to hereditary angioedema. Patients present with localized swelling and angioedema involving the subcutaneous tissue, the respiratory tract, and the gastrointestinal tract. These episodes may be severe enough to disfigure and may result in laryngeal edema and asphyxia. It is inherited in an autosomal dominant fashion, whereas most other complement factor deficiencies are inherited in autosomal codominant manner (heterozygotes have approximately one-half of the normal serum level). Two variants of hereditary angioedema are recognized: 85 percent of patients have very low or absent C1 inactivator protein (type I), and the other 15 per-

cent have a structurally abnormal, functionally inactive protein that is present in normal quantities (type II). Diagnosis is confirmed by finding low levels and/or function of C1 inhibitor. The patient may also have low C4 levels. During attacks of angioedema both C2 and C4 are further decreased. Treatment with impeded androgens (e.g., danazol) can prevent attacks of angioedema and may increase both the level and functional activity of C1 inactivator and C4. Purified human C1 inactivator is available for intravenous administration during acute severe attacks.

Deficiency of C2 is the most common complement deficiency. A lupus-like disease occurs in about 40 percent of patients. Other patients present with other collagen vascular diseases such as rheumatoid arthritis, Henoch-Schoenlein purpura, dermatomyositis, Crohn's disease, cutaneous vasculitis, or membranoproliferative glomerulonephritis. In addition some patients have had recurrent infections, frequently due to *S. pneumoniae, H. influenzae,* or *Neisseria meningitidis.*

Treatment of C2 deficiency as well as other complement component deficiencies is directed toward therapy of the associated autoimmune or collagen-vascular disorder. Antibiotics are given as indicated for specific infectious illnesses.

SUGGESTED READING

Barrett DJ, Ammann AJ, Waru DW, et al. Clinical and immunologic spectrum of the DiGeorge syndrome. J Clin Lab Immunol 1981; 6:1.

Cunningham-Rundles C. Clinical and immunologic analyses of 103 patients with common variable immunodeficiency. J Clin Immunol 1989; 9:22.

Ezekowitz RA, Newburger PE. New perspectives in chronic granulomatous disease. J Clin Immunol 1988; 8:419.

Lederman HM, Winkelstein JA. X-linked agammaglobulinemia: an analysis of 96 patients. Medicine 1985; 64:145

Moen RC, Horowitz SD, Sondel PM, et al. Immunologic reconstitution after haploidentical bone marrow transplantation for immune deficiency disorders. Blood 1987; 70:664.

Mouy R, Fischer A, Vilmer E, et al. Incidence, severity, and prevention of infections in chronic granulomatous disease. J Pediatr 1989; 114:555.

Ostrer H, Hejtmancik JF. Prenatal diagnosis and carrier detection of genetic diseases by analysis of deoxyribonucleic acid. J Pediatr 1988; 112:679.

Rosen FS, Cooper MD, Wedgwood RJP. The primary immunodeficiencies. N Engl J Med 1984; 311:235.

Schur PH. Inherited complement component abnormalities. Ann Rev Med 1986; 37:333.

Stiehm ER, ed. Immunologic disorders in infants and children. 3rd ed. Philadelphia: WB Saunders, 1989.

CHILDHOOD EXANTHEMS

ANNE A. GERSHON, M.D.

MEASLES AND RUBELLA

Measles and rubella have become uncommon diseases in many developed countries today owing to widespread use

of live attenuated measles and rubella vaccines introduced in 1963 and 1969, respectively. Perhaps because of the emphasis on prevention, specific antiviral therapy has never been developed for these diseases. Treatment for both thus remains symptomatic only and would include an antipyretic if indicated. Aspirin may be used to treat arthritis that often accompanies rubella in the adult. The cough of measles can be troublesome, but cough suppressants should be avoided. Prophylactic antibiotics are not indicated for either disease. Bacterial superinfections following measles, such as pneumonia and otitis media, are common, and if a superinfection has developed, it should be promptly treated with antimicrobials.

Because measles and rubella are so uncommon, it is useful to discuss diagnosis. Measles resembles a severe upper respiratory infection, such as influenza, during the first few days, with fever, cough, and coryza with no skin manifestations. Just prior to the development of rash, Koplik's spots, the pathognomonic enanthem of measles, may be seen on the buccal mucosa, usually opposite the molar teeth. The rash, which is morbilliform and then becomes confluent, begins on the face and moves down the body. Not all cases of measles fit the classic description, and since many younger physicians are unfamiliar with the disease, it is best to confirm the diagnosis serologically. To do this, 5 to 10 ml of clotted blood should be obtained as early as possible in the illness and again after 10 to 14 days. A fourfold or greater rise in serum antibody titer is, as with other viral infections, considered diagnostic. Both sera must be run simultaneously for accurate interpretation of the results.

Rubella is a milder illness than measles; as many as half the cases are subclinical. The major symptoms are a maculopapular rash, low grade fever, and cervical lymphadenopathy. Other illnesses may mimic rubella, so that the diagnosis should also be made serologically. It is particularly important to make the correct diagnosis if a woman in the first trimester of pregnancy either is the patient or has been exposed to the patient.

Congenital rubella has become a rare disease in the United States, but at one time it was a major cause of fetal malformations. The decrease in incidence of congenital rubella has been attributed to improvements in diagnostic procedures, abortion policies, and live attenuated rubella vaccine. No cases of the congenital rubella syndrome as a result of inadvertent vaccination of a pregnant woman have been reported, although the vaccine virus may reach and cross the placenta. Women who have been immunized inadvertently while pregnant require careful counseling. Although at one time abortion was considered mandatory, the fetal risk appears to be so small (1.4 percent or less) that each situation should be judged independently.

The best indication of immunity to rubella today is a history of receipt of live attenuated vaccine in the past. Standard serologic tests are often not sensitive enough to identify all immunes. To be safe, women of childbearing years who require immunization should refrain from becoming pregnant for at least 3 months after vaccination.

Measles, unlike rubella, poses a risk for susceptible immunocompromised patients, particularly those deficient in cellular immunity. Since measles vaccine is usually administered at 15 months of age, a situation of risk rarely arises. When there is a potential problem, however, immune serum globulin (ISG), 0.25 to 0.5 ml per kilogram intramuscularly, should be administered to the patient as soon as possible after the exposure. Neither measles nor rubella vaccine should be administered to immunocompromised patients. Passive immunization with ISG modifies measles; it does not prevent the congenital rubella syndrome, however, and

therefore ISG is not recommended for rubella susceptible pregnant women who have been exposed to rubella.

Individuals who have received killed measles vaccine in the past are at some risk to develop the atypical measles syndrome if they are exposed to wild measles. This hypersensitivity reaction may on occasion be more severe than measles itself. Killed measles vaccine has not been available since 1968, so that persons born after that time cannot be at risk. As of 1987, the Centers for Disease Control recommends that persons who received killed vaccine in the past be reimmunized with live vaccine, although fever and sore arm may develop. These risks would seem to outweigh the risks of developing atypical measles.

Most index cases of measles in the United States are "imported" and may be the source of mini-outbreaks in unvaccinated persons. When normal, previously unvaccinated individuals have been exposed, ISG, 0.25 mg per kilogram intramuscularly, should be administered promptly.

VARICELLA

Varicella (chickenpox) and zoster are both caused by varicella-zoster (VZ) virus. Varicella is the primary infection; zoster results when latent VZ virus acquired as a result of varicella is reactivated. A vesicular skin rash is characteristic of each illness, that of varicella being generalized and zoster localized. Low-grade to moderate fever may also occur. The rash of varicella is characteristically itchy and that of zoster painful. Both diseases are usually self-limited and rarely require more than symptomatic therapy.

Immunosuppressed patients are at risk to develop severe or fatal varicella with dissemination of the virus to lungs, brain, and liver. Adults who contract varicella and newborn infants whose mothers have developed chickenpox in the 5 days before or 2 days after delivery are also at some increased risk. Passive immunization with varicella-zoster immune globulin (VZIG) can clearly modify the course of varicella. Following an intimate exposure to the virus, VZIG should be administered to varicella-susceptible, immunocompromised individuals as soon as possible (within 3 days) or, in the case of infants, at birth. An intramuscular dose of 1.25 ml (125 units) per 10 kg is used, with a maximum of five vials (625 units). Adults, including pregnant women, should be passively immunized only if they are serologically proven to be susceptible to varicella, because most adults with no history of varicella are actually immune. VZIG, which contains about 20 times the amount of VZ antibody as ISG, may be obtained through local branches of the American Red Cross. VZIG is not effective for prevention of zoster in patients at high risk to develop the disease.

Pregnant women who contract varicella or zoster are at some increased risk to deliver a malformed fetus. The so-called congenital varicella syndrome, with eye, central nervous system, and limb defects, is so rare, however, that most experts do not advise mandatory interruption of pregnancy after maternal VZ infection. It is a situation that requires careful weighing of the potential risks and benefits to the family involved.

Once varicella or zoster has developed, VZIG is of no therapeutic value. The antiviral drug acyclovir (ACV) has been employed successfully to treat VZ infections. ACV must be phosphorylated by a thymidine kinase present only in virus-infected cells in order to interfere with DNA synthesis. Therefore, ACV has little effect on host DNA synthesis, and it is less toxic for the host than is adenine arabinoside (Ara-A), which was formerly employed. ACV is available in topical, oral, and intravenous formulations. Topical ACV is of no use for treatment of VZ infections. Orally administered ACV has been used successfully in high dosage (800 mg five times per day orally for 10 days) to treat immunocompetent patients with zoster, particularly those with ocular involvement. There are some indications that in addition to decreasing acute pain there may be a reduced incidence of posttherapeutic pain as well. For immunocompromised patients and those with varicella or severe zoster, intravenous therapy is preferred. A dose of 1,500 mg per square meter per day, divided in three doses, or 10 mg per kilogram every 8 hours is suggested if renal function is normal. Lower doses should be employed in the face of renal insufficiency. This is higher than the dose usually employed for herpes simplex viral infections. The duration of therapy is dependent upon the condition of the patient; usually a week to 10 days is adequate. Toxicity is limited to phlebitis and transient increases in serum creatinine levels.

Treatment with an antiviral should begin within 3 days of onset of VZ infection for best results. Whether or not to institute antiviral chemotherapy is often a difficult decision. In many instances the illness does not become severe until a week after onset, and at that time it may be too late to institute successful therapy. The question frequently asked is whether one ought to treat all immunosuppressed patients who develop varicella or zoster. Treatment is usually recommended for varicella in immunocompromised patients who have not been passively immunized. It is wise to treat before the illness becomes severe. For zoster, no general recommendations can be given, and the decision must be made on an individual basis. It would seem prudent to be liberal in the use of antivirals in patients thought to be highly immunocompromised. It is not considered necessary to study individuals with zoster for occult malignancy. An antiviral should be used to treat primary VZ pneumonia, which may be seen in the immunocompromised patient and occasionally in an otherwise normal adult who contracts varicella. An antiviral is of questionable use for varicella encephalitis, and it is not clear whether it is of benefit in treating encephalitis that may accompany zoster. The diagnosis of VZ encephalitis may be made by demonstrating antibody to VZ virus in cerebrospinal fluid.

Bacterial superinfections may follow varicella and should be suspected if there is a resurgence of fever or suspicious skin lesions, especially during convalescence from the illness. Prophylactic antibiotics, however, are not indicated. Superinfections are likely to be due to staphylococci or group A β-hemolytic streptococci. Reye's syndrome rarely may follow varicella in children. Since there is increasing evidence that aspirin may also be somehow related to development of Reye's syndrome, it is recommended to refrain from treating the fever of varicella with aspirin in children under 18 years of age.

A live attenuated varicella vaccine is currently being studied for prevention of varicella. It has been highly effective in normal children, adults, and immunocompromised children. It is currently under consideration for licensure in the United States.

SUGGESTED READING

Centers for Disease Control. ACIP:Measles prevention. MMWR 1987; 36:409–425.
Centers for Disease Control. Rubella vaccination during pregnancy. MMWR 1987; 36:457–461.
Leitman PS, Fiddian P, Chapman SK, eds. Symposium on antivirals. Am J Med 1988; 85(2A)1–213.
Markowitz L, Preblud S, Orenstein W, et al. Patterns of transmission of measles outbreaks in the US, 1985–1986. N Engl J Med 1989; 320:75–81.
Straus S. The management of varicella and zoster infections. Infect Dis Clin North Am 1987; 1:367–382.

KAWASAKI SYNDROME

JANE C. BURNS, M.D.

Kawasaki syndrome is an acute vasculitis of unknown etiology that occurs predominantly in infants and young children. The syndrome is characterized by a constellation of clinical findings that include persistent fever, rash, bilateral nonexudative conjunctivitis, cervical lymphadenopathy, edema and erythema of the extremities, and erythema of the lips and oral mucosa. The most serious complication is damage to the coronary arteries, which results in aneurysms or ectasia in 15 to 25 percent of children with the disease. Myocardial infarction, sudden death, or chronic coronary or valvular insufficiency may ensue. Kawasaki syndrome is currently the leading cause of acquired heart disease in children in the United States.

EPIDEMIOLOGY

The syndrome was first described by Tomisaku Kawasaki in Japanese children in 1967 and has now been reported throughout the world and can occur in all racial groups. As of the end of 1984, more than 60,000 patients with the syndrome had been recognized in Japan. Annual rates for the United States are gathered through a passive reporting system and therefore underestimate the true occurrence of the disease. Data from the Centers for Disease Control suggest that there are at least 3,000 to 4,000 cases per year in the United States and that the syndrome is most common in Orientals, intermediate in blacks, and least common in Caucasians.

The peak age incidence is during the second year of life, with 85 percent of cases occurring in children under 5 years of age. Boys are affected 1.5 times more frequently than girls. The disease occurs both sporadically and in community-wide outbreaks that are most common in the winter and spring months.

Although the clinical features and course of the disease and the seasonality suggest an infectious agent, investigation of outbreaks has failed to yield an etiologic agent. An association between exposure to freshly cleaned carpets and the onset of Kawasaki syndrome in the subsequent 2 weeks has been noted. Residence near a body of standing water has also been identified as a risk factor in some epidemiologic investigations. Cultures and serology for a variety of bacteria, rickettsiae, spirochetes, chlamydiae, and viruses have been negative. A possible retroviral etiology for Kawasaki syndrome has been suggested by the association of reverse transcriptase activity with cultured peripheral blood mononuclear cells from Kawasaki patients but not controls. There is no evidence of person-to-person spread of clinically overt disease. In Japan, Kawasaki syndrome is reported to recur in 3.9 percent of patients, and the attack rate among siblings is 1.4 percent. The case-fatality rate in Japan is 0.3 percent and is exclusively due to cardiac complications of the disease.

PATHOPHYSIOLOGY

The most significant vessel inflammation in Kawasaki syndrome occurs in medium-sized, extraparenchymal muscular arteries. Although the disease process may involve the microvasculature initially, the long-term sequelae are related to damage that occurs in these medium-sized vessels, particularly the coronary arterial bed. There may be an associated myocarditis, pericarditis, inflammation of the atrioventricular conduction system, and endocarditis. Although the coronary arteries are universally involved in autopsy cases, aneurysms and ectasia have also been noted in the femoral, iliac, renal, hepatic, axillary, and brachial arteries.

CLINICAL ASPECTS

The diagnosis of Kawasaki disease is entirely based on clinical criteria. As outlined by Dr. Kawasaki, the patient must have fever lasting more than 5 days without other cause, accompanied by the following features: (1) bilateral, nonexudative conjunctivitis; (2) at least one change in the mouth, including red, fissured lips, red oral mucosa without discrete lesions, or prominent fungiform papillae on the tongue with loss of the filiform papillae (strawberry tongue); (3) cervical lymphadenopathy of more than 1.5 cm; (4) at least one change in the extremities, including red palms and soles, swelling of the dorsa of the hands and feet, or

periungual desquamation in the early convalescent period; and (5) a polymorphous exanthem. These signs of systemic inflammation may be accompanied by aseptic meningitis, hydrops of the gallbladder, arthritis, anterior uveitis, and urethritis. Virtually all patients have some element of myocarditis although this problem may not be clinically apparent. Without treatment, the fever lasts from 5 to 21 days, with a mean of 11 days. Laboratory parameters of inflammation persist well beyond the period of acute systemic illness. Coronary artery aneurysms and ectasia first become evident by echocardiogram in the second week after onset of fever. Roughly 50 percent of these coronary artery abnormalities will resolve, as assessed by angiography during the first year after onset of the disease. These vessels, however, are persistently abnormal because of the scarring and fibrosis in the vessel wall. The long-term cardiac sequelae have not yet been adequately assessed.

DIFFERENTIAL DIAGNOSIS

Kawasaki disease must be differentiated from other rash and fever illnesses of infancy and early childhood. The disease shares many common features with streptococcal and staphylococcal toxin-mediated diseases, viral illnesses (adenovirus, enterovirus, and measles infection), and Stevens-Johnson syndrome. A slit lamp examination for anterior uveitis by a pediatric ophthalmologist and an echocardiogram to detect subclinical myocarditis may be useful in differentiating Kawasaki syndrome from these other illnesses.

Evaluation of the patient suspected of having acute Kawasaki syndrome is delineated in Figure 1.

LABORATORY FINDINGS

There is no single laboratory test that is diagnostic of Kawasaki syndrome. The laboratory profile is one of a systemic acute-phase response with an elevated white blood cell count with left shift, a normocytic, normochromic anemia, thrombocytosis that peaks by the third to fourth week of illness, an elevated erythrocyte sedimentation rate, and elevated C-reactive protein and α-1-antitrypsin. Mild elevation of hepatic transaminases is common, and a biochemical profile of cholestasis may accompany hydrops of the gallbladder. A mild cerebrospinal fluid (CSF) pleocytosis with occasional neutrophils may be present. The CSF protein and glucose levels are usually normal. Sterile pyuria with predominantly mononuclear cells is common; this finding will be missed if standard dipstick methods are employed to screen for white cells, as these tests detect only polymorphonuclear neutrophils.

THERAPY

Clinical trials executed in the United States and Japan have established intravenous gamma globulin in conjunction with aspirin as the treatment of choice for patients with Kawasaki syndrome who are diagnosed within the first 10 days after onset of fever. In the U.S. multicenter trial of intravenous gamma globulin (400 mg per kilogram daily

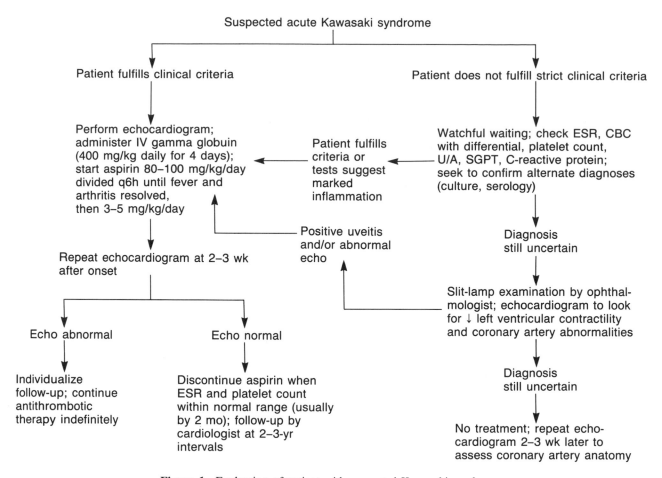

Figure 1 Evaluation of patient with suspected Kawasaki syndrome.

for 4 days) plus aspirin (80 to 100 mg per kilogram per day through the 14th day of illness, then 3 to 5 mg per kilogram per day until evaluation of coronary arteries is complete) compared to aspirin alone, the prevalence of coronary artery abnormalities at 7 weeks after onset of illness was 18 percent (14 of 79 patients) in the aspirin alone group versus 4 percent (three of 79 patients) in the group treated with intravenous gamma globulin plus aspirin. No patient suffered serious adverse effects from receiving gamma globulin. No formal comparison of different preparations of gamma globulin has been undertaken. Until the mechanism of action is better understood, there is no rational basis for choosing among the currently available commercial preparations of gamma globulin for intravenous administration. Studies are currently in progress to compare the 4-day regimen with a single infusion of 2 g per kilogram of gamma globulin. Until these data are analyzed, we recommend the use of intravenous gamma globulin at a total dose of 1.6 g per kilogram (400 mg per kilogram daily for 4 days) in conjunction with high-dose aspirin (80 to 100 mg per kilogram per day divided every 6 hours) to be initiated as soon as the diagnosis is secure and preferably within the first 7 days of illness. Aspirin at this dose should be continued until the fever and arthritis have resolved. Patients should then continue on low-dose aspirin (3 to 5 mg per kilogram per day) for the antiplatelet effect until evaluation

of the coronary arteries is completed and the sedimentation rate and platelet count have returned to normal (usually 2 months into the illness). Use of gamma globulin therapy beyond 10 days after onset of fever has not been studied. It is our practice to treat any patient with Kawasaki disease who has persistent clinical signs of continued inflammation such as fever and rash regardless of the day of illness at presentation. Some patients (fewer than 20 percent) do not respond to treatment or experience recrudescent fever in the 10 days following initiation of intravenous gamma globulin. No data are available to guide in the decision to administer additional gamma globulin to these patients. Gamma globulin treatment results in cessation of fever and rapid overall clinical improvement in the majority of patients within days of starting therapy. The large-joint arthritis that may develop in approximately 35 percent of patients in the second week of illness is ameliorated only slightly by gamma globulin administration. The arthritis may respond to continued high-dose aspirin or addition of a nonsteroidal anti-inflammatory agent.

All patients with suspected Kawasaki syndrome should be evaluated with a complete blood count, differential, erythrocyte sedimentation rate, platelet count, liver transaminase studies, and a urinalysis. Exclusionary serologic studies (e.g., ASLO titer, leptospiral and rickettsial antibodies) and cultures (viral, bacterial) should be obtained when clinically appropriate. A baseline echocardiogram to assess the coronary artery anatomy, left ventricular function, and valvular competence should be performed as soon as the diagnosis is established. An electrocardiogram should also be obtained. These studies should be repeated 2 or 3 weeks into the illness and again at 7 or 8 weeks into the illness. More frequent monitoring is appropriate for patients with coronary artery abnormalities. Aspirin therapy is discontinued at the 8-week visit unless there are coronary artery abnormalities, in which case therapy is continued indefinitely. Addition of other antiplatelet agents, such as dipyridamole and systemic anticoagulation, may be considered in patients with large aneurysms, although there are no clinical data to support this practice. All patients should be followed by a pediatric cardiologist.

The appropriate follow-up for patients with no detectable coronary artery abnormalities has not yet been established. It is our practice to screen all individuals for risk factors for coronary artery disease by assessing the family history for ischemic heart disease and measuring a serum lipid profile in patients and parents at least 2 months after the acute illness. Dietary counseling is provided for families with significant risk factors. We follow patients with no apparent coronary artery lesions every 2 to 3 years with repeat echocardiograms and electrocardiograms. Treadmill testing may be performed when the patient reaches 6 to 7 years of age.

SUGGESTED READING

Kato H, Ichinose E, Kawasaki T. Myocardial infarction in Kawasaki disease: clinical analyses in 195 cases. J Pediatr 1986; 108:923–927.

Kawasaki T, Kosaki F, Okawa S, et al. A new infantile acute febrile mucocutaneous lymph node syndrome prevailing in Japan. Pediatrics 1974; 54:271–276.

Newburger JW, Takahashi M, Burns JC, et al. Treatment of Kawasaki syndrome with intravenous gammaglobulin. N Engl J Med 1986; 315:341–347.

Rowley AH, Gonzalez-Crussi F, Shulman ST. Kawasaki syndrome. Rev Infect Dis 1988; 10:1–14.

TOXIC SHOCK SYNDROME

JEFFREY PARSONNET, M.D.

Despite significant advances in our understanding of the epidemiology, pathogenesis, and treatment of toxic shock syndrome (TSS), this disease continues to strike patients of both sexes, of all ages, and in a variety of clinical settings. TSS remains a clinical diagnosis, defined by the presence of fever, hypotension, rash with late desquamation, and multiple organ system dysfunction. The diagnosis must be made on the basis of clinical criteria alone, without the benefit of diagnostic cultures, antibody titers, or toxicologic studies. The disease is eminently treatable, however, and patients treated early in the course of illness usually recover without sequelae. The burden on the practicing physician is to maintain an awareness of TSS in order to facilitate early recognition, after which options of management are finite and straightforward.

Optimal therapy for TSS is grounded upon an understanding of its epidemiology and pathogenesis, for which reason attention must be directed to these aspects of the disease.

EPIDEMIOLOGY AND PATHOGENESIS

The classic association recognized by most physicians is that between tampon use during menstruation and the development of TSS. This is unfortunate, because it obscures an equally important, and probably more frequent, association between other types of staphylococcal infection and TSS. It is difficult to estimate the relative frequencies with which menstrual and nonmenstrual TSS occur, because of underreporting of the former, underrecognition of the latter, and the absence of a definitive diagnostic test for either. TSS has been reported to occur as a complication of the use of barrier contraceptives, childbirth (by cesarean and vaginal delivery), infections of the upper and lower respiratory tract, infections of prosthetic devices, and a variety of soft tissue and postoperative wound infections. The incidence in men is roughly the same as that in women, if menstrual, postpartum, and contraceptive-associated cases are excluded.

The common denominator in all cases of TSS is infection with a toxin-producing strain of *Staphylococcus aureus* in the absence of protective antibody at the time of infection. In 1981 two groups of investigators independently identified the most common TSS toxin, TSS toxin-1 (TSST-1). Formerly called pyrogenic exotoxin C and staphylococcal enterotoxin F, TSST-1 is now known to cause more than 90 percent of cases of menstrual TSS and about 40 to 60 percent of nonmenstrual cases. Although there is less certainty about what other staphylococcal products cause TSS, it appears that enterotoxins A through E, which heretofore have been recognized only as causing food poisoning, are the most likely candidates to be alternative TSS toxins. This conclusion is based upon the high frequency with which one or several enterotoxins are produced by TSST-1-negative, TSS-associated strains of *S. aureus*, certain biologic properties shared by TSST-1 and the enterotoxins in vitro and in animal models, and serologic data from patients with TSS. Enterotoxin B appears to be the most common TSS toxin among TSST-1-negative strains from cases of nonmenstrual TSS.

Reports of TSS occurring as a consequence of infection with coagulase-negative staphylococci have not been confirmed; only *S. aureus* produces the toxins implicated in TSS, making infection with this organism necessary. The presence of other bacteria, particularly gram-negative bacilli, at sites of infection or mucosal colonization may influence production of toxin or the severity of its effects, but bacteria other than *S. aureus* are not required.

Regardless of the causative toxin, susceptibility to disease correlates with absence of a protective level of antibody to that toxin. The likelihood of an individual having antibody to TSST-1 is a function of age: by age 10 years, about half of all individuals have what is considered to be a protective antibody titer; by age 20, three-quarters of individuals exceed this titer; and by age 30, more than 90 percent of all people are immune. These data suggest that colonization or subclinical infection with TSST-1-producing strains of *S. aureus* is adequate to induce the development of antibody. Antibody to TSST-1 is present at birth (unless the mother is lacking such antibody), making TSS uncommon in infancy. TSS is most common during adolescence, when there is still a relatively large population at risk (by virtue of seronegativity) and health practices come into play that promote infection or enhance production of toxin.

Conditions favoring colonization and infection with toxigenic strains of *S. aureus* have not been identified. At any time, 10 to 20 percent of all individuals are colonized with *S. aureus* at mucosal sites, and about 20 percent of these strains produce TSST-1. On the other hand, factors have been identified that enhance production of TSST-1 at sites of infection; these include an aerobic environment (oxygen being required for production of toxin); a neutral pH; and a low concentration of magnesium ion. The relation of these factors to the development of clinical disease is readily apparent. For example, insertion of a tampon introduces sufficient oxygen to the vagina (which is normally anaerobic) to allow production of TSST-1; vaginal pH, which is acidic in the interval between menses, rises closer to neutrality during menstruation; and certain tampons have been shown to bind magnesium ion, thereby lowering that which is available to the organism to a range that enhances production of TSST-1 in vitro. The relative contribution of each of these factors remains the subject of intense investigation, and the degree to which they apply to nonmenstrual disease and to production of staphylococcal enterotoxins is not known.

Although TSST-1 is potent in its ability to cause disease, it exerts virtually no direct toxicity on human cells. Rather, it appears to act by initiating a cascade of immunologic and nonimmunologic events that centers on binding to and stimulation of mononuclear cells, particularly circulating monocytes and lymphocytes and tissue macrophages. Purified TSST-1 is a potent inducer of interleukin-1 (also known as endogenous pyrogen) production by human monocytes. It also induces production by monocytes of tumor necrosis factor (also known as cachectin), now known to be an important mediator of the lethal effects of endotoxin. Production of these cytokines could account for many of the signs and symptoms of TSS, including fever, shock, and multiple organ system dysfunction, by virtue of direct effects on host cells or by induction of secondary mediators of inflammation. TSST-1 itself is rapidly cleared from the bloodstream when the nidus of infection is removed or drained (which is usually possible) and can be neutralized in vivo by the administration of antibody to the toxin, which may have clinical implications for some patients.

CLINICAL MANIFESTATIONS

The clinical manifestations of TSS are largely encompassed by the case definition, which has remained essentially unchanged over the past decade (Table 1). Fever is invariable. The rash is typically a diffuse, blanching, macular erythroderma, but it may be patchy in distribution. Petechial and papulopustular eruptions have been reported but are distinctly uncommon. The rash is usually present within 48 hours of the onset of illness but may be evanescent and may be mistaken for the flush that may accompany fever. Involvement of the hands and feet is common and is often associated with peripheral edema, which may be severe. Hypotension, defined as a systolic pressure of 90 mm Hg or less or an orthostatic decrease in diastolic pressure of 15 or more mm Hg, is usually present, but a history of orthostatic dizziness or syncope is sufficient to fulfill this criterion. Full-thickness desquamation, especially of the palms, soles, and fingertips, occurs during convalescence, usually 5 to 12 days after onset of illness. (Absence of desquamation at the time of presentation is often mistakenly interpreted as being inconsistent with TSS.) Finally, the diagnosis is contingent on there being "reasonable evidence" for absence of other causes of illness, a criterion satisfied in most cases by a careful epidemiologic history, complete physical examination, and routine cultures, particularly of blood.

TABLE 1   Case Definition of Toxic Shock Syndrome

Fever: temperature $\geq 38.9\,°C$

Rash: typically a diffuse macular erythroderma

Hypotension: systolic blood pressure ≤ 90 mm Hg for adults or below fifth percentile by age for children < 16 yr, orthostatic drop in diastolic blood pressure ≥ 15 mm Hg, orthostatic syncope, or orthostatic dizziness

Multisystem involvement—three or more of the following:
Gastrointestinal: vomiting, diarrhea
Muscular: severe myalgia or CPK $\geq$ twice the upper limit of normal
Mucous membrane: vaginal, oropharyngeal, or conjunctival hyperemia
Renal: BUN or creatinine at least twice the upper limit of normal, or pyuria (≥ 5 leukocytes per high-power field) in the absence of urinary tract infection
Hepatic: total bilirubin or serum transaminase at least twice the upper limit of normal
Hematologic: platelets $\leq 100,000/mm^3$
CNS: disorientation or alterations in consciousness without focal neurologic signs when fever and hypotension are absent

Desquamation: 1–2 weeks after onset of illness

Negative results on the following tests, if obtained; blood, throat, or CSF (blood culture may be positive for *S aureus*); rise in titer to Rocky Mountain spotted fever agent, leptospirosis, or rubeola

From Reingold AL, Hargrett NT, Shands KN, et al. Toxic shock syndrome surveillance in the United States, 1980 to 1981. Ann Intern Med 1982; 96(part 2):875–880.

Multiple organ-system dysfunction is one of the hallmarks of TSS. Table 2 reflects the frequency with which specific symptoms, signs, and laboratory abnormalities have been noted by various authors. Of note is the nonspecific nature of many features of TSS, including the most frequently reported symptoms of myalgia, vomiting, diarrhea, and headache. In addition to demonstrating signs of illness that are integral to the case definition, physical examination usually reveals a toxic-appearing patient with conjunctival and pharyngeal injection (or a "strawberry tongue"), diffuse abdominal tenderness, muscle tenderness, and peripheral edema. Disorders of the central nervous system, particularly disorientation and a depressed level of consciousness, may be disproportionate to the degree of hypotension. In cases of menstruation-related disease, the pelvic examination is most often normal, with no pelvic tenderness, signs of vaginal inflammation, or purulent discharge, although all have been reported. In nonmenstrual TSS, it is common for the usual signs of pyogenic infection to be lacking; infected surgical wounds, for example, often appear remarkably benign, but nonetheless yield toxigenic *S. aureus* upon culture. Typical manifestations of staphylococcal infection of skin and soft tissues may be evident, but subtle infections are more common. This disparity between the mildness of the local inflammatory response and the severity of systemic toxicity, while not universal, can be an important clue to the diagnosis.

Several aspects of multisystem dysfunction are distinctive enough to serve as diagnostic clues. Myalgias are common and may be severe, for which reason the "influenza-like" features of TSS may predominate. The creatine phosphokinase (CPK) level is often elevated and the degree of elevation may be extreme, with resultant myoglobinuria. The author has treated a young woman with menstrual TSS whose CPK level rose as high as 46,000 units per milliliter, despite rapid correction of what had been relatively mild hypotension. Abnormal clotting parameters and thrombocytopenia are common, which may be useful in distinguishing TSS from Kawasaki disease (in which platelets are either normal or increased) and other disorders. Bleeding is uncommon, however. Hypocalcemia is almost invariable, to the extent that a normal calcium value should prompt reconsideration of the diagnosis. Although the mechanism of hypocalcemia is not known, it appears that both ionized and total calcium are depressed, the latter in part because of hypoalbuminemia. Hypomagnesemia probably occurs more commonly than has been recognized, and hypocalcemia may be refractory to therapy until magnesium stores have been repleted. Despite renal insufficiency, hypophosphatemia is also common, which may be another useful clue to the diagnosis.

The most serious complications encountered in TSS are adult respiratory distress syndrome (ARDS) and progressive renal insufficiency, the pathogeneses of which are multifactorial. The severity and duration of hypotension are probably important determinants of whether these complications ensue, making rapid reversal of hypotension imperative. Cases not associated with a removable focus or with infections amenable to surgical drainage may be associated with an increased rate of complications, presumably because of a longer duration of toxemia. Unfortunately, the ultimate course of the disease is unpredictable in its early stages, making close observation obligatory in all but the mildest cases. Invasive monitoring is useful in guiding early resuscitative measures, particularly when use of a vasopressor is being considered. Consumptive coagulopathy is often present at the time of presentation, the pathogenesis of which is unknown. Rhabdomyolysis, possibly related to massive release of interleukin-1, may be present at the time of presentation or develop subsequent to initiation of therapy. Alopecia and loss of fingernails and toenails 2 to 3 months after the acute illness, a late rash, and persistent neuromuscular and neuropsychiatric abnormalities are commonly seen but ultimately resolve without residual deficits.

Recurrent TSS results from persistent colonization with a toxin-producing staphylococcus in the continued absence of antibody. Before the epidemiology and pathogenesis of menstrual TSS had been elucidated, recurrence rates as high as 66 percent were seen among women who continued to use tampons and were not treated with an antistaphylococcal agent. Some women have a brisk antibody response following an episode of menstrual TSS and are thereby protected from recurrent disease. Unfortunately, some women do not develop protective antibody for several months, and a num-

TABLE 2 Clinical Manifestations and Laboratory Abnormalities in Toxic Shock Syndrome

	Estimated Frequency of Occurrence (%)
Symptoms*	
Myalgia	92
Vomiting	90
Diarrhea	86
Headache	72
Dizziness	70
Sore throat	65
Signs†	
Abdominal tenderness	83
Pharyngitis/strawberry tongue	81
Peripheral edema	73
Conjunctivitis	65
CNS dysfunction	60
Vaginal inflammation	47
Laboratory abnormalities	
Anemia (within first 24 hours)	66
Leukocytosis	70
Thrombocytopenia	52
Increased prothrombin time	70
Increased partial thromboplastin time	43
Increased BUN	68
Increased serum creatinine	69
Increased SGOT	73
Increased total bilirubin	66
Increased CPK	66
Hypocalcemia	80
Hypophosphatemia	60
Hypoalbuminemia	81
Pyuria	77
Hematuria	46

The data are compiled from six reviews of clinical manifestations of TSS.
* Other reported symptoms: chills, cough, dyspnea, arthralgia, abdominal pain, vaginal discharge.
† All patients fulfilled criteria of fever, hypotension, rash, and desquamation. Other reported signs: joint effusion, meningismus, muscle tenderness.

ber have been shown to be antibody-negative a year or more after the first episode (during which time they may have had multiple recurrences). The reasons for this variability are not certain, but failure to develop antibody does not appear to have a hereditary basis nor does it signify a more general immunodeficiency state. As a potent immunomodulator, TSST-1 may actually suppress development of antibody to itself under some circumstances. For reasons that are unclear, recurrent nonmenstrual TSS is uncommon. Regardless of the clinical setting, the risk of recurrence can be determined and influenced by diagnostic and therapeutic measures, as discussed below.

DIAGNOSIS

The diagnosis of TSS is supported by laboratory studies performed at the time of presentation showing evidence of multiple organ–system dysfunction. Routine hematologic and chemistry profiles are usually sufficient for this purpose. For diagnostic purposes, particular attention should be directed to the platelet count; prothrombin time; urinalysis (microscopic and dipstick examinations); tests of renal and hepatic function; serum calcium, magnesium, and phosphate; and CPK—the sum of which often paints the distinctive picture of this syndrome. These data may also have important therapeutic implications for initial management, particularly the coagulation profile, serum electrolytes, and renal parameters. A chest radiograph and electrocardiogram should be performed. Routine cultures of blood and urine, as well as of other appropriate sites (such as the genital tract, throat, respiratory secretions, wounds, or other skin lesions) should be obtained. The isolation of S aureus is not an official criterion for diagnosing TSS, but failure to do so should prompt reconsideration of the diagnosis, unless there are mitigating circumstances. There are three reasons why S. aureus may not be cultured from a patient with TSS: first, the organism may be overgrown in culture by other organisms, which are often present in abundance; second, TSS-associated strains of S. aureus may be misidentified as coagulase-negative staphylococci because they are often not β-hemolytic or pigmented; and third, S. aureus may not be sought until after initiation of antimicrobial therapy.

Specialized tests related to detection of TSS toxins and antibody to these toxins are available and can serve three general purposes: first, to support or oppose the diagnosis of TSS in the acute setting, thereby guiding initial management; second, to establish the diagnosis with greater certainty after resolution of the acute process; and third, to provide guidelines for the patient and physician as to the risk of recurrence and the safety of contraceptive and catamenial product use. Such tests are performed by several clinical and research laboratories around the country, including the author's (Channing Laboratory, 180 Longwood Avenue, Boston, MA 02115). Three studies have proved to be of particular utility in the management of patients:

1. Testing for production of toxin by incriminated strains of S. aureus. This is especially useful in menstrual TSS, most cases of which are caused by TSST-1, making routine testing advisable. The finding of a TSST-1-positive strain of S. aureus in the setting of a compatible clinical illness is moderately supportive of the diagnosis.

2. Testing of acute serum for antibody to TSST-1. This test is also of greater utility in the setting of menstrual illness, in which a low antibody level indicates susceptibility to TSST-1 and a high titer connotes immunity. Some cases of menstrual and many cases of nonmenstrual TSS are caused by other toxins, however, again relegating this analysis to a supportive but nondiagnostic role.

3. Testing of convalescent serum for antibody to TSST-1. When paired with an acute serum sample, this test is of diagnostic utility if seroconversion to TSST-1 (or one of the enterotoxins) is demonstrated. The prognostic and therapeutic implications with regard to the risk of recurrence, and prevention of same, are readily apparent. It is appropriate to obtain a convalescent sample for testing 1 month after the acute illness and thereafter at monthly intervals if necessary.

Some laboratories may also be able to measure TSST-1 in serum and urine samples obtained during the acute illness. These studies (which remain investigational) are of potential diagnostic utility, particularly if arrangements can be made to obtain results quickly. It should be emphasized, however, that the diagnosis of TSS must still be made on clinical grounds and that the greatest utility of specialized testing is to assist the physician in counseling the patient about the risk of recurrence.

The differential diagnosis of TSS includes a large number of disease entities, especially if one considers all illnesses characterized primarily by fever and rash. Many such diagnoses can be effectively ruled out by a careful history, physical examination, and routine laboratory studies. Of prime consideration at the time of initial evaluation are the patient's age, the gynecologic history (including use of tampons and contraceptives), any unusual epidemiologic features, the presence of a possible focus of staphylococcal infection, and, of course, fulfillment of the diagnostic criteria of high fever, rash, hypotension, and multisystem disease. In most instances, these factors will narrow the differential diagnosis to a short list of disease entities (Table 3).

Differentiating between TSS and Kawasaki disease in young children can be difficult, particularly within 24 hours of admission. Like TSS, Kawasaki disease is diagnosed on the basis of clinical criteria, and these criteria are similar in many respects to those of TSS. In the author's experience, the presence of a lesion that could be infected with S. aureus (such as a recent burn, wound, or other skin lesion), the pace of the illness, the nature of the rash, the platelet count, and the serum calcium level are useful discriminating parameters in the acute setting. It is not uncommon, however, for patients to be treated for both illnesses while cultures and results of special studies are pending.

Streptococcus pyogenes (group A streptococcus), the etiologic agent of scarlet fever, can cause an illness that is virtually indistinguishable from staphylococcal TSS. This illness, which is mediated principally by streptococcal pyrogenic toxin A, appears to have been increasing in frequency over the past several years. In the author's experience, staphylococcal TSS in children tends to be milder than in adults, thus mimicking scarlet fever, whereas streptococcal infections in adults involving toxigenic strains may be every bit as severe as staphylococcal TSS. It is prudent, therefore,

TABLE 3 Differential Diagnosis of Toxic Shock Syndrome at the Time of Presentation

Disease	Comments
Kawasaki disease	Can closely resemble TSS in young children. Uncommon in individuals aged >4 yr. More of a subacute illness, with fever ≥5 days required for diagnosis. Swollen, fissured lips, prominent polymorphous rash, adenopathy, cardiac involvement, normal serum calcium level and platelet count, and absence of hypotension may help distinguish from TSS.
Scarlet fever	Exudative pharyngitis (rarely seen in TSS) suggests streptococcal infection. Rash prominent, less evanescent. Severe forms of scarlet fever ("septic scarlet fever," "toxic scarlet fever," "toxic strep syndrome") can be indistinguishable from TSS on clinical grounds.
Staphylococcal scalded skin syndrome	Exudative, bullous lesions with sloughing of skin in acute setting. Leaves extensive denuded areas that are red, raw, and wet. Positive Nikolsky sign (wrinkling of skin in response to gentle friction). Absence of multisystem disease.
Septic shock	Must be considered, for sake of empiric antibiotic coverage, unless clinical setting is classic for TSS or staphylococcal infection is evident (e.g., by Gram stain).
Rocky Mountain spotted fever	Merits consideration because of severe consequences of withholding therapy. Usually distinguishable on epidemiologic grounds or by nature of rash.
Meningococcemia	Merits consideration because of severe consequences of withholding therapy. Petechiae and purpura are uncommon in TSS, but maculopapular eruptions are occasionally seen in meningococcemia.
Viral illness with exanthem	Hypotension uncommon unless patient severely dehydrated.
Drug reactions	Careful history required. May be superimposed on viral or bacterial infection, making distinction from TSS difficult.

to culture appropriate sites for *S. pyogenes* if staphylococcal infection is not apparent at the time of presentation.

TREATMENT

Regardless of the clinical setting, the critical therapeutic measures in TSS are (1) removal of any nidus of infection or surgical drainage of pus; (2) administration of intravenous fluids (the requirements for which may be massive); (3) repletion of serum calcium and magnesium, if necessary; and (4) administration of an antibiotic active against *S. aureus*. When hypotension is severe, vasopressors may be required, but fluids should be considered the mainstay of therapy. In most cases antibiotics should initially be given intravenously, but an oral agent may suffice from the outset in mild cases, particularly if there is a foreign body that can be removed (thereby blocking further absorption of toxin). In such cases, the main rationale for antibiotic use is reduction of the risk of recurrent TSS by eradication of the infecting strain. The response to these measures is usually rapid, unless there has been a prolonged period of hypotension prior to institution of therapy.

The antibiotic used should be the narrowest-spectrum agent having good antimicrobial activity against the infecting strain of *S. aureus*. In most cases oxacillin (or nafcillin) would best meet these criteria at a dose of 6 to 12 g per day, depending on severity of illness (200 mg per kilogram per day for children), given every 4 hours. Penicillin should be used if the organism is shown to be susceptible to it. Cefazolin or vancomycin should be given to patients known to be allergic to penicillin. Vancomycin should be used before sensitivity data are available when there is a higher-than-usual likelihood of infection with a methicillin-resistant strain. Intravenous therapy can be discontinued in favor of an oral antibiotic following resolution of the acute illness, which is usually within 3 days. When TSS complicates a deep-seated focus of infection, intravenous therapy should be continued as long as would otherwise be necessary to treat that infection. Dicloxacillin is the oral drug of choice, assuming the most common susceptibility profile, with a variety of other drugs available for penicillin-allergic patients. A total duration of therapy of 2 weeks is recommended, although this has not been studied systematically.

Two additional forms of therapy, immunoglobulin and corticosteroids, merit consideration under some circumstances. All commercial preparations of immunoglobulin contain high levels of antibody to TSST-1 (and presumably to alternative TSS toxins). The rationale for using immunoglobulin would be to specifically neutralize circulating toxin. In the author's opinion, this treatment is justifiable when there is an undrainable or irremovable focus of infection, such as pneumonia or endometritis, that would result in ongoing toxemia for a considerable period after initiation of therapy. This treatment has not been critically evaluated and should be reserved for the sickest patients. A dose of 400 mg per kilogram, given as a single intravenous infusion over 2 to 3 hours, is reasonable based upon experience with use of immunoglobulin for other diseases (such as Kawasaki disease). A relative contraindication to this mode of therapy is cost; for an average-sized adult, the cost to the patient of immunoglobulin therapy would be more than (U.S.) $2,000.

In a retrospective study, corticosteroids were shown to have a favorable impact on severity of illness and duration of fever if administered within the first few days of illness. In the author's opinion, however, use of steroids on a routine basis cannot be recommended. Unless there is evidence of adrenal insufficiency, steroids should be considered only when a patient's hypotension is not responsive to removal or drainage of the focus of infection and several hours of fluid administration.

The risk of recurrence is low, probably less than 10 percent, among women who are treated with antibiotics for 2 weeks and who refrain from using tampons or barrier contraceptives. Recurrence of nonmenstrual TSS is unusual under any circumstances. The risk of recurrence can be gauged by testing convalescent serum for antibody to TSS toxins, particularly if TSST-1 (about which the most is known) is the causative toxin. If antibody testing is not performed, patients should probably refrain from using tampons or barrier contraceptives for 4 to 6 months, the rationale being that most recurrences take place within several months of the first episode. It may be useful, under some circumstances, to determine whether the patient is still colonized with *S. aureus* and to retreat with antibiotics if it is found, but this course of action is often problematic (and unsuccessful). A sounder approach, in the author's opinion, is to test for the development of antibody and to let these results guide long-term management.

SUGGESTED READING

Chesney PJ, Davis JP, Purdy WK, Wand PJ, Chesney RW. Clinical manifestations of toxic shock syndrome. JAMA 1981; 246:741–748.

Davis JP, Chesney PJ, Wand PJ, et al. Toxic-shock syndrome; epidemiologic features, recurrence, risk factors, and prevention. N Engl J Med 1980; 303:1429–1435.

Parsonnet J. Mediators in the pathogenesis of toxic shock syndrome: overview. Rev Infect Dis 1989; 11:S263–S269.

Reingold AL, Hargrett NT, Dan BB, et al. Nonmenstrual toxic shock syndrome: a review of 130 cases. Ann Intern Med 1982; 96(part 2): 871–874.

Todd J, Fishaut M, Kapral F, Welch T. Toxic-shock syndrome associated with phage-group-I staphylococci. Lancet 1978; 2:1116–1118.

INFECTION COMPLICATING IMMUNOSUPPRESSION

LOWELL S. YOUNG, M.D.

Patients may become immunosuppressed by two mechanisms: first, they may have an underlying condition with a defect in immune recognition or response. Secondly, they may receive medication or treatment such as x-rays which suppresses the immune system. Often both mechanisms contribute to a patient's susceptibility to infection. One may have a disorder such as a lymphoma or a leukemia and then receive treatment consisting of cytotoxic agents, anti-inflammatory agents such as corticosteroids, or radiation therapy, each of which can have a deleterious effect on the host immune response.

Table 1 lists examples of immunosuppressed states. This list is by no means all-inclusive, but it summarizes the major disorders associated with a blunted immune response and risk of developing opportunistic infection. It should be emphasized that increasing numbers of patients are receiving some type of medication that will impair humoral antibody synthesis, cellular immunity, or even the function of granulocytes. Many steroidal and non-steroidal anti-inflammatory agents will inhibit white cell mobilization; this defect is prominent in some of the collagen vascular disorders as well as in advanced alcoholic liver disease. Among the most commonly used medications that impair host defenses are adrenal corticosteroids. Their effect, fortunately, is dose dependent, and the risk of infection is small with doses equivalent to 100 mg of hydrocortisone per day or less.

CLINICAL SYNDROMES AND TYPES OF INFECTING ORGANISMS

Not surprisingly, microorganisms that cause serious infection in normal subjects, such as pneumococci, staphylococci, *Haemophilus influenzae*, and *Neisseria* species, can cause fulminant disease in immunosuppressed patients. Patients who are functionally asplenic or who are splenectomized (individuals, for instance, with Hodgkin's disease) are particularly susceptible to pneumococcal infections. Organisms of low intrinsic virulence, such as *Staphylococcus epidermidis*, may cause serious disease in immunosuppressed patients when associated with a foreign body such as an indwelling vascular catheter. Thus, the pathogenesis of disease in immunosuppressed patients is related to the intrinsic virulence of a potential pathogen and the degree to which host defenses are compromised. In the highly immunosuppressed patient, we see infections, such as disseminated aspergillosis and intestinal cryptosporidiosis, that are rarely if ever encountered in individuals with normal immune responses. In contrast, other processes that are quite common in the normal population, such as mycoplasmal pneumonia, are a rather infrequent problem in immunosuppressed subjects.

Clinical observations over the last two decades suggest that certain organisms are more likely to cause serious infections in immunosuppressed patients, and a background knowledge of the link between a clinical syn-

---

TABLE 1   Examples of Immunosuppressed States

Collagen vascular disease

Congenital immunodeficiency

Medications
    Corticosteroids
    Cyclosporine
    Azathioprine
    Alkylating agents
    Antimetabolites

Neoplastic disease

Recipients of organ transplants

TABLE 2 Suggested Pathogens in Immunosuppressed Patients by Site of Involvement

Meningitis	*Listeria monocytogenes, Cryptococcus neoformans*
Esophagitis	*Candida sp., Herpes simplex,* cytomegalovirus
Necrotizing vasculitis	*Pseudomonas aeruginosa, Aeromonas* sp., noncholera vibrios
Septic emboli	*Candida* sp., *Aspergillus* sp., *Staphylococcus aureus*
Pneumonia	
Diffuse	*Pneumocystis carinii,* cytomegalovirus
Segmental, lobar	*Legionella pneumophila,* pneumococcus
Cavitary	*Aspergillus* sp., *Nocardia, Mucor* sp.
Diarrhea	*Salmonella*
	Giardia lamblia
	Antibiotic side effects
	Cryptosporidia
	Isospora belli

drome and a specific pathogen may be of some help in the early stages of clinical decision making. Table 2 summarizes some of these associations, but the list is not intended to be comprehensive.

Central nervous system infections result from bloodstream spread or by direct extension from infected sites adjacent to the brain, such as sinus cavities or the middle ear. The usual causes of meningitis in the normal population are group B streptococci, *Escherichia coli*, meningococci, and *H. influenzae* (often depending on age). In contrast, *Listeria monocytogenes* is the most common cause of bacterial meningitis in the immunosuppressed patient, and *Cryptococcus neoformans* is the most common fungal pathogen isolated from the spinal fluid. This is not to exclude a wide variety of other bacterial and fungal processes that usually result from bloodstream seeding, but these are rather less common than listeriosis and cryptococcosis. Among the most common causes of infection around the oropharynx in immunosuppressed patients are *Candida* species. Oral thrush is common but it may progress to a severe esophagitis that may necessitate systemic therapy. The association between esophagitis and *Candida* infections is well known, but two other organisms are gaining increasing prominence as causes of esophagitis: *Herpes simplex* virus and the cytomegalovirus.

One of the most dramatic clinical presentations in immunosuppressed patients is the sudden appearance of necrotizing vasculitis or cutaneous lesions that represent septic emboli. Perhaps best known are the cutaneous lesions of *Pseudomonas aeruginosa* septicemia, so-called ecthyma gangrenosum. Similar appearing lesions, however, may be caused by other gram-negative rods, particularly two other groups of organisms, the *Aeromonas* species and noncholera vibrios. *Staphylococcus aureus* has classically been associated with peripheral emboliza-

tion, in which case one should strongly suspect an underlying bacterial endocarditis. Additionally, septic emboli and macronodular skin lesions are now well recognized as manifestations of the dissemination of *Candida* infections. *Aspergillus* species and other filamented fungi (*Mucor* species) can cause peripheral embolic lesions.

One of the greatest challenges in managing infectious complications in immunosuppressed subjects is the diagnosis and treatment of pneumonia. Although radiographs may readily identify lung infiltrates and the presence of pneumonia is further corroborated by physical findings, it is often difficult to establish the nature of a parenchymal lung abnormality without an invasive procedure. Sputum examination may be helpful in the patients who can cough and produce good material, but frequently contamination of respiratory secretions with oropharyngeal flora makes interpretation of culture results difficult. Two very important pulmonary pathogens in the immunosuppressed host, *Pneumocystis carinii* and *Legionella pneumophila*, may not be diagnosed by examination of expectorated sputum. The pattern of lung abnormality as suggested in Table 2 may occasionally be helpful in pointing toward diagnostic possibilities, but "pattern recognition" should not be relied on too heavily. *P. carinii* and cytomegalovirus are among the best appreciated causes of diffuse interstitial pneumonia, although technically *Pneumocystis* infection is usually a dense intra-alveolar inflammatory process. Lobar consolidation should still lead one to suspect pneumococcal disease, but *L. pneumophila* should now be high on the list of causes of a consolidative pulmonary process that develops in an immunosuppressed subject. The appearance of cavitary pneumonia in a patient who is severely neutropenic should lead to the suspicion of infection caused by a filamented fungus, such as one of the *Aspergillus* species. However, other fungi besides *Aspergillus* can cause an identical picture. These fungi belong to the *Mucor* group or are *Petriellidium boydii*. As organism now classified as a higher bacterium, *Nocardia asteroides*, can cause lung abscess plus multiple abscesses elsewhere in the body, such as in subcutaneous regions and the brain.

A wide variety of bacterial pathogens that cause diarrhea in normal hosts must be considered in evaluating diarrhea in immunosuppressed hosts. Outbreaks of salmonellosis have occurred among hospitalized immunosuppressed patients exposed to a common food source. Parasitic pathogens are increasingly recognized, including *Strongyloides stercoralis, Giardia lamblia*, and most recently, cryptosporidiosis or *Isospora* infection (the latter two now strikingly associated with the acquired immunodeficiency syndrome). Clinicians should not overlook the fact that diarrhea in immunosuppressed subjects is commonly a complication of antimicrobial therapy. The diarrhea and possible associated colitis may be the results of a toxin-producing *Clostridium* species.

DIAGNOSTIC APPROACHES

One of the cardinal errors in the management of immunosuppressed patients is the hasty administration of antimicrobial agents before appropriate diagnostic studies, including cultures, are done. Aggressive intervention with antibiotics may be lifesaving, but careful sampling of blood and body fluids prior to antibiotic intervention should be strongly emphasized. In the case of lung infections, premature or hasty intervention with antimicrobial agents may interfere with ability to diagnose an intrapulmonary process such as *Pneumocystis* infection. The care of immunosuppressed patients requires a well-organized team effort. The team should include specialists of many disciplines, including surgery. Invasive operation procedures such as organ biopsy sampling may be necessary to obtain a definitive diagnosis. Skilled laboratory workers are also required to perform special studies on any material obtained by an invasive procedure.

THERAPEUTIC SELECTIONS

While I have emphasized the need for appropriate diagnostic studies, the decision to initiate antimicrobial therapy may have to be made very rapidly. Those factors that must be considered are the patient's underlying disease and stage of underlying disease, physical findings, blood pressure, magnitude of body temperature, respiratory rate, and any clue to a rapidly progressing infectious process. If sepsis, meningitis, or severe pneumonia is diagnosed, therapeutic intervention should be considered within a matter of minutes.

Table 3 lists suggested choices for the initial therapy of suspected bacterial septicemia, meningitis, pneumonia, and intra-abdominal infection. The choices are conventional, and the reader should consult more detailed sources for further information on dosages and dose adjustments. For the neutropenic patient, my preference is to give an aminoglycoside such as gentamicin or tobramycin (5 mg per kilogram per day) or amikacin (15 mg per kilogram per day) combined with an antipseudomonal penicillin such as mezlocillin (16 g per day) or piperacillin (12 g per day). Alternatively, ceftazidime (6 g per day) plus an aminoglycoside may be used. The neutropenic patient is defined as an individual with a white count of 1,000 normal neutrophils per cubic millimeter or less, or one whose white count is progressively falling by a factor of ½ on successive days as a result of immunosuppressive and/or cytotoxic chemotherapy. For the non-neutropenic patient in whom staphylococci may be a stronger consideration, the combination of an aminoglycoside plus a first-generation cephalosporin or vancomycin is preferred. Alternative antistaphylococcal medications include first-generation cephalosporins and vancomycin.

Any immunosuppressed patient who develops evidence of meningitis but in whom spinal fluid examination fails to identify the cause should be empirically treated with a regimen that includes ampicillin, 12 g per day, until results of cultures are known. Ampicillin will be effective against *L. monocytogenes* and pneumococci but is now less reliable against *H. influenzae*. Suspicion of *H. influenzae* should lead to a prescription of a third-generation cephalosporin such as cefotaxime in a dose of 12 g per day; alternatively, ceftriaxone in a dose of 2 g

TABLE 3   Recommended Antimicrobial Therapy for Infection Developing During Immunosuppression

Bacterial Sepsis

Neutropenic patient (neutrophil count < 1000 mm³): anti pseudomonal penicillin plus aminoglycoside or antipseudomonal cephalosporin plus aminoglycoside

Non-neutropenic patient third-generation cephalosporin or imipenem

Meningitis

Ampicillin plus third generation* cephalosporin

Pneumonia

Same for bacterial sepsis unless *Staphylococcus aureus* isolated (then use oxacillin)

Trimethoprim-sulfamethoxazole for *Pneumocystis carinii* infection

Erythromycin for *Legionella* infection

Intra-abdominal Infection

Aminoglycoside plus clindamycin, metronidazole, cefoxitin, or broad-spectrum penicillin

Fungal Infection

Amphotericin B ± flucytosine

---

* Cefotaxime or ceftriaxone

intravenously every 12 hours one day, followed by 2 g per day, may be substituted. If *P. aeruginosa* is the central nervous system pathogen, ceftazidime in a dose of 4 g every 8 hours (12 g total) should be combined with an intravenous aminoglycoside. Although chloramphenicol has traditionally been cited as an effective agent against gram-negative bacillary infections of the central nervous system, the activity of the newer cephalosporins and related compounds is broader.

Treatment of pneumonia is a complex subject that is covered in other chapters of this book. In the immunosuppressed patient, the likelihood of gram-negative infection is high. Combination therapy with an aminoglycoside and a beta-lactam agent is recommended. Choices include an antipseudomonal penicillin or one of the newer cephalosporins such as ceftazidime that is active against *Pseudomonas*, *Klebsiella*, and *Serratia* species. Trimethoprim-sulfamethoxazole is the initial agent of choice for the treatment of *P. carinii* pneumonia. It is also effective against a wide variety of bacteria, including most of the gram-negative bacilli except *P. aeruginosa*. This agent should be used at an initial dose of 10 to 15 mg per kilogram per day (calculated in terms of trimethoprim).

Intra-abdominal infections are not particularly common in immunosuppressed patients unless there is trauma, tumor, or some other "mechanical" disruption that results in sudden soilage of the abdominal or pelvic cavities with fecal contents. Therapeutic regimens should include an aminoglycoside for the gram-negative rods and clindamycin, chloramphenicol, metronidazole, or one of the newer penicillins or cephalosporins that are active against the abundant anaerobes in bowel flora.

The choice of agents for treatment of fungal infection is extremely limited. Amphotericin B is the only broadly active antifungal agent that might be used for empiric therapy, and there are serious untoward effects associated with use of the compound. Amphotericin B is usually recommended in a dosage of 1 mg per kilogram per day, but this dosage can rarely be tolerated for a long period of time; a more realistic dosage is 0.7 mg per kilogram per day. The latter target dosage cannot be used initially, but a daily dosage is achieved by successive incremental doses of 5 mg of intravenous amphotericin (for example, a test dose of 1 mg followed daily by 5, 10, 15 mg, and so on until the target dosage is reached). The total recommended dose of amphotericin B for systemic infection if often given as 2 g, but patients with hematologic malignancies who achieve remission can be treated with less. The addition of flucytosine may be beneficial in cases of yeast infection, such as those caused by *Candida* species and *C. neoformans*. A new azole, fluconazole, appears effective against central nervous system cryptococcis and other systemic yeast infections; the maximal dose may be up to 400 mg per day orally. Some viral infections, such as those due to *Herpes simplex* or varicella-zoster, may be treated with acyclovir or adenine arabinoside.

Preventive regimens vary from the well accepted to the controversial. Any immunosuppressed patient who has a history of old tuberculosis (untreated) or a positive tuberculin test and Ghon complex on chest x-ray film should be a candidate for isoniazid prophylaxis. Trimethoprim-sulfamethoxazole is effective prophylactically against *P. carinii* in leukemics. There have been many studies of the use of trimethoprim-sulfamethoxazole for the prevention of bacterial infection in neutropenic patients. The results have been quite variable, and the agent could not be expected to prevent *P. aeruginosa* infection. In institutions where the incidence of resistance to trimethoprim-sulfamethoxazole is low and relatively few *P. aeruginosa* infections occur, prophylactic use may be efficacious. The usual adult dosage is 160 to 320 mg of trimethoprim (with a comparable five times that amount of sulfamethoxazole) given twice daily. Alternatively, a quinolone such as ciprofloxacin, 500 mg orally trice a day, or norfloxacin, 400 orally twice daily, provides effective suppression of the gastrointestinal flora and can minimize the development of bacterial infection. Topical nystatin is often used to prevent localized (upper gastrointestinal tract) and vaginal candidal colonization, but patient compliance may be poor. Ketoconazole is a systemically absorbed oral agent that is fungistatic and exerts a satisfactory long-term suppressive effect in patients with chronic mucocutaneous candidiasis (in a dosage of 200 to 600 mg daily). Its efficacy when used prophylactically in severely immunosuppressed patients is unclear.

A small proportion of patients who are immunosuppressed have quantitative or qualitative defects in circulating immunoglobulins. Patients with congenital hypogammaglobulinemia or acquired hypogammaglobulinemia have benefited from routine monthly or twice monthly injections of intramuscular gammaglobulins. Preparations of IgG that have been modified for intravenous use have become available, but their prophylactic role has been best established in a limited number of diseases such as chronic lymphatic leukemia where hypogammaglobulinemia is to be expected.

OTHER ASPECTS OF THE PROBLEM

This short review cannot provide an adequate discussion of the role of "protected environments" in preventing infections, nor the use of therapeutic or prophylactic granulocyte transfusions in immunosuppressed patients. In summary, it can be stated that both are rarely indicated in the management of immunosuppressed patients. In the case of prophylactic granulocyte transfusions, the evidence suggests that the complications far outweigh the anticipated benefits. Use of granulocyte transfusions does not appear to be indicated in the neutropenic patient unless there is a documented bacterial infection that fails to respond to appropriate antimicrobial therapy. Recombinant cytokines, such as the granulocyte or granulocyte-macrophage colony-stimulating factors may be more effective in restoring circulating neutrophil counts. "Protected environments" may be defined in many ways, but most are designed as strict isolation units with filtered air. Although it is associated with reduced rates of infection, patient management in a protected environment seems to have had little impact on treatment of the underlying disease.

A final point for emphasis is that the outcome of the management of infection in immunosuppressed patients is critically related to control of the underlying disease. Thus, the onset of infection in cancer patients should not deter appropriately designed antineoplastic therapy as long as adequate treatment of the infectious complication is also given. On the other hand, a documented infection complicating therapeutic immunosuppression, such as that given to a renal transplant recipient to prevent graft rejection, is the signal for temporary reduction in the immunosuppressive treatment.

SUGGESTED READING

EORTC International Antimicrobial Therapy Cooperative Group. Ceftazidime combined with a short or long course of amikacin for empirical therapy of gram-negative bacteremia in cancer patients with granulocytopenia. N Engl J Med 1987; 317:1692.

Rubin RH, Young LS. Clinical approach to infections in the compromised host. 2nd ed. New York: Plenum, 1988.

Young LS. Empirical antimicrobial therapy in the neutropenic host. N Engl J Med 1986; 315:580–581.

ACQUIRED IMMUNODEFICIENCY SYNDROME

MARTIN G. TÄUBER, M.D.

The acquired immunodeficiency syndrome (AIDS) is the result of a chronic viral infection. The causative agent, the human immunodeficiency virus (HIV), is transmitted by sexual contacts, by parenteral exposure to infected blood and other infected fluids, and from infected mothers to their infants in utero, during birth, or by breast milk. Subsequent to a serologically silent period of weeks to months, the HIV infection can easily be diagnosed using commercially available serologic tests that detect serum antibodies to viral epitopes.

PATHOGENESIS

HIV belongs to the family of retroviruses, containing an RNA genome. Once the virus has invaded a host cell, its genome is transcribed into DNA by a reverse transcriptase and is then integrated into the host cell's genome. Entry of the virus into cells occurs primarily by interaction between virus surface structures and the CD4+ epitope on cells. The CD4+ epitope is most abundant on T helper lymphocytes, and these cells are an important target of the HIV infection. Profound functional impairment and progressive depletion of these cells ultimately leads to the characteristic susceptibility of AIDS patients to a variety of opportunistic infections. HIV also infects macrophages and other cell types. Macrophages appear to transport the virus to the central nervous system, where HIV can cause an encephalopathy.

CLINICAL MANIFESTATIONS

Recent acquisition of HIV can lead to a self-limiting viral syndrome with fever, lymphadenopathy, rash, and in some cases aseptic meningitis or meningoencephalitis. In more than 50 percent of the patients, however, the infection does not cause early symptoms, and infected patients remain well for months to years. More than 50 percent of chronically infected patients will develop some degree of persistent, generalized lymphadenopathy before becoming otherwise symptomatic. The term AIDS designates the later stage of the disease, which is characterized by the occurrence of recurrent opportunistic infections and some tumors. Prior to AIDS, many patients develop the so-called AIDS-related complex (ARC) with fever, weight loss, chronic diarrhea, oral thrush, and oral hairy leukoplakia. The median time between the initial acquisition of the HIV and the development of AIDS is somewhere between 5 and 10 years.

TREATMENT OF THE HIV INFECTION

Zidovudine (azidothymidine or AZT) is the first and so far only drug licensed for the treatment of HIV. The beneficial effect of the drug appears to derive from its ability to inhibit the viral reverse transcriptase. The drug's ability to reduce the frequency of opportunistic infections and to prolong survival has only been well documented in ARC patients and in patients having recovered from a first episode of *Pneumocystis carinii* pneumonia. Nevertheless, treatment with zidovudine should be considered in all patients with symptomatic HIV infections (ARC and AIDS, including HIV-associated encephalopathy). Recent studies indicate that zidovudine is also beneficial to asymptomatic patients with low helper T cell counts. Its usefulness in other settings is still being evaluated.

Zidovudine's major toxicity consists of a bone marrow suppression that spares the platelets. Preexisting anemia results in the reduced tolerance of zidovudine but, if corrected by transfusions, is not a contraindication for therapy with zidovudine. Severe leukopenia does, on the other hand, preclude the use of zidovudine. Preexisting renal failure also makes treatment with zidovudine difficult because of drug accumulation and enhanced toxicity.

After institution of therapy, patients often complain of nausea, vomiting, headache, fatigue, and other constitutional symptoms, but these symptoms tend to disappear over time with continued therapy. Zidovudine-induced anemia is often megaloblastic and can develop as early as 4 to 6 weeks into therapy. If severe, it may require transfusions unless zidovudine is stopped. Leukopenia usually develops a few weeks later and is, with rare exceptions, reversible with dosage reduction or discontinuation of zidovudine.

Except for small children, zidovudine is administered orally as capsules containing 100 mg. The optimal dosing of zidovudine has not been established. In view of the short (less than 1 hour) serum half-life of zidovudine, a regimen of six daily doses given every 4 hours is advocated in the United States. Because of the inconvenience of this regimen, four daily doses during waking hours are frequently prescribed in Europe. In patients without preexisting bone marrow depression, a total daily dose of 20 to 30 mg per kilogram can be given during the first 4 to 6 weeks; later the daily dose is reduced to 15 mg per kilogram. Further reduction is often required because of toxicity. Daily doses of less than 400 mg are not recommended, though the lowest daily dose that maintains some efficacy is currently unknown.

MANAGEMENT OF OPPORTUNISTIC INFECTIONS IN AIDS PATIENTS

The severe immunodeficiency caused by the advanced HIV infection allows the development of a variety of opportunistic infections. Some of the pathogens encountered in AIDS patients (e.g., *Pneumocystis carinii*, *Mycobacterium-avium* complex) rarely cause disease in immunocompetent hosts. More commonly, the organisms recovered from AIDS patients are also pathogens in immunocompetent hosts but cause unusually severe disease in the immunodeficient patient (e.g., herpesviruses, *Toxoplasma gondii*, *Isospora belli*, *Cryptosporidium*, *Strongyloides*, *Mycobacterium tuberculosis*, *Candida albicans*, *Cryptococcus neoformans*). Besides these opportunistic infections, common bacterial pathogens (e.g., *Streptococcus pneumoniae*, *Salmonella*) cause recurrent, bacteremic infections in HIV-positive patients.

Some diagnostic and therapeutic principles apply for most infections in AIDS patients. In general, early diagnosis and treatment will improve the short-term outcome and will increase the patient's quality of life. Therefore, signs and symptoms indicative of an infection should be evaluated promptly. The presentation of most opportunistic infections is quite typical. Nevertheless, microbiologic confirmation of the diagnosis should be sought, since unexpected pathogens having therapeutic implications may be recovered in some patients. Even though adequate treatment can improve the patient's condition readily, many of the opportunistic organisms are difficult or impossible to eradicate. Recurrence rates are high and prophylactic posttreatment suppression should be considered after initial recovery from these infections.

Pneumocystis carinii

P. carinii pneumonia is by far the most common life-threatening infection in AIDS patients. The clinical picture consists of dry cough, fever, and progressive dyspnea. A diffuse interstitial pattern on the chest radiograph, a reduced PaO_2, and an increased uptake of radionuclide on gallium scan support the diagnosis. Even in suggestive cases, microbiologic confirmation should be attempted. This is best done by microscopic examination of sputum that is recovered after induction with inhalation of 3 percent saline (sensitivity 70 to 80 percent) or of bronchoalveolar lavage fluid (sensitivity more than 95 percent).

The three treatment regimens in Table 1 show comparable efficacy. Dapsone-trimethoprim is an oral regimen that is suited for outpatient treatment of moderately ill patients and has relatively few adverse effects, the most serious being methemoglobinemia. The other two regimens are used for more severely ill inpatients. Trimethoprim-sulfamethoxazole is often used as initial therapy in patients without known allergy to sulfonamides. Severe side effects, which are frequent, or failure to respond to therapy within 7 to 10 days are reasons to switch to pentamidine. The two regimens should not be combined. Treatment of *P. carinii* pneumonia must be followed by a prophylactic regimen. Weekly pyrimethamine-sulfadoxine is attractive, because it is easy to take. The monthly inhalation of pentamidine (300 mg)

TABLE 1 Therapy of Opportunistic Infections in AIDS

Pathogen or Disease	Drug	Usual Dose and Route in Adults	Duration	Adverse Effects	Prophylaxis
P. carinii pneumonia	TMP-SMZ	5 mg/kg 25 mg/kg IV or PO q6h	21 days	Rash, fever, GI symptoms, leuko-/thrombocytopenia	TMP-SMZ 160 mg/800 mg PO q12h
	or Pentamidine isethionate	3–4 mg/kg IV (slowly) q24h	21 days	Nephro-/hepatotoxicity, hypoglycemia, hypotension, leuko-/thrombocytopenia	Inhalation 300 mg/4 wk *or* Pyrimethamine 25 mg/wk PO *and*
	or Trimethoprim dapsone	5 mg/kg PO q6h 100 mg PO q24h	21 days	Methemoglobinemia, rash, GI symptoms	Sulfadoxine 500 mg/wk PO
T. gondii brain abscess	Pyrimethamine sulfadiazine *and* Folinic acid	75 mg PO q24h 1.0–1.5 g PO q6h 10 mg PO q24h	6 wk	Leuko-/thrombocytopenia, rash, nephro-/hepatotoxicity	25 mg/day PO 2 g/day PO
Isospora belli enteritis	TMP-SMZ	160 mg/800 mg PO q6h	10 days	As for *P. carinii*	Pyrimethamine 25 mg/wk PO; sulfadiazine 500 mg/wk PO
Candida esophagitis	Ketoconazole	400 mg q24h PO	21 days	Hepatitis, drug interactions	Not routinely
Oral thrush	Clotrimazole oral troche	10 mg PO q4h	21 days	GI symptoms	Not routinely
C. neoformans meningitis, brain abscess, pulmonary	Amphotericin B	0.4–0.6 mg/kg IV	6 wk	Fever, anemia, nephrotoxicity, pancytopenia, hepatotoxicity	100 mg/wk IV
H. simplex mucocutaneous	Acyclovir	5×200 mg/day PO or 10 mg/kg IV q8h	10 days	Pancytopenia, hepatotoxicity	None
H. zoster	Acyclovir	5×800 mg/day PO	10 days	As for H. simplex	None
Cytomegalovirus retinitis colitis	Ganciclovir (investigational)	2.5 mg/kg IV q8h	21 days	Neutropenia, hepatotoxicity, myalgias, spermatogenesis ↓	5 mg/kg IV q24h
M. tuberculosis pulmonary and extrapulmonary	Isoniazid, rifampin, pyrazinamide	300 mg/day PO 600 mg/day PO 25 mg/kg/day PO	9 mo	Neurotoxicity, hepatotoxicity	?
M. avium-complex disseminated	Rifampin, ethambutol, ansamycin, clofazimine *? plus* amikacin	600 mg/day PO 15 mg/kg/day PO 300 mg/day PO 100 mg/day PO 7.5 mg/kg IV q12h	9 mo	Hepatotoxicity N. opticus neuritis Skin discoloration Nephro-, ototoxicity	?

Abbreviations: TMP-SMZ=trimethoprim-sulfamethoxazole; GI=gastrointestinal.

has recently been found also to be effective, but a specified aerosolizer has to be used.

Toxoplasma gondii

T. gondii causes multiple brain abscesses in AIDS patients. Headaches and focal neurologic deficits should suggest this infection and prompt computed tomography or a magnetic resonance imaging of the brain. The lack of serum IgG antibodies to *T. gondii* makes the diagnosis unlikely, but serology, including cerebrospinal fluid (CSF) serology, cannot be used to confirm the diagnosis. The diagnosis is proved by demonstration of tachyzoites in brain tissue, but it is justified in clinically suggestive cases to start empiric treatment (see Table 1) and to perform a brain biopsy only if the patient does not respond to therapy within 2 weeks. In patients who cannot tolerate sulfadiazine because of allergic reactions, clindamycin (600 mg orally every 6 hours) may be used in combination with pyrimethamine. After 6 weeks of therapy, doses of the antibiotics should be reduced (e.g., to 25 mg pyrimethamine plus 2 g sulfadiazine daily), but treatment should be continued indefinitely to prevent recurrences.

Cryptosporidiosis and *Isospora belli*

Both organisms cause severe, watery diarrhea, and a clinical distinction between the two pathogens is not possible. However, there is no effective antimicrobial therapy for cryptosporidiosis, whereas *Isospora belli* infections respond well to trimethoprim-sulfamethoxazole (see Table 1). Therefore, microbiologic examination of feces (in addition to routine bacterial cultures) or small-bowel biopsy is mandatory in patients with severe diarrhea.

Candida albicans

C. albicans is a common pathogen in AIDS patients that primarily causes infections of the upper gastrointestinal tract (oral thrush, esophagitis). It can be diagnosed macroscopically (direct inspection or endoscopy) and by Gram stain or histology (cultures should not be used to make the diagnosis). Symptoms (burning sensation, dysphagia) should lead to treatment (see Table 1). Recurrences are common after successful therapy, but the usually benign course of these infections makes routine prophylaxis unnecessary.

Cryptococcus neoformans

Meningitis is the usual presentation of cryptococcal infections in AIDS patients, with fever, headache, and nausea as the most prominent symptoms. Only about one-third of the patients present with meningismus or photophobia. Rarely, cryptococcal infection can present as a brain abscess or as pulmonary disease. The diagnosis of cryptococcal meningitis is based on detection of the cryptococcal antigen in CSF and on CSF cultures. The CSF often shows only a mild pleocytosis in these patients, while the protein concentration is typically elevated.

Treatment should be instituted promptly and consists primarily of amphotericin B (see Table 1). 5-Fluorocytosine, which has been shown to exhibit synergism with amphotericin B against *C. neoformans* in patients not infected with HIV, produces bone marrow toxicity in AIDS patients too frequently. The drug should be reserved for cases that do not respond to amphotericin B alone, and these patients should be given lower doses than other patient populations (e.g., 20 mg per kilogram every 6 hours). Prevention of recurrence is necessary after successful treatment (see Table 1). Fluconazole may be useful in some settings.

Herpesviruses

In patients with AIDS, herpes simplex virus causes chronic, painful ulcerating infections in the genital, perianal, and perioral region. The infections may also extend to the rectum or the oropharynx. The diagnosis can be established by direct visualization of the virus in vesicular fluid or by culture. Prompt treatment is essential to improve the quality of life in these patients (see Table 1).

Herpes zoster tends to occur at an increased frequency in HIV-positive patients. The infection often involves several dermatomes, resolves less promptly than in immunocompetent patients, and disseminates at increased frequency. Herpes zoster infection is therefore considered an indication for therapy in an HIV-positive patient (see Table 1).

Cytomegalovirus (CMV) can often be recovered from various organs in severely ill AIDS patients. Its role in causing disease is, however, not well established when the virus is recovered from the lung or the brain together with a second pathogen. Retinitis and colitis, on the other hand, are well-established diseases caused by CMV in these patients. Retinitis is manifested by blurred vision. It can progress to progressive visual impairment and blindness and should prompt the institution of therapy (see Table 1). Funduscopic examination revealing multiple, hemorrhagic exudates along the retinal vessels is relatively typical. Colitis is associated with ulcerations, manifests itself with bloody diarrhea and fever, and often responds only partially to ganciclovir. Prolonged treatment is therefore usually necessary. However, long-term therapy is difficult because the drug can only be administered parenterally and has adverse effects, primarily neutropenia.

Mycobacteria

M. tuberculosis (MTB) and *M. avium-* complex (MAC) both play an important role in AIDS patients. MTB often presents as the first opportunistic infection and tends to cause focal infections that involve the lungs as well as extrapulmonary sites, such as lymph nodes. MAC is typically isolated from patients with advanced AIDS and other opportunistic infections. The organism can be recovered from blood, feces, and other organs, but its pathogenic role is not firmly established. As a consequence, while the necessity to treat a newly diagnosed MTB infection is unequivocal (see Table 1), this is not true for MAC infections. The decision to treat MAC infections is further complicated by the facts that the optimal drug regimen has not been established and response to therapy is often slow and transient. A therapeutic trial seems justified in a patient with severe constitutional symptoms (and diarrhea) in whom MAC is the only potentially treatable pathogen recovered. The optimal duration of therapy for both MTB and MAC has not been determined, but treatment for at least 6, and if possible 9 months should be attempted. There is currently no proof of the need to prolong treatment beyond the time needed to treat the acute infection. Also, even though advocated by some experts, there is no proof of the benefit of prophylactic isoniazid treatment of HIV-positive patients.

SUGGESTED READING

Fishl MA, Richman DD, Grieco MH, et al. The efficacy of azidothymidine (AZT) in the treatment of patients with AIDS and AIDS-related complex. N Eng J Med 1987; 317:185–191.
Glatt AE, Chirgwin K, Landesman SH. Treatment of infections associated with human immunodeficiency virus. N Eng J Med 1988; 318:1439–1448.
Kaplan LD, Wofsy CB, Volberding PA. Treatment of patients with acquired immunodeficiency syndrome and associated manifestations. JAMA 1987; 257:1367–1374.
Richman DD, Fishl MA, Grieco MH, et al. The toxicity of azidothymidine (AZT) in the treatment of patients with AIDS and AIDS-related complex. N Engl J Med 1987; 317:192–197.

INFECTION FOLLOWING BURN INJURY

JEFFREY A. GELFAND, M.D.

Infection is the leading cause of death in the hospitalized burned patient. In previous years, burn wound sepsis was the leading cause of infectious mortality; pneumonia is now the commonest life-threatening infection. The types of infections typically seen in severely burned patients are listed in Table 1.

Burn injury destroys local host defenses, converting the anatomic barriers of skin into culture media. Characteristic of all burn injury is ischemia, which impairs the delivery of both systemic antibiotics and phagocytic cells. In addition, burn injury produces profound abnormalities in both local and systemic immunologic and host defenses. These changes are generally proportional to the degree of burn injury (surface area and burn depth). With large burns, complement is consumed, reducing alternative pathway function, thus impairing resistance to gram-negative bacteria. Neutrophil numbers and function are abnormal, macrophage function is impaired, and cell-mediated immune responsiveness is diminished.

The development of burn infection is a function of the burn surface area and depth and the age of the patient. Burn depth will determine how much vascular supply remains, and this is a critical determinant of infection. In general,

TABLE 1 Infection in Burned Patients

Burn wound infection
Burn wound sepsis
Cellulitis
Pneumonia
Septicemia
Suppurative thrombophlebitis
Suppurative chondritis
Pyelonephritis
Endocarditis
Miscellaneous (fungal, viral)

partial-thickness wounds rarely become severely infected with good supportive care, whereas full-thickness wounds, being avascular, are readily infected. In addition, life-threatening burn wound infection is uncommon with full-thickness burns of less than 30 percent of the body surface area.

Ward nursing procedures, wound excision, and grafting, as well as topical therapy are all carried out with the recognition that complete sterility is practically impossible; the aim is to keep wound colonization at low levels (≤ 100 colony-forming units, or cfu, per gram of tissue). In contrast, lethal burn wound sepsis is usually seen with colony counts of more than 100,000 cfu per gram of tissue.

GENERAL MEASURES

More than any single factor, improved survival from burns has resulted from the creation of specialized burn units. The combination of a physical environment designed to isolate patients from exposure to bacteria in the environment with intensive care by personnel experienced in dealing with burns and their complications has vastly improved survival figures. Thus, the first step in management of burned patients after resuscitation ought to be transferral to a specialized burn unit. The bacteria-controlled nursing unit, in which patients are barrier-isolated in a plastic-film-contained area with positive pressure and bacteria-free air to prevent cross-contamination, has resulted in a marked reduction of burn infections. Aggressive fluid and nutritional support, early excision of full-thickness wounds, and early wound closure with skin grafts are crucial. Wound closure is the definitive therapy of burn infection.

MICROBIOLOGY OF BURN WOUNDS

Currently, gram-negative bacilli predominate. The bacteriology of wound infections in any particular burn unit is constantly changing, reflecting local antibiotic use and resistance patterns. *Enterobacter, Escherichia coli, Pseudomonas aeruginosa, Acinetobacter, Proteus, Klebsiella,* and *Serratia* have in general predominated, often with high levels of antimicrobial resistance. Methicillin-resistant *staphylococcus aureus* has emerged at a number of burn units and is a major consideration. Fungal infections with *Candida* species, *Mucor,* and *Aspergillus* species are increasingly encountered. Finally, herpes zoster, herpes simplex, and even systemic cytomegalovirus infections are being recognized with increasing frequency, as they are in other groups of immunosuppressed patients.

Surveillance surface cultures of the burn wound provide information on the patient's flora and its antimicrobial sensitivity. Weekly surveillance cultures of wound(s), urine, and respiratory tract should be obtained. Blood cultures should be routinely performed following extensive surgical debridement or with the development of fever, hypothermia, altered mentation, hypotension, hypoglycemia, acidosis, respiratory distress, oliguria, or ileus (all cardinal signs of burn wound invasion or sepsis). Routine wound biopsy with quantitative culture is controversial—the reliability of the technique has been questioned. We make the rapid diagnosis of suspected burn wound sepsis by biopsy and examination by frozen section for both bacteria and fungi, followed by reexamination of permanent sections coupled with culture, an alternative to quantitative culture. Invasion of unburned tissue is a sign of burn wound sepsis.

PROPHYLACTIC MEASURES

A tetanus booster with the adult Td (tetanus/diphtheria) toxoids (0.5 ml) is given to all patients without a history of immunization in the past year. If the state of tetanus immunity is unknown or if the wound has been grossly contaminated, human tetanus immune globulin TIG(H) (250 to 500 U) is administered intramuscularly at a site distant from the Td booster.

Topical therapy is begun immediately. The aim of topical therapy is not sterility but reduction of wound colony counts. A list of the major agents in wide use in topical burn care is given in Table 2, along with attributes and side effects.

We prefer to use silver nitrate 0.5 percent, which has a wide antibacterial spectrum and is bacteriostatic for gram-positive and gram-negative organisms as well as fungi. Resistance is extremely rare but has been reported. Silver nitrate does not cause pain on application and is also relatively inexpensive. There are some major drawbacks,

however. Silver nitrate 0.5 percent penetrates the eschar poorly, making it more useful in preventing wound infection than in treating established wound infection. Silver nitrate discolors everything it contacts (skin, dressings, linen, floors), and dressings must be re-wet every 2 hours to maintain bacteriostatic activity at the wound surface. Dressings are changed every 12 to 24 hours. This restricts the utility of the agent to burn units prepared to deal with these considerable logistic drawbacks. Hyponatremia is a significant threat but is readily detectable and preventable. Methemoglobinemia is a rare complication.

Silver sulfadiazine (Silvadene) 1 percent cream is the most commonly used topical burn agent. It is active against gram-negative rods, gram-positive organisms, and fungi. However, the development of resistance, especially by staphylococci, *Providencia*, *Pseudomonas*, and *Enterobacter*, has been described. Silver sulfadiazine penetrates the eschar, though not as well as mafenide, is painless on application, and does not discolor skin or linen. Transient leukopenia, appearing usually between days 3 and 5 and resolving despite continued use of the agent, is common. It is advisable to discontinue the drug when the leukocyte count falls below 3,000 cells per microliter. Hypersensitivity reactions, methemoglobinemia, and crystalluria are also potential adverse effects.

Mafenide acetate (11 percent cream) is bacteriostatic against gram-positive cocci, especially clostridia, and gram-negative bacilli. It has minimal activity against fungi. Superinfection by resistant gram-negative bacteria and fungi occurs with significant frequency. Mafenide readily penetrates the burn wound and is therefore most useful for treating established wound infection. This results in its being absorbed, where its action as a carbonic anhydrase inhibitor can cause bicarbonate loss, hyperchloremic metabolic acidosis, and compensatory hyperventilation, sometimes leading to respiratory exhaustion. Extreme caution must be used when treating large burns with this agent. An additional, serious drawback is pain upon application. This, coupled with the metabolic side effects, limits its use by most burn centers to short-term prophylaxis, smaller wounds, or treatment of developing infection.

TABLE 2 Topical Agents for Burn Wound Care

	Silver nitrate 0.5% Soaks	Silver Sulfadiazine 1% Cream (Silvadene)	Mafenide Acetate 11% Cream (Sulfamylon)
Antimicrobial spectrum			
Gram-positive cocci	+++	++	++
Gram-negative rods	+++	+++	+++
Fungi	+++	+++	++
Development of resistance	−	++	−
Eschar penetration	−	±	+
Adverse effects			
Pain on application	−	−	+
Hypersensitivity	−	+	+++
Neutropenia	−	++	−
Acidosis	+++	−	++
Hyponatremia	+	−	−
Methemoglobinemia	−	+	−

Polymyxin-bacitracin-neomycin ointment (Neosporin) is costly and difficult to apply, but is useful for small burns and in specific regions like the periorbital area.

Systemic prophylactic antibiotics are useful for two additional situations. β-Hemolytic streptococci may inhabit hair follicles and persist despite topical therapy. We advocate low-dose penicillin G (1.2 × 10⁶ U IV) for 2 days in all patients; some units have abandoned this. Most centers would treat children, especially those with scalds, with penicillin.

Bacteremia is common during wound debridement. Prophylactic antibiotics are advocated immediately before, during, and after such surgery. The choice of drugs should be guided by wound cultures; in general, both gram-negative rods and staphylococci should be covered. A reasonable empiric regimen would be an aminoglycoside (gentamicin; amikacin when there is resistance) and cefazolin (vancomycin if methicillin-resistant *S. aureus* [MRSA] is suspected). Prophylaxis is initiated immediately before surgery and usually spans 24 hours.

TREATMENT OF INVASIVE INFECTION

Altered mentation, hypotension, acidosis, respiratory distress, fever, hypothermia, oliguria, and ileus all signal sepsis. Differentiating colonization from invasion clinically has been previously discussed, as has the issue of surveillance surface cultures versus biopsy and quantitative culture. Mafenide affords penetration of wounds and may be helpful in topical therapy of invasive infection. Surveillance cultures with sensitivity patterns should certainly guide systemic therapy. Initial therapy should cover both gram-negative organisms and staphylococci. A reasonable regimen might be to start with amikacin, ticarcillin, and vancomycin, and to drop the latter if staphylococci are not isolated. Cefazolin or oxacillin could be substituted for vancomycin if MRSA is not suspected. Gentamicin can be used if sensitivities permit. There are no studies comparing newer agents, such as ceftazidime, imipenem, or timentin, to established combinations in burned patients. While these new agents are theoretically attractive, both ceftazidime alone and timentin alone have had notably equivocal results in some studies involving patients undergoing chemotherapy for malignancies. *Pseudomonas* organisms resistant to imipenem have been isolated from several burn patients.

It is important to emphasize that serum levels of drugs must be monitored especially carefully in burned patients in order to prevent toxicity and ensure efficacy. Aminoglycoside and vancomycin half-lives are substantially reduced in burned patients with normal renal function, for example. Higher-than-normal doses may thus be required but should be based on monitoring of serum levels.

SUGGESTED READING

Durtschi MB, Orgain C, Counts GW, et al. A prospective study of prophylactic penicillin in acutely burned hospital patients. J Trauma 1982; 22:11–14.

Glew RH, Moellering RC, Burke JF. Gentamicin dosage in children with extensive burns. J Trauma 1976; 16:819–823.

Luterman A, Dacso CC, Curreri PW. Infections in burn patients. Am J Med 1986; 81:45–52.

Monafo WW, Freedman B. Topical therapy for burns. Surg Clin North Am 1987; 67:133–145.

INFECTION FOLLOWING TRAUMA

JOSEPH KOO, M.D.
ELLIOT GOLDSTEIN, M.D.

Trauma may be followed by infection if there has been contamination by exogenous microorganisms or the introduction of endogenous flora into previously sterile sites. In general, the likelihood of posttraumatic infection depends on the injury and its extent. For example, injuries resulting in open fractures in an extremity with embedded skin flora and foreign materials or abdominal wounds that penetrate the intestinal tract are more prone to infection than injuries in which the integument and intestine remain intact. Since the internist and general practitioner most often treat these infections as well as complicating soft tissue and head injuries, the following discussion confines itself to posttraumatic infections of these four sites.

GENERAL PRINCIPLES

Recognition of the role of exogenous and endogenous microorganisms, foreign material, and devitalized tissue in initiating posttraumatic infection has resulted in a few general principles for prophylaxis (Fig. 1). The wound is first washed free of bacteria with saline rather than with antibiotic solutions. Saline is chosen because comparative studies have shown that irrigation with antibiotics adds little to perioperative prophylaxis when parenteral therapy is also administered. Moreover, irrigation with antibiotics may increase the likelihood of colonization with resistant bacteria. Devitalized tissue is then debrided under sterile conditions. After debridement, drains are inserted to prevent blood and tissue fluids from accumulating in dependent wound spaces. If the wound is clear and fluid accumulation is unlikely, drains are contraindicated since they allow bacterial colonization, thereby increasing the possibility of infection.

Since all injuries, even minor ones, pose the threat of tetanus, every patient is considered for prophylaxis with tetanus toxoid (active immunization), with or without tetanus immune globulin (TIG) (passive immunization). This

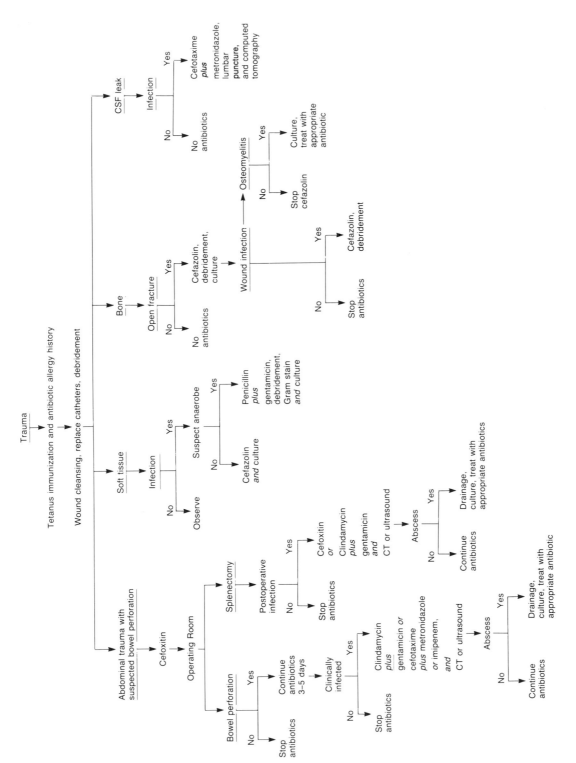

Figure 1 Management of infection in patients with trauma.

decision is determined by the patient's immunization history and the condition of the wound. Patients who have received a primary immunization series of three injections and who have not had a booster injection in 10 years are given absorbed tetanus toxoid, 0.5 ml intramuscularly (10Lf). The interval is shortened to 5 years for severe injuries likely to be contaminated by clostridial spores. Patients with minor injuries whose immunization is uncertain are treated with tetanus toxoid; if the wound is considered to be tetanus prone, 250 units of human TIG is given intramuscularly as well. When tetanus toxoid and TIG are given concurrently, separate syringes and sites should be used.

In this era of on-site care for trauma patients, intravenous catheters, urinary catheters, and chest tubes are often inserted during the initial management of these patients. These devices should be regarded as contaminated and removed or changed as soon as the patient's condition stabilizes.

ABDOMEN

Infection in 10 to 15 percent of patients is the major complication of abdominal trauma. Puncture of the gastrointestinal tract produced by gunshots, knives, or other causes permits gastrointestinal contents to leak into the peritoneum. Since the gastrointestinal tract is populated by large numbers of aerobic and anaerobic bacteria, the spill causes mixed infections with these bacteria. The gram-negative enteric aerobes—*Escherichia coli, Klebsiella* species, and *Enterobacter* species—and the gram-negative anaerobe—*Bacteroides fragilis*—are frequent causes of infection. Failure to eradicate gastrointestinal bacteria from the soiled peritoneum in the perioperative period may result in posttraumatic abdominal infections and abscess formation.

Clues to the presence of an abdominal infection are blood cultures containing commonly found abdominal pathogens and physiologic evidence suggesting sepsis, e.g., an unexplained anion gap of more than 20 mEq per liter, diminished systemic vascular resistance of less than 800 dynes sec cm^{-5}, unexplained hypotension, and a persistently positive fluid balance.

The diagnosis of abdominal infection, which was formerly a formidable clinical challenge, has been made considerably easier by advances in technology. The diagnosis is no longer limited to the interpretation of such tenuous findings as hiccups, abdominal tenderness, rebound tenderness, and ileus in a patient with fever and an elevated white blood cell count. Approximately 80 percent of abdominal abscesses are identifiable by radiographic or nuclear studies. Computerized tomography, which is the most sensitive and specific procedure for detecting abscesses, is the recommended initial investigation; it is only suitable for patients who can tolerate transfer to the radiology department. Ultrasonography can be performed at the bedside; however, it is less sensitive and specific, especially if ileus or anasarca is present (both are common in abdominal trauma, the former from the injury and the latter from fluid resuscitation to treat hypotension). Mag-

netic resonance imaging, the newest method of detecting intra-abdominal abscesses, enables better delineation of the abscess than does computerized tomography, but this procedure requires both transportation to the radiology department and considerable patient cooperation. Scintigraphy with indium 111–labeled leukocytes is rarely employed because of lower sensitivity and specificity than the other procedures and a waiting period of 24 hours before the scintiscans are evaluatable. Scintigraphy with gallium-67 is no longer considered of value in diagnosing abdominal abscesses because of its lack of specificity, especially in patients with recent abdominal operations.

The management of a patient with abdominal trauma begins at surgery, where hemostasis is effected, devitalized tissue and foreign materials are removed, damaged tissue is repaired, the wound area is cleansed, and tetanus prophylaxis is ensured. The risk of posttraumatic infection is reduced by instituting antibiotic therapy with cefoxitin (100 mg per kilogram per day intravenously in four divided doses) or gentamicin (5.0 mg per kilogram per day intravenously in three divided doses) plus clindamycin (30 mg per kilogram per day intravenously in three divided doses) (Table 1). The newer third-generation cephalosporins or aminoglycosides combined with metronidazole, imipenem alone, or ticarcillin plus clavulanic acid may be equally efficacious in reducing the risk of posttraumatic abdominal infections. Our preference is to use cefoxitin (100 mg per kilogram per day in four divided doses) as this agent provides therapy with minimal toxicity. Cefotetan, a less expensive congener, may prove equally efficacious when more data become available. We continue cefoxitin for 3 to 5 days, depending on the extent and location of the bowel perforation.

Despite the above measures, abdominal infections occur in approximately 20 percent of patients with intestinal perforations due to abdominal trauma. The clinician

TABLE 1 Antibiotic Choices for Immediate Treatment of Posttraumatic Infection

Site	Antibiotic*	Dosage
Abdomen	Gentamicin *plus* clindamycin or	5 mg/kg/day q8h 30 mg/kg/day q8h
	cefoxitin	100 mg/kg/day q6h
Spleen	Gentamicin *plus* clindamycin or	5 mg/kg/day q8h 30 mg/kg/day q8h
	cefoxitin	100 mg/kg/day q6h
Bone	Cefazolin	100 mg/kg/day q8h
Soft tissue, aerobic	Cefazolin	100 mg/kg/day q8h
Clostridial gangrene	Penicillin	16 × 10⁶ U/day q3h
Meningitis or brain abscess	Cefotaxime *plus* metronidazole	12 g/day q4h 30 mg/kg/day q6h

Note: Selections apply for cases in which antimicrobial sensitivity test results are either not available or support these choices. Other factors such as renal failure, penicillin hypersensitivity, or availability of aminoglycoside assays should be considered before applying these recommendations.
* In order of preference.

must be constantly aware of this possibility in patients with persistent low-grade fever and unexplained abdominal tenderness. We cannot overemphasize the importance of early diagnosis of abdominal infections in minimizing morbidity and mortality.

Once diagnosed, abscesses or collections of pus are drained percutaneously by use of ultrasonic or computed tomographic guidance or at laparotomy. Our preference is ultrasound for cases in which the abscesses are clearly defined and the drainage path avoids viscera. Laparotomy is recommended when percutaneous access is difficult or the possibility of undetected infection exists. Infected materials are removed and cultured. Adequate drainage is established by Penrose or sump drains attached to a vacuum pump. The antibiotic regimen is reevaluated, and agents are chosen on the basis of new culture and sensitivity results. While awaiting these results, we choose a regimen of an aminoglycoside (gentamicin, tobramycin, amikacin) plus clindamycin, cefotaxime, or ceftizoxime plus metronidazole, ticarcillin–clavulanic acid, or imipenem. These regimens have been successful in treating difficult abdominal infections, and none has been proved conclusively superior. Gentamicin plus clindamycin is our preference when renal failure is not a factor, and the third-generation cephalosporin plus metronidazole, if it is. Although the importance of *Streptococcus faecalis* is debated, we treat for this microorganism by adding ampicillin to the gentamicin regimen or using vancomycin. Ampicillin is preferred except when patients are allergic to penicillin. The duration of antibiotic therapy depends on the patient's course, which is monitored clinically and with repeated imaging procedures. In general, parenteral antibiotics are continued for 1 week after apparent clinical cure.

SPLEEN

Splenic abscess is a rare source of intra-abdominal infection. Direct extension from a contiguous source (such as a perforated bowel), hematogenous spread from septicemia, and direct trauma to the spleen are risk factors for this complication. Mortality remains high, especially in patients with silent or covert lesions. There are no pathognomonic findings associated with splenic abscess. Findings that suggest the diagnosis are fever with pain in the left upper quadrant, left flank, or left shoulder and chest roentgenographic abnormalities of left lower lobe atelectasis or left pleural effusion. Computed tomography, ultrasonography, or [^{99}Tc]sulfur colloid scintigraphy are used to establish the diagnosis. Frequently, distinguishing among splenic infarct, hematoma, and abscess is exceedingly difficult. Proof of infection is obtained by percutaneous aspiration using an imaging procedure or at laparotomy. Splenic abscesses are treated by splenectomy or percutaneous transabdominal catheter drainage and antibiotics chosen on the basis of culture results. Regimens of clindamycin and gentamicin are used empirically until a definitive pathogen(s) is isolated (unless renal failure is a concern, in which case cefoxitin is chosen).

Splenectomy following abdominal trauma presents special problems in regard to infection. First, a small percentage of patients develop subphrenic abscesses postoperatively. This incidence is increased in cases with associated bowel perforations, and it is reported that open drainage also enhances this incidence. When necessary, drainage is performed with a closed system using suction. Antimicrobial agents, either gentamicin and clindamycin or cefoxitin, are administered throughout the operative and immediate postoperative period (24 hours) in uncomplicated cases without bowel perforations. Cefoxitin is our choice in this situation because of its lower nephrotoxicity and the increased vulnerability of splenectomized patients to infection with encapsulated microorganisms. Chemotherapy is continued for longer periods in complicated cases or those with bowel perforations.

Second, because the spleen serves to filter bacteria, septicemia can be inordinately severe in the postsplenectomy period. Those infections that are due to encapsulated bacteria (pneumococcus, *Haemophilus influenzae, E. coli*) are frequently fulminant. Because septicemia can be overwhelming, treatment with cefuroxime, which has excellent activity against pneumococci and *H. influenzae*, at a dosage of 750 mg at 8-hourly intervals, together with gentamicin, 5 mg per kilogram per day, is begun at the first signs of sepsis. We no longer use ampicillin because of the possibility of β-lactamase-producing strains of *H. influenzae*.

The risk of fulminant septicemia in the years after splenectomy was first recognized in children but is now also known to occur, albeit at a much lower rate, in adults. Fulminant septicemia, the risk of which is highest in the first 2 years after splenectomy, is due to the pneumococcus in approximately one-half of cases, with other encapsulated bacteria accounting for the remaining cases. We vaccinate all patients with pneumococcal vaccine to minimize this risk. Children are also vaccinated with meningococcal vaccine, types A and C. In addition, children younger than 5 years receive oral penicillin VK (100,000 units per kilogram per day in twice-daily doses, to a maximum of 1.6 million units) as chemoprophylaxis. Chemoprophylaxis with oral penicillin VK (20,000 units per kilogram per day in twice daily doses) is also recommended for adults during the first 2 years after splenectomy even though the virtue of this prophylaxis is unproved. Patients who have had splenectomies are advised to seek prompt medical attention for respiratory illnesses or fever.

Third, patients who are splenectomized and receive multiple blood transfusions are prone to serious infections with cytomegalovirus. This illness is characterized by persistent fever, interstitial pneumonitis, and the presence of atypical lymphocytes. Definitive diagnosis depends on the identification of typical owl's eye cells in pulmonary lavage fluids or urine. The value of treatment with the experimental drug ganciclovir is uncertain.

BONE

Trauma that results in open fractures should be regarded as contaminated and likely to become infected. For this reason, many physicians add cephalosporins or aminoglycosides to irrigating fluids. We do not recommend this practice because its effectiveness is unproved and because locally administered antibiotics may promote superinfection with resistant bacteria. Debridement is of major importance, and, unless the surgeon is certain about its adequacy, the wound is left open.

Cultures obtained prior to completion of the surgical procedure are used to guide antimicrobial therapy in the postoperative period. Osteomyelitis secondary to trauma is usually polymicrobial. *Staphylococcus aureus, Staphylococcus epidermidis*, and the gram-negative enteric bacilli (*E. coli, Enterobacter* species, *Klebsiella* species, and *Pseudomonas* species) are often implicated in posttraumatic osteomyelitis. Anaerobes are less common pathogens, but recent studies suggest that they cause infection sufficiently often to warrant culturing for them. *Nocardia* and fungi are infrequent causes of infection.

Since infection is a common complication of severe fractures, systemic antibiotics are administered prior to surgery and in the postoperative period. Cefazolin, at a dosage of 100 mg per kilogram per day intravenously at 8-hour intervals, provides effective therapy for most staphylococci and gram-negative bacilli. Whether cephalosporins such as cefoxitin, ceftizoxime, or cefotaxime, which have additional activity against anaerobic bacteria, are better choices is an unsettled question. Combinations of an aminoglycoside—usually gentamicin—with clindamycin are also useful in the initial treatment of severely contaminated fractures. Because the combination is more toxic and of unproved advantage to the cephalosporins, we prefer the cephalosporins, even in severe injuries. We consider the differences that exist in the ability of antibiotics to penetrate bone to be of unproved clinical importance, and therefore this information is not used in deciding therapy.

The duration of therapy is unpredictable because it depends on the rate of wound healing. If the wound remains uninfected and heals appropriately, antibiotic therapy is discontinued before secondary closure. Wounds that become infected are recultured, and antimicrobial therapy is chosen on the basis of in vitro bacterial sensitivity results. When prolonged therapy is contemplated, an oral agent, such as ciprofloxacin, or a parenteral agent with a long half-life, like ceftriaxone, is used in outpatient therapy. If the isolate is sensitive to ciprofloxacin, this oral agent is preferred because it avoids the need for parenteral therapy.

Two potential causes for the persistence of posttraumatic infections of bone are unremoved sequestra and infected fixation devices. Sequestra, which are sometimes identifiable radiologically as opaque foreign bodies, serve as niduses for infection, often producing sinus tracts. Cure of these low-grade infections requires aspiration of the sinus tract, removal of the sequestra, and antimicrobial therapy. Antimicrobial therapy is based on cultures from the sequestra and not from the sinus tract.

Infected fixation devices pose a therapeutic dilemma. As a rule, cure is unlikely as long as the device is present. However, since alignment of the fracture is critical for future functional use, infected devices are left in place until the fracture is stable or the alignment can be maintained by external fixation. During this period, antibiotics are used to suppress the smoldering infection. As with wound infections, ciprofloxacin is preferred to ceftriaxone for prolonged therapy as long as the infecting microbes are sensitive. It is important to emphasize the need to remove the infected rod, plate, or screw as soon as the fracture is stable since these infections result in osteomyelitis, sequestra formation, and wound breakdown. Posttraumatic bone infections due to less common microorganisms such as *Actinomyces, Nocardia,* or fungi are treated with penicillin (*Actinomyces*), trimethoprim-sulfamethoxazole (*Nocardia*), or amphotericin B (fungi), according to the schedules recommended in the chapters pertaining to these infections.

SOFT TISSUE

Posttraumatic injuries of soft tissue are cleansed and treated with antibiotics in the aforementioned manner except for cases complicated by gas-associated myonecrosis, anaerobic cellulitis, necrotizing fasciitis, or synergistic fasciitis. These infections follow contamination of an inadequately debrided wound by enzyme, toxin, and gas-producing bacteria (*Clostridium* species, anaerobic streptococci, *Bacteroides* species, *E. coli, Enterobacter* species, *Klebsiella* species). Once within devitalized tissue, these microorganisms grow luxuriantly, rapidly destroying contiguous tissues. Because of their fulminant nature, these infections are medical emergencies requiring prompt diagnosis and therapy.

Diagnosis is suspected when soft tissue inflammation and necrosis progress rapidly, when crepitus is noted, or when a radiograph shows subcutaneous gas in an area of cellulitis. Findings of crepitus and subcutaneous air mandate immediate surgical exploration to determine the extent of tissue destruction and to identify the pathogens by Gram stain and culture. We cannot overemphasize the importance of debridement of necrotic muscle or fascia in managing these infections. Frozen sections sent from the operating room are helpful in ensuring that necrotic tissue is adequately resected. Although we are reluctant to recommend amputation, experience has taught us that the procedure is warranted if uncertainty exists regarding the vaibility of unexcised tissues.

With surgery, empiric antibiotic therapy is initiated with penicillin, 2 million units IV at 3-hourly intervals, and gentamicin, 5 mg per kilogram per day in 8-hourly doses. If a clostridial infection is proved, the gentamicin is discontinued. Penicillin is also used to treat nonclostridial anaerobic infections, except for those caused by *B. fragilis*. Nonclostridial infections tend to be confined to fascia and are less severe, requiring less-extensive surgery. Infections due to *Bacteroides* spp. are treated with cefoxitin, clindamycin, or metronidazole because these anaerobes are often resistant to penicillin. Infections with gram-negative Enterobacteriaceae are treated with gentamicin, which is continued unless in vitro sensitivity testing indicates resistance. If available, treatment with a hyperbaric oxygen chamber is helpful in retarding tissue necrosis in clostridial infections. Polyvalent gas gangrene antitoxins are no longer used because they did not prove to be effective.

CENTRAL NERVOUS SYSTEM

Although head injuries are common, infection of the central nervous system is infrequent because of the protection afforded by the skull and dura mater. For infection to occur, these barriers must be breached, permitting bacteria to enter the central nervous system. Fractures producing fistulae are those involving the frontal and ethmoid sinuses, the cribriform plate, and the temporal bone. Fractures that result in cerebrospinal fluid (CSF) rhinorrhea and otorrhea must be suspected in patients with severe paranasal injuries, bilateral orbital hematomas, mastoid bruising, or hemotympaneum.

The site of the fistula is often evident from the radiologic postion of the fracture. However, small fractures may elude radiologic detection, and in some cases, the diagnosis is difficult. In these instances, ^{99}Tc-labeled albumin or fluorescein dyes are injected intrathecally, and the fistula is identified by scintiscans showing radioisotope leaking from the anterior fossa or by demonstrating dye from small gauze packs placed within the nasal cavity. When the leakage is large, the clear nasal fluid is shown to be CSF by its high concentration of glucose. The origin of lesser discharges is exceedingly difficult to prove since the Dextrostix method, which is commonly used to detect small amounts of CSF, can be falsely positive because of the glucose content of nasal mucus.

The risk of bacterial meningitis is patients with a dural tear is estimated to be 5 to 25 percent. Meningitis is most likely in the first 2 weeks after trauma, but it can occur at any time as long as the leak is present. Patients with persistent or intermittent rhinorrhea are also prone to recurrent episodes of meningitis. A CSF fistula should be suspected in all patients who develop meningitis immediately after head trauma, who have had severe head trauma in the past, or who have had meningitis previously. The pneumococcus causes approximately 80 percent of posttraumatic meningitis. *H. influenzae* and *Neisseria meningitidis* are other important causes. Staphylococci and gram-negative bacilli infrequently cause posttraumatic meningitis. When these bacteria cause meningitis, it is usually the result of contiguous bone and soft tissue infection in patients with large cranial defects or penetrating wounds.

The initial management of a head injury is the same as that for other soft tissue and bone injuries, namely, wound cleansing, debridement, and the application of parenteral antibiotics, usually cephalosporins or penicillins. Whether chemotherapy is warranted is uncertain as its efficacy has never been documented. However, analogy with injuries at other sites suggests that chemotherapy with cefazolin is likely to minimize posttraumatic bone and soft tissue infections. Prevention of meningitis in patients with a CSF leak with either cephalosporin or penicillin is, however, unlikely to be successful because neither agent effectively penetrates into CSF in the absence of inflammation and neither reliably eliminates the pneumococcus from the nasopharynx. Because of these considerations, our practice is to treat patients with extensive head trauma with cefazolin, but not to use cephalosporins or penicillins as chemoprophylaxis in patients with closed fractures and CSF leak. Such patients are observed for signs of meningitis and treated promptly with large doses of cefotaxime (12 g per day) empirically. Lumbar puncture for CSF culture is essential and should be performed before antibiotics are administered. Further antibiotic adjustment is made after a specific pathogen is isolated.

Most tears of the dura heal spontaneously within 1 or 2 weeks following injury, obviating the need for surgical repair. Indications for surgery are persistence of the leak and the occurrence of meningitis. CSF otorrhea usually ceases spontaneously; operative repair is seldom required.

Infection of the brain after a compound fracture of the cranium more often results in brain abscess than meningitis. Brain tissue is relatively resistant to infection and in cases receiving early neurosurgical care, posttraumatic brain abscesses are uncommon. Such abscesses are usually due to contamination with *S. aureus*, Enterobacteriaceae, and anaerobes. These are treated with the aforementioned regimen of cefotaxime plus metronidazole, 30 mg per kilogram per day, pending indentification of the pathogens. In the event of life-threatening penicillin or cephalosporin allergy, chloramphenicol is a reasonable alternative. Abscesses that persist are drained and treated with antibiotics, on the basis of cultural results and according to the regimens detailed in the chapter *Localized Infection of the Central Nervous System*.

SUGGESTED READING

Caplan ES, Hoyt NJ. Identification and treatment of infections in multiply traumatized patients. Am J Med 1985; 79(Suppl 1A):68–75.
Durack DT. Prevention of central nervous system infections in patients at risk. Am J Med 1984; 76:231–237.
Nichols RL, Smith JW, Klein DB, et al. Risk of infection after penetrating abdominal trauma. N Engl J Med 1984; 311:1065–1070.

ANIMAL BITE INFECTIONS

CHARLES ELLENBOGEN, M.D.

About one million people suffer animal or human bites each year in the United States. Although most bite victims do not seek medical care, about 1 percent of all emergency room visits are for animal or human bites. About one-fourth of all such bites are human, and up to 90 percent of animal bites are from dogs and about 10 percent from cats. Almost one-half of domestic animal bites are in children aged 5 to 14 years. Dog and human bites are most likely to produce abrasions or lacerations, and dog bites may produce crush injuries. From 5 to 15 percent of dog bites become infected. About 15 percent of human bites become infected. Cat bites are more likely to result in puncture wounds, of which 20 to 50 percent may become infected.

Victims of animal bite appearing for care can be separated into two groups. In the first group, the patient appears within 8 to 12 hours of injury, rarely has evidence of established infection, and is mainly seeking wound management and rabies prophylaxis. In the second group, the patient appears more than 12 hours after injury, often with clinical signs of infection.

Among adults, about one-half of bite wounds are to the hand. Septic arthritis and osteomyelitis, especially from cat puncture wounds, though uncommon are more common in the hand. Facial wounds are most common in children but can be found in nearly 10 percent of adult victims.

Human bites tend to occur in adolescents or adults.

MANAGEMENT OF UNINFECTED WOUNDS

The management of human and animal bite wounds begins with examination of the wound. Catalog the number, size, shape, depth, and character of wounds and assess the integrity and function of underlying structures.

The next step is obtaining adequate anesthesia to permit careful and thorough cleansing and debridement of the wound. Where anesthesia is required, begin with antiseptic cleansing of the intact skin of the wound area with 1 percent povidone iodine or chlorhexidine scrub solution. Anesthesia with 0.5 percent or 1 percent lidocaine (Xylocaine) with epinephrine 1:200,000 prolongs anesthesia and reduces the risk of too rapid absorption of the lidocaine or toxicity associated with its use in large wounds. On the other hand, epinephrine should be avoided for anesthesia of digits or when blood supply to the local tissue is compromised.

After adequate anesthesia, wound cleansing should include thorough cleansing and lavage with an antiseptic solution. The best solution is 1 percent povidone iodine. It possesses both antibacterial and antiviral properties, and the 1 percent solution is more rapidly bactericidal than 10 percent povidone iodine because the free iodine release is greater. After initial wound cleansing and lavage with the antiseptic solution, follow with lavage with buffered Ringer's solution or commercially available balanced salt solution.

The process of wound cleansing is as important as the solution used. Beginning with the more shallow wound areas, use fine mesh gauze sponges for cleansing. This must be done gently because it can be damaging to exposed tissues. Then irrigate both shallow and deeper wounds using a 30- to 35-ml syringe and 18- to 19-gauge needle, which provide sufficient pressure to dislodge bacteria and debris from the deep lacerations and puncture wounds without forcing them into the tissue. A liter or more of antiseptic cleansing lavage solution is needed, especially for deep puncture wounds or lacerations. Alternative methods, such as simple soaking of the wound or irrigation with a bulb syringe, may be less effective for physically dislodging bacteria and debris. Moreover, injuries to extremities benefit from elevation and immobilization which may be delayed by soaking.

Debridement is performed along with irrigation, not as a separate step. High pressure irrigation with the antiseptic solution as described is, therefore, the first step in debridement. After initial irrigation, all devitalized tissue should be excised by a practitioner skilled in the procedure. Hand bites, especially cat bite puncture wounds or closed fist injuries from fist fights, should be debrided down to the bone by a hand surgeon immediately, due to the danger of osteomyelitis and septic arthritis.

As debridement proceeds, continue careful inspection and exploration of the wound to document damage to vascular or neural tissue, tendon, joint capsule, facial cartilage, or bone. Excision of a thin (e.g., 5-mm) margin of healthy dermis from the wound edge may improve outcome. Table 1 details the procedures to be used in management of the wound.

Wound closure can be a complex problem. Hand wounds may be best managed by delayed primary closure in 4 to 7 days. If the wound size permits, packing such a wound open with antiseptic soaked gauze is indicated. Facial bite wounds are more likely to require immediate closure for cosmetic reasons, especially if fresh (less than 12 hours old). Closure of uninfected wounds of less than 8-hours' duration can be successfully performed with a single layer of superficial sutures. If the possibility of contamination is high, wound tape closure may improve outcome. When deeper tissues are injured or casting is needed or functional impairment requires additional therapy, early involvement of an appropriate consultant is mandatory.

Some uninfected animal bite wounds deserve antibiotic prophylaxis in their management. Although published controlled studies of bite wound prophylaxis do not clearly document the benefit of such therapy, a number of such studies suggest that antibiotic prophylaxis results in a trend in the direction of benefit. Puncture wounds, especially common with cat bites, are at a particular risk of infection, at least partly because they are hard to irrigate and debride effectively. Wounds of the hand, likewise, are at an increased risk of infection as compared to other wound sites, especially if the source is a human bite.

The antibiotic to be prescribed for a prophylaxis of such wounds should be begun as soon as possible. The choice of antibiotic must be based on the bacteria that are likely to cause infection. *Pasteurella multocida* may be a pathogen in up to 50 percent of dog bites and an even higher percentage of cat bites. It is not seen in human bites. Other organisms that may be isolated include staphylococci, streptococci, and a spectrum of other gram-negative organisms, including species of *Pseudomonas*, *Moraxella*, and *Haemophilus*. In fact, more than half of infected animal bites may have multiple organisms. In addition to aerobic or facultive organisms as noted above, anaerobic isolates are also frequent. These include peptococci and peptostreptococci as well as *Fusobacterium* and *Bacteroides* species. Such anaerobes appear to be most common in human bite wounds but are seen also in cultures of infected wounds caused by dog and cat bites.

This lengthy list of possible pathogens, which often present in mixed infections, indicates that the prophylactic antibiotic regimen must have an appropriately broad spectrum. Likewise, failure of prophylaxis must be considered possible regardless of the antibiotic selected and close follow-up provided.

The prophylactic antibiotic of choice is the combination of amoxicillin and clavulanic acid (Augmentin) given

TABLE 1   Animal Bite Wound Care: Use Sterile Technique

Anesthesia

1. Disinfect skin through which injection to be given with povidone iodine scrub. Inject (Xylocaine) 0.5% or 1% combined with epinephrine 1:200,000. Do NOT use epinephrine in local anesthetic block of digits or thin skin flaps with compromised blood supply

2. Use small (25–30-gauge) needle for injection to minimize pain of skin penetration

Wound cleansing: use large volumes of solution (e.g., 1 liter)

1. 1% povidone iodine solution cleansing using fine mesh sponges

2. High-pressure irrigation (18–19-gauge needle and a large syringe, e.g., 30–35 ml) with 1% povidone iodine solution to all puncture wounds, deep lacerations, or other wound sites not cleanable with fine mesh sponge. After thorough irrigation with povidone iodine, repeat thorough high-pressure irrigation of entire wound with crystalloids such as buffered Ringer's solution or balanced salt solutions

3. If patient is at risk for rabies, use 20% soft soap solution for cleansing and irrigation; also cleanse puncture wounds with soap solution–impregnated cotton-tipped applicators

Debridement

1. To be performed by a skilled surgical specialist when appropriate, i.e., large or complicated wounds, wounds of hands or face, or when underlying structures require evaluation of repair

2. Debride visibly devitalized subcutaneous tissue and dermis; consider additional excision of a thin (5-mm) margin of dermis from nondevitalized wound margins

3. Carefully evaluate integrity and function of underlying structures

4. Repeat high-pressure irrigation of debrided wound with crystalloids.

---

orally in a dosage for adults of 250 mg of amoxicillin every 8 hours for 3 to 5 days. In children, prescribe as amoxicillin 25 mg per kilogram per day divided into three doses for 3 to 5 days. For patients allergic to penicillin, the combination trimethoprim-sulfamethoxazole (Septra, Bactrim) is the next best choice, with alternatives including a tetracycline (such as doxycycline) or an oral cephalosporin or erythromycin. Trimethoprim-sulfamethoxazole may be prescribed as 160 mg of trimethoprim and 800 mg of sulfamethoxazole administered orally every 12 hours for 3 to 5 days. In children, 10 mg per kilogram of trimethoprim and 50 mg per kilogram of sulfamethoxazole per day is prescribed in divided doses every 12 hours for 3 to 5 days.

MANAGEMENT OF INFECTED WOUNDS

When patients present with the animal bite wound already infected, they tend to present within 25 to 48 hours after the bite. Clinical presentations may include fever, with signs of local infection such as pain, purulent drainage, cellulitis, abscesses, lymphangitis, and lymphadenitis. Careful evaluation is needed to look for more extensive tissue involvement such as tenosynovitis, osteomyelitis, or septic arthritis. Even systemic infections such as gram-negative bacillary sepsis, endocarditis, or brain abscess must be considered as uncommon results of animal bite infections. *P. multocida* infections particularly may be characterized by a presentation within 24 to 36 hours of the animal bite. Streptococcal and staphylococcal infection may also be present (in some cases combined with *P. multocida*), presenting as abscesses, cellulitis, or lymphangitis.

Management of infected wounds must include drainage and debridement with an appropriate specialty surgical consultation. Gram stains and cultures, including anaerobic cultures, should be obtained. Since falsely negative Gram stains may occur, Gram-stain interpretation should only be used as a guide. The decision to hospitalize the patient depends on such considerations as the need for parenteral antimicrobial therapy or the need for debridement in the operating room. Thus, hospitalization may be needed in the presence of systemic symptoms or because of the rapidity and extent of the development of the infection and its resulting damage.

The same antibiotic choices suggested for prophylaxis apply to the initial choice of antibiotics for treatment. Parenteral therapy with the combination of ticarcillin–clavulanic acid (Timentin) in an intravenous dose of 3.1 g every 4 hours or 6.2 g every 6 hours is a good starting choice. Trimethoprim-sulfamethoxazole at an intravenous dose of 2.5 mg of the trimethoprim per kilogram administered every 6 hours is an alternative initial choice for the penicillin-allergic patient. The newer cephalosporin, ceftriaxone (Rochephin), in a dose of 25 mg per kilogram every 12 hours intravenously for children or 1 g every 12 hours for adults is an additional alternative for serious infections.

TETANUS

Although tetanus is a rare complication of animal bites, wound contamination by saliva places the wound in a category of high risk for tetanus. Additional factors placing the wound at higher risk include deep puncture wounds or wounds with devitalized tissue.

If the bite victim has completed at least a three-dose series of immunizations containing an adsorbed tetanus toxoid (such as DPT or DT for children younger than 7 years or Td for older children and adults), a booster dose of tetanus toxoid is required if the last dose was administered more than 5 years previously.

If the bite victim has an unknown history of tetanus toxoid immunization or has received fewer than three doses of toxoid, tetanus immune globulin (TIG) is administered as an intramuscular dose (deltoid, not gluteal) of 250 IU for a wound of average severity. Then tetanus toxoid should be administered to complete a primary series.

RABIES

Human rabies is rare in the United States, with only nine cases having been reported since 1980. Moreover, five of these nine cases were imported from countries where canine rabies is endemic. Thus, many if not most of the estimated 18,000 patients who receive antirabies prophylaxis in the United States each year may not need it.

Therefore, the determination of the risk of rabies for a patient presenting with an animal bite becomes the key to minimizing the need to administer this prophylaxis. Time is a significant factor, however, since delay in administration of antirabies prophylaxis may lessen its effectiveness.

The initial step in determining the risk of rabies is determination of the risk from the specific species of the biting animal. Dog and cat rabies is rare in the United States, with only 113 cases in dogs and 130 cases in cats reported in 1985. Farm animal rabies (260 cases in 1985) accounts for a majority of cases of rabies in domestic animals. Cases in wild animals account for the rest of the 5,607 cases reported in 1985 in the United States. The most common wild animals to have rabies are skunks, raccoons (mainly along the central and south Atlantic coast), foxes, and bats. Rodents, such as squirrels, hamsters, guinea pigs, gerbils, chipmunks, rats, and mice, and lagomorphs, such as rabbits or hares, are rarely infected with rabies. No person bitten by a rodent or lagomorph should receive antirabies prophylaxis

without consultation with the state or local health department. In fact, with any biting species, determine the likelihood or frequency of animal rabies identified in that species in your area by calling the local or state public health department. Wild animal bites should be assumed to put the patient at risk for rabies.

For domestic animals, the next step is to determine the behavior of the animal at the time of the bite injury. A majority of animal bites occur while the victim is playing or fighting or while the biting animal is feeding or being handled. Biting is a normal response in an animal that is excited or provoked because it perceives itself as cornered or under attack. Patients suffering from a provoked bite should not be given antirabies prophylaxis. An unprovoked bite or a bite related to abnormal or changed animal behavior should be assumed to be a sign of rabies, however.

Domestic animals immunized with an effective animal rabies vaccine within the accepted period of effectiveness for the vaccine are also unlikely to have or transmit rabies. However, you will often be unable to determine the animal's precise vaccination status, and in such a case an apparently vaccinated animal that otherwise is at risk for transmitting rabies according to species and behavior should be considered as rabid.

While domestic animals at low risk for transmitting rabies may be properly quarantined and observed for 10 days, wild animals and domestic animals that may be rabid should be humanely killed and the brain promptly examined for rabies antigen. However, delay in initiating antirabies prophylaxis may be dangerous. Once the clinical situation indicates that the patient is at risk for rabies (Table 2), therapy should be initiated immediately.

When a bite wound is sustained from an animal in a situation that places the patient at risk for rabies, thoroughly irrigate the wound with a 20 percent soft soap solution. Soap solution is the preferred disinfectant (as opposed to 1 percent povidone iodine) because soap solution is a highly effective antirabies solution. As previously noted, irrigation of puncture wounds or deep lacerations with a 19-gauge needle and a 30-mm syringe increases the effectiveness of

---

TABLE 2 **Assessing the Indication for Antirabies Postexposure Prophylaxis**

Biting animal species

    Have members of this species been diagnosed as rabid in your area?
    Assume bite of wild animal is rabid, except rodents, rabbits, or hares.

Biting animal behavior

    Was bite provoked, i.e., occurred during play or a fight when animal was excited or when animal was feeding or being cornered or territory invaded?

    Was bite unprovoked, i.e., deliberate attack in absence of discernible provocation?

    Has animal's behavior changed?

Biting animal rabies immunization (domestic animal only)

    Vaccine considered effective and administered within effective time prior to bite according to veterinarian or public health official.

    If a biting domestic animal's species behavior and absent or unknown vaccination status suggest the patient is at risk for rabies, do NOT postpone therapy while the animal is hunted or, if in custody, is observed in quarantine.

the step. In addition, deep wounds should be scrubbed using soap solution-impregnated cotton-tipped applicators.

Systemic antirabies prophylaxis consists of two steps. Human rabies immune globulin (RIG) is administered in a dose of 20 IU per kilogram or approximately 9 IU per pound of body weight. Up to half of the RIG should be thoroughly infiltrated in the area around the wound, based on the tissue volume of the area and the need to maintain normal tissue integrity. The remainder should be administered intramuscularly in the deltoid (not gluteal) area. After the RIG is administered, the first dose of human diploid cell rabies vaccine (HDCV) is administered in a 1.0-ml dose in the deltoid (not gluteal) region as soon as possible. Additional 1-ml intramuscular doses of HDCV should be given on days 3, 7, 14, and 28 after the first dose. In addition, a sixth dose is recommended by the World Health Organization on the 90th day. Unless the patient is immunodeficient, there is no reason to determine serum rabies antibody titers.

UNCOMMON INFECTIONS

Less common animal bite infections may include cat scratch fever, rat bite fever, brucellosis, tularemia, blastomycosis and, from human bites, syphilis. If the patient has had a splenectomy or is otherwise immunocompromised, in addition to all the previously described local infections, fulminant gram-negative bacterial sepsis is possible.

Herpesvirus simiae (B virus) infection may result from the bite of Asiatic monkeys, such as rhesus or cynomolgus monkeys of the genus *Macaca*. B virus infections in humans may produce encephalitis, which has been reported to have a high mortality rate. Although acyclovir (Zovirax) may be therapeutically beneficial in such patients, the danger of infection has prompted the publication by the Centers for Disease Control (CDC) of extensive precautions recommended to prevent bites for all macaque animal handlers. All macaque bites should be immediately scrubbed and cleansed with soap and water. When the animal handler has sustained a deep penetrating wound that is difficult to clean, investigation of the animal's infectious status is indicated. Acyclovir prophylaxis for macaque bite wound may be worth considering. For more information the physician should contact the Viral Exanthems and Herpes Virus Branch, Division of Viral Diseases, CDC (404–329–1338).

SUGGESTED READING

Aghababian RV, Conte JE Jr. Mammalian bite wounds. Ann Emerg Med 1980; 9:79–83.
Baker MD, Moore SE. Human bites in children. Am J Dis Child 1987; 141:1285–1290.
Jaffe AC. Animal bites. Pediatr Clin North Am 1983; 30:405–413.
Rest JG, Goldstein EJC. Management of human and animal bite wounds. Emerg Med Clin North Am 1985; 3:117–126.
Trott A. Care of mammalian bites. Pediatr Infect Dis 1987; 6:8–10.

RESPIRATORY TRACT INFECTIONS

OTITIS MEDIA

DAVID G. ROBERTS, M.D.
CANDICE E. JOHNSON, M.D., Ph.D.

EPIDEMIOLOGY

Acute or suppurative otitis media is primarily a disease of children under 2 years of age. It is usually defined as the presence of fluid in the middle ear, combined either with signs of inflammation (erythema, bulging, opacity of the drum) or with symptoms (fever, otalgia, irritability). Approximately two-thirds of infants will experience one or more episodes of acute otitis media within the first 2 years. Nonsuppurative otitis media, also known as otitis media with effusion, may follow suppurative otitis media or may be found incidentally during a routine examination. Nonsuppurative otitis media may be a cause of conductive hearing loss and speech delay in young children, although the significance of such problems remains controversial.

ETIOLOGY AND PATHOGENESIS

The etiology of otitis media is a complex interaction of eustachian tube dysfunction, viral upper respiratory tract infections, and bacterial agents. Viruses are rarely isolated from upper respiratory middle ear effusions but probably impair eustachian tube function, allowing nasopharyngeal flora to infect the middle ear. The risk of otitis media is high for several weeks after viral upper respiratory tract illness. The predominant bacterial organisms are listed in Table 1 and vary little with age except in neonates. In infants younger than 6 weeks, perinatally acquired organisms such as *Escherichia coli*, *Klebsiella*, *Staphylococcus aureus*, and group B *Streptococci* are seen in about 15 percent of cases.

With rare exceptions, *Streptococcus pneumoniae* remains sensitive to ampicillin, but the rate of β-lactamase-producing strains of *Haemophilus influenzae* has been increasing and now stands at around 25 percent (Table 1). *Branhamella catarrhalis* has been reported by several groups to be increasing in incidence, and 75 percent of isolates produce β-lactamase. Overall, the rate of in vitro resistance to ampicillin is approximately 21 percent. This does not mean that amoxicillin will fail in 21 percent of the children to whom it is given. In clinical trials in which the middle ear is retapped at 3 to 5 days, more than 80 percent of β-lactamase producing strains of *B. catarrhalis* are eradicated by amoxicillin.

DIAGNOSIS

Accurate evaluation of the tympanic membrane requires skill in pneumatic otoscopy (insufflation). A well-sealed otoscope with a speculum properly sized to occlude the ear canal painlessly is the only equipment needed. The presence of a fluid level or dampened mobility indicates effusion. In suppurative otitis media, effusion is usually accompanied by bulging of the pars flaccida and opacity of the drum; erythema is highly variable and may be due to fever or a screaming infant. Confirmation of the diagnosis is possible in cooperative children by tympanometry and acoustic reflex testing. In children under 7 months, however, special equipment and skill are needed for reliable results. Acoustic reflex measurements can be valuable in the child over 7 months, since they require less cooperation than tympanometry and uses less-expensive equipment.

TYMPANOCENTESIS

Tympanocentesis can be a valuable adjunct in planning therapy in select groups: infants under 6 weeks, immunosuppressed individuals, and children at risk of bacteremia. In infants under 6 weeks who are afebrile and have only upper respiratory tract symptoms, outpatient management

TABLE 1 Bacterial Pathogens Isolated From Suppurative Otitis Media

	Number of Ampicillin-Resistant Isolates/ Total Isolates (%) in Indicated Time Period	
Pathogen	*1979–1983*	*1984–1987*
Streptococcus pneumoniae	4/140 (2.9)	7/77 (9.1)
Haemophilus influenzae	9/127 (7.1)	15/60 (25)
Branhamella catarrhalis	61/75 (81.3)	25/33 (75.8)
Total pathogens	74/342 (21.6)	47/170 (27.6)
Number of cultures yielding no pathogen	151	90

Data are from Cleveland Metropolitan General Hospital.

is appropriate, provided that the parents are reliable. The infant should have tympanocentesis performed, particularly if he has had a sojourn in the intensive care nursery where enteric pathogens may have colonized the nasopharynx. All infants under 6 weeks presenting with otitis media accompanied by fever or systemic illness should be hospitalized and have an evaluation for sepsis performed. If the infant under 6 weeks is treated on an outpatient basis, broad-spectrum coverage with a drug such as amoxicillin-clavulanate that covers many neonatal pathogens is indicated while the results of the tympanocentesis are awaited.

Tympanocentesis is also indicated in all immunosuppressed individuals. Cultures for *Candida* and fungi should also be performed in these patients. A diagnostic tympanocentesis may also identify the course of infection in children with meningitis or sepsis and therefore should be part of the admission cultures of such children.

Tympanocentesis is rarely indicated in children who remain febrile while being treated with amoxicillin, since the cause is generally noncompliance, a β-lactamase-producing organism, or fever caused by another source. However, if the child is highly febrile or has any signs of mastoid involvement, tympanocentesis is indicated.

ANTIMICROBIAL TREATMENT AND FOLLOW-UP

Before selection of an antibiotic for otitis media, one further diagnostic step is needed in children under 2 years of age. Because the risk of bacteremia is high if the temperature exceeds 39°C rectally, a blood culture should be obtained. Those children with positive cultures should be reevaluated as soon as possible and admitted for intravenous therapy if still febrile or systemically ill.

The antibiotic used in the treatment of suppurative otitis media should be determined by the patient's age, clinical presentation, and history of adverse reactions to antimicrobial therapy. Figure 1 shows a recommended treatment protocol. In infants and children 6 weeks and older who present with acute otitis media, amoxicillin remains the drug of choice. Amoxicillin has been efficacious over many years against the common bacterial pathogens and has minimal adverse effects.

In patients in whom treatment failure is occurring on amoxicillin, another antibiotic should be given. Symptoms of treatment failure are fever, ear pain, or irritability after 48 hours on an antibiotic. Alternative drugs are erythromycin-sulfisoxazole (Pediazole), amoxicillin-clavulanate (Augmentin), trimethoprim-sulfamethoxazole (TMP/SMZ), and cefaclor. All of these antibiotics are effective against β-lactamase-producing organisms except for cefaclor, which has shown a high rate of bacteriologic failure when tympanocentesis was repeated 3 to 5 days into treatment. Children who are considered treatment failures on amoxicillin at 48 hours are candidates for tympanocentesis if they are very febrile or systemically ill; however, the possibility of other causes of persistent fever such as meningitis or bacteremia must also be considered.

Patients with suppurative otitis media who have been treated with an antibiotic with resolution of their symptoms, and then within 1 month develop signs and symptoms of otitis media, most likely have a new infection with a different organism and have not suffered a treatment failure. These patients can be treated successfully with the same antibiotic.

If a patient is allergic to penicillin, one may treat with erythromycin-sulfisoxazole, TMP-SMZ, or cefaclor, although one should be cautious with cefaclor as the patient may also manifest allergic symptoms to this antibiotic.

Patients should be treated for 10 days, and follow-up should be done approximately 1 month after diagnosis of the acute otitis media. At this time, pneumatic otoscopy should be used to assess the appearance of the tympanic membrane and to determine if middle ear effusion is present. Tympanometry is also a reliable method to determine the status of the middle ear. Persistent effusion following acute otitis media can be seen in 40 percent of children 1 month after diagnosis, in 20 percent after 2 months, and in 10 percent after 3 months. We do not recommend repeated courses of different antibiotics for asymptomatic effusions since 90 percent resolve within 3 months with one course of therapy. If middle ear effusion is present at 1 month, the patient should have monthly examinations with pneumatic otoscopy or tympanometry over the next 3 months to follow the effusion. If the effusion has resolved in this time, further follow-up is not necessary. However, in high-risk patients, such as those who have had three or more episodes of acute otitis media in an 18-month period, antimicrobial prophylaxis may be started after the 10-day antibiotic course for the acute otitis media is complete.

If after 3 months the effusion is still present, further treatment is indicated. If the child is not receiving antimicrobial prophylaxis at this point, a 10-day course of a drug effective against β-lactamase producers is indicated before referral to an otolaryngologist. As many as 50 percent of children with asymptomatic ear effusion have had pathogenic organisms isolated from an ear aspirate. If the child has had prophylaxis for 3 months, referral to an otolaryngologist is the best option. Serial audiologic assessment of children with middle ear effusion reveals an extremely variable degree of hearing loss from week to week, without concomitant changes in the appearance of the tympanic membrane. Therefore, a small degree of hearing loss on one examination is no guarantee that more substantial losses may not be present at other times. Children under 3 years are at a critical stage for language acquisition, when even small amounts of conductive hearing loss may be detrimental. Timely tympanostomy tube placement is indicated. Conversely, in older children, if audiologic assessment indicates normal speech development and only minor degrees of hearing loss, the otolaryngologist may follow the child without surgery. The natural history of most persistent ear effusions is to resolve in the summer months when fewer respiratory infections occur.

Table 2 lists the adverse effects of the oral antibiotics used to treat otitis media. Amoxicillin is a safe drug but has been noted to cause an erythematous maculopapular rash in as many as 10 percent of recipients. In addition, diarrhea is noted in approximately 3 percent of those receiving 40 to 50 mg per kilogram per day but in 9 percent of those receiving more than 50 mg per kilogram per day. Treatment does not have to be stopped if these side effects are mild.

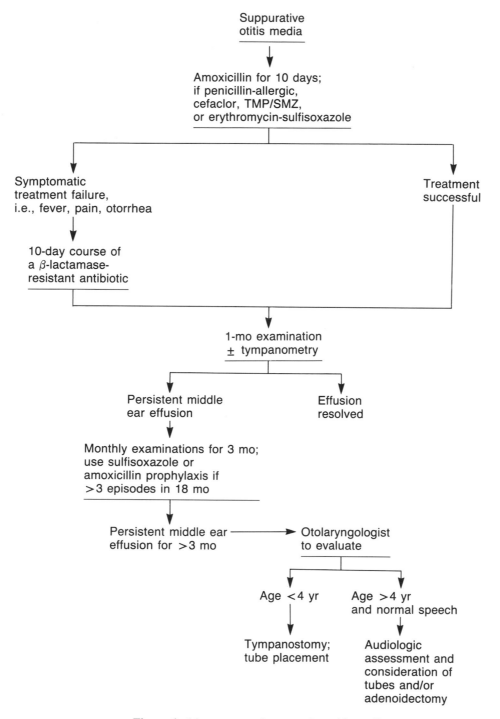

Figure 1 Management of suppurative otitis media.

Urticarial rashes require cessation of therapy. Amoxicillin-clavulanate can cause the same effects as amoxicillin, and the diarrhea has been noted to be more severe, but cessation of treatment is usually not required. The main disadvantage of sulfonamides is antibody-mediated reactions, the most frequent being erythematous maculopapular rashes. A rare occurrence is the Stevens-Johnson syndrome, exudative erythema multiforme bullosa. These rashes mandate stopping therapy at once. Bone marrow suppression has been reported with sulfonamides but does not appear to be clinically significant. In addition, before prescribing one of the sulfonamide antibiotics for more than 10 days, one should know the patient's glucose-6-phosphate dehydrogenase status, because in a patient who is deficient in this enzyme, treatment with a sulfonamide may induce hemolysis. Adverse effects associated with cefaclor include an erythematous maculopapular rash, erythema multiforme, and an infrequent serum-sickness–like reaction, characterized by arthritis and arthralgia with a rash or urticaria. Cefaclor has also been found to cause diarrhea in approximately 7 percent of patients. Erythromycin is associated with the development of anorexia, nausea, vomiting, and abdominal pain in up to 30 percent of patients.

ANTIMICROBIAL PROPHYLAXIS

Antimicrobial prophylaxis has been demonstrated in clinical trials to lower significantly the incidence of suppurative otitis media. Drug prophylaxis should therefore be instituted in children with three or more documented episodes of suppurative otitis media within an 18-month period. Prophylaxis should also be considered in children who have been on prophylaxis in the past and have again developed closely spaced episodes of suppurative otitis media. Sulfisoxazole can be used in a dose of 75 mg per kilogram per day divided twice daily. Amoxicillin, 20 mg per kilogram per day, once daily is an alternative. Drug administration should be during the time of year when upper respiratory tract infections and acute otitis media are commoner—generally from mid-October to mid-May.

TYMPANOSTOMY TUBES AND ADENOIDECTOMY

Controversy exists over the efficacy of tympanostomy tubes because of the small number of controlled clinical trials. However, tubes are probably indicated in several circumstances. Tympanostomy tubes should be considered in children who have a history of recurrent suppurative otitis media but have not responded to antimicrobial prophylaxis. Tympanostomy tube placement should be considered in infants and children with persistent middle ear effusion for a minimum of 3-months' duration, provided that there has been adequate antimicrobial therapy without otoscopic or tympanometric evidence of improvement. A recent clinical trial has, however, suggested that in children 4 to 8 years of age with persistent middle ear effusion, adenoidectomy plus bilateral myringotomy lowered the posttreatment morbidity (as measured by hearing acuity) and the number of surgical retreatments more than tympanostomy tubes alone and to the same degree as adenoidectomy with tympanostomy tube placement. Thus, adenoidectomy with myringotomy may be sufficient treatment for older children with persistent middle ear effusion, thereby avoiding the possible complications of tympanostomy tubes.

DECONGESTANTS AND ANTIHISTAMINES

Combinations of decongestants and antihistamines have been frequently prescribed in the therapy of both suppurative otitis media and persistent middle ear effusion; however, clinical trials have not supported their use. In a recent clinical trial comparing 4 weeks of daily pseudoephedrine hydrochloride plus chlorpheniramine maleate to placebo, there was no difference in the rate of resolution of middle ear effusion. Decongestants and antihistamines are not indicated in the treatment of otitis media and middle ear effusion.

STEROIDS

Steroid use in the treatment of persistent middle ear effusion has not received sufficient clinical evaluation. Clinical trials evaluating the efficacy of steroids in resolution of persistent middle ear effusion have had contradictory results, and at present, there appears to be no indication for the use of steroids.

TABLE 2 Oral Antibiotic Therapy for Suppurative Otitis Media

Drug	Recommended Dose	Advantages	Disadvantages
Amoxicillin	50 mg/kg/day divided q8h	Inexpensive; severe adverse effects rare	Increasing bacterial resistance; dose-related diarrhea
Trimethoprim-sulfamethoxazole	8 mg TMP and 40 mg SMZ/kg/day divided q12h	Inexpensive; active against β-lactamase-producing organisms in vitro	Sulfonamide-related allergic reactions
Erythromycin-sulfisoxazole	50 mg erythromycin ethyl succinate and 150 mg sulfisoxazole/kg/day divided q6h	Active against β-lactamase-producing organisms in vivo	Expensive; sulfonamide-related allergic reactions; frequent gastrointestinal adverse effects
Cefaclor	40 mg/kg/day divided q8h	Active against β-lactamase-producing organisms in vitro	Expensive; rare serious effects including erythema multiforme and serum-sickness-like reaction; bacteriologic failures reported
Amoxicillin-clavulanate	40 mg amoxicillin/kg/day divided q8h	Clavulanic acid inactivates β-lactamase, providing broad-spectrum coverage including neonatal middle ear pathogens; severe adverse effects rare	Expensive; diarrhea noted to be worse than with amoxicillin alone

PNEUMOCOCCAL VACCINE AND IMMUNOPROPHYLAXIS

Several well-controlled trials have evaluated pneumococcal vaccine for prevention of otitis media. However, a fundamental obstacle is the poor response of infants under 24 months to polysaccharide antigens. These trials have shown a modest reduction in total episodes of otitis media in older children but no effect in infants under 2 years. It appears that even though one can reduce type-specific pneumococcal episodes in infants, the total number of episodes is not affected. Therefore, use of pneumococcal vaccine for prevention of otitis media is not recommended.

SUGGESTED READING

Bluestone CD. Otitis media and sinusitis: management and when to refer to the otolaryngologist. Pediatr Infect Dis 1987; 6:100–106.
Bluestone CD, et al. Workshop on effects of otitis media on the child. Pediatrics 1983; 71:639–652.
Carlin SA, Shurin PA. Otitis media. In: Nelson NM, ed. Current therapy in neonatal-perinatal medicine. Toronto: BC Decker, 1985:270.
Paradise JL. Otitis media in infants and children. Pediatrics 1980; 65:917–943.
Shurin PA, Johnson CE, Wegman DL. Medical aspects of diagnosis and prevention of otitis media. In: Kavanagh JF, ed. Otitis media and child development. Fredericton, Canada: York Press, 1986:60.

PHARYNGITIS

MARK D. ARONSON, M.D.
ANTHONY L. KOMAROFF, M.D.

In the past 3 years there has been a resurgence of acute rheumatic fever in many areas in the United States. This resurgence should lead clinicians to be increasingly diligent in caring for patients with pharyngitis in attempts to identify and treat patients with group A β-hemolytic streptococcal (GABS) infection. Additionally, clinicians must be aware of other potentially treatable and clinically important organisms that may also cause pharyngitis.

GROUP A STREPTOCOCCAL PHARYNGITIS

Benefits of Treatment

Treatment speeds the relief of symptoms if it is begun early in the illness. Treatment probably further reduces the already low rate of suppurative complications and reduces the likelihood of spread to close contacts. However, treatment does not reduce with certainty the risk of acute glomerulonephritis. Delaying implementation of therapy by 24 to 48 hours may lower the risk of early and late recurrences of GABS.

Treatment does reduce the risk of acute rheumatic fever (ARF). Since initial reports from Utah of an ongoing outbreak of acute rheumatic fever (ARF), several other areas in the United States have also documented the resurgence of ARF. Most of the recent outbreaks of ARF have occurred in uncrowded, rural settings as opposed to previous outbreaks, which have generally occurred in poorer inner-city areas of developed countries. However, the degree of crowding within domiciles in the rural areas is still under study.

Strategy for Diagnosis and Treatment

We favor a strategy that individualizes diagnosis and treatment decisions. We recommend obtaining a specimen for culture or for a rapid diagnostic antigen test from any symptomatic patient who is at special risk for streptococcal infection (for example, patients with a history of acute rheumatic fever; school-aged children, including teenagers or young adults), from any patient in whom clinical findings suggest that the probability of streptococcal infection is relatively high (such as patients with fever, exudate, or anterior cervical adenitis), or in any community known to have a high rate of ARF or epidemic streptococcal infection. This strategy is summarized in Figure 3.

Several test kits are available that reliably detect group A streptococcal antigen. These are rapid assays and are being used increasingly in office settings as a substitute for or supplement to routine throat culture. Most reports suggest that these kits are extremely specific but variably sensitive. They may miss up to 10 or 15 percent of true positives. Adult patients can be categorized on clinical grounds as to the likelihood of GABS infection, and we prefer to decide, on that basis, whether treatment should be started at the time of visit. If a rapid screening test is used and is positive, that constitutes reliable evidence of GABS pharyngitis, and the patient should be treated accordingly. If the rapid test is negative, a throat culture should be done unless the kit is known to have a sensitivity exceeding 95 percent.

Acceptable treatment regimens that are therapeutically equivalent for streptococcal pharyngitis include benzathine penicillin G, 1.2 million units intramuscularly once for patients not likely to comply with an oral regimen; oral penicillin VK, 250 mg four times per day for 10 days; or, for penicillin-allergic patients, oral erythromycin, 250 mg four times per day, 500 mg twice a day, or 333 mg three times a day for 10 days, in that order of preference. (For true treatment failures, dicloxacillin is occasionally effective.) If compliance in children is a problem, once-a-day cefadroxil is effective.

MYCOPLASMAL PHARYNGITIS

Accumulating evidence suggests that pharyngitis from infection with *Mycoplasma pneumoniae* may be as common as or more common than streptococcal pharyngitis, particularly in young adults. Also, the presence of bronchopulmonary symptoms (such as cough or wheezing) along with pharyngitis suggests pharyngitis due to *M. pneumoniae*. Rapid detection of *M. pneumoniae* may be feasible soon with

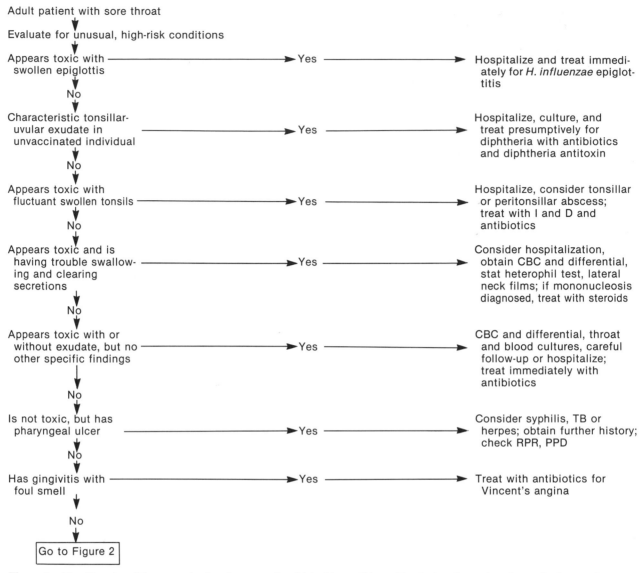

Adult patient with sore throat
↓
Evaluate for unusual, high-risk conditions
↓
Appears toxic with ───────────────────→ Yes ───────────────→ Hospitalize and treat immedi-
swollen epiglottis   ately for *H. influenzae* epiglot-
                                                                titis
↓
No
↓
Characteristic tonsillar-
uvular exudate in ─────────────────────→ Yes ───────────────→ Hospitalize, culture, and
unvaccinated individual   treat presumptively for
                                                                diphtheria with antibiotics
                                                                and diphtheria antitoxin
↓
No
↓
Appears toxic with
fluctuant swollen tonsils ─────────────→ Yes ───────────────→ Hospitalize, consider tonsillar
                                                                or peritonsillar abscess;
                                                                treat with I and D and
                                                                antibiotics
↓
No
↓
Appears toxic and is
having trouble swallow- ───────────────→ Yes ───────────────→ Consider hospitalization,
ing and clearing   obtain CBC and differential,
secretions   stat heterophil test, lateral
                                                                neck films; if mononucleosis
                                                                diagnosed, treat with steroids
↓
No
↓
Appears toxic with or
without exudate, but no ───────────────→ Yes ───────────────→ CBC and differential, throat
other specific findings   and blood cultures, careful
                                                                follow-up or hospitalize;
                                                                treat immediately with
                                                                antibiotics
↓
No
↓
Is not toxic, but has
pharyngeal ulcer ──────────────────────→ Yes ───────────────→ Consider syphilis, TB or
                                                                herpes; obtain further history;
                                                                check RPR, PPD
↓
No
↓
Has gingivitis with ──────────────────→ Yes ───────────────→ Treat with antibiotics for
foul smell   Vincent's angina
↓
No
↓
Go to Figure 2

Figure 1 Algorithm describing an evaluation for unusual or high-risk conditions. The designation *toxic* refers to findings such as high fever, prostration, tachycardia, and thready pulse.

kits using DNA probes. We have had variably reliable results with these probes in our practice thus far.

Because erythromycin is effective in eradicating the streptococcus as well as *M. pneumoniae*, we recommend treatment with erythromycin, 250 mg four times a day for 10 days, for patients with pharyngitis and bronchopulmonary symptoms or for any patient whose pharyngitis has not responded promptly. It should be pointed out, however, that this recommendation is not based on evidence that erythromycin is efficacious in such cases; no studies of this question have yet been conducted. The various enteric-coated forms of erythromycin may be less likely to produce gastrointestinal effects, but 1 g per day is usually tolerated in adults.

INFECTIOUS MONONUCLEOSIS

Pharyngitis often occurs with infectious mononucleosis. It may be worth making the diagnosis of infectious mononucleosis (as contrasted with other forms of viral pharyngitis) to alert the patient to symptoms suggesting complications, particularly ruptured spleen and upper airway obstruction.

Heterophil antibody is found in approximately 2 to 6 percent of patients younger than the age of 40 years seeking care for pharyngitis but is extremely uncommon in patients over 40 years of age. Most cases of pharyngitis associated with positive heterophil antibody are mild and may not have the characteristic hematologic findings (lymphocytosis with greater than 10 percent atypical lymphocytes) or the full-blown clinical picture of infectious mononucleosis.

We recommend obtaining a differential white blood cell count and a heterophil test in patients with even one of the findings shown in Figure 2 because the presence of these findings greatly raises the probability of infectious mononucleosis. Rapid differential slide tests (spot tests) for heterophil antibody have largely replaced the original Paul-Bunnell heterophil test. The characteristic hematologic and serologic abnormalities of infectious mononucleosis often

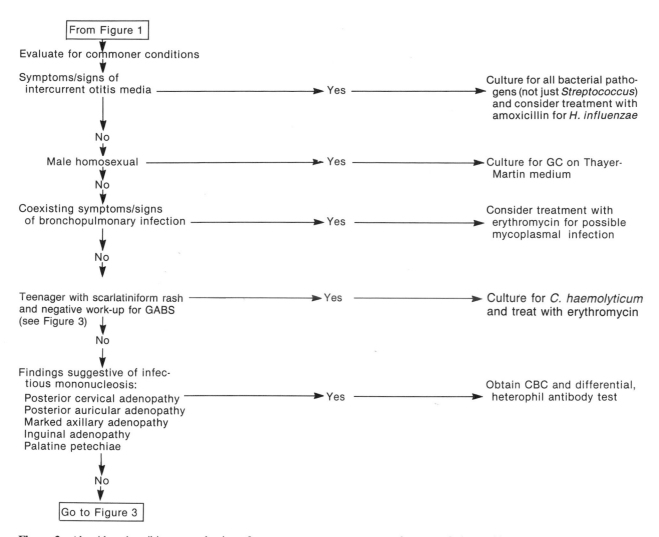

From Figure 1

Evaluate for commoner conditions

Symptoms/signs of intercurrent otitis media ——————→ Yes ——————→ Culture for all bacterial pathogens (not just *Streptococcus*) and consider treatment with amoxicillin for *H. influenzae*

No

Male homosexual ——————→ Yes ——————→ Culture for GC on Thayer-Martin medium

No

Coexisting symptoms/signs of bronchopulmonary infection ——————→ Yes ——————→ Consider treatment with erythromycin for possible mycoplasmal infection

No

Teenager with scarlatiniform rash and negative work-up for GABS (see Figure 3) ——————→ Yes ——————→ Culture for *C. haemolyticum* and treat with erythromycin

No

Findings suggestive of infectious mononucleosis:
Posterior cervical adenopathy ——————→ Yes ——————→ Obtain CBC and differential, heterophil antibody test
Posterior auricular adenopathy
Marked axillary adenopathy
Inguinal adenopathy
Palatine petechiae

No

Go to Figure 3

Figure 2 Algorithm describing an evaluation of more common nonstreptococcal causes of pharyngitis.

occur within 1 week of onset of symptoms in the majority of patients, but either of these may be absent in a patient or may not appear until 2 or 3 weeks after onset.

OTHER CAUSES OF PHARYNGITIS

Pharyngeal gonorrhea, although usually an asymptomatic infection, may be the cause of pharyngitis in 1 percent of patients seeking care. It should always be suspected—and pharyngeal cultures on appropriate media obtained—when the patient is known or thought to be a male homosexual. Obtaining a gonococcal culture might also be wise for patients with intercurrent symptoms of genitourinary infection with rectal sores or pain or with persistent pharyngitis.

We recommend culture on appropriate media for meningococci or *Corynebacterium diphtheriae* when a known epidemic raises the possibility of these otherwise rare pharyngeal pathogens. A diphtheritic membrane may be absent in cases of diphtheria, and a pseudomembrane may be seen in infectious mononucleosis and illnesses other than diphtheria. Nevertheless, an apparent membrane, especially when covering the uvula or soft palate, should be cultured for *C.*

diphtheriae. Corynebacterium haemolyticum causes pharyngitis in teenagers and young adults and is frequently accompanied by a rash resembling scarlet fever. Erythromycin is an effective treatment for this infection.

A swollen, red epiglottis indicates epiglottitis. This condition, rare in adults, is a medical emergency. Sore throat, hoarseness, and stridor, along with direct visualization of an inflamed epiglottis on depression of the tongue, are the key symptoms and signs. Lateral neck films may be diagnostically useful. The patient should be treated immediately for presumed epiglottitis. *Haemophilus influenzae* is the usual pathogen. A third-generation cephalosporin such as cefotaxime (up to 2 g every 4 hours for life-threatening infections) or chloramphenicol would be an appropriate antibacterial agent. The patient should be kept under constant observation for respiratory obstruction, a life-threatening event. Manipulation of the epiglottis by a swab or endoscope may provoke laryngeal spasm and should be avoided. *H. influenzae* may also be a cause of pharyngitis, sometimes with concurrent otitis media. When the patient has concurrent otitis media, a throat culture for all bacterial pathogens (not just GABS) should be obtained. When the throat culture demonstrates a heavy and predominant growth of *H. influenzae*,

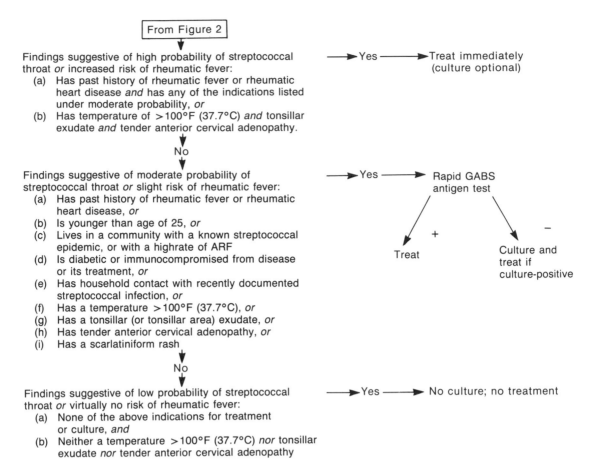

Figure 3 Algorithm describing an evaluation of the probability of group A streptococcal pharyngitis and the risk of developing acute rheumatic fever. Immediate treatment is preferred for those individuals whose throat culture results will not be complete for 9 days into the illness, since treatment after that time has not been shown to be protective against rheumatic fever.

appropriate treatment should be initiated: ampicillin, 500 mg every 6 hours, or amoxicillin, 500 mg every 8 hours. In settings with known high rates of ampicillin resistance or if the organism is shown to be ampicillin-resistant, trimethoprim-sulfamethoxazole (one double strength tablet twice a day), cefaclor (250 to 500 mg every 8 hours), or amoxicillin-clavulanate (250 to 500 mg every 8 hours) are appropriate oral substitutes.

Several viruses cause pharyngitis. Perhaps the commonest are the respiratory viruses (influenza virus, parainfluenza virus, adenovirus, respiratory syncytial virus, rhinovirus, coronavirus, and enterovirus). The primary infection with herpes simplex virus type 2 is associated with pharyngitis. An important cause of pharyngitis and stomatitis, particularly in the summer, is herpangina, a viral syndrome caused primarily by coxsackievirus A. No specific therapy exists for these viral infections, but preparations containing hydrogen peroxide in a glycerin base can be prescribed to relieve symptoms. One recent report suggests that human immunodeficiency virus infection may initially begin with pharyngitis and lymphadenopathy.

Notable gingivitis in association with pharyngeal inflammation suggests Vincent's angina, a mixed infection with a spirochete and fusiform gram-negative bacillus that responds

to penicillin therapy. A single pharyngeal ulcer is most often caused by a fusobacterial infection. However, such an ulcer can be a primary chancre or a tuberculous granuloma; serologic testing for syphilis and an evaluation for tuberculosis should be undertaken. Several ulcers, especially in association with a rash, may represent secondary syphilis and should lead to serologic testing. Unilateral tonsillar swelling, if fluctuant, suggests a peritonsillar abscess requiring incision and drainage; on rare occasions, a hard, nonfluctuant, unilateral tonsillar mass may be a carcinoma or lymphoma. In patients with a sore throat and a prominent headache, the possibility of meningitis must be considered. Patients with acute leukemia may present with pharyngitis and characteristically have a foul, necrotic exudate. Those patients with symptoms of severe chronic fatigue of greater than 6 months' duration who also have pharyngitis may have chronic fatigue syndrome, formerly called chronic Epstein-Barr viral infection.

The evaluation of patients for these unusual, high-risk conditions is summarized in Figure 1. Figures 1, 2, and 3 describe a sequential consideration of (1) the unusual or high-risk conditions, (2) the commoner forms of nonstreptococcal pharyngitis, and (3) an evaluation of possible group A streptococcal pharyngitis and the risk of acute rheumatic fever.

FOLLOW-UP ISSUES

A patient with a throat culture positive for GABS who has a sore throat unresponsive to penicillin for 1 week suggest several possibilities: poor compliance, true treatment failure, mycoplasmal pharyngitis, infectious mononucleosis, gonococcal pharyngitis, or, possibly, other forms of nonviral pharyngitis. Cervical adenopathy should remit within 1 month in streptococcal pharyngitis and within 2 months in infectious mononucleosis; failure to remit suggests lymphoma, leukemia, granulomatous diseases, or a malignant neoplasm of the head, neck, or chest. People in contact with patients who have streptococcal pharyngitis or living mates of those patients who are at high risk for infection (for ex-

ample, those with a history of acute rheumatic fever or indigent people living in crowded conditions) should have cultures performed and receive treatment if the culture is positive.

SUGGESTED READING

Bisno AL, Shulman ST, Dajani AS. The rise and fall (and rise) of rheumatic fever. JAMA 1988; 259:728–729.
Burke P, Bain J, Lowes A, et al. Rational decisions in managing sore throat: evaluation of a rapid test. Br Med J 1988; 296:1646–1649.
Editorial. Bacterial pharyngitis. Lancet 1987; 1:1241–1242.
Hillner BE, Centor RM. What a difference a day makes: a decision analysis of adult streptococcal pharyngitis. J Gen Intern Med 1987; 2:244–250.

PNEUMONIA

JAMES R. TILLOTSON, M.D.

Never forget that it is not a pneumonia, but a pneumonic man who is your patient
Sir William Withey Gull, 1816–1890

Sir William recognized the importance of dealing with the patient with pneumonia individually even prior to the availability of antimicrobial therapy and the recognition of the variety of causes seen today. The disease has not lost its distinction as "captain of all these men of death," at least among infectious diseases, but its character depends on the vantage point of the observer. To the pathologist, pneumonia is an inflammatory reaction in the lung often categorized as consolidating, interstitial, or necrotizing, usually without regard to cause. The radiologist attempts to correlate shadows with anatomic structures but cannot prove these changes are inflammatory let alone establish the cause of the inflammation. To the epidemiologist, pneumonia is the fifth leading cause of death in the United States and a major cause of nosocomial infection; but his diagnosis of pneumonia lacks specificity and emphasizes quantity rather than etiology. To the patient, pneumonia is a much greater problem, causing more morbidity and mortality than realized by any of the above, but the patient's concern for health does not include a consideration of etiology or specific therapy.

To the clinician, however, pneumonia is a common disease affecting many patients, with a variety of presentations and almost countless causes (Table 1). In fact, virtually all microorganisms known to be human pathogens have been associated with pneumonia. Therefore, the establishment of an etiologic diagnosis is the most important, but often the most difficult, aspect in the management of patients with pneumonia, but once a diagnosis is established, therapy can be relatively easy.

ETIOLOGY

The diagnostic features and the natural course of typical cases of the common infectious and noninfectious pneumonias will be described and specific treatment recommendations will be given. Since treatment, if required, cannot usually be delayed until results of definitive diagnostic tests are available, the approach to therapy proceeds by careful evaluation of the meaning and significance of each of the presenting manifestations, logical choice of appropriate diagnostic studies, offering safe and effective therapy based on a presumptive initial diagnosis, and reevaluation of this therapy at frequent intervals on the basis of the results of diagnostic studies and the course of the illness. The classic textbook approach of describing the manifestations and treatment of a number of specific causes of pneumonia is unrealistic in the real world since it assumes that a specific diagnosis has been made early, which is often not true. An alternative approach is shown in Figure 1.

A set of symptoms, limited findings on examination, and an abnormal roentgenogram of the chest usually provide sufficient information to diagnose "pneumonia." Little effort is required to divide the population into three groups based on preexisting health and thus begin to establish the cause of a patient's pneumonia (Fig. 1, steps 1 to 4).

Pneumonia in the Previously Healthy

Pneumonias in previously healthy persons in most age groups are caused by viruses and mycoplasmas, bacteria being likely pathogens only in the newborn and adults over 30 years of age (Figure 1, step 5; Table 2). Since erythromycin is the drug of choice for *Chlamydia trachomatis*, *Mycoplasma pneumoniae*, and *Legionella pneumophila* and is as effective as penicillin against *Streptococcus pneumoniae* as well as being active against many anaerobic and other upper respiratory tract bacteria, there is no logical alternative if empiric therapy is used in any previously healthy patient with pneumonia beyond the neonatal period. Most children and many adults, however, require no therapy and should not be subjected to the cost and toxicity of erythromycin or any other antibiotic. Therefore, antibiotic treatment

TABLE 1 Some Causes of Pneumonia

Common (and Uncommon)	Rare	
	Localized to Lung	Systemic Disease
Bacteria		
Anaerobic bacteria	*Acinetobacter* species	*Brucella* species
(*Branhamella catarrhalis*)	*Actinomyces israelii*	*Campylobacter fetus*
Escherichia coli	*Aeromonas hydrophila*	*Francisella tularensis*
Haemophilus influenzae	*Bacillus* species	*Leptospira* species
(*Klebsiella pneumoniae*)	*Bordetella* species	*Listeria monocytogenes**
Legionella pneumophila	*Corynebacterium* species	*Pasteurella multocida*
(*Mycobacterium tuberculosis*)	*Eikenella corrodens*	*Pseudomonas mallei*
(*Neisseria meningitidis*)	*Morganella morganii*	*Pseudomonas pseudomallei*
(*Nocardia asteroides*)*	*Mycobacterium* species	*Salmonella* species
(*Pseudomonas aeruginosa*)	*Proteus* species	*Treponema pallidum*
(*Staphylococcus aureus*)	*Streptococcus pyogenes†*	*Yersinia pestis*
Streptococcus pneumoniae	*Streptococcus* species	*Neisseria gonorrhoeae*
Bacteria-like		
Chlamydia trachomatis†	*Chlamydia psittaci*	
Mycoplasma pneumoniae	*Coxiella burnetii*	
Viruses		
Adenovirus 1, 2, 3, 5†	Adenovirus 4, 7‡	Epstein-Barr virus
(Cytomegalovirus)	Enterovirus†	Herpes simplex virus
Influenza virus A	Influenza virus B	Varicella-zoster virus
Parainfluenza 1, 2, 3†	Measles virus†	Rabies virus
Respiratory syncytial†	Rhinovirus†	
	Reoviruses†	
Fungi		
(*Aspergillus* species)*	*Blastomyces dermatitidis*	
(*Candida* species)	*Coccidioides immitis‡*	
(*Cryptococcus neoformans*)	*Histoplasma capsulatum‡*	
(*Mucor, Rhizopus, Absidia*)†	*Paracoccidioides* species	
	Sporothrix schenckii	
	Torulopsis glabrata	
Parasites		
(*Pneumocystis carinii*)*	Several	*Toxoplasma gondii**
Noninfectious pneumonias		
Aspiration: gastric, food/feedings, other	Interstitial pneumonia usual; granulomatous,	Collagen-vascular disease, rheumatoid
(Chemical/drug induced)	lymphoid, desquamative	arthritis, polyarteritis, other vascu-
(Hypersensitivity)	Radiation	litides
Noninfectious conditions often misdiagnosed		
as pneumonia		
Atelectasis	Alveolar proteinosis	
Heart failure	Pneumoconioses	
Oxygen toxicity	Pulmonary fibrosis	
Pulmonary infarction	Sarcoidosis	
Respiratory distress syndrome	Tumors	

* Primarily or exclusively an opportunistic pathogen.
† Occurs primarily or exclusively in infants and children.
‡ May be more common in specific epidemiologic circumstances.

is begun only if the patient manifests chills, evidence of pulmonary consolidation, leukocytosis with an increase of immature neutrophils, or other evidence suggestive of a bacterial infection.

Pneumonia With Preexisting Chronic Diseases

In patients with chronic disease, the incidence of pneumonia is greater, the variety of common causes is broader, and the case fatality rate is higher. While relatively fewer infections due to *Mycoplasma* and respiratory viruses (except influenza) occur in these patients, there is a striking increase in bacterial infections, especially those due to *S.*

pneumoniae and gram-negative bacilli, such as *Haemophilus influenzae, Pseudomonas aeruginosa*, and several members of the family Enterobacteriaceae (*Escherichia coli, Klebsiella, Proteus, Serratia*).

To some extent these organisms are disease related (Fig. 1, step 5; Table 3). Specific diagnosis, however, is much more important in this group because of the greater variety of organisms and the higher morbidity and mortality. While chronic diseases are more common with advanced age, age per se has little effect on the incidence or specific etiology, except for tuberculosis. Without a diagnosis erythromycin remains an important part of therapy, treating not only infection due to *Legionella, Mycoplasma*, and streptococci,

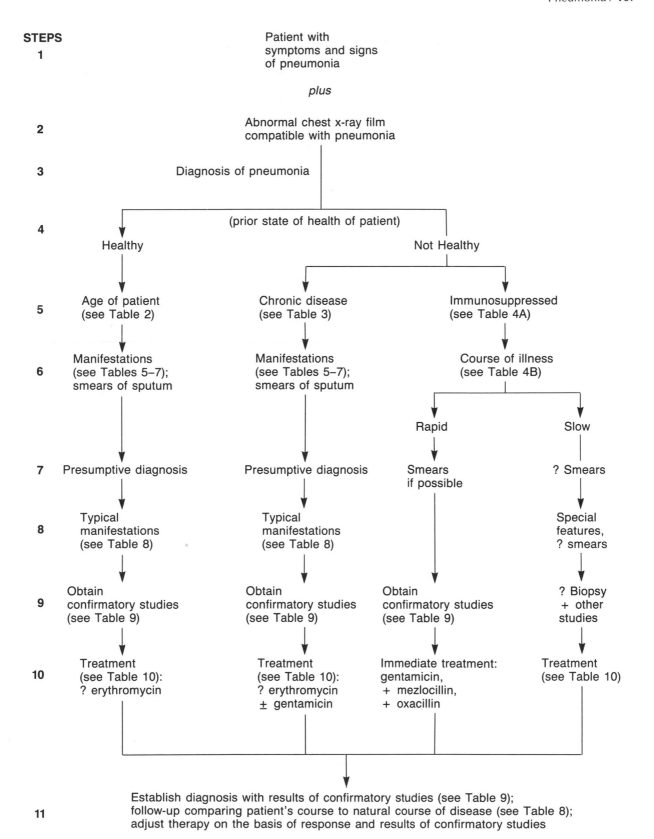

Figure 1 Treatment of pneumonia.

TABLE 2   Causes of Pneumonia in Healthy Individuals at Various Ages

Age	Common Causes	Less Common Causes	Rare Causes
<1 mo	Escherichia coli	Other gram-negative bacteria	Staphylococcus aureus
	Streptococcus agalactiae (B)	Respiratory syncytial virus	Streptococcus pneumoniae
1–12 mo	Respiratory syncytial virus	Adenovirus 1, 2, 3, 5	S. pneumoniae
	Chlamydia trachomatis	Parainfluenza virus	
1–5 yr	Parainfluenza virus	Respiratory syncytial virus	Adenovirus 1, 2, 3, 5
		Influenza virus A	
5–10 yr	Influenza virus A	Adenovirus 1, 2, 3, 5	Mycoplasma pneumoniae
10–30 yr	M. pneumoniae	Influenza virus A	S. pneumoniae
≥ 30 yr	S. pneumoniae	Influenza virus A	M. pneumoniae
	Legionella pneumophila	Anaerobic bacteria	

but also many strains of *Haemophilus*, *Branhamella*, *Staphylococcus*, and anaerobic bacteria. Empiric therapy for this group of patients may also need to include treatment of gram-negative bacillary infection, which plays an increasingly important role. Aminoglycosides remain the most effective therapy for pneumonias due to facultative (aerobic) gram-negative bacilli, but third-generation cephalosporins may be effective alternatives. First-generation cephalosporins such as cephalothin, cephapirin, and cefazolin—while effective against streptococci, staphylococci, and at times *Haemophilus*

(cefazolin)—are not useful in the treatment of pneumonias caused by gram-negative bacilli (or anaerobes) and do not offer any benefit in combination with aminoglycosides.

Opportunistic Pneumonias

Diagnosis of the cause of pneumonia in a patient with significant immunosuppression is particularly challenging. Many organisms that are not pathogenic under other circumstances assume importance when normal defenses are sig-

TABLE 3   Some of the More Common Pathogens Associated With Common Chronic Diseases

Type of Disease	Explanation	Likely Causes
Neurologic	Primarily due to aspiration because of altered mentation or swallowing dysfunction	Anaerobic bacteria Streptococcus pneumoniae Aspiration of food, gastric contents
Pulmonary	Altered pulmonary defenses, ineffective cough, defective ciliary action, alveolar macrophage dysfunction	S. pneumoniae Haemophilus influenzae Legionella pneumophila Klebsiella pneumoniae Influenza virus A Pseudomonas aeruginosa Branhamella catarrhalis
Cardiac	Secondary pulmonary disease, wet alveoli	S. pneumoniae Influenza virus A L. pneumophila Pulmonary emboli, infarcts
Gastrointestinal	Bacteremia	Escherichia coli Anaerobic bacteria
	Esophageal dysfunction	Aspiration of secretions Anaerobic bacteria
Liver (alcoholism)	Defective leukocyte function	S. pneumoniae K. pneumoniae
	Life style/contacts	Mycobacterium tuberculosis Anaerobic bacteria Aspiration of food, gastric contents
Renal failure	Cell-mediated immune defects	M. tuberculosis Influenza virus A S. pneumoniae
Malignancy	See Table 4B	
Lung cancer	Obstruction of airway	Anaerobic bacteria S. pneumoniae

TABLE 4A   Diagnosis of Pneumonia in Immunosuppressed Patients

Type of Immune Defect	Examples of Causes	Common Causative Organisms

Cell-mediated immunity (T lymphocytes)	Corticosteroids
	Hodgkin's disease
	AIDS (see text)
		Viruses:
		  varicella zoster
		  cytomegalovirus
		  herpes simplex
		  Pneumocystis carinii
		  Toxoplasma gondii
		Intracellular bacteria:
		  Mycobacterium species
		  Listeria monocytogenes
		  Salmonella species
		Fungi

Humoral immunity (B lymphocytes)	Hypogammaglobulinemia: congenital, acquired Chronic lymphatic leukemia	*Haemophilus influenzae* *Streptococcus pneumoniae*
Neutropenia	Cancer chemotherapy Cyclical neutropenia Drug-induced Neutrophil dysfunction	*Staphylococcus aureus* *Pseudomonas aeruginosa* Enterobacteriaceae *Aspergillus* species
	Chronic granulomatous disease of childhood	*S. aureus* *Serratia marcescens*
Complement	Deficiency of terminal components	*Neisseria meningitidis*

nificantly depressed. Space does not allow for lists of specific disease-microorganism relationships (e.g., multiple myeloma and *S. pneumoniae*, acute myelocytic leukemia and *Aspergillus* species), but opportunistic infections occur because of the type of defect in the immune system, which may be quite specific (Fig. 1, step 5; Table 4A). Neutropenia predisposes the patient primarily to infections with pyogenic bacteria, whereas encapsulated bacterial species predominate as pathogens when B cell function is defective. The large group of organisms seen when cell-mediated immunity is affected have one feature in common—they are intracellular pathogens. Two other aspects are characteristic of opportunistic pneumonias: manifestations are often atypical and the usual diagnostic tests are often not informative. Pneumonias that depend on a cellular inflammatory response in the lung are often difficult to diagnose in the neutropenic patient because no pulmonary infiltrate or sputum will develop in the absence of neutrophils, and typical granuloma formation and skin test reactivity require an intact cell-mediated immunity. Antibody response is often inhibited or delayed, and cultural results are often negative or too late to be of assistance.

Even opportunistic infections have a natural course, however (Fig. 1, step 6; Table 4B). Rapidly progressing

TABLE 4B   Characteristics of the Course of Pneumonia Associated With Opportunistic Pathogens

Abrupt/Rapid (hours)	Less Abrupt/Slow (over several days)	Insidious/Very Slow (over weeks)
S. pneumoniae *H. influenzae* *S. aureus* *P. aeruginosa* Enterobacteriaceae	*L. monocytogenes*	*Mycobacterium tuberculosis* *Nocardia asteroides*
Cytomegalovirus	Varicella-zoster	—
Candida species	*Aspergillus* species *Candida* species *Cryptococcus neoformans* *Mucor, Absidia, Rhizopus*	*Candida* species
	P. carinii	*P. carinii* (in AIDS) *T. gondii*
Gastric aspiration Atelectasis Pulmonary infarct	Other aspiration Congestive heart failure	Antineoplastic drug reactions Neoplasms

illness, characteristic of extracellular bacteria and some viruses, is seen most commonly in patients with neutropenia or hypogammaglobulinemia. The rapidity of onset and progression demands prompt treatment, and thus immediate decisions must be made regarding likely causes. Empiric therapy should include antibiotics effective against *Streptococcus* and *Haemophilus* (ampicillin or cefuroxime), if the patient has a humoral immune defect, or *Staphylococcus* and gram-negative bacilli (gentamicin, mezlocillin, and oxacillin) for the neutropenic patient.

Intracellular bacteria, fungi, parasites, and most viruses generally have a slower course. Unless antigen detection or cultural techniques that will provide early results are available, biopsies are often necessary to establish a diagnosis. Empiric antibiotic therapy begun early in this group of patients often results in a delay in proper diagnosis and should be withheld in favor of a more aggressive diagnostic approach. The time lost in looking for a response to (often inappropriate) therapy is better spent carrying out a logically designed plan to establish the cause in patients whose disease is progressing at a slower pace.

DIAGNOSIS

General Considerations

Empiric treatment has significant limitations. Rather than succumb to the temptation of using empiric therapy, one should attempt to establish a more precise presumptive diagnosis. Variation in the presentation of pneumonia provides clues to the cause of the pneumonia (Fig. 1, step 6; Tables 5, 6, and 7) that are available early, when therapeutic decisions must be made.

No single manifestation should be considered diagnostic, and, more important, the absence of any feature should not be used to exclude a diagnosis. Some clues are more specific than others, but few are pathognomonic. The typical clinical presentation of *S. pneumoniae* or *M. pneumoniae* or the classical chest roentgenogram of *Klebsiella pneumoniae* or *Pneumocystis carinii* (in the appropriate clinical setting) is generally sufficient to make a presumptive diagnosis and initiate therapy, but few diseases present with the typical or classical pattern. In fact, the term *atypical*

TABLE 5 Interpretation of Common Symptoms and Signs of Pneumonia

Causes of Illness	Explanation	Likely Organisms
Onset/progression		
Sudden/rapid	Rapid multiplication and/or toxins	*Streptococcus pneumoniae, Legionella pneumophila, Neisseria meningitidis, Streptococcus pyogenes*
Insidious/slow	Minimal tissue injury	*Mycoplasma pneumoniae, Chlamydia trachomatis*
	Slow multiplication	*Mycobacterium tuberculosis*, many fungal pneumonias
Prodrome		
Upper respiratory tract infection	Site of initial infection	Respiratory viruses, *M. pneumoniae*
	Alteration of flora/defenses (especially with influenza)	*S. pneumoniae, N. meningitidis, S. pyogenes Staphylococcus aureus*
Sinusitis	Aspiration of infected matter	*Proteus, Morganella*, anaerobic bacteria
Bacteremia	Metastatic infection to lung	
	Skin	*S. aureus*
	Burns	*Pseudomonas aeruginosa*
	Intravascular device	*S. aureus, Candida* species
	Genitourinary/gastrointestinal	Anaerobic bacteria, *Escherichia coli, Klebsiella pneumoniae, Salmonella* species *Brucella* species
Symptoms		
Chills (rigors)	Bacteremia or toxemia	Bacterial pathogens
Myalgias	Unknown	Viruses, *Mycoplasma, Haemophilus, Neisseria*
Sputum		
None	Interstitial disease	Viruses, early *M. pneumoniae, Legionella pneumophila*
	No airway communication	Hematogenous (early), *S. aureus, E. coli*
	Dehydration	*S. pneumoniae*, other
Purulent	Neutrophilic inflammation	Most bacterial pathogens, later *M. pneumoniae*
Foul	Fatty acid byproducts	Anaerobic bacteria
Red/blood	Red blood cell diapedesis (rusty)	*S. pneumoniae*
	Tissue destruction (red)	Necrosis, especially *S. aureus, Klebsiella, M. tuberculosis*
	Cough-induced (streaking)	Any
	Pigment from organism	*Serratia marcescens*
Chest pain	Retrosternal	*M. pneumoniae*
	Lateral, pleuritis	Empyema (see Table 7)

TABLE 6 Diagnostically Helpful Laboratory Studies in Pneumonia

Laboratory Result	Explanation	Likely Organisms
Leukocyte count:		
<5,000	Typical of disease	Occasionally viruses
	Folate deficiency	*Streptococcus pneumoniae,* *Klebsiella pneumoniae*
	Overwhelming infection	Bacteria, especially *Staphylococcus, Streptococcus, Klebsiella, Pseudomonas*
	Preexisting neutropenia	See Table 4A
>10,000	Bone marrow stimulation	Many bacterial pathogens, influenza virus A
>50,000	Leukemoid reaction	*Mycobacterium tuberculosis* (miliary)
Sedimentation rate		
<20 mm/h		Viruses, *Mycoplasma pneumoniae*
>100 mm/h		Legionella pneumophila, *M. tuberculosis* (miliary)
Chemistries		
Hyponatremia	SIADH	*L. pneumophila, M. tuberculosis*
	Intracellular shift	*S. pneumoniae*
Hypophosphatemia	Unknown	*L. pneumophila*
		Bacteremia (gram-negative bacilli > gram-positive cocci)
Liver dysfunction	? Toxemia	*S. pneumoniae, L. pneumophila, Escherichia coli, K. pneumoniae*
	Hepatic infection	*M. tuberculosis* (miliary), *Staphylococcus aureus, E. coli,* other gram-negative bacilli
	Preexisting liver disease	*S. pneumoniae, K. pneumoniae* anaerobic bacteria
Renal dysfunction	? Toxemia, ? myoglobinuria	*L. pneumophila*
	Preexisting renal disease	*S. pneumoniae,* influenza virus A
	Shock with acute tubular necrosis	Many bacteria (especially gram-negative)
	Acute glomerulonephritis	*S. aureus, S. pyogenes*
Elevated creatine phosphokinase	? Myositis	*L. pneumophila,* influenza virus A

pneumonia has little meaning today because most pneumonias are atypical. Nevertheless, the nonspecific symptoms and signs of pneumonia have diagnostic significance.

Of all the items listed in Tables, 5, 6, and 7, the microscopic examination of sputum often is most helpful but most likely to be misinterpreted. For these reasons, it deserves special attention. Contamination of sputum by oral or pharyngeal secretions is invariable unless the sputum is collected by transtracheal aspiration or bronchoscopy, but few of us will subject our patients to the danger and discomfort of these procedures unless absolutely necessary. Consequently, the smears must be interpreted in the light of ever-present contamination. Initially, the presence, number, and type of inflammatory cells on the slide should be determined by examining the smear under low- and high-power magnification. Unless there is obvious suppuration of the mouth or throat (e.g., dental abscess, exudative tonsillitis), inflammatory cells in the specimen connote lower respiratory tract inflammation, indicating that the specimen contains lower respiratory tract secretions and that there is inflammation within the lower respiratory tract. With few exceptions (e.g., commonly *Legionella*, occasionally *Mycobacterium*, rarely *Klebsiella*), bacterial pathogens will be present in abundance on stained smears and uniformly distributed in the inflammatory exudate when the pneumonia has a bacterial cause. Therefore, the absence of a particular organism that should be visible virtually eliminates that species as the cause. The presence of the organism, however, does not exclude the mouth or upper respiratory tract as the source or distinguish the bronchi from the lung as the site of inflammation. Thus, contamination of sputum is often easy to detect (presence of epithelial cells, mixed flora, or clumped organisms; nonuniform distribution of the microorganisms) but difficult to exclude. Certain types of organisms (gram-positive bacilli, yeasts) should also suggest contamination, and, contrary to statements commonly found in the literature, intracellular bacteria that have been phagocytosed by polymorphonuclear leukocytes are usually not pathogens.

The most complex, but often the most specific, clues may be found in the x-ray film. Virtually any pathogen can produce any radiologic pattern, the lists in Table 7 being only suggestive of likely pathogens. Carefully analyzed, however, the patterns, timing, and complications can be among the most helpful in diagnosis. While there is a definite relation between pathologic and radiologic characteristics, this should not be considered absolute. Of all the possible changes on x-ray film, only necrosis is reasonably specific for an infectious (bacterial or fungal) cause. The timing of the appear-

TABLE 7   Diagnostic Aspects of Radiologic Characteristics

Previously Healthy	Chronic Disease	Immunosuppressed
Interstitial		
Many viruses	Influenza virus A	*Pneumocystis carinii*
Streptococcus pyogenes (early)	*Mycobacterium tuberculosis* (miliary)	Cytomegalovirus
Hypersensitivity pneumonia	Congestive heart failure, pulmonary fibrosis	Drug toxicity, radiation
Patchy		
Mycoplasma pneumoniae	*Escherichia coli*, aspiration/atelectasis	*Aspergillus* species
		Nocardia asteroides
Nodular		
Staphylococcus aureus	*S. aureus, Klebsiella pneumoniae, Pseudomonas aeruginosa,* metastatic carcinoma	Neoplasms, *N. asteroides,* many fungi, lymphoma
Lobar/segmental		
S. pneumoniae	*S. pneumoniae*	*Aspergillus* species
Anaerobic bacteria	*K. pneumoniae*	*N. asteroides*
Fungi	Anaerobic bacteria	Other fungi
Actinomyces israelii	*S. aureus* (bronchogenic)	Lymphomas, neoplasms
	Fungi	
"Pseudolobar"		
M. pneumoniae	*L. pneumophila*	Cytomegalovirus
Legionella pneumophila	*Haemophilus influenzae*	Amphotericin + white blood cell transfusion
Adenovirus	Oxygen toxicity, acute respiratory disease syndrome, influenza virus A	
Necrosis		
Early pneumonic		
Anaerobic bacteria	*Pseudomonas* species	
Midpneumonic		
S. aureus	*K. pneumoniae*	*K. pneumoniae*
Anaerobic bacteria	Anaerobic bacteria	
	Proteus, Morganella	
Late pneumonic		
Anaerobic bacteria	Anaerobic bacteria	Anaerobic bacteria
S. pneumoniae	*S. pneumoniae*	*N. asteroides*
M. tuberculosis	*M. tuberculosis*	*M. tuberculosis*
	Pulmonary infarcts	Neoplasms
Pleural effusions		
Nonpneumonic		
Anaerobic bacteria	*M. tuberculosis*	*Cryptococcus neoformans*
Coccidioides imitis		Neoplasms
Prepneumonic		
Streptococcus pyogenes		
Early pneumonic		
S. pneumoniae	*S. pneumoniae*	*L. pneumophila*
M. pneumoniae	*K. pneumoniae*	*K. pneumoniae*
Anaerobic bacteria	*P. aeruginosa, H. influenzae*	*S. pneumoniae, H. influenzae*
Meta(mid)pneumonic		
S. aureus	*S. aureus*	*N. asteroides*
Anaerobic bacteria	*P. aeruginosa*	
Late pneumonic	*E. coli*	
Postpneumonic		
S. pneumoniae	*S. pneumoniae*	

ance of the necrosis or of a pleural effusion in relation to the parenchymal infiltrate is helpful in suggesting specific diagnoses (see Table 7).

An epidemiologic history should also be obtained, particularly if the pneumonia does not seem to fit into any pattern. Too much emphasis can be placed on circumstantial epidemiologic facts, however. Most patients in California with pneumonia do not have coccidioidomycosis, and alcoholics who occasionally use intravenous drugs are still more likely to have pneumonia due to pneumococcus or anaerobic bac-

teria than to either *Klebsiella* or *Pneumocystis*. Inquiring about the patient's occupation, hobbies, habits, travel, and contacts, including pets, may provide important clues to a diagnosis that would have otherwise been overlooked. Of greatest importance is contact with other persons with the same or similar illness. Most patients with viral and mycoplasmal pneumonias will give such a history, but common-source outbreaks can be seen with *Legionella*, *Histoplasma*, and *Mycobacterium tuberculosis*, to name a few.

To use Tables 5, 6, and 7, carefully evaluate the patient to determine symptoms, physical findings, laboratory abnormalities, and roentgenographic patterns to determine which of the numerous causes might be implicated. Note that the diagnosis of opportunistic pathogens and the evaluation of the immunosuppressed host (see Table 4) do not depend as heavily on these findings since the causes are different and the manifestations atypical.

Once a presumptive diagnosis is made (Fig. 1, step 7), the patient's manifestations should be compared with the typical findings of that disease (Fig. 1, step 8; Table 8), recognizing, of course, that typical diseases rarely occur. This assists in confirming the presumptive diagnosis and directs the obtaining of appropriate specimens (Fig. 1, step 9; Table 9) to eventually confirm the diagnosis, if possible, before therapy is initiated (Fig. 1, step 10; Table 10).

The importance of limiting the number of likely diagnoses, and thus the number of antibiotics used, cannot be overemphasized. Use of high-dose, broad-spectrum combination antibiotics to cover all possible pathogens not only results in unnecessary allergy and toxicity, but, more important, can cause significant mortality due to suprainfection. This is most likely to occur in patients with underlying associated diseases and may result in mortality exceeding that due to the primary infection.

Special Situations

Hospital-Acquired Pneumonia

Pneumonia occurring after hospital admission is most commonly caused by aspiration of oropharyngeal contents, feedings, or gastric secretions or by bronchogenic spread of respiratory flora. The establishment of a diagnosis is made particularly difficult by the frequently occurring noninfectious conditions presenting as pneumonia and the difficulty in interpreting sputum cultures (if sputum is available) contaminated by altered upper respiratory tract flora. Many characteristics of hospitalized patients predispose them to aspiration. Acute or chronic pulmonary diseases common in hospitalized patients adversely affect local pulmonary defenses, and patients with systemic diseases are often given a variety of therapies that inhibit the lung's ability to resist lower respiratory tract colonization and subsequent infection. Disease, antibiotics, manipulation of the tracheobronchial tree, and exposure to nosocomially transmitted pathogens produce colonization of the pharynx with gram-negative bacilli.

Bacteremia from intravascular lines and from gastrointestinal or genital and urinary tract infections or manipulations also occurs more commonly in the hospital setting and

TABLE 8 Confirmatory Diagnostic Studies

Suspected Pathogen	Test(s)	Comments

Pyogenic bacteria
  Streptococcus
  Staphylococcus
  Haemophilus
  Enterobacteriaceae
  Anaerobic bacteria
	Blood cultures (3)
	Aerobic sputum culture
	Serology for antigens
	Pleural fluid analysis, smears and cultures
	Anaerobic cultures of pleural fluid and transtracheal sputum
		Also smears and cultures of suspected secondary sites (e.g., CSF, joints, urine) or of primary sites (e.g., urine, skin, stool) if a hematogenous pneumonia

Legionella pneumophila	Direct fluorescent-antibody test (FA) of sputum Sputum culture Serology (antibody)	Several serotypes Requires special media Often late (3–4 wk) response
Mycobacterium species	Ziehl-Neelson or FA of sputum Sputum culture for acid-fast bacilli	Urine smears/cultures if *Mycobacterium tuberculosis* Stool smears/cultures and blood cultures if *Mycobacterium avium* complex in AIDS
Mycoplasma pneumoniae	DNA probe or other antigen tests, culture, serology (antibody)	Cold agglutinin test; high rate of false-negative and false-positive results
Chlamydia trachomatis	Sputum cytology, FA, culture, serology (IgG, IgM)	FA and culture often not available Present at onset (maternal antibody)
Respiratory virus	Throat culture Indirect FA, other rapid tests Stool culture (enterovirus) Serology (antibody)	? Not effective unless rapid and treatment available
Cytomegalovirus	Sputum, urine cytology (IgM and IgG) Sputum, urine culture Monoclonal antibodies	IgG antibody detection of limited value—most patients have antibodies, limited response in compromised host
Pneumocystis carinii	Toluidine blue or silver stain of sputum, bronchial washings, and/or lung biopsy Gallium scan if x-ray film is negative/normal	Direct smears more likely positive in AIDS Transbronchial biopsy/washing usually positive
Fungus	Antigen: *Cryptococcus, Aspergillus* Antibody: *Histoplasma, Cryptococcus, Coccidioides* Culture of sputum, blood, urine, biopsy Biopsy: lung, nodes	CSF examination, culture, antigen if diagnosis of cryptococcosis Skin tests of little value

TABLE 9 Specific Features of Some Common and Uncommon Pneumonias

Adenoviruses: Insidious onset with conjunctivitis, pharyngitis (with or without rhinitis), and bronchitis; white blood cell count often elevated; benign, often lower lobe interstitial infiltrates (types 1, 2, 3, 5) in children; may be fulminant (type 7) in infants; may be consolidating and severe (type 3, 4, 7) in adults, especially military recruits; slow resolution.

Anaerobic bacteria (variable course and manifestations): Acute or insidious onset following period of unconsciousness or genital > gastrointestinal infection; foul-tasting or smelling sputum in 50%; hemoptysis; patchy, nodular or lobar infiltrates with early or late necrosis; lung abscess with air-fluid levels; empyemas commonly large with large loculations.

Aspergillus fumigatus and other species: Several pulmonary syndromes including hypersensitivity pneumonia with fleeting or more-persistent infiltrates, "fungus balls" in preexisting cavities, miliary infiltrates following massive inhalation by healthy children, and fairly rapidly progressively consolidating (or occasionally patchy) infiltrates in immunosuppressed patients. The last spreads contiguously, with sharply defined advancing borders, and occurs in the absence of neutrophils usually required to develop infiltrates.

Branhamella catarrhalis: In patients with chronic lung disease, progressive illness with bronchitis and low fever; copious sputum; patchy infiltrates; good response to therapy. In other patients abrupt onset following upper respiratory tract infection with chills, fever, cough, pleuritic chest pain; lobar consolidation; occasionally bacteremia and empyema; slow response to therapy.

Candida albicans and other candidal species: Following (persistent) fungemia, usually in an immunocompromised host; large nodular infiltrates (similar to metastatic neoplasms); endophthalmitis and other organ involvement common; blood cultures may be negative.

Chlamydia trachomatis: Insidious onset at 3–16 weeks of age with progressive cough (terminated by vomiting but without a whoop) and respiratory distress; afebrile and otherwise appears well; conjunctivitis common; eosinophilia; patchy infiltrates with hyperinflation; therapy slightly shortens duration of illness.

Cytomegalovirus: Congenital infection with fulminant multisystem illness consisting of jaundice, hepatosplenomegaly, petechiae, microcephaly, motor disability, chorioretinitis, cerebral calcifications, lethargy, convulsions, and respiratory distress; diffuse interstitial-alveolar infiltrate. Occasionally a benign interstitial pneumonia in a healthy child or adult with an acute cytomegalovirus infection such as cytomegalovirus mononucleosis. In immunocompromised, abrupt onset of mild to severe illness with fever, nonproductive cough, and dyspnea; often with mononucleosis or hepatitis; diffuse interstitial infiltrate that becomes nodular.

Escherichia coli: Prior gastrointestinal or genitourinary infection or manipulation with bacteremia, chills and fever; minimal cough, sputum; nonspecific lower lobe infiltrates; late empyema.

Haemophilus influenzae: Most commonly with chronic lung disease; insidious onset with bronchitis, copious sputum, myalgias and arthralgias; diffuse miliary pattern on x-ray film. With diabetes, alcoholism and hypogammaglobulinemia, and in young children onset is abrupt; high fever and chills; bacteremias and empyemas common; lobar pneumonia.

Influenza virus, type A: Influenza begins with dramatic onset with fever, malaise, myalgias, and severe anorexia; systemic >respiratory symptoms; respiratory signs (pharyngitis, conjunctivitis) > symptoms; epistaxis; leukopenia; short incubation period and duration of high fever (2 days). Viral pneumonia begins as influenza is starting to resolve (2–3 days after onset) with persistent or increased cough and continued fever; white blood cell (WBC) count, 15,000–18,000; sputum with many leukocytes and tracheal cells; benign course with diffuse reticular interstitial infiltrate in children; progressive cyanosis and respiratory distress with obliteration of lung on x-ray film in patients with chronic diseases (especially cardiac, renal, pulmonary). Bacterial pneumonia begins very abruptly with chills, fever, increased sputum production, and toxicity (2–10 days after influenza); WBC count often <5,000 or >25,000; nonspecific infiltrates lacking typical characteristics of pathogen (commonly *Staphylococcus aureus* > *Streptococcus pneumoniae*, *Haemophilus influenzae*, *Streptococcus pyogenes* [*Proteus* species or *Klebsiella pneumoniae* if prior antibiotics]).

Klebsiella pneumoniae: In alcoholics, rapid onset with fever, chills, cough, bloody sputum, and early nonlocalized pleuritic chest pain; leukopenia; abnormal liver function, bacteremia, empyema common; dullness without egophony, pectoriloquy, or bronchial breath sounds on examination; dense homogenous lobar consolidation (often posterior segment of upper lobes, with bulging fissure) without air bronchograms; contiguous spread to adjacent lobes; necrosis in 4–7 days; slow response to therapy. With other chronic diseases, insidious onset with bronchitis; localized central nodular (secondary lobules) infiltrate.

Legionella pneumophila: Abrupt onset with fever and chills followed by confusion, diarrhea, abdominal pain, and nonproductive cough leading to respiratory distress; no prodromal upper respiratory tract illness; tender hepatomegaly; erythrocyte sedimentation rate > 100 mm/h; hyponatremia (inappropriate antidiuretic hormone); hypophosphatemia; abnormal liver and kidney function; homogeneous lower lobe infiltrate on x-ray film.

Mycobacterium tuberculosis: Primary tuberculous pneumonia is usually asymptomatic, being detected by a chance x-ray film; sympotomatic disease has acute onset with fever and cough (often brassy); homogeneous mid- or lower lung consolidation with hilar lymphadenopathy; late hilar calcifications. Secondary or chronic tuberculosis develops over weeks or months with late afternoon or evening fever, night sweats when fever subsides, cough with slightly bloody sputum (occasionally exsanguination occurs), fatigue, and anorexia; lymphocytosis or monocytosis; hyponatremia; fibrotic and cavitating infiltrates involving more than one lobe, usually including at least one of the apical segments. Miliary tuberculosis has insidious or more acute onset with systemic symptoms; elevated canalicular > parenchymal liver enzymes; anemia with abnormal WBC counts (leukopenia, leukemoid reactions, eosinophilia, etc.); hyponatremia; abnormal urine and CSF; diffuse nodular interstitial infiltrate (50% of x-ray films erroneously read as negative initially).

Mycoplasma pneumoniae: Long (1–3 week) incubation period with isidious onset with "scratchy" throat (often without rhinitis), tinnitus or decreased hearing, and progressive cough, initially nonproductive and later with mucoid sputum; cough is paroxysmal and predominantly nocturnal, often precipitated by recumbency or exposure to cold, and causes retrosternal pain and frontal headache; discrepancy between physical and radiologic examinations; small effusions common; pleural fluid is transudate; response to treatment at 36–48 hours with loss of systemic (fever, malaise, myalgias, anorexia) but not respiratory symptoms; cough and infiltrates may persist for weeks.

Neisseria meningitidis: Similar to *Branhamella catarrhalis* except more benign illness not limited to patients with chronic lung disease, and arthralgias and myalgias similar to a viral illness are prominant in both types.

TABLE 9 *(continued)*

Nocardia asteroides: Slow onset over weeks with progressive cough and fever; copious sputum; nodular infiltrates with late necrosis; slow responses to therapy.

Parainfluenza virus: Progressive illness with fever, cough following a febrile nasopharyngitis; may be associated with croup or bronchiolitis; diffuse finely reticular interstitial infiltrates; resolves quickly.

Pneumocystis carinii: Progressive (nonproductive) cough, dyspnea, and fever; tachypnea out of proportion to x-ray; few or no rales or rhonchi; diffuse interstitial infiltrate that becomes almost homogeneous with time, occasionally with air bronchograms.

Pseudomonas aeruginosa: Usually abrupt onset with chills, fever, cough, bloody sputum, and chest pain; normal or low WBC count; abnormal liver and kidney function; reversal of diurnal temperature pattern common; recurrent bacteremias; diffuse nodular infiltrates with early necrosis and small empyemas; slow response to therapy.

Respiratory syncytial virus: In infant abrupt onset of fever, cough, which may be paroxysmal and associated with vomiting following an upper respiratory tract infection; often with bronchiolitis (wheezing, prolonged expiration); diffuse interstitial infiltrates with hyperinflation, occasionally consolidation; slow resolution.

Staphylococcus aureus: Hematogenous with abrupt onset with fever, chills, pleuritic chest pain; peripheral nodular infiltrates that undergo necrosis at 5 days; pyopneumothorax late; often multiple organ disease. Bronchogenic in children or elderly adults with abrupt onset with or without preceding upper respiratory tract infection; lobar consolidation with late necrosis and empyema; pneumatocoeles in children (see influenza).

Streptococcus pneumoniae: In healthy person abrupt onset with fever, single chill, cough, rusty sputum and very well localized chest pain following nasopharyngitis; hyponatremia (with absent urine sodium); mild increase of bilirubin and alanine aminotransferase; occasionally lobar consolidation and empyema; bacteremia in 20%–40%; prompt response to therapy. With chronic diseases onset more insidious with bronchitis; lower lobe nonconsolidating pneumonia.

Streptococcus pyogenes: Dramatic onset following upper respiratory tract infection, influenza, or measles, with high fever, chills, severe toxicity, cough, and pleuritic chest pain; thin bloody sputum; diffuse interstitial infiltrates initially; early (prepneumonic) serosanguinous effusions; slow response to therapy.

---

are often associated with secondary pneumonia. *Staphylococcus aureus* (from intravascular devices or skin sites), *E. coli* (following urinary or intestinal manipulations), and anaerobic bacteria (from genital or intestinal sources) are the species most likely to seed the lung from the blood. Other gram-negative bacilli, especially *Pseudomonas aeruginosa* and *K. pneumoniae* may also produce metastatic pneumonias.

Management of nosocomial pneumonia requires careful attention to the precipitating events and a healthy skepticism of the significance of the results obtained from sputum cultures. Transtracheal aspiration presumably avoids contamination from the upper respiratory tract, but interpretation of the culture results of these specimens in this setting must include consideration of the fact that the hospitalized patient who is continually aspirating will also be continually contaminating a specimen obtained by the transtracheal route. Many hospitalized patients also have tracheobronchitis, making it difficult to distinguish the source of the organism found in specimens of lower respiratory tract secretions.

Empiric antibiotic therapy is often necessary. The absence of aerobic or facultative gram-negative bacilli or staphylococci on the smear or culture should exclude these organisms as a cause of the pneumonia, but their presence often reflects oropharyngeal or tracheobronchial colonization. The presence of large numbers of organisms of a single morphologic type on smears in a purulent specimen is suggestive of—but does not distinguish infection of the lung from—tracheobronchitis but should be considered adequate for initial therapy.

The most common causes of infectious nosocomial pneumonia in the absence of obvious aspiration or bacteremia are aerobic gram-negative bacilli. Treatment should include gentamicin (or another aminoglycoside). Large numbers of staphylococci on smear or culture in a patient with nosocomial pneumonia should prompt treatment since

staphylococci are not common colonizers of the oropharynx and tend to be even more invasive than gram-negative bacilli. Streptococci and *Haemophilus* are common causes of nosocomial pneumonia in patients who are not receiving antibiotics active against these species. Also organisms usually considered to be community acquired, such as *Legionella* and *M. tuberculosis*, can cause infections following hospitalization.

Aspiration and/or atelectasis are the most common causes of nosocomial "pneumonia." Most of these, however, are not infectious in origin. Atelectasis in the postoperative period is common. The early postoperative fever, linear densities and/or loss of volume on roentgenogram, and subcrepitant rales are readily distinguished from the changes in infectious pneumonia, but if untreated, secondary bacterial pneumonia can occur in the atelectatic segment. Altered states of consciousness and particulate aspiration also produce atelectasis.

Aspiration is universal, but the consequences vary with the amount and type of material aspirated and the ability of the defenses to handle it. Altered sensorium, neurologic diseases affecting swallowing, restrictive lung diseases, instrumentation of the airway or esophagus, tracheoesophageal fistulae, other esophageal disorders, and gastrointestinal obstruction in the hospitalized patient promote aspiration.

The management of aspiration depends upon the character of the material aspirated. Aspiration of acidic (pH < 2.0) gastric secretions produces diffuse infiltrates early, and these are associated with an intense inflammatory reaction but few or no bacteria on smear. The resultant pulmonary edema responds to positive end expiratory pressure (PEEP) and does not require antibiotics. Pneumonia due to aspiration of feedings, nonacid gastric secretions, or other noninfected materials develops more slowly and is associated with less fever and inflammatory response. The frequent use of H_2 block-

TABLE 10 Antimicrobial Therapy for Infectious Pneumonias

Causes of Pneumonia	Drug of Choice* (in order of preference)	Alternative Therapy
Bacteria		
Anaerobic bacteria	Clindamycin 10 mg/kg IV/IM q6h	Penicillin G 30,000 U/kg IV q4h
Branhamella catarrhalis	Cefuroxime 10 mg/kg IV q8h *or* Cefaclor 7 mg/kg PO q8h	Tetracycline 3 mg/kg PO q6h *or* Erythromycin 3 mg/kg PO q6h
Escherichia coli	Gentamicin 1.5 mg/kg IV q8h	Ceftizoxime 20 mg/kg IV q8h
Haemophilus influenzae	Ampicillin 15 mg/kg IV q6h	Cefuroxime 10 mg/kg IV q8h *or* Doxycycline 1.5 mg/kg IV q12h
Klebsiella pneumoniae	Gentamicin 1.5 mg/kg IV q8H *and either* Doxycycline 1.5 mg/kg IV q12h *or* Chloramphenicol 15 mg/kg IV q8h	Ceftizoxime 20 mg/kg IV q8h *or* Cefotaxime 20 mg/kg IV q6h *or* Ceftriaxone 20 mg/kg IV/IM qd
Legionella pneumophila	Erythromycin 15 mg/kg IV q6h	Rifampin 10 mg/kg PO q12h can be added for synergy
Mycobacterium avium–intracellulare	Ansamycin 3 mg/kg PO qd *and* Clofazimine 1.5 mg/kg PO qd	
Mycobacterium tuberculosis	Isoniazid 5 mg/kg PO/IM qd *and* Rifampin 10 mg/kg PO qd	Many other treatment regimens are available, depending on susceptibility studies
Nocardia asteroides	Sulfisoxazole 3 mg/kg IV q6h to maintain blood levels at 10 to 15 µg/ml	Ampicillin 15 mg/kg IV q6h *or* Erythromycin 7 mg/kg IV/PO q6h
Pseudomonas aeruginosa	Tobramycin 1.5 mg/kg IV q8h *and* Piperacillin 50 mg/kg IV q6h	Ceftazadime 30 mg/kg IV q8h *or* Imipenem 15 mg/kg IV q6h
Staphylococcus aureus	Oxacillin 30 mg/kg IV q4h *or* Nafcillin 30 mg/kg q4h	Cefazolin 15 mg/kg IV/IM q6h *or* Vancomycin 10 mg/kg IV q12h
Streptococcus pneumoniae	Penicillin G 10,000 µ/kg IV q4h *or* Penicillin V 5 mg/kg PO q6h	Cefazolin 5 mg/kg IV/IM q8h *or* Erythromycin 5 mg/kg IV/PO q6h
Other Microorganisms		
Chlamydia trachomatis	Erythromycin 10 mg/kg PO q6h	Sulfisoxazole 40 mg/kg PO q6h
Mycoplasma pneumoniae	Erythromycin 7 mg/kg PO q6h	Doxycycline 1.5 mg/kg PO q12h
Cytomegalovirus	DHPG 5 mg/kg IV q8h	None
Herpes simplex virus	Acyclovir 5 mg/kg IV q8h	None
Influenza virus, type A	Amantadine 3 mg/kg PO qd	None
Respiratory syncytial virus	Ribavirin 20 mg/ml aerosol qd	None
Varicella-zoster virus	Acyclovir 10 mg/kg IV q8h	None
Aspergillus, Mucor, Rhizopus	Amphotericin 1 mg/kg IV qd	None
Candida, Torulopsis glabrata	Amphotericin 0.5 mg/kg IV qd	Ketoconazole 6 mg/kg PO qd
Coccidioides, Histoplasma	Amphotericin 1 mg/kg IV qd	Ketoconazole 10 mg/kg PO qd
Cryptococcus neoformans	Amphotericin B 0.5 mg/kg IV qd *and* Flucytosine 25 mg/kg PO qid	None
Pneumocystis carinii	Trimethoprim-sulfamethoxazole 5 mg/kg (of TMP) and 25 mg/kg (of SMZ) IV q6h	Pentamidine 4 mg/kg IM/IV q24h
Toxoplasma gondii	Pyrimethamine 0.5 mg/kg qd *and* Sulfadiazine 50 mg/kg PO q12h	None

* Depending on susceptibility patterns and availability substitutions are as follows: (*1*) tobramycin 1.5 mg/kg IV q8h for gentamicin, (*2*) amikacin 7.5 mg/kg IV q12h for tobramycin, (*3*) cefotaxime 20 mg/kg IV q6h or ceftriaxone 20 mg/kg IV/IM q24h for ceftizoxime.

ers in hospitalized patients has reduced the incidence of chemical pneumonia but increased the frequency of bacterial infections. Without the protection of a low pH, microorganisms are able to survive in the stomach and gain entrance to the gastrointestinal tract or be aspirated into the lungs.

Oropharyngeal secretions, when aspirated, may produce secondary bacterial pneumonia that develops slowly over days and is most commonly due to anaerobic bacteria, although the colonization of the oropharynx with gram-negative bacilli in hospitalized patients results in increased incidence of gram-negative bacillary pneumonia, often mixed with anaerobes. A gram-stained smear will reveal a purulent exudate and abundant polymorphic bacteria. Treatment should be guided by the smear (or culture, if a smear is not done). There is no need to treat the patient for gram-negative bacilli if they are not present. Clindamycin alone, or with gentamicin if gram-negative bacilli are present, should be started immediately and continued until the x-ray film is clear or stable.

Acquired Immunodeficiency Syndrome (AIDS)

AIDS has rewritten the textbook on pneumonia. Infections caused by previously unknown pathogens, known pathogens causing previously undescribed syndromes, new clinical presentations so different from the above as to be unrecognizable, effective diagnostic tests that are negative in the face of active disease, and otherwise successful treatment regimens that fail are only some of the difficulties encountered by the physician dealing with patients infected with the human immunodeficiency virus (HIV). Fear of AIDS has also created a syndrome that may be as fatal for the individual as actually having HIV infection. Many patients without HIV infection but with an acute pneumonia are currently being subjected to invasive diagnostic tests, excessive and dangerous treatment, and at times neglect, because the physician, influenced by emotions rather than logic, erroneously assumes that the patient has AIDS.

The same logic described must be applied to patients who may, or do, have HIV infection, with or without AIDS, recognizing that the manifestations of pneumonia in this situation often differ significantly from the descriptions presented here. This subject is discussed elsewhere in this volume.

THERAPY

Only patients with uncomplicated viral and mycoplasmal pneumonias can be safely treated as outpatients, and patients must be hospitalized if they are in a toxic or hypoxic state or are suffering from other pulmonary or extrapulmonary complications. Alteration in mentation due to fever, toxemia, or early meningitis may result in failure to take oral antibiotics, with serious consequences. Hospitalization also provides a better setting for the nonspecific therapy of pneumonia. Clearance of secretions with adequate hydration, expectorants, and, if necessary, postural drainage, chest percussion, and/or bronchoscopy is essential for resolution of the pneumonia. Monitoring vital signs, correcting electrolyte abnormalities, and preventing decubiti and thromboembolic disease are important components of treatment. The availability of better- and longer-acting antibiotics and

better systems for nonhospital care will allow outpatient treatment of stable patients once an initial evaluation is completed and proper therapy initiated, but if hospitalization is the better alternative, there should be no hesitation in using it.

Parenteral antibiotics are generally preferred since absorption is ensured and higher doses can be given, if needed. The spectrum of activity of the initial antimicrobial therapy must be broad enough to cover the likely pathogens, balancing the risks of complications if certain microorganisms are not covered against the allergies, toxicities, and suprainfections of excessive antibiotics in the individual patient. Therapy must be constantly reevaluated and adjusted as diagnoses are made or excluded, clinical response occurs or not, and complications develop (Fig. 1, step 11).

Throughout the course of treatment, reevaluation of the patient is necessary as new information becomes available. A few rules are in order regarding the interpretation of the results obtained from confirmatory studies (see Table 8). The presence of antibodies or a positive skin test only means previous exposure, not causation; diagnosis is dependent on a rising antibody titer, the presence of IgM antibodies (recent infection), or the detection of antigen (active infection). Most pathogens also exist as normal flora or contaminants, so that isolation of *Klebsiella* or *Staphylococcus* from a sputum culture does not confirm a diagnosis. Isolation of organisms from blood or pleural fluid or the demonstration of tissue invasion by biopsy is generally adequate for diagnosis, however.

The appropriate duration of therapy for most pneumonias is not known. As a general rule, treatment should continue until the chest x-ray film has returned to the prepneumonic state or is stable and should be continued for at least 10 to 14 days for most bacterial pathogens. Exceptions include uncomplicated pneumonias caused by microorganisms that respond promptly and do not recur. Treatment of *S. pneumoniae*, *H. influenzae*, and *Neisseria meningitidis* or *Neisseria gonorrhoeae* can be stopped when the patient has been afebrile for 2 days. Continuing therapy for more than 5 days for *M. pneumoniae* is unnecessary. Early discontinuation of therapy of *S. aureus*, *L. pneumophila*, *P. aeruginosa*, *Nocardia asteroides*, *M. tuberculosis*, and *Actinomyces israelii* has been associated with frequent recurrences. In some situations, such as infections due to *Mycobacterium avium–Mycobacterium intracellulare* in patients with AIDS, treatment must be continued indefinitely.

Except for empiric therapy (which should be based on some logic), treatment of pneumonia depends on the establishment of an etiologic diagnosis since antimicrobial therapy is directed at the cause, not the pneumonia. If the cause is established, the treatment is fairly straightforward (see Table 10). Inadequate experimental experience is available, however, to determine the "drug of choice" for any pneumonia (including pneumococcal pneumonia), so the recommendations in Table 10 reflect personal experience over many years of treating patients with pneumonia.

SUGGESTED READING

Brown RB. Community-acquired bronchitis and pneumonia: presentation, pathogens, and therapy. Postgrad Med 1986; 79:241–250.

Committee on Diagnostic Standards in Respiratory Disease of the American Thoracic Society. Definitions and classifications of infectious reactions of the lungs. Am Rev Respir Dis 1970; 101:1–39.

Dorff GJ, Rytel MW, Farmer SG, Scanlon G. Etiologies and characteristic features of pneumonias in a municipal hospital. Am J Med Sci 1973; 266:349–358.

Putnam JS, Tuazon C, eds. Symposium on infectious lung diseases. Med Clin North Am 1980; 64:317–576.

Smith CB, Overall JC Jr. Clinical and epidemiologic clues to the diagnosis of respiratory infections. Radiol Clin North Am 1973; 11:261–278.

Toews GB. Southwestern internal medicine conference: nosocomial pneumonia. Am J Med Sci 1986; 291:355–367.

PLEURAL EFFUSION AND EMPYEMA

ALBERT S. KLAINER, M.D.

Pleural effusion is defined as the presence of excessive fluid. Empyema is defined as the presence of frank pus in the pleural space. When due to pulmonary infection, pleural effusions generally occur as a result of bacterial pneumonias, occasionally result from mycoplasmal pneumonia, but are seen uncommonly in viral pneumonia. Although pleural effusions of varying degree may also be seen in pulmonary tuberculosis and fungal infections of the lung, noninfectious causes are also prominent (Fig. 1). In general, empyema is associated only with infectious diseases, most commonly bacterial in origin. Appropriate treatment of pleural effusion and/or empyema essential for complete resolution is based upon an early diagnostic approach to the etiology of the effusion.

ETIOLOGY

Pleural effusions commonly accompany bacterial pneumonia, whereas true empyemas are uncommon in the antibiotic era.

Pleural effusions most commonly develop secondary to pneumonia caused by *Staphylococcus aureus*, *Streptococcus pneumoniae*, *Haemophilus influenzae*, group A β-hemolytic streptococci, and anaerobic and gram-negative bacteria as well as pulmonary tuberculosis. A pleural effusion may occasionally accompany mycoplasmal pneumonia. Pleural effusion occurring during the active phase of viral pneumonia is distinctly uncommon; however, postpneumonic effusions may be seen with viral as well as bacterial pneumonias.

True empyema is most commonly caused by *S. aureus* or anaerobic bacteria, usually the result of the formation of

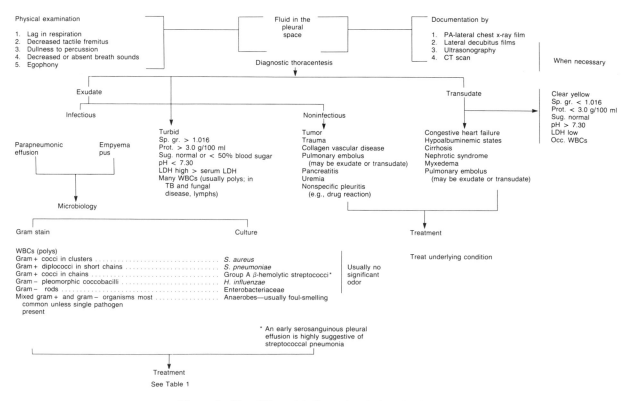

Figure 1 The differential diagnosis of pleural effusions.

microabscesses near the surface of the lung, which rupture through the pleural surface into the pleural space. Gram-negative bacteria such as *Klebsiella, Pseudomonas,* and some of the Enterobacteriaceae may also result in empyema. Post-pneumococcal empyema is now uncommon.

DIAGNOSIS

The diagnosis of pleural effusion is first made by physical examination. Signs include a lag in respiration on the involved side, a decrease in tactile fremitus, dullness to percussion, decreased or absent breath sounds, and egophony just above the effusion. In most immunocompetent patients, pleural effusion due to infection, especially empyema, is associated with significant fever and leukocytosis. At least 300 to 500 ml of fluid must be present to be detected by physical examination. Rapid respiration, shallow breathing, and a contralateral mediastinal shift may be seen with large effusions. Radiographic substantiation is desirable in most cases. Although the presence of fluid may be detected on a posteroanterior and lateral film of the chest, decubitus films are frequently helpful, especially in identifying small pleural effusions. Ultrasonography or computed tomography (CT) may be needed to identify loculated or small effusions.

Once a pleural effusion is identified, a diagnostic and/or therapeutic thoracentesis is mandatory. There is almost no contraindication to such; even thrombocytopenia and/or clotting abnormalities are rarely contraindications to a diagnostic thoracentesis. Since almost all antimicrobial agents diffuse well into pleural fluid, Gram stains, cultures, and other studies should be obtained before therapy is instituted.

If a pleural effusion is difficult to obtain, guiding the needle by ultrasound or CT may be helpful.

A diagnostic thoracentesis should be performed in all cases with enough fluid removed to suffice for the tests planned. In the case of large pleural effusions that compromise respiration, a therapeutic thoracentesis to permit expansion of the lung may be necessary. Although there is some variation in the number of tests to be obtained on the pleural fluid, those usually ordered are a white blood cell count, differential count, total protein, glucose, pH, specific gravity, LDH, Gram stain, and appropriate cultures. The use and significance of this information to differentiate between an exudate and a transudate is outlined in Figure 1. If tuberculosis is suspected, a pleural biopsy should be obtained since granulomata and acid-fast bacteria are usually not in the pleural effusion but reside in the pleura itself. Although infections may cause grossly bloody pleural effusions, their presence usually indicates tuberculosis, pulmonary infarction, trauma, or tumor. Parapneumonic effusion is particularly common in group A streptococcal infections. The diagnostic approach to pleural effusions is outlined in Figure 1.

TREATMENT

Table 1 lists my preference for antimicrobial therapy related to the etiology of the effusion and or empyema.

Antimicrobial agents should be given intravenously. In the case of parapneumonic effusions, the duration of therapy is dictated by that of the underlying pneumonia. The author treats true empyemas with 4 weeks of intravenous therapy,

TABLE 1   Treatment of Infectious Pleural Effusions and Empyema

Etiology	Preferred Antibiotics	Alternative Antibiotics (for Patients Allergic to Preferred Choice)
S. aureus (penicillin-sensitive)	Aqueous penicillin G 2.0×10^6 U IV q4h	Vancomycin 500 mg IV q8h
S. aureus (penicillin-resistant)	Oxacillin or nafcillin 2.0 g IV q4h	Vancomycin 500 mg IV q8h
S. aureus (methicillin-resistant)	Vancomycin 500 mg IV q8h	Clindamycin 900 mg IV q8h if sensitive
S. pneumoniae	Aqeous penicillin G 2.0×10^6 U IV q4h	Clindamycin 900 mg IV q8h
Group A β-hemolytic streptococci	Aqueous penicillin G 2.0×10^6 U IV q4h	Clindamycin 900 mg IV q8h
H. influenzae (ampicillin-sensitive)	Ampicillin 1.0 g IV q4h	Bactrim 8 mg/kg/day trimethoprim 40 mg/kg/day sulfamethoxazole
H. influenzae (ampicillin-resistant)	Cefuroxime 2 g IV q8h	Chloramphenicol 2 g IV q6h
Klebsiella pneumoniae	Tobramycin 5 mg/kg/day in 3 divided doses q8h IV	Ceftazidime 2 g IV q8h
Pseudomonas aeruginosa*	Tobramycin 5 mg/kg/day in 3 divided doses q8h IV	Ceftazidime 2 g IV q8h
Other Enterobacteriaceae*	Tobramycin 5 mg/kg/day in 3 divided doses q8h IV	Ceftazidime 2 g IV q8h
Anaerobes	Clindamycin 900 mg IV q8h	Aqueous penicillin G 2.0×10^6 U IV q6h

* Choice of antibiotic may vary according to sensitivities in individual hospitals.

but others prefer to change to oral therapy once the patient has been afebrile for 48 to 72 hours and drainage has been accomplished.

In infections of the pleural space, especially true empyemas, therapy includes specific antimicrobial agents given intravenously as well as removal of accumulated fluid. Since all antimicrobial agents diffuse well into pleural fluid, there is no need for the intrapleural injection of antimicrobial agents. The removal of accumulating fluid or pus not only hastens recovery, but is necessary to prevent "plastering" of the parietal to the visceral pleura with the production of an increasing "peel," which would require open thoracotomy and decortication for reexpansion of the involved lung. Complicated pleural effusions and all empyemas require total drainage by closed tube thoracostomy. The duration of closed thoracostomy tube drainage varies. I prefer to continue drainage until the effusion diminishes to less than 50 ml or has ceased for 48 hours. At such time, the chest tube is gradually withdrawn. It is not usually necessary to drain the small pleural effusions related to mycoplasmal pneumonia or the postpneumonic effusions related to viral disease.

SUGGESTED READING

Bartlet JG, Gorbach SL, Thadepalli H, Finegold SM. Bacteriology of empyema. Lancet 1974; 1:338–340.

Lerner AM, Jankauskas K. The classic bacterial pneumonias. DM 1975; Feb:32–38.

Levinson ME, Mangura CT, Lorber B, et al. Clindamycin compared with penicillin for the treatment of anaerobic lung abscess. Ann Inter Med 1983; 98:466–471.

Taryle DA, Potts DE, Sahn SA. The incidence and clinical correlates of parapneumonic effusions in pneumococcal pneumonia. Chest 1978; 74:170–173.

Thomas MJ, Taylor FH, Sanger PW, et al. Decortication in the management of the complications of staphylococcal pneumonia in infants and children. J Thorac Cardiovasc Surg 1965; 49:708–713.

Wallace RJ Jr, Musher DM, Martin RR. *Hemophilus influenzae* pneumonia in adults. Am J Med 1978; 64:87–93.

Weinstein LW, Fields BN, eds. Seminars in infectious diseases. V. Pneumonias. New York: Thieme-Stratton, 1983.

SINUSITIS

CARL B. LAUTER, M.D.

Inflammation of the paranasal sinuses is usually caused by infectious agents, most commonly, bacteria. The process is initiated, under most circumstances, as a complication of preceding viral upper respiratory tract infection. Allergic nasal disease may also predispose to sinusitis. Defects in mucociliary clearance that are part of cystic fibrosis or the immotile-cilia syndrome also may lead to bacterial sinusitis. Obstruction in the nasal passages by inflammatory edema or mass lesions such as polyps and tumors presumably leads to stasis, accumulation of secretions, and secondary bacterial infection. Other mechanisms that may lead to sinusitis include direct extension from an adjacent focus such as upper maxillary ridge dental infection or direct implantation of microorganisms after trauma or a surgical procedure.

The bacteriology of sinusitis varies with the presence or absence of underlying disorders such as cystic fibrosis, hypogammaglobulinemia, leukemia, or immunosuppressive drug therapy. Nosocomial sinusitis has a different clinical presentation and microbiology from sinusitis that develops out of the hospital. There are acute, subacute, and chronic forms of sinusitis. The differential diagnosis, microbiology, and treatment of these three forms of the diseases may at times be different from each other. The microbiology of acute flare-ups of chronic sinusitis is usually the same as the microbiology of acute sinusitis. Fungal sinusitis is relatively uncommon, and most cases have been described in patients with diabetes mellitus or who are immunosuppressed by certain hematologic malignancies or immunosuppressive medications.

Noninfectious causes of sinusitis may occur. Such vasculitic diseases as Wegener's granulomatosis, Goodpasture's syndrome, lethal midline granuloma, and polyarteritis nodosa may be complicated by or associated with sinusitis. Recent reports that the sinusitis of Wegener's granulomatosis may respond to trimethoprim-sulfamethoxazole (TMP/SMZ) suggests that this disorder may also be caused by an infectious agent. Allergic (or nonallergic) chronic rhinitis may be complicated by an apparently noninfectious low-grade form of sinusitis. Allergic fungal sinusitis is a nondestructive pansinusitis that usually occurs in atopic individuals. It appears to be analogous to allergic bronchopulmonary aspergillosis, although other fungi have also been implicated.

Neoplastic disorders may cause or mimic sinusitis. The commonest of these is squamous cell carcinoma. Cocaine abuse may lead to a particularly aggressive form of osteolytic sinusitis, not infrequently complicated by ocular and neurologic problems. A number of medications may be associated with rhinitis and sinusitis (aspirin and nonsteroidal anti-inflammatory drugs) or may lead to chronic rhinitis masquerading as sinusitis; a number of antihypertensive medications and estrogens produce the latter syndrome. Pregnancy and hypothyroidism may cause nasal stuffiness and obstruction and thus mimic chronic sinusitis.

Lastly, the clinical diagnosis of sinusitis may be imprecise, especially in the subacute and chronic forms. Roentgenographic observations show the best correlation with cultures obtained by direct sinus puncture. In practice, a "clinical" diagnosis is often adequate and roentgenographic studies may be reserved for acutely ill patients who fail to respond to initial therapy, those who require surgical intervention, or patients who suffer recurrences. A firm diagnosis, however, does rely on roentgenographic studies. Thorough roentgenographic study of the paranasal sinuses should include a Water's (occipitomental) view, a Caldwell (posteroanterior) view, and an erect lateral view. Nasopharyngeal cultures are neither sensitive nor specific; the predictive value of a positive test correlates poorly with results obtained simultaneously with direct maxillary antrum sinus puncture. This latter procedure is rarely indicated in standard office practice and should be reserved for complicated cases. Patients who fail to respond to conventional empiric therapy as well as immunocompromised patients in whom more resistant bacteria and fungi are suspected would be the ones who require more invasive diagnostic studies. In addition to direct sinus aspiration, specimens for culture and special stains may also be obtained during a sinus lavage or at the time of surgical exploration.

Transillumination is unreliable, and ultrasonography of the sinuses is both expensive and insensitive. Computed transaxial tomography is reliable and accurate; however, the expense, radiation exposure, and relative unavailability of this test precludes its frequent use in clinical practice. More recently, fiberoptic rhinopharyngoscopy studies have demonstrated grossly purulent and infected secretions draining directly from the sinus orifices in patients who have "normal" sinus radiologic films.

THERAPEUTIC ALTERNATIVES

The medical treatment of sinusitis takes two forms: antimicrobic and adjunctive. As noted earlier, an accurate microbiologic diagnosis is rarely available except in the acute form of sinusitis where a blood culture may be positive. The culprit bacteria may be isolated from the site of a metastatic complication such as the cerebrospinal fluid in a patient with meningitis. Antibiotic treatment is usually empiric and based on the data obtained from several studies that utilized sinus puncture to obtain their cultures.

In acute community-acquired sinusitis of both children and adults, the three commonest causative bacteria are *Strep-*

tococcus pneumoniae, *Haemophilus influenzae*, and *Branhamella catarrhalis*; these three organisms account for more than 50 percent of bacteria isolated. Although ampicillin or amoxicillin have been traditional agents of choice in the past, the increasing incidence of β-lactamase-producing bacteria (ampicillin-resistant) from patients with sinusitis suggests that alternative agents may soon be required in a significant number of patients. Alternative agents might include: amoxicillin-clavulanic acid, cefaclor, TMP/SMZ, and erythromycin-sulfisoxazole. In patients with anaphylactic (immediate type) reactions to penicillins, cefaclor should also probably not be used. My current approach is to use, in order of preference, amoxicillin-clavulanic acid, cefaclor, cefuroxime axetil, TMP/SMZ, and erythromycin-sulfisoxazole in all but the very mildest of cases. Regional differences in antibiotic susceptibility patterns may allow amoxicillin to remain a front-line therapy in some office situations. In patients with anaphylactic (immediate) reactions to penicillins, cefaclor and cefuroxime should probably not be used unless allergic skin testing is performed first. Some patients may at times respond to a tetracycline, especially doxycycline (not used for patients under the age of 8 years).

Subacute sinusitis frequently accompanies other upper respiratory tract problems in children. In one study, 27 percent of children who were being operated on for tonsillectomy and adenoidectomy or tympanostomy were found to have abnormal sinus roentgenograms and positive sinus-puncture cultures. The majority of these children had no symptoms. The microbiology was similar to that described above for acute sinusitis.

Chronic sinusitis is quite different. After 3 or more months, and perhaps lasting indefinitely, the chronic form of sinusitis is characterized by irreversible epithelial changes in the mucosa of the involved sinuses. The microbiologic flora in chronic sinusitis is often anaerobic; anaerobes have

TABLE 1 Antibiotic Treatment for Sinusitis

Organism	Antibiotic Choices (in order of preference)
Usual microbiologic findings	
1. *Streptococcus pneumoniae*	Penicillin V, ampicillin, amoxicillin, cephalexin, cephradine, erythromycin, TMP/SMZ
2. *Haemophilus influenzae*	
β-lactamase-negative	Ampicillin, amoxicillin, TMP/SMZ, cefaclor, cefuroxime axetil, erythromycin-sulfisoxazole, amoxicillin-clavulanic acid, chloramphenicol
β-lactamase-positive	All of above except ampicillin, amoxicillin
3. *Branhamella catarrhalis*	Amoxicillin-clavulanic acid, cefaclor, cefuroxime axetil, TMP/SMZ
4. Anaerobic bacteria (assume increasing β-lactamase production)	Amoxicillin-clavulanic acid, combination with clindamycin and second drug in 1, 2, 3 above. Tetracycline (age $\geq$ 8 yr), chloramphenicol
Less-usual Microorganisms	
1. *Staphylococcus aureus*	
Methicillin-sensitive	Dicloxacillin, cephalexin, amoxicillin-clavulanic acid, TMP/SMZ, erythromycin $\pm$
Methicillin-resistant	TMP/SMZ, ciprofloxacin, vancomycin IV
2. *Streptococcus pyogenes*	Penicillin V, ampicillin, cephalexin, erythromycin
3. Gram-negative rods	
Excluding *Pseudomonas aeruginosa*	Amoxicillin-clavulanic acid, cefaclor $\pm$, TMP/SMZ, tetracyclines $\pm$ according to susceptibility tests, chloramphenicol
Pseudomonas aeruginosa	Ciprofloxacin; others must be IV or IM: aminoglycosides, ticarcillin, newer antipseudomonal penicillins, ceftazidime, imipenem, aztreonam

TABLE 2   Doses of Commonly Used Oral Antibiotics in the Treatment of Adult Sinusitis

Antibiotic	Usual Dose
Ampicillin	500 mg q6h
Amoxicillin	500 mg q6–8h
Amoxicillin-clavulanic acid	500 mg amoxicillin + 125 mg clavulanic acid q6–8h
Cephalexin	500 mg q6h
Cephradine	500 mg q6h
Cefaclor	500 mg q6h
Cefuroxime axetil*	500 mg q12h
Trimethoprim-sulfamethoxazole (double-strength)	160 mg trimethoprim + 800 mg sulfamethoxazole q12h
Erythromycin	500 mg q6h
Doxycycline	100 mg q12h
Ciprofloxacin*	500 mg q12h

* Role in sinusitis not yet fully established.

been reported in as many as 100 percent of patients in some series. Among the aerobes, α- and β-hemolytic streptococci as well as *Staphylococcus aureus* predominate. Enteric gram-negative rods occur often in the acute and chronic forms of sinusitis that follow nasotracheal intubation, such as in the intensive care unit. It is not uncommon to find *Klebsiella*, *Enterobacter*, and *Pseudomonas aeruginosa* under such conditions. Both *S. aureus* and *Staphylococcus epidermidis* may be etiologic agents in such patients. The bacteriology of the sinusitis that occurs in patients with cystic fibrosis includes a significant number of isolates of *P. aeruginosa*. The isolation of *P. aeruginosa* from a patient with community-acquired sinusitis should suggest the diagnosis of cystic fibrosis. Acute flare-ups of sinusitis characterized by pain, fever, and other systemic symptoms in a patient with known chronic sinusitis should lead to treatment similar to that used for patients with new-onset acute sinusitis since the microbiology is similar.

Antibiotic treatment options for acute, subacute, and chronic sinusitis are outlined in Table 1. Suggested doses for adults for oral forms of the most commonly used antibiotics are listed in Table 2. Antibiotic therapy must be continued for at least a full 2 weeks. Parenteral therapy is necessary in any patient who is sick enough to be hospitalized or in whom the microbiology is not treatable by oral antibiotics.

Adjunctive measures that I have found to be useful in the treatment of sinusitis include nasal decongestants such as phenylephrine 0.5 to 1 percent nose drops or nasal sprays. These measures are effective in promoting drainage when used in conjunction with antibiotics. When drainage is spontaneous, these medications are not needed. Analgesics may be needed to control pain, but care must be taken not to overvigorously suppress fever or depress consciousness lest a metastatic complication such as brain abscess or meningitis be overlooked. The role of oral decongestants and/or antihistamines is still controversial, but I have found them to be helpful and use them. Steam appears to be helpful, and nasal irrigation with saline may be useful in some patients.

Surgical procedures that may be needed in patients who fail to respond to the medical treatment are outlined in Table 3. Minor procedures, including sinus lavage and astringent packs, should be attempted first except in an acute emergency. Detailed discussion of the major surgical procedures that may be required in such patients is beyond the scope of this review. The indications for more aggressive sinus surgery include chronic, recurrent sinusitis, sinusitis in the immunocompromised patient, sinusitis refractory to medical treatment, nasal polyps refractory to steroids and causing obstruction, suspected neoplasm, complications of sinusitis, osteomyelitis, mucocele or mucopyocele, and progressive pulmonary dysfunction, due to severe steroid-dependent asthma in association with sinusitis.

TABLE 3   Surgical Procedures in Sinusitis

Minor procedures
  Fiberoptic rhinopharyngoscopy (mostly for diagnosis)
  Sinus irrigation (lavage)
  Astringent nasal packing
Major Procedures
  Turbinate reduction
  Septoplasty
  Polypectomy
  Specific sinuses
    Maxillary
      Nasoantral window
      Caldwell-Luc
    Ethmoid
      Ethmoidectomy with polypectomy
    Frontal
      Rarely needed
    Sphenoid
      Needed more often when associated with CNS suppurative complication
      Sinus x-ray films insensitive for diagnosis, will need CT
Nasal endoscope (rigid, permits short-stay surgery, not in common use yet)

A.(1) <u>Community-acquired sinusitis</u>

Onset ≤ 1–3 wk. Facial pain, nasal obstruction, fever, other systemic symptoms. Nasal discharge may be present.

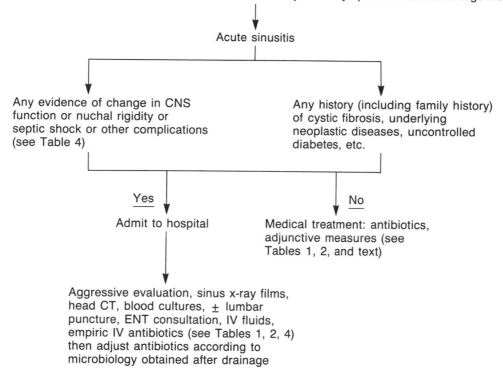

A.(2) <u>Community-acquired sinusitis</u>

Onset ≥3 wk–3 mo or >3 mo. Evidence of nasal obstruction and/or nasal discharge is primary.

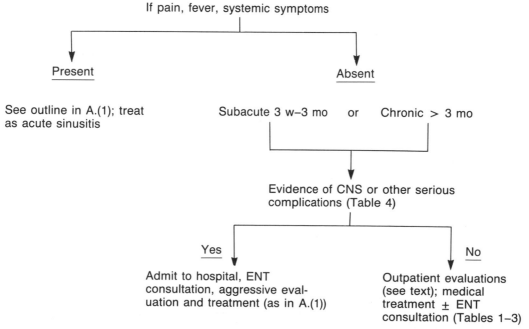

Figure 1 Evaluation and treatment of sinusitis. *Figure continues on following page*

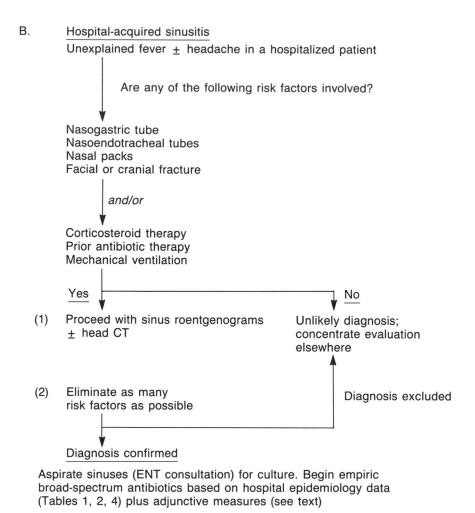

B.   Hospital-acquired sinusitis
     Unexplained fever ± headache in a hospitalized patient

          Are any of the following risk factors involved?

     Nasogastric tube
     Nasoendotracheal tubes
     Nasal packs
     Facial or cranial fracture

          and/or

     Corticosteroid therapy
     Prior antibiotic therapy
     Mechanical ventilation

     Yes   No

(1) Proceed with sinus roentgenograms   Unlikely diagnosis;
     ± head CT   concentrate evaluation
                                                 elsewhere

(2) Eliminate as many   Diagnosis excluded
     risk factors as possible

     Diagnosis confirmed

Aspirate sinuses (ENT consultation) for culture. Begin empiric
broad-spectrum antibiotics based on hospital epidemiology data
(Tables 1, 2, 4) plus adjunctive measures (see text)

Figure 1   *continued*

PROS AND CONS OF TREATMENT

Since many patients have mild and nonspecific signs and symptoms of sinusitis (or none at all), a therapeutic plan in the ambulatory setting must include a high index of suspicion for the diagnosis. Nasal obstruction and/or nasal discharge may be the only findings in patients with chronic sinusitis, whereas pain, fever, and systemic symptoms may accompany the nasal symptoms listed above. Many patients may cure themselves with nasal decongestant drops or sprays and steam, if they can relieve the obstruction. A flow diagram is outlined in Figure 1 as a suggested algorithm for the evaluation and treatment of such patients.

COMPLICATIONS OF SINUSITIS

These can be divided into three main categories in addition to bacteremia and sepsis—osteomyelitis, orbital complications, and intracranial complications—and are listed in Table 4. These are often preventable by early diagnosis and treatment of the underlying sinusitis.

TABLE 4   Complications of Sinusitis

Local or contiguous spread
  Frontal bone osteomyelitis
  "Potts' puffy tumors"

Orbital
  Frequently from ethmoid and/or frontal sinuses
  Stages
    Inflammatory edema
    Orbital cellulitis
    Cavernous sinus thrombophlebitis
    Subperiosteal abscess
    Orbital abscess

Intracranial
  Epidural abscess
  Subdural empyema
  Brain abscess
  Thrombosis of the dural sinus
  Meningitis

Adapted from Baker AS. Sinusitis. Medical Grand Rounds 1984; 3:154–165.

SUGGESTED READING

Baker AS. Sinusitis. Medical Grand Rounds 1984; 3:154–165.
Caplan ES, Hoyt NJ. Nosocomial sinusitis. JAMA 1982; 247:639–641.

Daley CL, Sande M. The runny nose: infection of the paranasal sinuses. Infect Dis Clin North Am 1988; 2:131–147.
Fisher SR, Newman CE. Surgical perspectives on allergic airway disease. J Allerg Clin Immunol 1988; 81:361–375.
Kuhn JP. Imaging of paranasal sinuses: current status. J Allerg Clin Immunol 1986; 77:6–8.

CHRONIC BRONCHITIS

IRA B. TAGER, M.D., M.P.H.

Chronic bronchitis (CB) refers to the presence of cough and phlegm for 3 months out of the year for more than 2 consecutive years. This definition was developed on the basis of epidemiologic studies performed in the 1950s to provide more precise meaning to a constellation of respiratory symptoms observed in clinical practice and in epidemiologic studies. From its inception, the term CB became synonymous with a disease spectrum that ranged from simple hypersecretion of mucus to airflow obstruction. Although evidence now suggests that the presence and course of mucus hypersecretion are unrelated to long-term deterioration of lung function and mortality, in this chapter, the specific term CB refers to the entire spectrum of illness that includes obstructive lung disease.

EPIDEMIOLOGY

Chronic bronchitis is a common disease that increases in prevalence with age. As a cause of death, CB ranks fifth among all causes and has been rising over the past 25 years. Cigarette smoking is the most important factor that is associated with occurrence of mucus hypersecretion and airflow obstruction. Current estimates indicate that 80 to 90 percent of CB can be attributed to cigarette smoking. Among the number of other factors that have been investigated as causes of CB (Table 1), only the Pi ZZ genotype of α_1-antitrypsin and possibly male sex have been associated with the occurrence of CB. Of note, episodes of acute infection in adult life have not been definitively associated with CB (see below).

PATHOGENESIS

Two epidemiologically derived hypotheses related to the occurrence of CB have dominated the thinking about this disease spectrum. In the "British" hypothesis, mucus hypersecretion results from exposure to a variety of inhaled irritants, which leads to obstructed airways and the occurrence of recurrent infections. These recurrent infections, in turn, were thought to result in further damage to pulmonary airways and parenchyma. A landmark test of this hypothesis has refuted this basic pathophysiologic sequence. The "Dutch" hypothesis proposes that mucus hypersecretion is

TABLE 1 Risk Factors for Mucus Hypersecretion and/or Chronic Airflow Obstruction in Adults

Clearly established factors
   Cigarette smoking (active)
   α_1-antitrypsin deficiency

Factors for which some data suggest increased risk
   Age
   Air pollution
   Alcohol
   Atopy, allergy or hypersensitivity (bronchial hyperreactivity)
   Childhood respiratory illness
   Environmental pollution
   Familial and/or household
   Genetic
   Lower social class
   Male sex
   Occupational exposures
   Respiratory illness history in adulthood

a manifestation of an allergic hypersensitivity to a variety of environmental insults. Recurrent infections are thought to be a secondary consequence of airways that are already constricted and have a decreased ability to clear microbial insults. Although much indirect evidence has provided support for this hypothesis, a definitive test of its applicability has yet to be completed.

In contrast to the above epidemiologic hypotheses, the protease-antiprotease hypothesis derives from the specific pathologic lesion found in patients with CB. In this hypothesis, cigarette smoke is seen as disrupting the normal homeostatic mechanisms that protect the lung from damage by proteolytic enzymes. The role of pulmonary infection is not addressed specifically, but its role can be inferred to be minor relative to the effect of cigarette smoke. Although this hypothesis has a reasonable body of laboratory data to support it, nonetheless, at present it offers incomplete insight into the considerable variability of risk for CB among smokers.

CLINICAL MANIFESTATIONS AND MANAGEMENT

Patients with CB are most likely to present with complaints of shortness of breath with or without complaints of wheeze, cough, and phlegm. Symptoms typically are episodic, especially those related to worsening cough, phlegm, and wheeze (so-called acute exacerbations). In this context, decisions about the management of acute respiratory infections in the context of acute exacerbations of CB require consideration of four issues: (1) the extent to which infections are the cause of acute exacerbations; (2) the susceptibility of patients with CB to respiratory infection and the types of infections involved; (3) the efficacy of antimicrobial therapy; and (4) the relationship of acute infectious exacerbations and their treatment to the long-term course of chronic airflow obstruction.

Although early investigations suggested a unique pathophysiologic role for *Haemophilus influenzae* and *Streptococcus pneumoniae* in the lower respiratory tract secretions of patients with CB, subsequent prospective studies have failed to support such a relationship or have suggested a complex interaction between the occurrence of viral infections and serologic evidence of infection with these bacterial organisms. No consistent associations between other bacteria and acute exacerbations of CB have been identified.

Viruses and *Mycoplasma pneumoniae* also have been implicated as causes of acute exacerbations of CB. Overall, evidence does suggest that patients with CB are somewhat more susceptible to infection with common respiratory viruses and possibly with *M. pneumoniae*. Viral infections are far more common than infections with *M. pneumoniae*, and, together, they account for less than one-half of all exacerbations in patients under the care of physicians. The cause(s) of acute exacerbations in patients without evidence of infection remains unknown, as does the specific role of cigarette smoking in the episodic nature of the clinical manifestations of CB.

Since antiviral agents have been and remain generally unavailable for therapy (with the exception of amantadine/rimantadine for influenza A infection), virtually all of the data that relate to the utility of antimicrobial agents for the treatment of acute exacerbations of CB concern the use of antibacterial agents. These data, and the recommendations that follow, are based on the assumption that radiographically confirmed pneumonia is not present as the cause of the acute exacerbation. During outbreaks of influenza A infection, amantadine/rimantadine can be used in accordance with the usual recommendation for the therapy with these agents.

Until recently, the evidence that antibacterial agents provided a meaningful clinical benefit in the management of acute exacerbations of CB (including those that require hospitalization) was marginal. However, a recent, large placebo-controlled study has suggested that a 10-day course of an antibacterial agent (doxycycline, amoxicillin, or trimethoprim-sulfamethoxazole) in patients with significant airflow obstruction does lead to significantly more rapid resolution of symptoms in exacerbations characterized by increased dyspnea, sputum volume, and sputum purulence. Other types of exacerbations, including those with wheeze in the absence of increased cough and phlegm, were not so benefitted. Peak flows also recovered faster in patients with "responsive" exacerbations, but the effect was observed only for the first 2 weeks of the exacerbation.

Data from well-controlled studies of the prophylactic use of antibacterial agents to suppress the occurrence of acute exacerbations of CB have been uniform in their failure to show any meaningful clinical benefit in terms of the number of such episodes and/or on the rate of deterioration of lung function.

Table 2 provides a suggested approach to the use of antibacterial agents for the management of acute exacerbations of CB. Since only erythromycin and tetracyclines have proven efficacious against *M. pneumoniae* and are also active against *Streptococcus pneumoniae* (both agents) and *H. influenzae* (tetracyclines), no other alternatives are identified in the table. For patients who cannot be given these agents, any antibiotic with activity against the pneumococcus and *H. influenzae* may be given. Since β-lactamase-producing strains are infrequent among the unencapsulated strains of *H. influenzae* found in patients with CB, ampicillin (amoxicillin) should be used in preference to more expensive and/or toxic alternatives, including trimethoprim-sulfamethoxazole (sulfonamide toxicity). Recommendations on the role of corticosteroids and bronchodilators in exacerbations of CB are beyond the scope of this chapter.

TABLE 2   Suggested Approach for the Use of Antibacterial Agents in the Management of Acute Exacerbations of Chronic Bronchitis

General
  Routine Gram stain and culture are not necessary
  Advice on smoking cessation and reduction is essential

Specific
  Exacerbations characterized by new or increased dyspnea with increased cough and purulent sputum: 7–10-d course of a tetracycline or erythromycin (250 mg qid for both; 100 mg bid for doxycycline) (if patient cannot take these agents, choose ampicillin [amoxicillin] (250 mg q4h) or trimethoprim-sulfamethoxazole [80:400 ī]

  All other types of exacerbations:
  Observe patient 3–5 d to determine if improvement occurs without antibacterial therapy

  If, during observation period, exacerbation meets criteria above or there is clinical deterioration ($\downarrow PaO_2$ or $\downarrow O_2$ saturation, $\uparrow PaCO_2$, onset or worsening of systemic signs/symptoms), begin 7–10-d course of antibacterial agent as above

  For all exacerbations treated with antibacterial agents, discontinue after 7–10 d and reevaluate if no improvement or continued worsening

Note: This approach assumes that there is no clinical suspicion of pneumonia and/or that pneumonia has been ruled out by radiographic evidence.

SUGGESTED READING

Anthonisen NR, Manfreda J, Warren CPW, et al. Antibiotic therapy in exacerbations of chronic obstructive pulmonary disease. Ann Intern Med 1987; 106:196–204.

Gump DW, Philips CA, Forsyth BR, et al. Role of infection in chronic bronchitis. Am Rev Respir Dis 1976; 113:465–474.

Johnston RN, McNeill RS, Smith DH, Legge JS, Fletcher F. Chronic bronchitis-measurements and observations over ten years. Thorax 1976; 31:25–29.

Monto AS, Higgins MW, Ross HW. The Tecumseh Study of respiratory illness. VIII. Acute infection in chronic respiratory disease and comparison group. Am Rev Respir Dis 1975; 111:27–36.

Nicotra MB, Rivera M, Awe JR. Antibiotic therapy of acute exacerbations of chronic bronchitis. Ann Intern Med 1982; 97:18–21.

LUNG ABSCESS

BURT R. MEYERS, M.D.

Lung abscess can be defined as either a single or multiple area(s) of pulmonary suppuration with necrosis, manifested radiologically by cavitary formation. Primary lung abscess follows aspiration of oropharyngeal organisms and secretions; in some cases gastroesophageal reflux followed by pulmonary aspiration may occur. Predisposing factors for this aspiration are a decrease in consciousness related to a cerebrovascular accident, seizure disorder, alcoholism, drug overdose, or general anesthesia. Patients with indwelling nasogastric or gastrostomy tubes or esophageal disorders of either intrinsic or neurologic origin are prone to aspiration. Other predisposing factors include gingivodental suppuration as well as immunosuppressive therapy with corticosteroids. Lung suppuration and abscess may follow a necrotizing pneumonia or localized obstruction from an endobronchial lesion (benign or malignant) or carcinoma of the lung. Septic pulmonary emboli, often associated with tricuspid valve endocarditis, may present as lung abscess. Other secondary factors include the association of lung abscess with cystic fibrosis, bronchiectasis, and infected lung cysts.

DIAGNOSIS

Lung abscess should be suspected in any patient with fever, a productive cough (often with a fetid smell), malaise, weight loss, and radiographic evidence of cavitary disease, which is often associated with empyema. Studies of the primary microbiology of the lung abscesses reveal that 80 to 90 percent of the isolates are anaerobic, ranging from two to six species per patient (see Fig. 1). Transtracheal aspiration reveals the commonest organisms to be *Bacteroides melaninogenicus*, *Peptostreptococcus* or *Peptococcus* species, and *Fusobacterium nucleatum*. Other *Bacteroides* strains, including *Bacteroides fragilis*, and microaerophillic streptococci are often isolated; the commonest aerobes are *Staphylococcus aureus*, enteric gram-negative bacilli, including *Klebsiella pneumoniae*, *Haemophilus influenzae*, and *Serratia* species. A variety of other organisms have been associated with abscess formation, and these include *Legionella* species and *Actinomyces* species. In certain immunocompromised patients receiving corticosteroids, lung abscess may occur secondary to infection with *Nocardia asteroides* and *Strongyloides stercoralis*. In patients with acquired immunodeficiency syndrome (AIDS), *Corynebacterium equi* has been noted with increased frequency. In severely granulocytopenic patients or transplant recipients on immunosuppressive therapy, the rapid development of a necrotizing cavitary pneumonia should lead one to consider such organisms as *Aspergillus* species, *Pseudomonas aeruginosa*, and phycomyces (i.e., *Mucor*); these are often associated with hemoptysis and pleural symptoms.

THERAPY

All patients should be considered for treatment of primary lung abscess as soon as the diagnosis is made; in addition to antimicrobial therapy, attempts to prevent further deterioration from decreased sensorium should be instituted (e.g., when necessary, patients should be intubated, the nasogastric tube withdrawn and seizure disorder treated). Cultures of oropharyngeal secretions are an unreliable indicator of lower respiratory tract pathogens. In a stable patient, an attempt at transtracheal aspiration to determine microbiology may be carried out; this procedure is not without adverse effects and should be performed only by skilled physicians. A transtracheal aspirate or protected specimen brush should be used for the patient who fails to respond to standard therapy. At least two blood samples taken from peripheral sites should be cultured; if pleural fluid is present, a thoracentesis for Gram stain and diagnostic microbiology for aerobic and anaerobic organisms should be performed.

It is important to assess whether the patient is allergic to antibiotics and, specifically, whether a type I allergy to penicillin is present. In the absence of this allergy, therapy for primary lung abscess may be begun with either intravenous penicillin or clindamycin. It is generally accepted that although both aerobic and anaerobic organisms are associated with lung suppuration, treatment of the anaerobes is usually all that is necessary for cure.

The older literature suggested that penicillin therapy was associated with clinical cure even when isolates included *B. fragilis* and Enterobacteriaceae. In a prospective study in 1983 comparing penicillin to clindamycin, clindamycin was found to be more effective in shortening febrile days and fetid sputum production; some patients receiving penicillin had clinically significant extension of their pulmonary infection. Overall, only one-half of the patients treated with penicillin were cured, compared with all patients treated with clindamycin. This suggested to the authors that penicillin was not optimal therapy for the treatment of anaerobic lung abscess. It should be noted that in that study no diagnostic microbiology was obtained.

Clindamycin (600 mg every 8 hours) could be the initial therapy for primary lung abscess in seriously ill patients; an alternative dose of penicillin (1 to 3 $\times$ 10^6 units every 4 hours) in the patient at less risk may be given. These drugs are administered intravenously for 2 to 4 weeks, at which time therapy can be switched to the oral route if clinical improvement is noted: penicillin V, 500 to 750 mg every 6 hours, or clindamycin, 300 mg every 6 hours. Clindamycin offers other potential advantages; it is not susceptible to β-lactamase produced by the anaerobic species and has been noted in certain studies to accumulate within alveolar macrophages. The exact significance of this finding has never been established.

Patients should be followed with regard to their general well being and temperature as well as by serial roentgenograms. Postural drainage with pulmonary physical therapy may be of some benefit. The clinical response may be prolonged during the initial 2 weeks of therapy and radiographic changes may show deterioration even in patients who are destined to improve. However, the presence of clinical

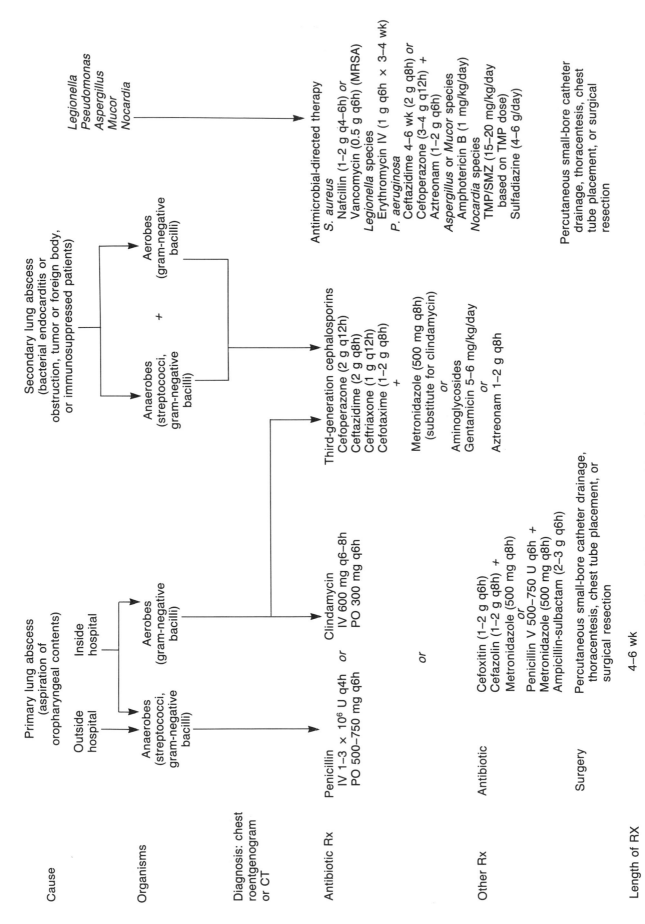

Figure 1 Lung abscess: etiology and therapy.

deterioration or failure to defervesce or an increase in pleural fluid should lead to further considerations. When pleural fluid is noted, thoracentesis should be carried out; in the presence of thick secretions and pus, an indwelling thoracotomy tube or a surgical procedure (i.e., decortication) may be necessary. For patients with pyogenic lung abscesses who do not respond clinically within 10 to 14 days or who show signs of clinical deterioration, percutaneous small-bore catheter drainage has been associated with prompt clinical improvement. Potential risks associated with this drainage include empyema, hemorrhage, and bronchopleural fistula. Literature review reveals that these complications have been found more commonly in patients who have undergone pulmonary resection.

Computerized tomography (CT) has yielded more diagnostic information than conventional radiographs and may be a more accurate method to delineate radiographic response than conventional X-ray films. Radiolabeled scanning techniques with either indium or gallium have been used for diagnosis in some reported cases.

In the penicillin-allergic patient with type I allergy, clindamycin is the drug of choice. Metronidazole is highly effective against *Bacteroides* species and other gram-negative anaerobic bacilli; it has less activity against microaerophilic streptococci and *Actinomyces*. Two published reports revealed poor response rates with metronidazole and suggested it should not be used as monotherapy in the treatment of lung abscess. Other parenteral agents that are available are cefoxitin, which has good activity against *B. fragilis* as well as other anaerobes, including those that produce β-lactamases. This drug could be used in a dose of 4–8 g per day although there are few published reports documenting clinical efficacy. While other cephalosporins have activity in vitro against most oral anaerobic isolates, clinical data are limited in regard to their clinical efficacy. As cost-effective therapy we have often used a first-generation cephalosporin, cefazolin (1 g every 8 hours), in combination with metronidazole (500 mg every 8 hours). Recently β-lactam antibiotics have been combined with β-lactamase inhibitors: ticarcillin with clavulanic acid, ampicillin with sulbactam—both to be administered intravenously—and amoxicillin-clavulanate, a new oral combination. On the basis of its in vitro spectrum, ampicillin-sulbactam could be given as initial therapy, followed by oral amoxicillin-clavulanic acid. This may represent an alternative to the above-mentioned therapies, but clinical studies are needed to determine whether these combinations are efficacious and cost effective when compared with either clindamycin or cefoxitin. Imipenem-cilastatin, a broad-spectrum antimicrobial agent, has in vitro activity against most isolates, but this drug should be reserved for use in nosocomial infection after other agents have been employed.

The treatment of hospital-acquired lung abscess should be more intense. Studies have shown that the oropharynx of such patients is colonized with aerobic gram-negative bacilli. It is generally believed that following aspiration these organisms, as well as oral anaerobes, may be synergistically pathogenic. Therapy should be directed against both components. Clindamycin (600 mg every 6 hours, or 900 mg every 8 hours) should be supplemented with antimicrobial agents that are active against aerobic gram-negative bacilli.

We would add a third-generation cephalosporin to clindamycin—either ceftazidime, 2 g every 8 hours, or cefoperazone, 2 g every 12 hours, if *Pseudomonas* is suspected. Otherwise, ceftriaxone, 1 g every 12 hours, or cefotaxime, 1 to 2 g every 8 hours or aztreonam, 1 to 2 g every 8 hours, may be administered. These β-lactam agents penetrate well into lung secretions and are not affected by the acidic endobronchial pH. Some have suggested that aminoglycosides be given; these agents have been found to bind to pus, are inactivated by low pH that is often found in abscesses, and penetrate poorly into lung secretions. Aminoglycosides are associated with both oto- and nephrotoxicity; both are increased in the seriously ill patient. One clinical study has shown that efficacy in the treatment of gram-negative bacillary pneumonia correlates with serum levels, but no studies have addressed the treatment of lung abscess. Although gentamicin is an inexpensive agent, the cost of determining serum levels, as well as biweekly renal function studies and on occasion audiometric determinations, would markedly raise the cost of aminoglycoside therapy. Studies have shown that gentamicin is taken up poorly by alveolar macrophages.

In a patient with known predisposition to staphylococcal lung abscess (i.e., intravenous drug addicts or patients with bacterial endocarditis or indwelling catheters), therapy should include a penicillinase-resistant penicillin, either nafcillin (8 to 12 g per day) or oxacillin (8 to 12 g per day). In the hospital setting where methicillin-resistant *S. aureus* (MRSA) strains have been reported, it is prudent to begin therapy with vancomycin (500 mg every 6 hours) until the sensitivity of the staphylococci is determined. The dose of vancomycin should be adjusted, depending on renal function. For the treatment of pneumonia with lung abscess secondary to *P. aeruginosa* we prefer combined therapy with double β-lactam agents, such as ceftazidime (2 g every 8 hours) or cefoperazone (3 to 4 g every 12 hours) combined with aztreonam (2 g every 8 hours). Other alternatives to aztreonam may include aminoglycosides, such as amikacin (15 mg per kilogram daily) or tobramycin (1.5 mg every 8 hours) plus a third-generation cephalosporin.

Adverse effects of β-lactam antibiotics include rash, occasional gastrointestinal upset, and neutropenia (in less than 1 percent of patients), and elevation of liver enzymes (in less than 5 percent). In patients who are elderly or those with evidence of renal insufficiency, dosage adjustments are necessary for ceftazidime and cefotaxime. Ceftriaxone and cefoperazone may be given in usual doses for patients with mild renal insufficiency; vitamin K (10 mg biweekly) should be given with cefoperazone to patients over 65 years and to those with renal insufficiency in order to prevent an increase in prothrombin time or clinical bleeding. Imipenem-cilastatin, a new carbapenem derivative, has been associated with seizures, especially in patients with evidence of renal insufficiency; therefore, this drug should be used with caution in patients with decreased renal function.

When clindamycin is combined with a third-generation cephalosporin, the risk of superinfection with enterococcus is somewhat increased since clindamycin and ceftazidime have poor activity against this agent; both cefotaxime and cefoperazone show some in vitro activity against enterococccus and have been infrequently associated with superinfection with this organism.

The mortality from lung abscess is approximately 22 to 28 percent and has remained stable from the 1960s to the mid-1980s. The risk factors associated with this mortality are older age and concomitant underlying disease. It is hoped that with the availability of newer, safer, broad-spectrum antimicrobial agents and their better penetration into pulmonary tissue (compared with aminoglycosides), mortality will decrease in the future. The use of percutaneous small-bore catheter drainage in the high-risk, nonresponding patient may offer an alternative to pulmonary resection and the morbidity and mortality associated with this surgery.

If CT reveals an obstructive lesion, bronchoscopy will usually be necessary to diagnose an endobronchial or infiltrative lesion and even possibly to relieve an obstruction secondary to a foreign body. Radiation of infiltrative lesions may be beneficial in shrinking tumor size and allowing for better drainage. In patients who do not respond, the small-bore percutaneous drainage catheter has been effective, as described above. In some cases neither antimicrobial therapy nor localized drainage is effective, and surgical extirpation is required.

The treatment of lung abscess in the granulocytopenic and/or immunocompromised patient requires selection of specific antimicrobial agents. For the treatment of lung abscess secondary to *Aspergillus* or *Mucor* species, the drug of choice is amphotericin B; in some cases surgical extirpation is curative. Lung abscess secondary to *Nocardia* species is often multifocal; the treatment of choice is either trimethoprim-sulfamethoxazole (TMP/SMZ) or sulfadiazine.

Legionella species on rare occasions in an immunocompromised host have been associated with abscess formation. The recommended treatment is erythromycin (1 g every 6 hours) intravenously for at least 4 to 6 weeks; oral rifampin (600 to 1,200 mg every 12 hours) may be helpful in the patient not responding to monotherapy. Both of these agents penetrate alveolar macrophages and are effective in an animal model.

A new class of oral antimicrobial agents, the quinolones, have recently been marketed. Although these agents have poor activity against anaerobic organisms and some streptococcal strains, they do penetrate into lung secretions and have activity against Enterobacteriaceae and *P. aeruginosa*. These agents should have a role in the follow-up therapy for necrotizing gram-negative pneumonia and lung abscess but should be given with other oral agents such as penicillin or clindamycin. Further studies to determine the clinical efficacy of the quinolones are needed.

SUGGESTED READING

Bartlett JG. Penicillin or clindamycin for primary lung abscess? Ann Intern Med 1983; 98:546–548.

Bartlett JG, Finegold SM. Anaerobic infections of the lung and pleural space. Am Rev Respir Dis 1974; 110:56–77.

Levison ME, Mangura CT, Lorber B, et al. Clindamycin compared with penicillin for the treatment of anaerobic lung abscess. Ann Intern Med 1983; 466–471.

Meyers BR. Pulmonary phycomycosis. In: Samty AH, Smith L, Wyngarden JB, Braude E, eds. Infectious diseases and medical microbiology, 2nd ed. Philadelphia: WB Saunders, 1986.

Parker LA, Melton JW, Delany DJ, Yankaskas BC. Percutaneous small-bore catheter drainage in the management of lung abscesses. Chest 1987; 92:213–218.

EPIGLOTTITIS (SUPRAGLOTTITIS)

GERALD W. FISCHER, M.D.

Epiglottitis is an acute life-threatening infection that can cause sudden, fatal airway obstruction. Epiglottitis occurs in both children and adults and may be confused with other infections such as laryngotracheobronchitis and bacterial tracheitis. Although epiglottitis and supraglottitis are almost exclusively caused by *Haemophilus influenzae* type b, other organisms such as *Streptococcus pneumoniae*, group A β-hemolytic streptococci, and *Staphylococcus aureus* have been implicated in this disease as well. The devastating potential of this disease is related to the anatomic location of the infection. The inflamed and swollen supraglottic tissues impede efficient inspiratory air flow. Inflammation and edema may also involve the hypopharynx and may extend down the trachea for several centimeters. This infection represents a true emergency since airway obstruction may occur abruptly. Immediate attention is required to ensure that an alternative airway is secured by intubation or tracheotomy as quickly as possible.

CLINICAL PRESENTATION

The clinical course of epiglottitis is one of progressive respiratory distress due to tissue inflammation and swelling that impedes effective air intake. Although the child may initially only complain of a mild sore throat (or have pharyngeal inflammation such as uvulitis), in the typical case dysphagia, drooling, and breathing difficulties become apparent within a short time (minutes to hours). The voice is often muffled. Fear and anxiety are apparent by the child's facial expressions. An upright posture is preferred (generally sitting) with the mouth open and the chin extended forward. Although the child is febrile, the degree of toxicity and prostration are out of proportion to the infection. The physician must realize that complete airway obstruction may occur at any time and take immediate steps to ensure that an alternate airway is provided in a safe and expedient manner. The child should not be laid down but should be allowed to remain upright to maximize air exchange. Oxygen is given by mask and held by the parent in a manner that does not disturb the child. A written protocol that defines the actions and responsibilities of each service is advised to minimize wasted time and effort.

DIAGNOSIS

Once the diagnosis of epiglottitis is suspected, a physician must stay with the child and be prepared to provide an alternative airway should the airway suddenly obstruct. The senior anesthesiologist or otolaryngologist on call, the radiology department, and the operating room are notified immediately. The child should not be examined further except to record and monitor vital signs. A tongue blade should not be used to examine the mouth or pharynx since this activity may precipitate obstruction. In addition, invasive procedures, such as the drawing of blood or insertion of an intravenous catheter, should be avoided until the airway is secured. In many hospitals lateral and anteroposterior neck roentgenograms can be rapidly and safely obtained without delaying the child's move to the operating room. Children with airway obstruction and severe respiratory distress should be taken directly to the operating room and the diagnosis established by direct visualization of the epiglottis. If the child has mild respiratory distress or the clinical presentation suggests laryngotracheobronchitis or bacterial tracheitis (Table 1), the anteroposterior and lateral neck x-ray films may be valuable to rule out other causes of airway obstruction and to confirm the diagnosis of epiglottitis. Portable roentgenograms should be obtained in a setting where emergency airway management can be provided, such as an intensive care unit, and a physician must be present at all times. The child should be kept calm and sitting comfortably on the parent's lap. The x-ray films should be immediately processed and interpreted by experienced physicians.

MANAGEMENT IN THE OPERATING ROOM

The anesthesiologist, otolaryngologist, and pediatrician should confer on the management, and the child should be taken to the operating room at the earliest possible moment. During transport, the child should not be laid down but should be allowed to remain upright. A physician should remain with patient at all times during transport, and appropriate airway management equipment must accompany the child. This includes: laryngoscope with proper blade size and a light that works; appropriate-sized endotracheal tube (Table 2) and stylet; self-inflating bag and adapter that fits the endotracheal tube. A smaller endotracheal tube should be available in case edema is more severe than anticipated. Scalpel and cannulae for tracheotomy should be available. The parent should be allowed to stay with the child until the operating room is entered. The anesthesiologist should meet the child before entrance to the operating room and should speak with calm, soothing tones. The conversation should provide reassurance and explain to both the parents and the child what is about to happen. The conversation is continued until induction has been successfully accomplished.

An array of endotracheal tubes (internal diameter, 3.0 mm to 5.0 mm), laryngoscope blades (Miller 1 to 3), a rigid bronchoscope, and materials to perform an emergency tracheostomy (appropriate-sized tracheostomy cannulae and tubes) should all be present in the operating room. Personnel experienced in the delivery of anesthesia and intubation of infants are ideal members of the team caring for these patients. The otolaryngologists should be prepared to perform an immediate emergency tracheostomy should intubation and rigid bronchoscopy fail.

Once the team is ready to secure the airway, induction is begun with the child in the preferred position for maximal air exchange. Movement should remain slow and gentle,

TABLE 1 Differential Diagnosis of Acute Airway Obstruction

Disease	Onset of Symptoms	Fever	Cough	Dysphagia	Toxicity	Neck Roentgenogram
Most common						
Epiglottitis	Rapid and progressive (often 24 h)	Yes (103–104 °F)	Occasionally	Yes	Yes	Loss of vallecula and swollen epiglottis and supraglottic structures
Bacterial tracheitis	1–3 days	Yes (103–104 °F)	Yes	No	Yes	Pus in trachea and subglottic narrowing on AP films
Laryngotracheobronchitis	1–3 days	Variable (103–104 °F)	Yes	No	Generally mild	Subglottic narrowing on AP films
Spasmodic croup	Sudden (often minutes)	No	Yes	No	No	Not useful
Less common						
Retropharyngeal abscess	3–5 days	Yes (102–104 °F)	Variable	Yes	Yes	Widened retropharyngeal space on AP films
Laryngeal diphtheria	2–3 days	Generally (101–102 °F)	Yes	Common	Generally mild	Not useful
Acute angioneurotic edema	Sudden	No	No	Yes	No	Swollen supraglottic structures
Foreign body	Sudden	No	Variable	Variable	No	May reveal foreign body

AP = anteroposterior.

TABLE 2   Sizes of Nasotracheal Tubes Recommended for Children with Acute Supraglottitis

Age	Size* (mm)
Birth to 6 months	3.0
6 months to 2 years	3.5
3 years to 5 years	4.0
Older than 5 years	4.5

From Cherry JD. Croup. In: Feigin RD, Cherry JD, eds. Textbook of pediatric infectious diseases. Philadelphia: WB Saunders, 1981. Reprinted with permission.
* Inner diameter

and muscle relaxants should be avoided if possible. Halothane and 100 percent oxygen have provided successful anesthesia in epiglottitis. Atropine, 0.02 mg per kilogram intramuscularly, may be given prior to anesthesia to reduce bradycardia due to halothane, hypoxia, and intubation-induced vagal stimulation. Some experienced pediatric anesthesiologists prefer to use nitrous oxide (50/50 with oxygen) for induction since it is more acceptable to the child and, if the child is stable, quickly to insert an intravenous catheter and infuse atropine (0.01 to 0.02 mg per kilogram) intravenously before starting halothane anesthesia.

The expertise available at each hospital will determine whether intubation or tracheostomy is the procedure of choice. Where there are experienced personnel, nasotracheal intubation is generally preferred. Generally, the child should be intubated first with an orotracheal tube, and when this is established the oral tube can be safely replaced with a nasotracheal tube of appropriate size. Since edema may be severe and extend down the trachea for several centimeters, a tube of 0.5 mm to 1.0 mm smaller than predicted for age should be utilized (see Table 2), and a smaller tube should be available for emergency use. If the tube is too large and impinges on the tracheal wall, it may increase complications such as subglottic stenosis.

Once the nasotracheal tube is properly positioned, it is held in place and tincture of benzoin is applied from ear to ear and over the tube segment just outside the nostril. Dried strips of half-inch adhesive tape are applied over the benzoin and around the tube and secured over the occiput. A number 20 or 22 teflon intravenous catheter is inserted, and blood is obtained for blood culture, white blood cell count, and differential count.

A nasogastric tube is generally placed before leaving the operating room, and cultures of the epiglottis are obtained. The child's arms are restrained at the elbows to prevent the hands from reaching the nose and pulling out the nasotracheal tube.

MANAGEMENT IN THE INTENSIVE CARE UNIT

The child should be admitted to the intensive care unit during the period of intubation and sedated as necessary with 0.1 to 0.2 mg of morphine sulfate per kilogram every 2 to 4 hours. Nasal intubation is generally well tolerated, and sedation is often not necessary. However, morphine sedation will decrease anxiety and movement that may trauma-

tize the trachea or dislodge the airway. In addition, morphine sedation can be rapidly reversed with naloxone. Since sedation may depress the agitation that occurs with hypoxia, it is critical to ensure that the endotracheal tube does not become plugged or dislodged. Oxygen saturation monitoring will allow continuous noninvasive assessment of oxygenation. The physical examination and history should be completed with special attention to other potential foci of infection such as the lungs, joints, and meninges (sedation will alter the signs and symptoms of meningitis). Nursing care is the most important factor in managing the child with epiglottitis. Tube placement should be checked by auscultation and x-ray films, and the tube should be marked so that inadvertent movement can be easily detected. Adequate warmed humidified air should be delivered via T-tube every 1 to 2 hours, followed by suctioning as needed (at least every 2 hours) to prevent blockage of the tube by secretions. The child is given nothing by mouth until 3 hours after intubation. During the period of intubation the parents should be encouraged to remain with the child to provide reassurance that this situation is temporary and to reduce fear and anxiety. Both nurses and parents must be observant to ensure that the child does not extubate himself.

Antibiotic therapy should be started to cover *H. influenzae* type b, streptococci, and *S. aureus*. Appropriate antibiotics are listed in Table 3. Cephalosporins such as cefuroxime are now commonly used to treat epiglottitis since they are active against all of the pathogens cited, have good cerebrospinal fluid (CSF) penetration, and have less toxicity than chloramphenicol. However, if meningitis is suspected clinically, once the tube is secured and the patient sedated, a lumbar puncture should be carefully performed. If meningitis cannot be excluded, meningitis doses should be given until the CSF cultures are known to be negative. Rifampin prophylaxis should be given to household contacts if a sibling younger than 4 years of age resides in the house (20 mg per kilogram per day; maximum, 600 mg for 4 days). Since many children with uncomplicated epiglottitis will be discharged from the hospital after 3 to 5 days, oral antibiotics should be given to complete the course of therapy. Oral antibiotic therapy should be based on the sensitivity of the bacteria isolated from the blood. When no pathogen is identified, Augmentin (50 mg per kilogram per day [amoxicillin] every 8 hours) or Pediazole (40 mg per kilogram per day [erythromycin] every 6 hours) should provide effective coverage.

The epiglottis should be visualized by the otolaryngologist every 12 to 24 hours to determine when the edema has resolved. Generally, fever and toxicity are reduced and

TABLE 3   Recommended Antibiotics in the Treatment of Epiglottitis

Antibiotic	Dose	Interval	Route
Cefuroxime	75–100 mg/kg/day	q8h	IV, IM
Cefotaxime	100–150 mg/kg/day	q6h	IV
Ceftriaxone	50–75 mg/kg/day	q12h	IV, IM
Chloramphenicol *plus*	50–75 mg/kg/day	q6h	IV
Ampicillin	150 mg/kg/day	q6h	IV, IM

Antibiotics are listed in order of preference.

supraglottic edema has resolved within 24 to 48 hours after the child has been intubated and antibiotic therapy has been instituted. The endotracheal tube can be safely removed when the edema has decreased, the child is breathing around the tube, and the supraglottic structures such as the arytenoid cartilages are clearly identifiable. The otolaryngologist and anesthesiologist should determine when extubation is safe. Dexamethasone (0.6 mg per kilogram intravenously) can be used to prevent the development of postintubation croup. The child should be observed in the intensive care unit for 4 to 6 hours after extubation, and preparations should be made to reintubate the child should this be required (correct size of tubes, laryngoscope, and blades should be at the bedside). Thereafter, the child can be transferred to the general ward for 24 hours of observation before discharge.

COMPLICATIONS

Many patients with epiglottitis are bacteremic or septic, and heart rate, respiratory rate, and blood pressure should be closely monitored. Associated meningitis is rare, and other septic complications such as pericarditis, pneumonia, and septic arthritis are also uncommon. In some children pulmonary edema may develop when the airway obstruction is relieved. Arterial blood gases, chest roentgenogram, and respiratory rate will be helpful in detecting developing pulmonary edema. If pulmonary edema develops, assisted ventilation with positive end-expiratory pressure, fluid restriction, and diuretics may be used to reverse the process. Auscultation for pericardial rub, an electrocardiogram, and chest roentgenograms should be helpful to diagnose pericarditis. Echocardiography may also demonstrate pericardial fluid.

Antibiotics should be given for a total of 7 to 10 days. If bacteria are isolated from blood, appropriate antibiotics should be selected based on sensitivities and the sites of infection identified.

MILD OR ATYPICAL PRESENTATION

Some children present with mild symptoms of respiratory obstruction, and the differential includes viral croup, bacterial tracheitis, and early epiglottitis. Less than one-third of children with epiglottitis present with hoarseness and croupy cough, but in these children with increasing respiratory distress, a specific diagnosis is critical. The lateral and anteroposterior neck film may be helpful in identifying subglottic edema in croup or tracheal edema and exudate in bac-

terial tracheitis (pus in the trachea may look like mucosal irregularities). If toxicity is present the child should go immediately to the operating room and the epiglottis should be visualized and oral endotracheal intubation performed as previously described. If there is no supraglottic swelling, bronchoscopy or intubation is still important to determine if purulent exudate is present in the trachea.

PREVENTION

New conjugated polyribose phosphate (PRP) *H. influenzae* type b vaccine is now available for use in children 18 to 60 months of age. This vaccine is more immunogenic than the older unconjugated PRP vaccine and has the potential to prevent the majority of cases of epiglottitis. If the conjugate vaccines are sufficiently immunogenic in infants under 6 months of age, most of the infections caused by *H. influenzae* type b may be prevented. This vaccine should be given to all children at 18 months of age.

ADULT EPIGLOTTITIS

Epiglottitis may be more common in adults than previously recognized, and *H. influenzae* type b is a commonly identified pathogen. The risk of acute airway obstruction may be as high as that observed in children. A mortality rate of 7 percent has been reported in adults. Sudden death has also occurred in adults with epiglottitis who were admitted to the hospital for observation. Since fatal airway obstruction can occur in adults without warning, adults with epiglottitis should also have an airway secured as quickly as possible.

SUGGESTED READING

Bass JW, Fajardo JE, Brien JH, Cook BA, Wiswell TE. Sudden death due to acute epiglottitis. Pediatr Infect Dis 1985; 4:447–449.

Bass JW, Steele RW, Wiebe RA. Acute epiglottitis: a surgical emergency. JAMA 1974; 229:671–675.

Gonzalez C, Reilly JS, Kenna MA, Thompson AE. Duration of intubation in children with acute epiglottitis. Otolaryngol Head Neck Surg 1986; 95:477–481.

Mayosmith MF, Hirsch PJ, Wodzinski SF, Schiffman FJ. Acute epiglottitis in adults: an eight-year experience in the state of Rhode Island. N Engl J Med 1986; 314:1133–1139.

Rothstein P, Lister G. Epiglottitis—duration of intubation and fever. Anesth Analg 1983; 62:785–787.

Schloss MD, Gold JA, Rosales JK, Baxter JD. Acute epiglottitis: current management. Laryngoscope 1983; 93:489–493.

THE COMMON COLD

BARRY M. FARR, M.D.
JACK M. GWALTNEY Jr., M.D.

The common cold remains the most frequent cause of acute morbidity and of visits to physicians in the United States. Adults average two to four colds per year, while children suffer six to eight colds per year.

The disease is actually a syndrome of symptoms produced by respiratory infections with any one of more than 100 antigenically distinct viruses (Table 1). A viral etiology has been determined in two out of three colds by currently available cultural and serologic techniques; the remaining one-third of colds are presumed to be caused by currently unidentified viruses. Colds caused by the various etiologic agents are usually indistinguishable from one another except by viral isolation or serology, but viral culture and serology are both unavailable and unnecessary for routine patient care.

DIAGNOSIS

The manifestations of the common cold are so characteristic that the patient's self-diagnosis is usually correct. The key symptoms are nasal discharge, nasal obstruction, sneezing, sore throat, and cough. Recent studies suggest that cold symptoms may be caused by the release of inflammatory mediators secondary to the viral infection. High concentrations of kinins and lysylbradykinins have been measured in the nasal mucus of patients with rhinovirus colds. Similar symptoms due to allergic conditions are usually easily distinguished by their chronic or recurrent pattern and also by a relation to allergen exposure. Fever is usually absent except in the colds of infants or young children. The median

duration of symptoms is 1 week, but colds last for up to 2 weeks in 25 percent of patients. The severity and duration of cough is often increased in cigarette smokers with a cold.

Physical examination is usually unrevealing except for the occasional presence of visible rhinorrhea or of nasal voice. The physician's most important challenge is to differentiate the uncomplicated cold from the 2 percent of cases accompanied by otitis media (mostly children) and the 0.5 percent of patients who develop secondary bacterial sinusitis (mostly adults) requiring antimicrobial therapy. A history of change in auditory acuity or earache should be evaluated with pneumatic otoscopy. Pain or tenderness in the maxillary or frontal bones suggests the need for sinus transillumination and/or radiography. Severe sore throat or tonsillar pharyngeal exudate indicates the need for throat culture to exclude streptococcal pharyngitis.

TREATMENT

The uncomplicated cold is self-limited and best treated by reassuring the patient and prescribing only those medications needed to relieve the patient's symptoms. Combination products containing remedies for all possible symptoms are usually less effective and cause more adverse effects than specific therapy.

Nasal congestion is best treated with topical vasoconstrictors, such as 0.25 to 0.5 percent phenylephrine or 1 percent ephedrine drops or sprays. These nasal drops or sprays must be used regularly every 4 hours for 3 to 4 days. Longer-acting compounds, such as oxymetazoline (Afrin) drops or spray, may be used twice daily. Oral administration of decongestants, such as pseudoephedrine (Sudafed) 60 mg orally four times a day, offers an alternative that is less effective than topical therapy and may be complicated by increased blood pressure. This may be a significant hazard in patients with prior hypertensive or cardiac disease. Patients should also be warned about the danger of rhinitis medicamentosa following prolonged usage of decongestants. Antihistamines have not been shown to relieve the nasal congestion of colds, which correlates with recent research finding no elevation of histamine in the nasal secretions of patients with experimentally induced rhinovirus colds. The drying effect of some antihistamines on nasal secretions is due to an anticholinergic side effect that is absent in some of the newer antihistamines, such as terfenadine. This slight benefit must be weighed against antihistamines' other frequent adverse effect of drowsiness.

Malaise, aches, and low-grade fever are best treated with bed rest and analgesics or antipyretics, such as aspirin or acetaminophen. Sore throat is relieved by warm saline gargles and mild analgesics. Cough usually does not require treatment, but moderate to severe coughing may be suppressed with codeine, 15 to 30 mg orally every 4 to 6 hours, after excluding the possibility of pneumonia by history, physical examination, and if necessary, chest radiography. The patient should be warned that this dosage of codeine may result in constipation, which may be counteracted by increasing dietary bulk. Proprietary cough syrups containing dextromethorphan are also effective. The usual adult dose is

TABLE 1   Causes of the Common Cold

Agent	Number of Antigenic Types	Approximate Percentage of Cases
Rhinovirus	89 numbered (plus 20 more awaiting enumeration)	30
Coronavirus	≥ 3	≥ 10
Respiratory syncytial virus	1	
Influenza virus	3	10–15
Adenovirus	33	
Parainfluenza virus	3	
Other viruses (enterovirus, varicella, rubeola)		5
Presumed undiscovered viruses		30–40
*Streptococcus pyogenes**		5

* Streptococcal pharyngitis is not always clinically distinct from viral pharyngitis.

15 to 30 mg three to four times daily. Smokers should always be advised to stop smoking.

Antibiotics should never be prescribed prophylactically for a patient with an uncomplicated cold. They have no effect on the natural course of the viral infection, they alter the patient's flora to more resistant bacterial species, and they expose the patient to unnecessary risks ranging from mild side effects such as rash and diarrhea to more severe, life-threatening complications such as pseudomembranous colitis and anaphylaxis.

Large-dose therapy with vitamin C has not been shown to be effective as either prophylaxis or therapy for the common cold. Zinc gluconate has also been touted as a possible cure of the common cold, but carefully controlled studies have shown no efficacy. No specific antiviral agent is yet available for prophylaxis or therapy, and vaccines have proven impractical because of the many different viruses involved. Since some cold viruses may be spread by direct hand contact and self-inoculation, hand washing and avoidance of finger-to-nose or finger-to-eye contact is recommended after exposure to a cold sufferer.

SUGGESTED READING

Farr BM, Conner EM, Betts RF, et al. Two randomized controlled trials of zinc gluconate lozenge therapy of experimentally induced rhinovirus colds. Antimicrob Agents Chemother 1987; 31:1183–1187.

Gwaltney JM Jr. Rhinoviruses. In: Evans AS, ed. Viral infections of humans. 3rd ed. New York: Plenum Publishing, 1989.

Gwaltney JM Jr, Hendley JO, Simon G, Jordan WS Jr. Rhinovirus infections in an industrial population. II. Characteristics of illness and antibody response. JAMA 1967; 202:494–500.

Nacleno RM, Proud D, Hendley JO, et al. Kinins are generated during experimentally induced rhinovirus colds. J Infect Dis 1988; 157:133–142.

INFECTION OF THE MOUTH, SALIVARY GLANDS, AND NECK SPACES

JAMES P. DUDLEY, M.D.

SALIVARY GLAND INFECTION

There are six major salivary glands: two paired parotid glands, two paired submaxillary glands (also called submandibular glands), and the sublingual glands that occupy the area of the floor of the mouth just under the tongue on each side. The sublingual glands are not involved by infection.

Parotid Infection

There are three presentations of parotid gland infections (parotitis): viral infection (usually mumps), recurrent swelling and tenderness of the gland associated with eating, and cellulitis and/or abscess.

The most frequent of these is mumps. This occurs chiefly in children but can occur in adults.

Recurrent swelling following eating can be as painful as that seen with mumps. Parotid enlargement subsides over several hours but usually occurs again with the next meal; it is probably secondary to obstruction of one or more of the salivary ducts within the gland. The walls of the ducts become inflamed, swell, and obstruct. The microorganisms inducing this inflammatory response are from the oral cavity. This kind of infection is probably similar to that occurring in severe cases of bronchitis or bronchiectasis. This kind of limited parotid gland infection may be an initial step toward parotid cellulitis or abscess.

The third kind of parotitis—cellulitis and/or abscess formation—occurs in both children and adults. This type of infection is usually associated with a fever, an elevated white blood cell count, and an increase in the numbers of neutrophils and band forms. The gland itself is usually tender and swollen. This swelling may be accompanied by fluctuance and/or the presence of purulent secretions from the parotid duct (Stenson's duct), which is located on the buccal mucosa opposite the second upper molar on each side. In this kind of parotid infection, the patient is generally ill. The skin overlying the gland may be erythematous. Microorganisms responsible for this kind of parotitis are oral flora, including anaerobes. Other organisms may be responsible, e.g., *Streptococcus pneumoniae* and *Eikenella corrodens*. Although *Staphylococcus* has been associated in physicians' minds with this kind of infection, normal oral flora, including anaerobes, is a more likely cause. A needle aspirate of the infected gland may provide further information by either Gram stain or culture of the aspirate.

Treatment of Viral Infections

Analgesics may or may not be needed, depending on the severity and extent of parotid edema. Usually acetylsalicylic acid or acetaminophen should be satisfactory for this purpose. A bland diet is also a must in viral parotitis as well as all other kinds of parotitis. Any increased production of saliva tends to make the glands more swollen and thus increase pain.

Treatment of Recurrent Parotid Swelling

An antibiotic should be used. Amoxicillin–clavulanic acid (250 mg three times a day) is preferred, or, alternatively, a drug such as cefaclor (250 mg four times a day) may be used. An antibiotic should be given for about 2 to 3 weeks. Subsequently, it should be continued in a prophylactic dosage (250 mg once daily) for 4 to 8 additional weeks. Obviously, if the gland is not severely involved (i.e., does not produce severe pain), a bland diet alone, in which foods that the patient reports increase the production of saliva are avoided, might be all that is necessary. Usually, however, it is not. In a penicillin–allergic patient, tetracycline (250 mg four times daily), trimethoprim–sulfamethoxazole (80 mg trimethoprim and 400 mg sulfamethoxazole twice daily), or clindamycin (150 mg four times daily) can be administered.

If diet and antibiotic therapy fail, the patient should have a roentgenologic evaluation of the gland by computed tomography (CT). Sialograms provide information about the status of the ductal system, but they are infrequently done today. After CT, a needle aspirate should be done to determine the kind of tissue causing parotid enlargement. Surgical removal of the gland may be indicated if antibiotics and diet fail to bring an end to this kind of swelling. There is, however, significant risk in surgery on a gland that is chronically infected, for the facial nerve runs through the center of the gland. An adjunctive surgical procedure with minimal risks is a tympanic neurectomy on the ipsilateral side. This surgical procedure, which cuts the tympanic nerve in the middle ear cavity, has had some reported success. The rationale for the procedure is to cut the parasympathetic (secretory) fibers to the parotid gland. If secretion is either slowed or stopped by this nerve transection, discomfort of the gland should cease.

Treatment of Parotid Cellulitis or Abscess

This kind of infection needs to be treated more vigorously. If there is an abscess present, aspiration of the abscess can be done safely. Aspiration can be done with a 20- or 22-gauge needle, and it provides great relief. Pus should be cultured for aerobes and anaerobes. These patients may need repeat aspiration and in rare instances surgical incision and drainage. Intravenous antibiotics can be given on an outpatient basis. Antibiotics such as ceftazidime, 1 to 2 g, can be given every 8 hours. Although either cefazolin or clindamycin may be used in the hospital, ceftriaxone or ceftazidime is more practical when patients are receiving antibiotics at home because they can be given at 8-hour or 12-hour intervals. The duration of intravenous antibiotic therapy should be at least 1 week, but it may be necessary to continue antibiotic therapy for as long as 3 weeks. At the end of that time, antibiotics should be given by mouth for an additional 2 to 3 weeks. The ultimate duration of antibiotic therapy will have to depend upon the gland size and the reduction in induration. A good oral antibiotic to use is amoxicillin–clavulanic acid (500 mg three times a day).

Submaxillary Gland

Submaxillary gland infections are more common than parotid infections. Unlike parotid gland infections, they are more likely to be associated with stones, and abscess formation is less likely to occur. Mumps seldom involves this gland. Glandular swelling and pain are made worse by eating. As is the case in parotitis, mouth flora, including anaerobes, produce this infection. Actinomycetes are probably also responsible for some of these. It is important to detect *Actinomycetes* because of the time required for eradi-

cation of this organism by antibiotics. Amoxicillin–clavulanic acid should be given (250 mg three times daily). Antibiotics should be given until swelling of the gland and pain subside. Symptoms sometimes subside in 1 to 2 weeks, only to recur with cessation of antibiotic therapy. Antibiotic therapy for relapsed patients should continue for 4 weeks at full dose followed by a prophylactic dose for 3 months (e.g., amoxicillin–clavulanic acid 250 mg daily). In penicillin–allergic patients, tetracycline (250 mg four times daily), trimethoprim–sulfamethoxazole (80 mg trimethoprim and 400 mg sulfamethoxazole every 12 hours), or clindamycin (150 mg four times daily) could be substituted; tetracycline is preferred. A bland diet is also helpful in these infections.

If antibiotic therapy fails or there are frequent recurrences, surgical excision is indicated. The gland can be removed under local or general anesthesia. There is a risk of damage to the lower branch of the facial nerve (the marginal mandibular branch), which is responsible for contraction of the lower lip depressor muscle; the hypoglossal nerve (or cranial nerve XII), which provides motor innervation to the ipsilateral tongue; or the lingual nerve (branch of cranial nerve V), which provides sensation to the ipsilateral tongue. Since the gland has a capsule and the nerves do not cross through the gland, the risk of damage to these nerves is slight in contrast to the risk of damage to the facial nerve, which travels through the center of the parotid, a gland that has no capsule.

If a stone can be palpated in the duct of the gland (Wharton's duct), a simple intraoral removal of the stone will effect a cure unless there are other stones in the gland or unless glandular infection is severe.

CERVICAL INFECTIONS

Actinomycosis

Actinomycosis is not so common as it was 20 years ago. It is characterized by virtually no systemic symptoms or induration and minimal erythema. The indurated mass is usually confluent with and attached to the mandible. Infection usually arises from a tooth root and involves the soft tissues overlying the mandible. Although a biopsy or aspiration should reveal "sulfur" granules (i.e., collections of organisms), they may be absent. Culture of this tissue should be positive for an actinomycete, but that test too may be negative. It is, however, the only infection that fixes itself so firmly to the mandible and produces so few symptoms.

Actinomycosis should be treated with intravenous antibiotics for at least 3 weeks (1 to 2 million units of penicillin every four hours). Follow-up is with orally administered penicillin (penicillin V, 500 mg three times a day for 6 more weeks). If the patient will not cooperate with the intravenous administration of penicillin or is allergic to penicillin, clindamycin (30 mg per kilogram daily) can be given.

Necrotizing Fasciitis

Infections of the neck often traverse fascial planes. All of the significant neck structures are enveloped in fascia. This anatomic necessity provides many parallel planes in a cephalad to caudad direction. How microorganisms gain entrance to all of these areas is not entirely clear. Lymph nodes that drain tonsillar fossae and infected tooth roots may be a source. Blows to the neck may cause this kind of problem without any break in the integrity of overlying skin. The hallmark of this infection is severity of illness (elevated temperature and white blood cell count) and minimal neck findings (lack of erythema; some swelling; minimal induration; minimal to absent erythema overlying the swollen or slightly swollen neck tissue). It may take 24 hours or 4 weeks for infection to progress, but as it does so, neck pain becomes worse, crepitus may be felt, and bullae may be seen on the skin. CT will often reveal air in soft tissues of the neck.

The microorganisms associated with this process are many: anaerobes (*Peptostreptococcus, Bacteroides, Fusobacterium), Streptococcus pyogenes* (group A β–hemolytic), *Actinomyces*, and even *Haemophilus influenzae* type b. Anaerobes are present 100 percent of the time. A needle aspiration can be done to obtain neck contents for culture. A standard–length 22–gauge needle or a 3½–inch (spinal) needle can be used for this purpose. Although biopsy accompanied by a frozen section has been touted as a way of making a diagnosis by showing the presence of necrotic muscle tissue in the biopsy specimen, this method probably is not of value in the neck.

Treatment has two arms, medical and surgical. In the early phase of the disease, treatment with intravenous antibiotics is the starting point (penicillin, 2 million units every 4 hours). Although penicillin may be excellent against *Streptococcus*, it may not be effective against β–lactamase producers. There is increasing evidence that a large percentage of head and neck anaerobes fall into this category. Consequently, clindamycin (600 mg every 6 hours IV) or metronidazole (500 mg every 8 hours) can be used as an adjunct to penicillin. These antibiotics will provide coverage for any β–lactamase–producing anaerobes. If metronidazole is used, penicillin should be used as well.

If there is no improvement in neck swelling, fever, or white blood cell count, surgical drainage should be done. This is especially true if CT shows more than a small amount of air. Surgical drainage consists of raising a large neck flap, exposing the deep neck tissues to air, irrigating the area with hydrogen peroxide, and packing the entire wound open. If tissue swelling begins to approach the midline, a tracheotomy should be done to guarantee the safety of the airway.

These infections are potentially fatal. Although most respond to antibiotic therapy alone, the patient and the patient's family need to be made aware that surgical drainage may be needed. The patient should know that the scar of any surgical drainage will be a rather prominent one and will be visible in the lower and mid neck.

Ludwig's Angina

This is a peculiar infection that has features of both neck abscess or cellulitis due to actinomycosis and anaerobic– or streptococcal–induced necrotizing fasciitis. It is limited to the submaxillary–submandibular area on one or both sides. The induration produced is similar to that seen in ac-

tinomycotic infections but is usually not as hard. Edema is described as "brawny"—firm but not hard.

The process begins in an infected tooth root, breaks through the mandibular cortex, and insinuates itself beneath the mylohyoid muscle (this is the muscle that demarcates the floor of the mouth). Edema and induration follow. Even though laryngeal structures are not involved with edema, infection produces swelling in the floor of the mouth. The swelling forces the tongue in a posterior direction endangering the integrity of the airway. Consequently, every patient in whom the diagnosis of Ludwig's angina is made should have a tracheotomy or a nasotracheal tube put into place. Since an airway has to be put into place, all of these patients need hospitalization.

While in the hospital intravenous antibiotics are given. In this strictly tooth root–derived anaerobic infection, intravenous penicillin is the drug of choice (2 million units every 4 hours).

Surgical drainage may need to be done. Needle aspiration may suffice to remove pus if there is a collection, but an actual surgical drainage with raising of a flap and emplacement of multiple drains may be required.

The most important aspect of this kind of infection is that the airway must be established before anything else is done. Airway compromise can occur very quickly, and this is virtually the only cause of death in this infection.

Atypical Mycobacterial Infections

Atypical mycobacteria are a frequently identified cause of infections in the neck. This is true in nonimmunocompromised as well as in immunocompromised patients. True tuberculous infections (*M. tuberculosis*) are exceedingly rare today. The term scrofula has been associated with these now nearly extinct cervical infections. The swelling in neck nodes can be discrete. Diagnosis is usually made by failure to respond to antibiotics that would be effective against staphylococcal or streptococcal cervical adenitis. With atypical mycobacterial adenitis (single–lesion disease of atypical mycobacteria) patients generally are not ill. Diagnosis may be made by aspiration of the node. Contents should be sent for culture. Gram staining may fail to reveal any abnormality if it is an atypical mycobacterial infection. Acid–fast stain may reveal the characteristic appearance of atypical organisms. An experienced mycobacteriologist is often able to make the diagnosis of an atypical mycobacterial infection on the basis of a positive stain.

Most physicians give antituberculous therapy despite the fact that atypical mycobacterial organisms are resistant to the commonly used antituberculous agents. We prefer to use isoniazid (10 mg per kg per day in children; 4 mg per kg per day in adults, up to 300 mg per day). Although nearly every physician will give antituberculous chemotherapy, the effectiveness of these drugs in these cervical infections is uncertain. The duration of therapy is shorter rather than longer (e.g., 3 to 6 months rather than 6 to 12 months).

Surgical excision of these nodes provides an ideal way to cure single–lesion disseminated disease. However, because these nodes sometimes produce an enormous amount of surrounding edema and cellulitis, surgical excision may not be easy if the node is located in the area of the facial nerve or just below the mandible. This paramandibular position is a common place for this infection in young children. In instances such as this, multiple aspirations provide the ideal minisurgical treatment, for they avoid the possible damage to the facial nerve that may occur in resection of an infected node in this particular location. Damage to this nerve would be a big price to pay for curing a very benign disease.

INFECTIONS OF THE MOUTH

Infections of the Gingiva (or Gums)

Gingivitis is common if cleansing measures are not used to clean debris from gingival surfaces (i.e., Water–Pik; dental floss). It is common in childhood and adolescence. Some patients may be unaware of the disease. Foul breath is one of the manifestations of this problem. Patients may become aware of this infection when bleeding occurs after tooth brushing. The etiology of this inflammatory process is the presence of debris and trapped bacteria on the gingiva around the tooth base. Since it is superficial, simple cleansing with floss or a Water–Pik usually clears up the problem.

Persistent gingivitis results in periodontitis. Since this is an infection of an important tooth appendage, the periodontium, tooth loss can result. Antibiotics should be used to treat it. Penicillin V (500 mg three times daily) can be used.

Periodontal abscess can develop when a periodontal infection is unable to drain into the oral cavity. Pus from such an abscess must be drained, and the patient placed on penicillin (penicillin V 500 mg three times daily).

Aphthous Ulcers

These are common intraoral lesions of uncertain etiology, and they are among the least amenable to therapy. They have a characteristic "punched out" appearance, with virtually no surrounding erythema. There may be a single ulcer or several. They also may be confluent. Although they can occur anywhere on the buccal (or cheek) mucosa, and their most common site is the sulcus between the buccal (or cheek) mucosa and the mucosa of the gingiva (the gums). The base of the ulcer is filled with necrotic debris.

Although no microbial cause has ever been found, they are usually considered to have an infectious component. Despite this assumption, no antibiotic appears to have any effect on their course. Except for one report of an outbreak among institutionalized adults, they are not infectious. Each ulcer lasts 7 to 14 days.

Pain relief is virtually impossible. All topical analgesics have been touted as effective at one time or other, but there is none lasting beyond a few minutes. Orally administered analgesics (e.g., acetaminophen with codeine) are virtually the only way to provide prolonged relief, but since the lesions are usually single, such drugs are seldom required. Colchicine (0.6 mg three times daily) has been suggested for recurrent aphthous ulcers, but diarrhea and abdominal discomfort may be unpleasant side effects, necessitating discontinuation of this medication.

Herpes Simplex

Each individual initial challenge with herpes simplex type 1, whether in a child or an adult, should produce a gingivostomatitis (i.e., inflammation of the gums and other areas of the oral mucosa). Although vesicles are part of the disease process, they are rarely seen in the mouth in healthy children or adults. When they do occur, they and the resultant desquamative, erythematous, ulcerative process may also involve the oropharynx, hypopharynx, and esophagus. This initial contact with virus in most individuals induces limited disease for which the patient may not seek professional help. However, dysphagia caused by this erosive infectious process can be so marked that intravenous fluids may be required.

The diagnosis can be suspected from the clinical picture alone, but if confirmation is desired, cells for viral culture or for a stain (Tzanck stain) can be obtained from the base of one of the ulcers (wipe away exudate overlying ulcer first).

Most of the time analgesics such as acetaminophen or acetaminophen with codeine will be satisfactory unless the pain is severe, in which case intravenous narcotics will be required. Subsequent attacks of herpes simplex do not induce oral disease, but they do produce lip ulcerations—the typical "cold sores."

Herpes Zoster

This virus affects only the hard and soft palate and only one side of the palate at a time. The pain is usually severe and is not altered by any topical therapy. There is no information about the effectiveness of antiviral agents in otherwise healthy patients in this extremely rare infection. In immunocompromised patients, however, intravenous acyclovir may shorten the infection (800 mg five times daily).

Herpangina

This is the term given to ulcerations seen on the posterior end of the soft palate and the tonsillar pillars (these are the mucous membrane flaps that lie in front of the tonsil). The ulcers are shallow, about 1 mm to 2 mm in diameter, and have an erythematous margin. There may be fever and malaise. There is always a sore throat, which can be as severe as that seen in a case of exudative tonsillitis. These ulcerations are enteroviral in origin and are thus untreatable. Fortunately, infection is self-limited (7 to 10 days).

Hand, Foot, and Mouth Disease

This is similar to herpangina except that this vesicular disease involves only parts of the mouth as well as the hands and feet. It is caused by coxsackieviruses and is also self-limited, i.e., it lasts 7 to 10 days.

Thrush and Oral Candidal Infections

Candida albicans is the best known and most frequent fungal pathogen in the oral cavity. However, not all mucosal infections due to this fungus are the same. The most famous is thrush, which occurs in healthy and unhealthy infants and in unhealthy (immunocompromised) adults. In this disease process, fungus invades underlying epithelium and causes desquamation. This results in a white plaque, which is semifirmly attached to the underlying mucosa. If removal is attempted, a bleeding mucosal surface will be found underneath. Although the diagnosis can be made on clinical grounds in infants, it may be necessary to examine plaque in older children and adults to ensure the diagnosis. If that is done, numerous hyphae will be seen amidst nephrotic debris. Pain may be nearly absent or mild to moderate.

Treatment consists of nystatin in infants, older children, and adults (100,000 units four times daily in infants and younger children, and 500,000 to 1 million units four times daily in adults). In immunocompromised patients treatment may have to be repeated as the disease returns. In infants, the source of the fungus is presumed to be the birth canal. Once the fungus is eradicated, the infant will probably be free of infection.

A second kind of candidal infection is that which occurs under dentures. This mucositis, which can be very uncomfortable, is characterized by erythematous and atrophic membranes. Histologically, no hyphae can be identified, but surface cultures should be positive for the yeasts. It is always difficult to ascribe an inflammatory process to an organism that may be present in asymptomatic individuals. It is thought that increased fungal growth or strain–related differences in *C. albicans* may account for this particular kind of pathogenicity in some denture wearers and not in others.

A similar form of mucositis may also be seen in users of aerosolyzed cortisone. Mucosa may be erythematous but is usually not as "atrophic" or thinned out. The use of an antifungal agent (nystatin) may allow continued use of the aerosol.

Other Mucosal Fungi

Other fungi that can produce disease in the oral cavity (*Histoplasma capsulatum, Blastomyces dermatitidis, Blastomyces brasiliensis*) will all produce exophytic lesions resembling tumor. Consequently, they will all be biopsied and the diagnosis made at that time.

SUGGESTED READING

Alessi DP, Dudley JP. Atypical mycobacteria–induced adenitis. Arch Otolaryngol Head Neck Surg 1988; 114:664–666.

Dierks EJ, Meyerhoff WL, Schultz B, Finn R. Fulminant infections of odontogenic origin. Laryngoscope 1987; 97:271–274.

Dudley JP. Ear, nose, throat, and sinus infections. Top Emerg Med 1989; 10:43–51.

Matlow A, Korentager R, Keystone E, Bohnen J. Parotitis due to anaerobic bacteria. Rev Infect Dis 1988; 10:420–423.

Stiernberg CM. Deep neck space infections. Diagnosis and management. Arch Otolaryngol Head Neck Surg 1986; 112:1274–1279.

INTRA-ABDOMINAL INFECTIONS

INFECTIOUS DIARRHEAS

RONICA M. KLUGE, M.D.

Infectious diarrhea is the second most common infection for which medical attention is sought in the United States. It accounts for approximately 20 percent of adult office visits and for nearly one-third of pediatric office visits and admissions to the hospital. From a practical standpoint, it is useful to distinguish noninflammatory from inflammatory diarrhea. The noninflammatory forms are more common, usually arise in the upper small bowel as a result of the effects of enterotoxin or other alterations of absorptive physiology, cause watery diarrhea with or without nausea and vomiting, produce minimal or low-grade fever, and tend to be self-limited, requiring fluid replacement therapy only. The inflammatory forms arise as a consequence of mucosal invasion involving the colon or distal small bowel; cause an inflammatory bloody diarrhea, accompanied by tenesmus, high fever, and abdominal cramps; and generally require specific antimicrobial agents in addition to rehydration.

DECISIONS

Evaluation of the patient should be directed initially toward two critical decisions: first, whether the patient can be managed as an outpatient or will require hospitalization, and second, whether specific antimicrobial treatment will be needed, in addition to supportive measures. The majority of patients with acute diarrhea of infectious origin can be managed satisfactorily as outpatients and require supportive therapy only. Information gained from a detailed history, a thorough physical examination, and examination of a fresh stool for white blood cells will help to differentiate between inflammatory and noninflammatory forms of infectious diarrhea and allow the critical decisions to be reached swiftly.

The age of the patient, season of the year, clinical presentation, and history of specific exposures are helpful clues to the most likely etiologic agent. Exposure history should include facts about foreign travel, antibiotic usage, animals, mountain streams, ingestion of crusta-ceans, picnics, sexual preferences, and illness in family members or close friends. Such clues can guide early therapy before the causative agent is identified. A summary of the clinical and epidemiologic features of acute infectious diarrheas is provided in Table 1.

A number of factors enter into the decision to hospitalize a patient with acute infectious diarrhea. In general, very young and very old patients with severe diarrhea and patients of any age who manifest significant toxicity, hyperpyrexia, or dehydration require in-hospital management. Some authorities recommend that patients with serious underlying diseases also be hospitalized for management of severe diarrhea. Hospitalized patients with diarrhea thought to be infectious in origin should be placed in enteric isolation.

The presence or absence of stool leukocytes is often of assistance in differentiating the patient who requires antimicrobial therapy from the patient in whom only supportive measures are indicated. The test is easy to perform: Place a small fleck of mucus or a drop of liquid stool on a microscope slide. Add an equal volume of methylene blue to the slide and mix thoroughly with a wooden applicator stick. Place a coverslip over the mixture and examine under high power (not oil) with a simple light microscope. Most bacteria that invade the colonic mucosa are accompanied by stool leukocytes. One toxin-related diarrhea, that due to *Clostridium difficile*, also produces fecal leukocytes. In general, these are the infectious diarrheas that may require specific antimicrobial therapy. Although patients with noninfectious inflammatory bowel disease (Crohn's disease, ulcerative colitis) may have stool leukocytes, their symptoms are more likely to be chronic and/or intermittent rather than acute and isolated. Stool leukocytes are not associated with diarrheal disease due to viruses, most toxigenic bacteria, and parasites. Unless parasites are involved, only supportive therapy is required.

The presence of fecal leukocytes or bloody diarrhea indicates the need for stool cultures and examinations for parasites. The toxic febrile patient should also have blood obtained for culture. Most laboratories prefer a stool specimen to a rectal swab for optimal recovery of pathogens, except in the case of viruses. Special media and/or incubating conditions are required for certain pathogens such as *Campylobacter, Yersinia, Vibrio parahaemolyticus*, and *C. difficile* to grow optimally, so the laboratory must be alerted to your suspicions.

TABLE 1 Clinical and Epidemiologic Features of Acute Infectious Diarrheas

Agent	Age Group Most Affected	Associated Symptoms			Stool Character			Stool Leukocytes	Epidemiologic Characteristics				Therapy
		Fever	Vomiting	Cramps	Watery	Mucoid	Bloody		Season	Foreign Travel	Food/Water-Borne	Incubation Period	
Noninflammatory													
Rotavirus	6 mo–2 y	+++	++	++	+	±	0	0	Winter	+/0	0	2–4 days	Supportive
Norwalk virus–like agents	School-aged children, adults	+	++++	++	+	0	0	0	Year-round	+/0	0	1–2 days	Supportive
S. aureus, toxin	Any	0	++++	++	+	0	0	0	Summer	0	+	1–6 h	Supportive
B. cereus, diarrheal	Any	0	+	++	+	±	0	0	Year-round	0	+	8–16 h	Supportive
E. coli, toxic	Any	0	+	++	+	+	0	0	Year-round	+/0	+	1–2 days	Supportive
C. perfringens	Any	0	0	+++	+	0	0	0	Year-round	0	+	8–24 h	Supportive
V. cholerae	Any	0	+	+	+	0	0	0	Year-round	+/0	+	2–5 days	Specific*
E. histolytica	Any	++	0	++	+	+	+	0	Year-round	+	+	3 days–3 wk	Specific*
G. lamblia	Any	0	0	++	+	±	0	0	Year-round	+/0	+	3 days–3 wk	Specific*
Cryptosporidia	Any	0	0	+	+	0	0	0	Year-round	0	0	Unknown	Supportive
Inflammatory													
S. aureus, overgrowth	Any	+++	±	+++	+	+	±	Many polys†	Year-round	0	0	1–2 wk	Specific*
Nontyphoid salmonellae	<5 y	++	0	++	+	±	±	Occasional polys, monos‡	Summer	+/0	+	1–2 days	Specific*
Shigellae	<5 y	+++	0	+++	+	+	+	Many polys	Summer	+/0	+	1–3 days	Specific*
Campylobacter	< 5 y, young adults	+++	+	+++	+	+	+	Many polys	Summer	0	+	3–5 days	Specific*
E. coli, invasive	Any	+	+	+++	+	+	+	Many polys	Year-round	+/0	0	8–24 h	Specific*
Y. enterocolitica	5–20 y	++	0	++	+	±	0	Many polys	Winter	+/0	+	1–2 days	Specific*
V. parahaemolyticus	Any	+	+	++	+	±	±	Occasional polys	Summer	0	+	1–4 days	Supportive
C. difficile	Any	++	0	++	+	±	+	Many polys	Year-round	0	0	4–10 days	Specific*

* Specific: may be specific in all or only some instances; see text.
† Polymorphonuclear cells.
‡ Monocytes.

TREATMENT OPTIONS

Fluid and electrolyte replacement therapy is of benefit to most patients with infectious diarrhea, whether administered as the sole means of treatment or in conjunction with specific antimicrobial therapy. The decision to administer oral or parenteral therapy rests on the patient's state of hydration and ability to tolerate oral fluids. Because the oral route offers the most cost-effective method of treating acute infectious diarrhea, its use should be encouraged unless vomiting is a problem or the patient is moderately or severely dehydrated.

In the patient with minimal dehydration, fluid and electrolyte balance can be maintained by intake of fruit juices, caffeine-free soft drinks, and salted crackers. Salty broths should be recommended only for the patient who has had significant vomiting. Milk products, except for breast milk, should be avoided. If the dehydration is more advanced, oral replacement with commercially available Pedialyte is optimal, as it is low in solute and thus avoids the possibility of hypertonicity. Pedialyte contains 25 g of glucose per liter, 45 mEq of sodium per liter, 20 mEq of potassium per liter, 35 mEq of chloride per liter, 30 mEq of citrate per liter, and 100 calories per liter. The World Health Organization's oral fluid replacement has a similar make-up but contains 90 mEq of sodium per liter.

For patients with moderate to severe dehydration, parenteral fluids are indicated. The type of fluid depends on the patient's particular deficits; however, most respond well to an initial solution of 5 percent dextrose with 35 to 40 mEq of potassium per liter and 40 to 50 mEq of sodium per liter. Close monitoring of the patient's electrolytes and fluid status will allow appropriate changes to be made. The total amount of fluid required to replace deficits can be calculated by use of standard formulas.

As indicated in Table 1, the noninflammatory diarrheal diseases require only supportive therapy except in the case of cholera and the protozoal diarrheas. In addition, specific therapy is indicated for each of the inflammatory infectious diarrheas except for that due to *V. parahaemolyticus*. Table 2 outlines the antimicrobial agent(s) of choice and alternatives against those microbes for which specific treatment is required. In general, gastroenteritis caused by the nontyphoidal salmonellae is treated only with supportive measures. However, in a patient with a compromised immune system, foreign bodies such as grafts in place, a known aneurysm, extremes of age, hemolytic anemia, or signs of extreme toxicity, specific

TABLE 2 Specific Antimicrobial Therapy for Acute Infectious Diarrheas

Agent	Drug(s) of Choice	Alternatives
Noninflammatory		
V. cholerae	Tetracycline 40 mg/kg/day in 4 divided doses × 2–5 days	Ampicillin, chloramphenicol, or trimethoprim-sulfamethoxazole
E. histolytica	Metronidazole 750 mg t.i.d. × 10 days *followed by* iodoquinol 650 mg t.i.d. × 20 days	Diloxanide furoate (from CDC only) or paromomycin
G. lamblia	Quinacrine 100 mg t.i.d. × 5–7 days	Metronidazole or furazolidone
Inflammatory		
S. aureus, overgrowth	Vancomycin 250 mg q.i.d. × 5–7 days *or* parenteral antistaphylococcal penicillin	Cephalosporin, first-generation
Nontyphoid salmonellae*	Ampicillin 0.5–1.0 g q.i.d. × 10–14 days	Trimethoprim-sulfamethoxazole
Shigellae	Trimethoprim 160 mg *and* sulfamethoxazole 800 mg b.i.d. × 5 days	Tetracycline, ampicillin, or newer quinolone
Campylobacter*	Erythromycin 250–500 mg q.i.d. × 7 days	Newer quinolone
E. coli, invasive	Trimethoprim 160 mg *and* sulfamethoxazole 800 mg b.i.d. × 5–7 days	Ampicillin
Y. enterocolitica	Gentamicin 3–5 mg/kg/day in 3 divided doses × 7 days	Tetracycline, chloramphenicol, or trimethoprim-sulfamethoxazole
C. difficile*	Vancomycin 125 mg q.i.d. × 10 days *or* metronidazole 250–500 mg q.i.d. × 10 days	

* See text for additional information.

antibiotic treatment is recommended. For optimal effect, *Campylobacter* diarrhea must be treated within the first 4 days of symptoms. There is considerable controversy about the effectiveness of antibiotic therapy for diarrheal illness caused by *Yersinia*. In spite of this, specific therapy with an aminoglycoside is suggested in the more toxic-appearing patient. In a patient with *C. difficile* toxin-induced diarrhea without pseudomembrane formation, some success with bismuth subsalicylate has been reported. In every instance of antibiotic-associated diarrhea, it is essential to discontinue the offending antibiotic.

In selected patients, other therapies may be useful. Adsorbents such as Kaopectate act to firm up the stool and may be viewed as important by the individual patient. The patient with a toxin-related diarrhea (except *C. difficile*) may benefit from the administration of bismuth subsalicylate, which has antisecretory properties. Antimotility drugs are used rather indiscriminately for all types of diarrhea. In the presence of an infectious diarrhea, the antimotility drugs are best avoided in children less than 2 years of age and in any patient with high fever or bloody diarrhea.

SUGGESTED READING

Breeling JL. Newly recognized bacterial causes of infectious diarrhea. Infect Dis Pract 1989; 12:1–7.

Cantey JR. Infectious diarrheas. Pathogenesis and risk factors. Am J Med 1985; 78(suppl)6B:65–75.

Consensus conference: Travelers' diarrhea. JAMA 1985; 253:2700–2704.

DuPont HL, Ericsson CD, Johnson PC, et al. Prevention of travelers' diarrhea by the tablet formulation of bismuth subsalicylate. JAMA 1987; 257:1347–1350.

Gorbach SL. Bacterial diarrhoeae and its treatment. Lancet 1987; 2:1378–1382.

Guerrant RL, Wanke CA, Barrett LJ, Schwartzman JD. A cost effective and effective approach to the diagnosis and management of acute infectious diarrhea. Bull NY Acad Med 1987; 63:484–499.

Smith PD, Lane D, Gill VJ, et al. Intestinal infections in patients with acquired immunodeficiency syndrome (AIDS). Etiology and response to therapy. Ann Intern Med 1988; 108:328–333.

TYPHOID FEVER AND ENTERIC FEVER

MYRON M. LEVINE, M.D., D.T.P.H.

Typhoid fever is an acute generalized infection of the reticuloendothelial system, intestinal lymphoid tissues, and gallbladder due to *Salmonella typhi*. A similar disease, paratyphoid fever, follows infection with *S. paratyphi* A and B. These generalized salmonella infections are referred to as enteric fever. Rarely, other serotypes, such as *S. typhimurium*, can cause enteric fever if they infect compromised hosts, young infants, or the elderly.

Humans are both the only natural host and the reservoir of *S. typhi*, and infection is acquired by ingestion of contaminated food or water. Typhoid and paratyphoid bacilli rapidly pass through the intestinal mucosa and reach the systemic circulation by means of lymphatic drainage and the thoracic duct. As a consequence of this primary bacteremia, the fixed phagocytic cells of the reticuloendothelial system become seeded with *S. typhi* as they ingest the bacilli. Following an incubation period of 9 to 14 days, clinical illness appears, accompanied by the characteristic secondary bacteremia of enteric fever. The clinical picture is typified by fever (which increases in stepwise fashion), malaise, headache, and abdominal pain. In adults, constipation is often present, whereas in children diarrhea may occur. Typhoid and paratyphoid infections exhibit a spectrum of clinical illness that includes asymptomatic infection, mild illness with low-grade fever and minimal malaise, or a severe syndrome of very high fever (up to 105 °F to 106 °F), toxemia, and even delirium.

There are many complications that can follow acute enteric fever, but the most important are intestinal perforation and intestinal hemorrhage (which occur in approximately 0.5% of cases) and the chronic biliary carrier state (which occurs in 3% to 5% of cases and is more frequent among females and older patients). In certain areas of the world, such as Indonesia, some patients present with a particularly severe clinical picture of typhoid infection marked by delirium or obtundation.

DIAGNOSIS

Transmission of typhoid or paratyphoid infections within the United States is rare, although occasional outbreaks and sporadic cases still occur. In contrast, enteric fever is a risk for US citizens who travel to less developed areas of the world where these infections are still highly endemic. Microbiology technicians in clinical laboratories comprise another high-risk group because they can acquire the infection while processing cultures. When enteric fever occurs in a very young child in the United States, one should look for a carrier within the household.

If the clinical picture is suspicious, appropriate cultures should be performed. The highest yield of positivity is obtained with a bone marrow culture. This should always be obtained for suspect patients who have had some prior antibiotic therapy; bone marrow cultures in such patients are often positive when blood cultures may be negative. For patients who have not had prior antibiotic therapy, properly performed blood cultures give a high rate of positivity. Three specimens for culture should be obtained, 30 minutes apart, with at least 5 ml of blood per specimen. The blood should be inoculated into a flask containing at least 50 ml of broth to obtain a blood-to-broth ratio of at least 1:10. This dilutes out the factors in blood that may be inhibitory to the salmonellae. Any broth routinely used for blood culture will support the growth of *S. typhi*, but medium containing sodium polyanethol sulfonate is preferred.

Because infection of the gallbladder is usual in acute typhoid fever, culture of bilious duodenal fluid is almost as sensitive as a bone marrow culture. This can easily be accomplished by means of a string-capsule device, the Enterotest (Hedeco; Mountain View, Calif). The string device contained within a gelatin capsule is ingested in the morning by a fasting patient and is removed by gentle traction 3 to 4 hours later. Fluid for culture is expressed from the bile-stained distal 15 cm, using two fingers of a gloved hand. String capsule cultures should be obtained on 2 consecutive days, even if antibiotics have already been started.

Three stool cultures should also be performed as an adjunct to bone marrow, blood, and bile cultures, although they are positive in only about 50 percent of cases (higher if diarrhea is present).

The Widal test, which measures O and H antibodies to *S. typhi*, is not of much practical value. If proper reagents are available and quantitative tube dilutions are performed, elevated titers may be helpful in the non-vaccinated traveler or in children younger than 10 years of age, in endemic areas. However, such Widal serologic techniques are not widely available. Healthy adults in endemic areas often have elevated titers, as do recipients of parenteral typhoid vaccine in the United States; in such patients the Widal titers have no value. Aggressive collection of proper culture specimens should preclude the need for a Widal test.

THERAPY

Historically, the therapy of typhoid fever can be divided into three eras: (*1*) prior to 1948, when effective antibiotic therapy did not exist and the case fatality rate was approximately 10 percent; (*2*) the period from 1948 to 1972, during which oral chloramphenicol was shown to be highly efficacious, practical, and economical, particularly in less developed areas of the world; (*3*) from 1973 to the present, when, as a result of some epidemics due to chloramphenicol-resistant strains of *S. typhi* and the advent of trimethoprim-sulfamethoxazole and amoxicillin, alternative drugs appeared to challenge the pre-eminent role of chloramphenicol as the mainstay of therapy for typhoid fever.

It is helpful to divide the management of acute typhoid fever into three categories: specific antibiotic therapy, general supportive measures, and treatment of the commoner life-endangering complications.

Antimicrobial Agents

Chloramphenicol has been the mainstay of specific therapy of typhoid fever since its first demonstration of efficacy in 1948. Although many other antibiotics of the 1950s and 1960s (such as tetracycline, streptomycin, kanamycin, and colistin) had impressive in vitro activity against *S. typhi*, only chloramphenicol was clinically effective. Chloramphenicol remains the drug of choice in less developed countries because of its practicality, inexpensiveness, and effectiveness when administered orally. Chloramphenicol had reduced typhoid fever from a 3- to 4-week illness with 10 percent case fatality to an illness of 1 week (or less) with a case fatality well below 1 percent. However, a number of observations make chloramphenicol a less-than-ideal drug: (*1*) relapse occurs in approximately 8 to 15 percent of patients; (*2*) it causes irreversible aplastic anemia in approximately 1 in 40,000 to 100,000 recipients; (*3*) occasional patients treated with this drug develop "toxic crises" (Herxheimer-like reactions); (*4*) in recent years the duration of therapy necessary to achieve an afebrile state has increased; (*5*) the drug is not impressive in preventing development of chronic carriers; and (*6*) epidemics caused by chloramphenicol-resistant strains have occurred (as in Mexico in 1972, in Vietnam in 1973, and in Peru in 1980).

The recommended regimen is 750 mg of chloramphenicol every 6 hours to adults (50 mg per kilogram for children) until the fever subsides (usually 3 to 7 days), followed by 500 mg every 6 hours for adults (50 mg per kilogram for children); the drug is given for a total of 14 days. If the patient is unable to take oral medication, the drug should be given intravenously until the switch to oral medication can be made. Chloramphenicol should not be given intramuscularly because only poor blood levels are achieved. Occasional patients develop a "toxic crisis" following the first doses of drug; it is postulated that this may result from a sudden release of endotoxin secondary to death of the bacteria.

If the *S. typhi* isolate is known to be resistant to chloramphenicol or if epidemiologic data make such infection likely, there are two highly effective alternatives, trimethoprim-sulfamethoxazole and amoxicillin, both of which are administered orally.

Amoxicillin, a congener of ampicillin, shows superior intestinal absorption. Adults are given 1.0 g (children, 100 mg per kilogram) every 6 hours for 14 days. During the 1972 Mexican epidemic caused by chloramphenicol-resistant *S. typhi*, strains began to appear that bore plasmid-mediated resistance to amoxicillin as well. Infections with such strains can be successfully treated with oral trimethoprim-sulfamethoxazole. The dose is 1 tablet of 160 mg trimethoprim and 800 mg sulfamethoxazole twice daily for 14 days. Children should receive 8 mg per kilogram of trimethoprim and 40 mg per kilogram of sulfamethoxazole daily in two divided doses. A large experience with trimethoprim-sulfamethoxazole therapy for typhoid fever caused by chloramphenicol-sensitive strains has shown that it is comparable in efficacy to chloramphenicol in approximately 90 percent of cases. In 8 to 10 percent of infected persons, however, the therapeutic response is retarded, requiring 10 or more days for the body temperature to become normal.

Irrespective of the aforementioned antibiotics selected, the clinical response in typhoid fever is not dramatic. Usually 2 complete days of therapy are required before the fever begins to abate, and a normal temperature is usually not reached for 5 to 7 days.

General Supportive Measures

Because of the high fever, maintenance requirements for water and electrolytes are greatly increased, so the patient should be encouraged to drink fluids liberally. If the patient is too ill to maintain hydration via oral fluids, intravenous fluids must be given; daily maintenance requirements should be increased by 10 percent for each degree of fever above 99 °F (37.2 °C).

Salicylates should not be given to patients with typhoid fever, since they can induce abrupt changes in temperature, hypotension, and even shock. The temperature should be lowered by sponging with tepid water.

Laxatives and enemas should, in general, not be employed because of the danger of precipitating intestinal hemorrhage. If constipation requires relief, oral lactulose should be used; this nonabsorbable disaccharide is a gentle physiologic softener of stool.

COMPLICATIONS

In the preantibiotic era, typhoid fever was a disease marked by a wide array of complications involving virtually every organ system and including intestinal perforation, intestinal hemorrhage, myocarditis, empyema of the gallbladder, encephalopathy, bronchitis, pneumonia, parotitis, osteomyelitis, hepatitis, meningitis, septic arthritis, and orchitis. Since the advent of specific antimicrobial therapy, most of the complications are still encountered with some frequency and are discussed below.

In some areas of the world, such as in Djakarta, Indonesia, an exceptionally virulent form of typhoid fever is seen in a small percentage of patients. These patients with acute typhoid fever present with severe toxemia, delirium, and obtundation and proceed to coma and shock. The case fatality rate in these patients is 55 percent with chloramphenicol alone. However, two days of high-dose dexamethasone drastically reduces the case fatality (to 10%) as the fever and toxemia are reduced. An initial dose of dexamethasone of 3 mg per kilogram should be given intravenously, followed by 1 mg per kilogram every 6 hours for a duration of 48 hours. The use of steroids should be reserved for this rare situation only and otherwise plays no role in the treatment of typhoid fever.

Despite adequate therapy with appropriate antibiotics, 5 to 15 percent of patients manifest relapse. In general, all signs and symptoms are milder in nature than the initial clinical episode, and the treatment is the same as for the initial episode.

Two dreaded complications of typhoid fever are still encountered in approximately 1 percent of cases: intestinal hemorrhage and perforation. When a definitive diagnosis of typhoid fever is made, a unit of blood should be typed and cross-matched as a precaution. Hemorrhage occurs late in the course, often in the second or third week, when the patient is often feeling better. The management of hemorrhage is conservative, utilizing repeated transfusion unless there is evidence of intestinal perforation. In the preantibiotic era, intestinal perforation was almost always fatal. Current consensus favors a combination of medical treatment and surgical intervention. Most surgeons experienced in the treatment of typhoid fever complications favor simple closure of the ulcer. This must be accompanied by additional antibiotics, such as gentamicin, tobramycin, or amikacin (in that order of preference) plus cefoxitin or clindamycin to treat peritoneal contamination by normal enteric flora.

CARRIER STATE

Approximately 3 to 5 percent of persons with acute typhoid fever become chronic biliary carriers. The propensity to carriage increases with age at the time of initial *S. typhi* infection and is greater in females. Most chronic carriers have cholecystitis with stones; occasional carriers lacking gallbladders manifest chronic pathology and infection in the intrahepatic biliary system.

If indicated because of economic or social factors and if the patient is sturdy enough to withstand surgery, cholecystectomy accompanied by 4 weeks of combined intravenous ampicillin and oral amoxicillin therapy can cure the carrier state in approximately 85 percent of instances. When this is not feasible, 3 weeks of high-dose intravenous ampicillin therapy has also shown promising results. Most recently, a moderate success rate has been reported by long-term (at least 4 weeks) oral therapy with ciprofloxacin (750 mg every 12 hours) or norfloxacin (400 mg every 12 hours).

PREVENTION

In multiple controlled field trials in endemic areas, acetone-killed *S. typhi* parenteral vaccine has been shown to confer 75 to 90 percent protective efficacy against typhoid fever. The protection afforded to persons from nonendemic areas appears to be somewhat less. However, the parenteral vaccine causes fever or adverse local reactions (heat, swelling, erythema) in 15 to 25 percent of recipients. Nevertheless, for persons traveling to highly endemic areas, immunization with two 0.5-ml doses 1 month apart is recommended.

A new, live, oral attenuated *S. typhi* vaccine (strain Ty21a) is becoming available in many countries. Three doses of lyophilized vaccine in enteric-coated capsules was recently shown in field trials in Santiago, Chile, to provide approximately 65 percent protection without causing adverse reactions. This vaccine will be licensed in the United States in 1990.

SUGGESTED READING

Avendano A, Herrera P, Horwitz I, et al. Duodenal string cultures: practicality and sensitivity for diagnosing enteric fever in children. J Infect Dis 1986; 153:359–362.
Ferreccio C, Morris JG Jr, Valdivieso C, et al. Efficacy of ciprofloxacin in the treatment of chronic typhoid carriers. J Infect Dis 1988; 157:1235–1239.
Levine MM, Taylor DN, Ferreccio C. Typhoid vaccines come of age. Pediatr Infect Dis 1989; 8:374–381.
Snyder MG, Perroni J, Gonzalez O, et al. Comparative efficacy of chloramphenicol, ampicillin and co-trimoxazole in the treatment of typhoid fever. Lancet 1976; 2:1155–1157.

INTRA-ABDOMINAL ABSCESS

DORI F. ZALEZNIK, M.D.

Intra-abdominal abscesses, either peritoneal or visceral, usually arise as a subacute complication of intra-abdominal sepsis. The most common inciting event for an intra-abdominal abscess is appendicitis with perforation. However, any disruption of the normal integrity of the bowel, for example, surgery, trauma, eroding tumor, diverticulitis, or perforated ulcer, may result in peritonitis and eventual localization into an abscess. Abscesses may arise in an area contiguous to the perforated viscus; may collect in organs such as liver (most common), kidneys, or spleen; or may be located in the subphrenic regions, attached to the peritoneum or within the omentum. Gallbladder perforation may result in peritonitis or liver abscesses via contiguous spread. Abscesses, particularly visceral collections, also may occur following bacteremia.

As will be considered in greater detail below, it is important to consider the origin of peritonitis or bacteremia that has led to abscess development because diagnostic approaches, the need for surgical correction, and the choice of antimicrobial therapy all will be influenced by the initiating events of the infection. Typically, intra-abdominal abscesses represent infections from which many bacterial species are isolated. Anaerobic organisms are found in 96 percent of cases of intra-abdominal sepsis. Knowledge of the normal flora of the human intestine, female genital tract, and gallbladder is helpful in determining likely bacterial species to be involved. Several organisms figure especially prominently in intra-abdominal abscesses, however, and more commonly than one would predict from their numerical representation in the normal flora. The most important of these organisms is *Bacteroides fragilis*, a gram-negative anaerobe which is the most common anaerobic species found in abscess contents and in bacteremia. Among aerobic species, *Escherichia coli* is the most common organism isolated. An exception to the usual polymicrobial content of abscesses may occur when a visceral abscess results from hematogenous spread. A single organism such as *Staphylococcus aureus* or even a viridans streptococcal strain such as *Streptococcus milleri* may cause abscesses under those circumstances. Empiric therapy of suspected intra-abdominal abscess should be directed at both anaerobic and aerobic organisms.

In experimental animal systems mortality in intra-abdominal sepsis is caused by aerobic gram-negative bacilli in the bloodstream. While *B. fragilis* bacteremia is common, mortality from bloodstream infection is rare presumably because the lipopolysaccharide (LPS) component of this anaerobe does not induce the same endotoxin manifestations as gram-negative aerobic LPS. In both animal and human infections, the later manifestation of intra-abdominal sepsis is abscess formation, which usually requires the presence of an anaerobic species. *B. fragilis* given experimentally can cause abscesses, but other anaerobic and aerobic species require a synergistic combination of both anaerobes and aerobes to produce abscesses. For successful antimicrobial prophylaxis against intra-abdominal sepsis in colonic surgery, antibiotics must be active against both aerobic gram-negative bacilli (to prevent gram-negative rod sepsis) and against anaerobes (to guard against later abscess development).

DIAGNOSIS

The presentation of an intra-abdominal abscess may be subtle. Acute peritonitis generally is readily recognized with dramatic abdominal findings of rebound tenderness or guarding. In cases of intra-abdominal abscess, however, physical findings may be absent. Occasionally patients note pleuritic pain from diaphragmatic irritation or shoulder discomfort. Fever and constitutional symptoms, such as malaise or anorexia, suggest a more chronic process and may indicate abscess without any localizing manifestations. Liver abscesses, particularly in elderly patients, may be especially subtle and present only as a fever of unknown origin (FUO). Abdominal findings or antecedent abdominal complaints may be absent. The only abnormal laboratory finding may consist of an elevated alkaline phosphatase. Leukocytosis and other abnormal liver function tests may be absent. An unexplained unilateral pleural effusion can sometimes precipitate an evaluation of the abdomen. Fever is common, and in one-third of patients with a liver abscess, concomitant bacteremia will be found.

In a suspected case of intra-abdominal abscess, several radiologic evaluations are helpful. The most useful specific and sensitive test is computed tomography (CT), which provides a view of the abdomen and pelvis previously obtainable only by exploratory laparotomy. Intravenous or, in the case of examining the bowel, oral contrast enhances the lesions to differentiate from hematomas or tumors. If readily accessible, CT is the single test by which most intra-abdominal abscesses will be diagnosed. Ultrasound studies, if thorough, also can frequently detect abscesses, particularly those in the pelvis. The presence of internal echoes helps to distinguish abscesses from cysts, for example in liver or kidneys. The exact nature of the lesion on ultrasound is more difficult to diagnose than by CT, however. Gallium scans are useful as a broad screen for the evaluation of a patient with an FUO. In the abdomen, however, a gallium scan will never be diagnostic because tumors and other collections take up gallium as well as abscesses, and the bowel concentrates the material, leading to the potential for diagnostic confusion. The test requires a minimum of 48 to 72 hours to perform, limiting its acute diagnostic utility. Gallium can help to pinpoint an area for more specific assessment with CT or ultrasound. On occasion, a single study, even CT, will be negative. If the clinical suspicion for an intra-abdominal abscess is high, a second study should be pursued. The most problematic situation for establishing the diagnosis of intra-abdominal abscess is diverticulitis with abscess. Diverticulitis is a common clinical diagnosis. When perforation occurs, the process will frequently wall off locally rather than causing distant peritonitis. The diagnostic modalities cited above are not ideal for imaging the bowel and a collection contiguous to the bowel may be missed.

Diverticula may be seen on CT, but an abscess may not be visualized. In some instances, barium or gastrografin enemas may be necessary to diagnose a diverticular abscess. In rare cases of diverticular abscess, in which the patient experiences recurrent gram-negative bacillary bacteremia without an established focus, exploratory surgery may be required.

TREATMENT

Therapy for intra-abdominal abscess may be divided into two parts. While choice of antimicrobial agents is important, particularly with a number of newer products available, the mainstay of treatment remains drainage of the walled-off pus. In the past, surgical drainage was required. With skilled diagnostic radiologists using CT or ultrasound, however, surgery frequently can be avoided. Percutaneous drainage even of large collections of pus can be performed under CT or ultrasound guidance with insertion of small pigtail catheters that can be left in place to drain and can later be manipulated. There are several clinical situations in which drainage is not required routinely. Diverticulitis with a small, localized abscess can usually be cured medically. The occasional patient with multiple, small liver abscesses not amenable to drainage also may be cured with prolonged antibiotic therapy. Liver abscesses caused by the parasite *Entamoeba histolytica* usually do not require drainage. If an amebic abscess is suspected clinically in a patient, for example, with a travel history, blood serology, which is positive in more than 90 percent of patients with extraintestinal amebiasis, may be diagnostic without aspiration of the lesion. In some patients, mixed amebic and bacterial abscesses occur. In such situations, however, the patients do not respond to therapy for amebiasis alone. Some pelvic collections, such as tubo-ovarian abscesses, may be cured medically without surgical intervention as well.

Some current literature advocates medical therapy of other intra-abdominal abscesses, particularly liver abscesses. While certain patients may be unable to tolerate surgery and have lesions not amenable to the percutaneous approach, the literature is difficult to evaluate. Patients in these studies frequently undergo diagnostic aspiration which may, in some instances, be the equivalent of drainage. While other patients are cured, the length of antibiotic course usually is measured in months rather than weeks. In general, the preferred approach to an intra-abdominal abscess, including liver abscesses, is to establish drainage and use antimicrobial therapy as an important adjunct. Lengthy courses of antibiotics are not without hazard, and patients with prominent constitutional symptoms and fever may take much longer to feel better with a medical approach alone.

As stated above, antimicrobial therapy of intra-abdominal abscesses must be directed at both anaerobic and aerobic species. In general, this dictates combination therapy. It is useful to discuss therapy directed at anaerobes separately as the literature may be confusing and sensitivity testing of anaerobes in most clinical laboratories is not performed routinely. First-line therapy for anaerobes in intra-abdominal sepsis includes three potential choices for which considerable in vitro and clinical data are available. In 1989, the first

among these three antibiotics is metronidazole. This agent has a broad anaerobic spectrum, including the more resistant members of the *B. fragilis* group, penetration into abscesses is excellent, and high blood levels can be achieved with oral as well as intravenous administration, raising the possibility of completing therapy with an oral agent. Resistance in clinical isolates has not been reported in the United States. Metronidazole is not active against any aerobic species. If infection with *Clostridium perfringens* is suspected, penicillin is the drug of choice, but that organism is rarely found in intra-abdominal abscesses.

Two other widely used antibiotics are clindamycin and cefoxitin. Both are active against the anaerobic flora below the diaphragm. Clindamycin does not cover aerobic gram-negative bacilli. Cefoxitin can be used as a single agent since it is active against many aerobic gram-negative bacilli as well as against anaerobes such as *B. fragilis*. In some areas of the country, however, there is growing resistance to second-generation cephalosporins among aerobic gram-negative bacilli. In these locales, another agent active against gram-negative organisms should be added to cefoxitin. In recent years reports of growing resistance to clindamycin or cefoxitin by *B. fragilis*, approaching 10 percent, have been published. While these trends are of interest, reports of well-documented clinical failures due to resistant organisms are scarce. Most experts in anaerobic infections still would include both of these antibiotics among first-line therapy. If an individual patient, however, seems to be failing therapy and there is no other focus of infection that needs to be drained, a change of therapy and attempts to perform sensitivity testing on anaerobic isolates are appropriate. There also has been concern that cefoxitin resistance may cross to other β-lactam agents, suggesting that another class of antibiotic should be chosen if cefoxitin resistance is suspected.

Chloramphenicol is another antibiotic that has been used for many years against anaerobes. While *B. fragilis* has not been found to be resistant to this agent in vitro, clinical failures with this drug in experimental and human infections may be as high as 40 percent. Many patients will respond to chloramphenicol, however, and if a patient is improving on the drug, there is no reason to change.

Third-generation cephalosporins, while popular and active against gram-negative aerobic bacilli, are not very effective against *B. fragilis*. Moxalactam displayed the greatest activity of this class of agents but because of bleeding problems is not in widespread use currently. *B. fragilis* has high resistance to cefoperazone and cefotaxime and even to an active metabolite of the latter drug. While there was some initial interest in ceftizoxime, in vitro testing of *B. fragilis* to this antibiotic makes it appear more sensitive than is reflected in clinical results.

The new oral antibiotic class of quinolone agents, such as ciprofloxacin, has a wide antibacterial spectrum but is notable for the absence of anaerobic coverage. Broader-spectrum penicillins, such as ticarcillin or piperacillin, are active against *Bacteroides* species, but the clinical utility of these drugs has not been evaluated widely. Cefotetan, a newer second-generation cephalosporin, is equivalent to cefoxitin in activity against *B. fragilis* but is not as active against other members of the *Bacteroides* group, such as *Bacteroides thetaiotaomicron*. While the half-life of cefotetan allows for less-frequent administration than cefoxitin, thereby decreasing costs, metronidazole is less costly than either of the cephalosporins and is generally preferred.

Several new types of antibiotics appear to be active against anaerobes and bear watching as large clinical trials of intra-abdominal sepsis are completed. These drugs include imipenem, ticarcillin-clavulanic acid, and ampicillin-sulbactam. All are broad-spectrum agents with potential use as monotherapy, although local resistance rates for aerobic gram-negative bacilli need to be assessed in determining the adequacy of single-drug therapy. While clinical trials in known infections involving anaerobic species are not extensive with any of these agents, they are likely to be promising additions in the future.

For treatment of the aerobic components of abscesses, metronidazole or clindamycin usually is used in conjunction with an aminoglycoside. Cefoxitin may be used alone with the proviso that local aerobic gram-negative bacilli are not highly resistant. Chloramphenicol has some aerobic gram-negative spectrum but, as a bacteriostatic antibiotic, generally should be combined with an aminoglycoside. Once the sensitivities of the aerobic species are known, less toxic agents such as cephalosporins can be substituted for the aminoglycoside. Ciprofloxacin also may be considered as oral therapy along with metronidazole, but there are no clinical trials of this regimen in intra-abdominal abscess.

As mentioned above, it is important to consider the site of origin of peritonitis or bacteremia in considering antibiotic coverage. For example, perforation of a duodenal or gastric ulcer or pancreatitis with abscess formation often produces substantial chemical irritation of the peritoneum with less prominent abscess formation.

Much of the consideration for therapy for intra-abdominal infections, usually arising from the colon, takes into account the sensitivities of the *B. fragilis* group. When treating pelvic abscesses arising from the female genital tract, consideration needs to be given to coverage of *Neisseria gonorrhoeae* and *Chlamydia*. When abscesses arise in the pelvic region, as opposed to pelvic inflammatory disease, *B. fragilis* figures prominently as a pathogen as well.

Another location of concern is the gallbladder. Except in cases of multiple episodes of cholecystitis or previous biliary tree surgery, anaerobic organisms do not figure prominently as flora of the gallbladder. Aerobic gram-negative bacilli are the most common organisms found, with enterococci also prominent. Many clinicians will treat to eliminate the enterococcus in intra-abdominal sepsis. Most of the regimens discussed, including metronidazole or clindamycin/gentamicin and cefoxitin, do not include enterococcal coverage. The importance of the enterococcus in mixed intra-abdominal processes has not been established. My practice is not to cover empirically for enterococci except in infections arising in the gallbladder and to consider broadening coverage to include enterococci if the organisms are isolated from blood or repeatedly from abscess contents. Ampicillin usually is added to eliminate the enterococcus (vancomycin in the case of penicillin-allergic patients).

Table 1 summarizes my recommendations about antibiotic regimens for intra-abdominal abscesses. Although an opinion, these recommendations reflect a review of anaerobic susceptibility patterns and the clinical literature at the present time. In general, the technology necessary to perform sensitivity testing on anaerobic species is not available in most clinical laboratories. This should not be viewed as a criticism, since the need for routine susceptibility testing has not been proved. In problematic individual cases, it is helpful to have sensitivity testing accessible. Most of the relevant information can be obtained from studies by experts who have the facilities for susceptibility testing of anaerobes.

TABLE 1   Antibiotics Useful in the Treatment of Intra-Abdominal Abscess

Anaerobic Coverage	*Aerobic Gram-Negative Coverage*
First-line therapy	
Metronidazole 500 mg q8h	Gentamicin 1.5 mg/kg q8h*
Clindamycin 600 mg q8h[†]	Gentamicin 1.5 mg/kg q8h*
Cefoxitin 2 g q4h	Cefoxitin[‡] 2 g q4h
Alternative regimen	
Chloramphenicol 500 mg q6h	Gentamicin 1.5 mg/kg q8h*
Newer antibiotics to be considered	
Imipenem 1 g q6h	Imipenem 1 g q6h
Ampicillin-sulbactam 3 g q6h[§]	Ampicillin-sulbactam[‡] 3 g q6h[§]
Ticarcillin-clavulanic acid 3.1 g q4h[#]	Ticarcillin-clavulanic acid[‡] 3.1 g q4h[#]

* Intervals should be adjusted based on creatinine and peak and trough drug levels in renal insufficiency.
† The pharmacokinetics of clindamycin suggest that every 8 hours is a more appropriate dosing interval than every 6 hours.
‡ In areas in which resistance of aerobic gram-negative bacilli to this agent is known to be fairly high, addition of an antibiotic such as gentamicin should be considered.
§ Ampicillin component is 2 g and sulbactam 1 g.
# Ticarcillin component is 3 g and clavulanic acid 100 mg.

SUGGESTED READING

Altemeier WA, Culbertson WR, Fullen WD, Shook CD. Intra-abdominal abscesses. Am J Surg 1973; 125: 70–79.

Cuchural GJ, Tally FP, Jacobus NV, et al. Susceptibility of the *Bacteroides fragilis* group in the United States: analysis by site of location. Antimicrob Agents Chemother 1988; 32:712–722.

Gerzof SG, Robbins AH, Johnson WC, Birkett DH, Nabseth DC. Percutaneous catheter drainage of abdominal abscesses. N Engl J Med 1981; 305:653–657.

Tally FP, Gorbach SL. Therapy of mixed anaerobic-aerobic infections. Am J Med 1985; 78:145–153.

Thadepalli H, Gorbach SL, Broido PW, Norsen J, Nyhus L. Abdominal trauma, anaerobes, and antibiotics. Surg Gynecol Obstet 1973; 137:270–276.

BILIARY TRACT INFECTION

HARRY E. DASCOMB, M.D.
DALE W. OLLER, M.D.

The liver, biliary tract, supportive tissue, and serosal membranes receive blood supply from the portal vein and the hepatic artery. Microorganisms that breech the intestinal mucosa from the esophagus to the middle region of the rectum gain access to the portal vein. Since the portal vein contributes two-thirds of the hepatic blood supply, portal vein–borne enteric bacteria or parasites cause the majority of intrahepatic or biliary tract infections. Although portal blood is usually sterile, portal blood cultures of humans and dogs with colitis frequently reveal bacteria. Similarly, patients with acute enteritis, Crohn's disease, ulcerative colitis, diverticulitis, and amebiasis have liver and biliary tract infections as complications. To a lesser extent, the liver, biliary tract, and gallbladder are exposed to systemic bacteremia and viremia conveyed by the hepatic artery or more rarely by the splenic vein (in event of a splenic abscess or septic splenic infarcts). Enteric bacteria also gain access to and colonize the biliary tract via the ampulla of Vater (duodenal papilla), particularly during duodenitis, intestinal obstruction, or common bile duct (CBD) stasis. Intestinal bacteria also gain access to the biliary tract through cholecysto- or choledocho-intestinal fistulae, endoscopic retrograde cholangiopancreatography (ERCP), and transendoscopic surgery. Palliative or diagnostic surgical procedures, such as cholecystotomy or percutaneous transhepatic cholangiography, may contaminate the biliary tract with skin bacteria.

Bile is usually sterile despite these potential sources of hepatic and biliary tract infection. Sterility of the biliary tract is dependent on the phagocytic efficiency of the hepatic Kupffer cells; the daily secretion of 600 to 800 ml of bile, which flushes the biliary system; and the maintenance of a critical balance of bile acids, pigment, cholesterol, and lecithin in the bile, which prevents formation of cholesterol and pigment stones. An imbalance of cholesterol, unconjugated bilirubin, or lecithin and bile acids, together with stasis, causes crystallization of cholesterol micellae or of bilirubinate salts. Bacteria present in the bile may be sequestered in the stones. Indeed, bacteria secreting β-glucuronidase may have a central role in pigmented stone production. Those bacteria capable of producing gas, particularly anaerobes, can cause radiolucent clefts within the stones, which are recognized radiographically as the "Mercedes Benz" sign. The sludge and stones resulting from crystallization usually appear first in the gallbladder and obstruct the cystic duct at the valves of Heister. Stones frequently migrate from the gallbladder (or occasionally from elsewhere) and obstruct the common or hepatic ducts. Biliary obstruction also may occur from primary inflammation and fibrosis as well as malignancy. Stasis due to obstruction permits casual biliary infectious contaminants to flourish, and inflammation results. The inflammatory swelling may cause ischemia, necrosis of adjacent tissue, and complete obstruction of a portion or all of the entire biliary tree; closed space infection can result. In this manner, biliary tract obstruction and infection are expressed in several syndromes: cholecystitis—acute and chronic or acalculous, acute; cholangitis—obstructive (ascending) pyogenic cholangitis, sclerosing cholangitis, and oriental or recurrent cholangitis; pancreatitis—secondary to biliary tract infection; liver abscess—cholangitic or hematogenous; and hepatitis—chronic, granulomatous or acute, nonbacterial. The effective management of biliary tract infections depends on:

1. Identification of the syndrome and specific etiology by clinical examination, clinical laboratory study of blood and urine, and aerobic and anaerobic cultures of venous blood collected from patients with current or recent fever and tissue and bile collected via endoscopy, percutaneous transhepatic aspiration during cholangiography, or cholecystotomy. Serum may be stored ($-20°C$) for possible subsequent antibody testing of acute phase and convalescent specimens against protozoa, bacteria, and viruses.

2. Investigation of the biliary tract radiographically for confirmation or exclusion of biliary tract obstruction or the presence of intrahepatic or extrahepatic fluid or abscess.

3. Estimation of the etiologic agent(s) based on clinical and initial laboratory findings.

4. Selection of antibiotics based on results of studies 1 through 3—for immediate therapy in acutely ill or septicemic patients or for perioperative prophylaxis against sepsis and wound infection resulting from surgical, endoscopic, or radiologic invasive procedures.

5. Correction or control of metabolic disorders prior to surgery.

6. Performance of surgical, endoscopic, or percutaneous procedures for the prompt removal of biliary tract obstruction, excision, or incision and drainage of localized infection; the collection of tissue, bile, and exudate by surgery or transendoscopic procedure for direct study (wet mount, Gram and special stains), culture for bacteria (identification and antibiotic sensitivity of isolates), culture for viruses when appropriate (e.g., patient with acalculous cholecystitis and sclerosing cholangitis), cytology (special stains for mycobacteria, fungi, protozoa), and histopathology.

7. Revision of the initial antibiotic therapy to attain specificity, optimal dosage, and cost effectiveness, based on the completed microbiologic study results of initial body fluid and surgical specimens, the anatomic diagnosis, and clinical response. Subsequent changes in therapy are determined by the clinical response and the microscopic and culture findings using interval specimens of tissue or exudate.

ACUTE CHOLECYSTITIS

Acute cholecystitis is an emergency that usually presents with symptoms of fever, persistent right upper-quadrant (RUQ) pain extending in a band-like fashion to the infra- or interscapular region, nausea, vomiting, and anxiety. Acute cholecystitis is heralded by fluctuating epigastric cramping pain or colic that persists, with increasing severity, and becomes localized in the right hypochondrium. Occasional episodes of postprandial or nocturnal epigastric pain may occur prior to the acute illness. Physical findings reveal an acutely ill person with elevated vital signs. There is voluntary guarding in the RUQ and tenderness to gentle palpation. Deep inspiration provokes a transient inspiratory arrest and complaint of pain in the subcostal region at the midclavicular line as the tender gallbladder descends against the examiner's hand (Murphy's sign). Gentle pressure with a finger may be required to elicit this sign but fist percussion of the costal margin is unnecessary and elicits excessive patient discomfort. Despite the abdominal muscle guarding, a tender mass or phlegmon may be palpated in the hypochondrium and extend below the paraumbilical line. The skin overlying the inflamed gallbladder radiates heat. Laboratory findings include leukocytosis with moderate left shift and slightly elevated concentrations of serum alkaline phosphatase, bilirubin, and aspartate aminotransferase (AST). Serum amylase elevation may be transient. Persistent serum amylase elevation suggests associated obstruction of pancreatic duct of Wirsung and pancreatitis. Bilirubinuria is frequently present.

Management

Fever or history of rigors, feverishness, and night sweating are indications for the prompt collection of blood and urine for culture. Although the clinical diagnosis of acute cholecystitis is 85 percent accurate, it is helpful to ascertain the gallbladder size and wall thickness and the presence of stones or dilated bile ducts. It is also important to exclude pancreatic, renal, and colonic disease and acute viral hepa-

titis. Ultrasonography provides excellent definition of the gallbladder, gallstones or bile sludge, and biliary tree dilatation and can exclude extrahepatic disease. Scintigraphy with technetium-99m iminodiacetic acid, such as [^{99m}Tc]Pipida permits visualization of the liver, of segments of the biliary tract, of the duodenum, and of the gallbladder (in the absence of disease). When utilized as an adjunct to ultrasonography, scintigraphy permits accurate diagnosis of gallbladder disease. In cholecystitis the cystic duct is occluded. This prevents or delays the entrance of radioactive bile and a gallbladder image. Radioactivity is apparent, however, in the liver, bile ducts, and duodenum. Scintigraphy may be diagnostic when bowel gas obscures ultrasonographic images. It is helpful also in differentiating acute cholecystitis from acute hepatitis and occasionally from cirrhosis of the liver. Unless ultrasound and scintigraphic findings are incompatible with cholecystitis, no further imaging is necessary. Computed tomography (CT) is considered if an intrahepatic lesion, extra biliary tract compression, renal infection, or pancreatic disease is suspected. Magnetic resonance imaging offers no further advantages over CT at present.

Early surgical correction of biliary tract obstruction is the most effective therapy and at the same time promptly confirms the diagnosis. Surgical removal of the diseased gallbladder and direct examination of the biliary tract usually prevent future problems from stones obstructing extrahepatic bile ducts, the common duct, or the ampulla of Vater. Fortunately, an early inflamed, edematous gallbladder usually presents no major technical difficulties in surgical removal. Surgery is best performed during the first 3 days of acute clinical symptoms. After 3 days of symptoms, inflammatory neovascularity develops, dissection about the gallbladder is more difficult, and the risk of surgical complications increases.

Immediate medical therapy is designed to prepare the patient for surgery. Cardiopulmonary, renal, hematologic, or metabolic diseases are excluded or treated. Nasogastric suction is given to relieve ileus, gastric distention, and vomiting. Meperidine is injected intravenously in doses sufficient to reduce pain and smooth muscle spasm. Intravenous fluids and electrolytes are provided to restore hydration and plasma osmolality.

After blood has been collected for aerobic and anaerobic cultures, antibiotics are initiated immediately if the patient has fever or recent history of fever with or without abdominal pain. A combination of ampicillin 200 mg per kilogram per day (in four divided doses at 6-hour intervals) together with gentamicin 4 mg per kilogram per day (in divided doses at 8-hour intervals) is preferred. These antibiotics give excellent tissue levels that inhibit enterococci as well as most aerobic and anaerobic bacteria associated with acute cholecystitis. If the patient is allergic to penicillin, cefazolin 1 g every 6 hours intravenously or cefoxitin 2 g every 6 hours (or cefotetan 2 g every 12 hours) is effective against *Escherichia coli* and non–hospital-acquired *Klebsiella* species, but these antibiotics are ineffective against enterococci. Adequate perioperative coverage of enterococci and enteric bacilli is accomplished in penicillin-allergic patients by vancomycin 500 mg every 6 hours with cefazolin or cefoxitin, as above. In our experience postoperative infections complicating biliary tract surgery are associated often with enterococci, particularly in patients given a cephalosporin alone perioperatively. For this reason we recommend vancomycin, together with perioperative gram-negative coverage, in patients who are allergic to penicillin. During the surgical procedure, specimens are collected for immediate study. The results of the examination of unstained and stained fresh preparations and the preliminary results of aerobic cultures are often sufficient for tentative identification of infection due to cocci or anaerobes likely to be resistant to the initial choice of antibiotics. For example, immediate identification of gram-negative and -positive pleomorphic rods and coccal bacteria in bile or gallbladder mucosa obtained during surgery suggests anaerobic infection. In this situation, metronidazole should be added to the perioperative antibiotic(s) and the duration of postoperative therapy is extended to prevent appearance later of anaerobic abscesses. When the gallbladder and biliary tract stones have been removed and there is no evidence of obstruction or infection, perioperative antibiotics may be stopped 1 day after surgery. However, if smears and cultures from specimens of bile and tissue collected during surgery contain bacteria, particularly enterococci or highly resistant gram-negative rods, prolonged specific therapy may be needed to eliminate the pathogens and prevent the inflammatory obstruction or extra- or intrahepatic abscess as a late complication. If fever persists or the patient fails to improve, further studies are indicated to exclude biliary obstruction, superimposed biliary tract infection, or a nosocomial infection elsewhere. The bacteria isolated from the T-tube in the common bile duct (CBD), from drainage of the gallbladder bed, or from transendoscopic aspirates of CBD may be colonizers only and should not be treated routinely. However, they should be considered in selecting adequate perioperative prophylaxis for any additional postoperative invasive procedure.

Patients with acutely inflamed gallbladders who receive no treatment during the first 10 days of fever may develop pericholecystitis, cholecystoenteritic fistulae, or gallstone ileus. The resulting local and generalized peritonitis and septicemia have a mortality exceeding 30 percent. The complications demand aggressive and often repeated surgical procedures as well as intensive and specific antimicrobial therapy against initial and superimposed pathogens. Piperacillin or imipenem with an aminoglycoside and metronidazole are empirically selected until microbiologic data suggest more effective combinations.

Persons with acute cholecystitis and recent myocardial infarction or other illnesses that increase the risk of immediate cholecystectomy should receive intravenous ampicillin and aminoglycoside or alternate antibiotics for 7 to 10 days or longer, depending on subsidence of symptoms and local signs of gallbladder or liver tenderness. If the operative risks for cholecystectomy or cholecystotomy remain high, surgery may be delayed indefinitely by continuing oral or intramuscular antibiotics. However, surgery should be rescheduled as soon as possible, because cholecystitis will recur until the gallbladder and stones have been removed or cholecystotomy and drainage have been accomplished.

ACUTE ACALCULOUS CHOLECYSTITIS

Acute cholecystitis may occur in the absence of gallstones during a systemic illness. Persons at risk are those with salmonellosis (particularly typhoid fever) and infections due to group A streptococci and disseminated cytomegalovirus (CMV). Acute cholecystitis and gallbladder distention due to insidious development of bile stasis are complications of total parenteral nutrition, acute pancreatitis, trauma, and Caroli's syndrome. Bile stagnation may result also from inanition, dehydration, fever, CBD obstruction from mesenteric lymphadenopathy due to malignancy or viral infection, or duodenal papillitis. The resulting syndrome of acalculous cholecystitis appears to be due to impaired biliary defenses by atonic smooth muscle, to intrahepatic bile duct dilatation, or to extrinsic or intrinsic CBD obstruction culminating in bile stasis. This permits hematogenous pathogens, indigenous enteric microorganisms, to breach the weakened barriers, to replicate prodigiously within the biliary tract and gallbladder, and to produce acute and chronic inflammation. The clinical and laboratory findings indicate cholecystitis with or without cholangitis.

Management

Successful management of acute acalculous cholecystitis is dependent upon prompt recognition of the etiology of systemic infection and gallbladder pathology, the use of specific antibiotics, and adequate drainage of the gallbladder and biliary tract. Peri- and postoperative antibiotic therapy is selected on the basis of all available clinical and laboratory data. Transendoscopic drainage of the CBD may provide specimens of tissue for parasitic, bacterial, and viral studies as well as relief of pain. Surgery is the most effective procedure to relieve pain and reduce danger of a ruptured gallbladder and peritonitis. When cholecystitis occurs with *Salmonella typhi* or other salmonellae postinfection carrier state often follows as a result of residual biliary tract or splenic foci of infection. This shedding of salmonellae in feces may persist indefinitely despite optimal antibiotic therapy and cholecystectomy. Public health assistance with these patients is required to protect against water and food contamination and community infection. When CMV is identified in symptomatic children or in persons with acquired immunodeficiency syndrome (AIDS), dihydroxypropoxyquanine (ganciclovir) 7.5 to 15 mg per kilogram per day in three divided doses should be considered for its antiviral effect. The appropriate indications for ganciclovir are still being developed.

CHRONIC SYMPTOMATIC CHOLECYSTITIS

Chronic inflammation of the gallbladder is usually associated with cholelithiasis. Complaints of flatulence, anorexia, nausea, hypogeusia, and epigastric abdominal discomfort or pain in the right hypochondrium are common symptoms but are not specific. There may be history of fatty food intolerance with postprandial exacerbation of abdominal colic-like pain and eructations. Usually fever is not present. Physical findings are limited to minimal tenderness in the right upper quadrant of the abdomen. The gallbladder is usually contracted, fibrosed, and not palpable. Occasionally, a palpable fluctuant mass is due to a noninflamed, noncalculous gallbladder that is obstructed and distended with clear to cloudy mucus (hydrops). This, according to Courvoisier's law, suggests carcinoma of the head of the pancreas but occurs in absence of malignancy. Laboratory studies give normal results except for a slight elevation in serum alkaline phosphatase. The differential diagnosis includes functional disorders, systemic diseases (including diabetes mellitus, megaloblastic anemia, myxedema, and malignancies of the biliary tract, pancreas or lymph nodes), or peptic ulcer disease and hiatal hernia.

Gallstones and gallbladder wall thickening are usually readily identified by ultrasonography. These ultrasonographic findings confirm chronic cholecystitis, and at the same time other organs can be visualized to help exclude renal and pancreatic disease. Cholecystography, using a double dose of oral contrast material, is diagnostic if radiolucent stones can be outlined. Cholelithiasis and chronic cholecystitis are confirmed also if the sonogram shows stones and the oral cholecystogram provides no opacification of the gallbladder. ERCP has no role in the diagnosis of confirmed stone-induced chronic cholecystitis, but transendoscopy may have a therapeutic role in removing small gallstones when these have been treated with litholytic chemicals or fragmented by extracorporeal lithotripsy. Stone fragments can be removed from the common duct endoscopically. Endoscopic sphincterotomy after lithotripsy may be a reasonable option in the elderly, poor-risk patient who has gallstones obstructing the duodenal papilla. The major complication of transendoscopic sphincterotomy is hemorrhage into the duodenum, requiring surgical hemostasis. Duodenal or CBD perforations are complications also. Endoscopy-laser fragmentation of stones in the common bile ducts appears to be a promising nonsurgical method of lithotripsy.

Management

Optimal therapy for the majority of patients with chronic symptoms and evidence of cholelithiasis is elective cholecystectomy and thorough exploration of the biliary tract for obscure gallstones. Recent evidence that 40 percent of gallbladders removed for chronic cholecystitis and 80 percent of pigmented stones contain bacteria supports the decision to use perioperative antibiotic prophylaxis for both endoscopic or surgical procedures. Debilitated persons particularly need this protection. Cefazolin is effective against normal skin flora and most aerobic bacteria that may colonize the biliary tract. Cefazolin is ineffective against hospital-acquired *Staphylococcus epidermidis*, all strains of *Enterococcus faecalis*, and most anaerobes. For this reason, ampicillin and gentamicin are preferred initial perioperative therapy and are continued or replaced as determined by the study of the surgical specimen and by the clinical events postoperatively. An alternate perioperative antibiotic is piperacillin in full therapeutic dosage intravenously (Table 1). In the event of penicillin allergy, cefoxitin and vancomycin or van-

TABLE 1 Antimicrobial Agents for Specific Problems in Biliary Tract Infections

Antibiotic	Dose (mg/kg/day)	g/h	Route	Total g/day	Indication*
Ceftriaxone	30	2/24	IV IM	2.000	Penicillin allergy; Prolonged therapy (3–21 days)
Cefoperazone	60	2/12	IV	4.000	As above; renal failure
Aztreonam	110	2/6	IV	8.000	Gram-negative bacteria, resistant to other antibiotics
Imipenem	50	1/6	IV	4.000	*Pseudomonas* species; *S. aureus*, enteric bacteria resistant to other antibiotics
Metronidazole	15	0.5/6	IV	2.000	Adjunctive therapy for anaerobic bacterial infection
Clindamycin	40	0.9/8	IV	2.700	Penicillin allergy; adjunctive therapy against anaerobes, *S. aureus*
Chloramphenicol	50	1.0/6 1.0/6	IV PO	4.000	Penicillin allergy; liver/renal failure; anaerobic/aerobic; enteric bacteria, enterococcal infection
Sulfamethoxazole-trimethoprim	50 10	1.0/6 0.2/6	IV PO	4.000 0.800	Therapy, penicillin allergy, gram-negative aerobic rods
Ciprofloxacin	21	0.750/12	PO	1.500	Penicillin allergy, prolonged suppressive therapy; *S. aureus, Pseudomonas, Salmonella*, aerobic enteric gram-negative rods
Ganciclovir (DHPG)	7.5	0.175/8	IV	0.525	Cytomegaovirus†
Amphotericin	0.35–1.00	0.025 to 0.075/24	IV	0.035	Systemic fungal infection
Ansamycin (investigational)	7–9	0.450/24	PO	0.450	*M. avium* complex

Average Adult Dose spans g/h, Route, Total g/day columns.

* When identity and in vitro sensitivity of pathogen are appropriate for prophylaxis and/or therapy.
† Specific indications for use in this setting are still being developed.

comycin with an aminoglycoside are options for perioperative prophylaxis against the most common bacterial colonizers of the biliary tract (Table 2).

If the patient is febrile, routine specimens are collected, and ampicillin and gentamicin or alternatives are selected empirically. Both antibiotics are continued postoperatively until the patient is afebrile or the ampicillin and gentamicin are replaced by a more specific single antibiotic or combination of antibiotics. Specificity is determined by in vitro sensitivity tests and by serum bactericidal effect against the isolates from the surgical specimen.

If specimens collected during surgery contain a polymicrobial flora in the stained smear suggesting mixed anaerobic-aerobic infection, and the patient's clinical status worsens, blood is recultured, and piperacillin should replace ampicillin or cefazolin. Aminoglycoside is continued until cultures of intraoperative tissue and bile show no aerobic enterobacteria and those present are sensitive to piperacillin. If *Bacteroides fragilis* or *Bacteroides melaninogenicus* groups are identified, metronidazole is combined with piperacillin.

Chloramphenicol is effective in treating biliary tract infections due to enteric bacteria, including anaerobes and enterococci. It is bacteriostatic and is only curative if drainage has been established. A total daily dose of 4 g is essential in an adult. Polymorphonuclear depression and moderate anemia occur with prolonged therapy but may be monitored by frequent examination of the peripheral blood for polymorphonuclear cells, platelets, and occasional serum iron levels. Chloramphenicol is an excellent choice in patients

with renal and liver failure and in β-lactam allergy. It is as effective orally as parenterally. As experienced in treating patients with typhoid fever, chloramphenicol orally has no different depressing effect on the bone marrow than does the intravenous route.

Third-generation cephalosporins should not be used against unidentified bacteria pre- or postoperatively since these may induce resistance in less than bactericidal concentrations. When bacteria in blood or bile are identified and the susceptibilities are known against ceftriaxone or cefoperazone, either is effective. Vitamin K should be given with cefoperazone to prevent prothrombin deficiency. Postoperative therapy with orally administered antibiotics is considered when results of microbiology studies confirm effectiveness of available drugs and as soon as alimentation is tolerated. Ciprofloxacin, ampicillin, clindamycin, metronidazole, and chloramphenicol, alone or combined with one another appropriately, may provide adequate specific therapy. Oral clindamycin has a greater propensity for producing pseudomembranous colitis. Chloramphenicol-treated persons require frequent monitoring of the peripheral blood polymorphonuclear cells and platelets. Chloramphenicol is indicated when biliary tract infection is complicated by renal and/or hepatic disease or in persons allergic to β-lactam antibiotics. Ciprofloxacin is well tolerated orally but has limited effect against anaerobes and enterococci. Specific antibiotic therapy orally or intramuscularly should be continued in patients with pre- or postoperative infection until signs of local and systemic infection have disappeared. An occasional patient may relapse, with anorexia, fever, weight loss, and anemia even after prolonged postoperative antibiotics. Intra-abdominal infectious complications must be then considered. Aggressive diagnostic studies are initiated. Frequently, exploratory surgery is necessary for both diagnosis and therapy.

TABLE 2 Perioperative Antibiotic Prophylaxis: Dosage and Rationale

Antibiotic	Dose (mg/kg/day)	Average Adult Dose g/h	Total g/day
Ampicillin*	200.0	3.0/6	12.0
Gentamicin	4.3	0.1/8	0.3
Tobramycin	4.3	0.1/8	0.3
Amikacin	15.0	0.5/12	1.0
Piperacillin†	340.0	6.0/6	24.0
Vancomycin‡	30.0	0.5/6	2.0
Cefazolin§	115.0	2.5/8	8.0
Cefoxitin‖	200.0	3.0/6	12.0
Cefotetan#	100.0	3.0/12	6.0

* Ampicillin plus gentamicin, tobramycin, or amikacin: effective against group D enterococci, gram-negative enteric bacteria (not hospital acquired or in a patient previously treated with antibiotics), clostridia and other anaerobes but not for *B. fragilis, B. melaninogenicus.*
† Piperacillin plus gentamicin, tobramycin, or amikacin: effective against the above plus nosocomial gram-negative bacteria and *B. fragilis, B. melaninogenicus.*
‡ Vancomycin, plus gentamicin, tobramycin, or amikacin: effective against enterococci, *S. aureus, S. epidermidis,* gram-negative enteric bacteria, and some anaerobes. Tolerated by persons allergic to β-lactam antibiotics.
§ Cefazolin: effective against *E. coli, Klebsiella* species, *S. aureus, S. epidermidis* (methicillin-sensitive), and some anaerobes. Tolerated by most persons allergic to penicillin.
‖ Cefoxitin plus gentamicin, tobramycin, or amikacin: effective (as are ampicillin and gentamicin) against gram-negative enteric bacteria and anaerobes. Less effective against enterococci. Tolerated by most persons allergic to penicillin. Cefoxitin and vancomycin: effective against enterococci, *S. aureus, S. epidermidis* (methicillin-resistant or -sensitive), gram-negative enteric bacilli, and anaerobes. Tolerated by most persons allergic to penicillin.
Cefotetan: alternative for cefoxitin.

CHOLANGITIS

The clinical syndromes of simple obstructive or ascending cholangitis, sclerosing cholangitis, and oriental recurrent cholangitis are the result of biliary tract obstruction. In each of these cholangitides, primary obstruction is due to different combinations of metabolic, infectious, or genetic etiologies.

Obstructive (ascending) pyogenic cholangitis is usually due to gallstones forming in or migrating to the common bile duct (CBD) or to strictures or diverticula of the bile ducts secondary to trauma or infection.

Sclerosing cholangitis is associated with the following conditions:

1. Immunopathy permits opportunistic chronic infection of the biliary tree by viruses, protozoa, bacteria, and fungi that result in biliary tract fibrosis and obstruction, e.g., papillary stenosis associated with cytomegalovirus alone or with protozoa causing CBD obstruction.
2. Viral infection of the ductal mucosa with or without immunodeficiency results in subepithelial fibrosis and obstruction of the CBD and its tributaries, eliminating the secondary and tertiary bile duct branches.
3. Duodenal parasitic infection occludes the distal CBD by periductal fibrosis and lymphadenopathy. The presenting

syndrome is intermittent because of acute and chronic pericholangitis resembling chronic active hepatitis.

4. Congenital multifocal dilatation of the segmental bile ducts, CBD and gallbladder, or Caroli's syndrome culminates in polycystic disease of the liver.

Oriental recurrent cholangitis is characterized by intrahepatic bile duct obstruction due to fibrosis. The patients with this impairment have lived in areas in which infection by liver flukes and *Ascaris* species is endemic.

Obstructive (Ascending) Pyogenic Cholangitis

Definition

Calculous biliary obstruction is complicated by a highly concentrated bacteriocholia with enteric, aerobic, and anaerobic bacteria. *E. coli, Klebsiella, Enterobacter, Bacteroides, Clostridium* species, and group D enterococci are most commonly isolated from the bile in pyogenic cholangitis. These pathogens are proteolytic and invasive, causing necrosis, fistulae, abscesses, strictures, and polymicrobial bacteremia.

The cardinal signs of obstructive cholangitis are intermittent pain, fever, and jaundice (Charcot's triad). The attacks are characterized by rigors, fever, moderate RUQ pain, and tenderness. Dark urine and jaundice follow within 3 or 4 days. A cholecystectomy scar is often present in the RUQ, and the liver is enlarged and tender. Clinical evidence of disseminated intravascular coagulation (DIC) may be present, particularly if medical care is delayed. Depending on the severity of the illness, laboratory studies reveal an elevated white blood cell count or leukopenia with granulocytic left shift, consisting of band-formed nucleated cells and metamyelocytes; hyperbilirubinemia; and elevated alkaline phosphatase and transaminases. Often an elevated level of serum amylase is transient. If serum amylase increases and is associated with signs of pancreatitis, obstruction of the duct of Wirsung and/or the CBD at the ampulla of Vater is likely. Increased plasma prothrombin time, partial thromboplastin time, and fibrinogen degradation products, blood urea nitrogen, and creatinine, as well as albuminuria and bacteriuria, confirm endotoxemia and DIC.

Management

Immediate intravenous infusions of fluids and electrolytes are given while blood is collected for hematology, chemistry, and culture. A urine specimen obtained by catheter should be submitted for analysis, Gram stain, and culture. Organisms that cause bacteremia are sometimes also present in the urine. Isolates from cultures of the urine sediment often appear within 18 hours of incubation, permitting antibiotic sensitivity results before positive blood cultures confirm the etiology. Piperacillin, metronidazole, and gentamicin or other aminoglycosides are initiated using one-third of the calculated daily dose of each antibiotic as an initial or loading dose. Piperacillin and metronidazole infusion every 6 hours and gentamicin every 8 hours are continued if results of BUN and creatinine are within normal limits and if there is no clinical or laboratory evidence of hepatocellular dysfunction. At 8 hours of antibiotic therapy, blood samples for trough and 1-hour postinfusion peak aminoglycoside levels are collected. A peak serum level less than 7 to 10 μg per milliliter necessitates a dosage increase. At 24 hours the gentamicin peak and trough levels are again determined, the former to assure continued therapeutic levels, the latter to assure adequate clearance. Piperacillin has been used alone successfully in patients with azotemia since enterococci and most anaerobes are susceptible to it. However, using piperacillin without an aminoglycoside increases the risk of including bacterial resistance, particularly in acute cholangitis. The addition of metronidazole enhances antianaerobe bactericidal activity and prevents persistence and later-appearing abscesses. If biliary obstruction is associated with hepatocellular dysfunction but renal function is normal, metronidazole daily dosage is reduced by 50 percent and divided into two infusions. Piperacillin serum levels are usually not affected during the first 24 hours of therapy in persons with rising BUN and creatinine levels. Dosage reductions of piperacillin recommended by established creatinine clearance nomograms for β-lactam antibiotics should be monitored with peak and trough serum antibacterial levels to assure adequate treatment of patients with severe septicemia. The triple combination of piperacillin, metronidazole, and gentamicin is preferred in severely ill persons to assure optimal bactericidal therapy, resolution of fever, and earliest surgical drainage.

If a patient is allergic to penicillins, cefoxitin or cefotetan may replace piperacillin. If there is allergy to all β-lactam antibiotics and the cephamycins, choramphenicol 1 to 1.5 g every 6 hours for a total daily dose of 4 to 6 g should be used along with metronidazole to prevent inactivation of chloramphenicol by *B. fragilis* or *Clostridium perfringens* that may occur in closed-space infection prior to surgical drainage. Chloramphenicol is also an excellent antimicrobial agent in patients with hepatic and renal impairment. Frequent monitoring of peripheral blood smears and occasionally determining serum levels of chloramphenicol are safeguards against a rapid decrease in leukocytes or platelets observed in occasional patients during therapy.

As the patient improves, further studies are necessary preoperatively to visualize the liver and adjacent organs. Ultrasonography, in the absence of a distended, gas-filled bowel, shows presence or absence of biliary duct dilatation. The site of obstruction is best located by direct visualization using radiopaque substances. If the biliary ducts are dilated, percutaneous transhepatic cholangiography (PTC) is an option. If no biliary tract dilatation is observed in sonograms, ERCP is indicated for diagnosis and occasionally therapy. Common duct stones lodged in the sphincter of Oddi may be removed transendoscopically. Surgery is mandatory if transendoscopic drainage fails. The obstruction may be due to CBD or proximal bile duct pathology such as diverticula, granulomas, extensive fibrosis, or malignancy with or without gallstone impaction. The diagnosis and treatment is best assured by exploration. After the obstruction has been removed or bypassed, a T-tube is emplaced to assure drainage, to provide access for contrast cholangiography and postoperative stone extraction, and to sample bile for bacterial colonization in the event of complications.

Occasionally, emergency measures to drain the biliary tract are necessary prior to definitive surgery when antibiotics fail to control fever and toxemia. This is accomplished by surgical placement of the T-tube in the CBD. Intensive antibiotic therapy is discontinued when the patient improves clinically and is afebrile and laboratory studies reveal no evidence of infection or biliary obstruction. The T-tube is retained for a variable period of time to maintain an access to the biliary tract until convalescence is secured. Occasionally fever persists for 10 or more days postoperatively, associated with anorexia, leukocytosis, and no signs of hospital-acquired infections of the urinary tract, lungs, intravenous access sites, or wounds. This may be due to delayed resolution of the pericholangitis or liver parenchymal infection that will respond to continued antibiotic therapy. Iatrogenic or drug fever must be considered if the persisting fever is unaccompanied by leukocytosis, granulocytic left shift, and toxemia. Effective and less costly antibiotic therapy may be considered for the delayed resolution of cholangitis. Ceftriaxone intramuscularly or ciprofloxacin orally are well tolerated and effective if either inhibits, in vitro, bacteria previously isolated. In most patients with cholangitis and prolonged postoperative fever, further studies are indicated to resolve the cause. These consist of a search for site and cause of intra- or perihepatic infection and biliary tract obstruction. A specimen of bile should be examined for presence of a newly acquired predominant pathogen. T-tube cholangiography is done to determine the existence and location of an obstruction. In the absence of biliary obstruction, CT is necessary to localize abscesses or cysts. Fever and toxemia should improve promptly with surgical or endoscopic relief of obstruction or abscess drainage and effective antibacterial therapy.

Sclerosing Cholangitis

Definition

Sclerosing cholangitis has been an uncommon disease that until recently was not associated with a specific infectious etiology. The biliary tract obstruction is due to subepithelial fibrous thickening of the CBD, gallbladder, and extra- and intrahepatic bile ducts and ductules. Contrast imaging of the biliary tree shows strictures, beading, and fistulae of the bile ducts and decreased arborization and terminal "pruning" of secondary and tertiary radicles. The fibrosis of the common bile duct and gallbladder results in reduced size and thickened walls. The process culminates in biliary obstruction, bacterial infection, and biliary and portal cirrhosis.

Sclerosing cholangitis occurs occasionally in persons with Crohn's disease, ulcerative colitis, Riedel's struma of the thyroid, and lymphoma, suggesting immunopathy as a factor in the pathogenesis. Persons with AIDS develop papillary stenosis and sclerosing cholangitis and present with acalculous cholecystitis. In addition to the immunopathy, CMV has been demonstrated within and isolated from the diseased mucosa cells of the biliary duct in patients with AIDS and sclerosing cholangitis. The localized biliary tract infection with CMV appears in AIDS accompanied by disseminated CMV infection. This complication of AIDS supports a pathogenic role of immunodeficiency in sclerosing cholangitis and suggests that other obligate intracellular pathogens also may

initiate damage in the biliary tract that terminates in sclerosing cholangitis. In order to unravel the pathogenicity of sclerosing cholangitis, specimens should be collected at the time of surgery or endoscopy for viral studies particularly in patients with atypical cholangitis and other disease, such as cholangiocarcinoma.

Sclerosing cholangitis also occurs in children following duodenal infection with *Giardia, Ascaris,* and *Strongyloides.* Inadequate antiparasitic therapy or reinfection causes chronic duodenitis, lymphadenitis, and an inflammatory mass adjacent to the duodenum and distal portion of the CBD. The resulting intermittent obstruction causes ascending cholangitis, pericholangitis, and fibrosis. The clinical manifestations are repeated episodes of fever, abdominal pain, hepatosplenomegaly, jaundice, and abnormal serum levels of hepatic enzymes. This syndrome resembles chronic active hepatitis. The diagnosis is usually made during surgery, which offers the most effective means of eliminating the obstruction—a choledochojejunostomy.

Caroli's disease is an autorecessive trait causing multifocal dilatations of the segmental bile ducts and resulting in ectasias and cysts. The biliary ectasia may be diffuse or localized. Spontaneous bacterial cholangitis is the presenting illness as late as 5 to 20 years of age. Prognosis is poor and death ensues 5 to 10 years after the onset of acute cholangitis.

Diagnosis and Management

The clinical and laboratory manifestations of sclerosing cholangitis vary considerably, depending on the underlying disease. In sclerosing cholangitis, Charcot's triad prevails, but gallstones are not the cause of biliary obstruction. Acute bacterial cholangitis frequently is precipitated by endoscopy or surgery, except in Caroli's disease when it may be the presenting illness. Liver enlargement or a palpable gallbladder is often present on examination. Abdominal tenderness in the epigastrium or RUQ of the abdomen is associated with elevated levels of serum bilirubin (direct), alkaline phosphatase, hepatic transaminases, and γ-glutamyl transpeptidase but normal bilirubinemia. Ultrasound study of the upper abdomen is most productive. In absence of signs of stones, grossly dilated bile ducts, or intrahepatic cysts, cholangiography is indicated along with antibiotic prophylaxis. Duodenal endoscopy and retrograde cholangiopancreatography evaluate ampulla of Vater, provide bile and biopsy tissue for study, as well as demonstrate patency or obstruction of the biliary tree. The specimens obtained should be studied for malignancy, bacteria, virus, and parasites.

If the endoscopy and cholangiogram reveal papillary stenosis, dilated CBD, and sclerosed cholangioles in a patient at risk for or proven to be a carrier of human immunodeficiency virus (HIV), a superimposed CMV infection should be considered. The subchondral pain and tenderness may be relieved promptly by biliary tract decompression accomplished by transendoscopic sphincterotomy of the distal CBD. If the gallbladder is distended, cholecystectomy provides permanent relief from pain. Antibiotics specific for bacterial opportunistic infections should be combined with ganciclovir (DHPG) when biopsy reveals cytopathology consistent with CMV or the patient has extensive retinitis. Initial therapy of 2.5 mg per kilogram every 8 hours for 10 to 20 days, followed by prolonged suppressant doses of 5 mg per kilogram per day for 5 to 7 days per week indefinitely are essential in a patient with AIDS. Patients receiving DHPG require monitoring for bone marrow suppression.

Children with symptoms resembling chronic progressive hepatitis, yet equivocal findings in needle biopsy, and previous intestinal parasites should be studied for distal CBD obstruction. Ultrasonography may reveal liver enlargement without dilated bile ducts or gallstones. Endoscopy and ERCP, with periprocedural antibiotic prophylaxis, may confirm obstruction or stenosis of the distal CBD and demonstrate irregular narrowing of its lumen proximally due to chronic inflammation. Choledochojejunostomy is the surgical procedure of choice. These children are acutely and chronically ill and need intensive supportive and antimicrobial therapy pre- and postoperatively. Piperacillin, aminoglycoside, and metronidazole initiated prior to surgery provide a synergistic effect against the most likely bacterial and protozoan pathogens until specific microbes are identified. The prognosis is excellent if biliary tract obstruction is relieved permanently.

Patients with Caroli's disease usually present with acute bacterial cholangitis. Ten to 20 recurrences each year may follow the initial episode. Intensive antibiotic therapy for the infection should be initiated and ultrasound studies of the abdomen should be done. The finding of multiple cysts of varying size and the history are diagnostic of Caroli's disease. Neither antibiotics nor surgical therapy is curative. Antibiotic effect is impaired by polymicrobial infection, multiple intrahepatic biliary tract obstructions, and multiple noncommunicating cysts. Many of the cysts contain stones. Surgery is only palliative and can only drain the larger cysts by converting them to bilioenterostomies. Gallstones in cysts adjacent the liver surface may be removed by transhepatic lithotomy. Although optimal surgical drainage is impossible, suppressant antibiotic using orally administered preparations such as ciprofloxacin, ampicillin, and trimethoprim-sulfamethoxazole reduces the frequency and severity of recurrent cholangitis attacks. These antibiotics are selected empirically due to the multiple sites of infection having no communication with the biliary tree.

When the cystic pathology is localized rather than diffuse, partial hepatectomy is the procedure of choice. Otherwise, total hepatectomy and liver homotransplantation are the only alternatives for cure.

Oriental Cholangiohepatitis

Definition

Oriental cholangiohepatitis is a form of recurrent pyogenic cholangitis that occurs in 20 to 40 year-old men and women in or from Hong Kong, Taiwan, and Southeast Asia. The etiology is not known. The initial pathology is obstruction by a fibrotic stricture of the intrahepatic bile duct near the junction of its right and left tributaries. This process may have been initiated earlier by infection or trauma. Dilatations of bile ducts, stasis, stones, and cysts are present above

and below the stricture. The common bile duct is thickened, dilated, and filled with stones. The ampulla of Vater and the sphincter of Oddi are patulous. This may be the reason for preclinical asymptomatic bacteriocholia and the prodigious bacterial counts during illness.

The clinical presentation is similar to that of recurring, simple, obstructive cholangitis. During an acute attack jaundice usually develops, and severe general abdominal tenderness and guarding prevent localization of the site of infection. Ultrasonography usually demonstrates biliary tree dilatation, stones, and gallbladder distention, but CT provides clearer definition of the hepatic pathology. Gas may be demonstrated in the biliary tract by abdominal x-ray films, particularly if anaerobes or *Proteus* species are present. Percutaneous transhepatic cholangiography should be avoided or delayed until signs of infection have subsided.

Management

Medical and surgical protocols for therapy are as described for ascending pyogenic cholangitis. Complications are more frequent than in simple obstructive cholangitis and include liver abscess, subphrenic abscess, empyema, ruptured gallbladder, bile peritonitis, biliary enteric fistulae, and thrombophlebitis of the hepatic vein.

Surgery should be delayed until toxemia and fever have been controlled, unless the patient continues to deteriorate. The location for emergent biliary drainage (stricture above the bile duct) should be decided from results of ultrasound or CT studies, but surgery may be required to localize obstruction in some cases in spite of the danger of contaminated bile spilling into the peritoneal cavity. The surgical objective is to obtain effective and permanent uninhibited bile flow. Choledochojejunostomy is the most effective surgical procedure. Strictures in bile duct should be dilated, and stones and sludge should be removed. Cholecystectomy is done to prevent further stone formation and perforation of the gallbladder. Transhepatic lithotomy, cyst drainage, and hepaticojejunostomy proximal to the bile duct obstruction are corrections required. Surgical access to the biliary tree via a biliary-enteric bypass should be made to provide endoscopic stone removal, stricture dilatation, or stenting if obstruction reoccurs.

Pancreatitis

Pancreatitis associated with biliary tract infection is usually less severe but as common as that associated with alcohol. In many instances the inflammation is transient, resulting from partial obstruction of the duct of Wirsung during passing of a stone via the ampulla of Vater. Occasionally, it may be chronic, associated with persisting infection about the distal CBD, as in a child with duodenal parasites. In the latter, the biliary tract obstruction, rather than mild pancreatitis, provokes most of the symptoms. Diagnosis is dependent on serum amylase elevations and the ultrasound image. ERCP is preferred by some as the diagnostic procedure since transendoscopic sphincterotomy may relieve the obstruction in the ampulla of Vater and the pancreatic duct. Surgery is the treatment of choice if granuloma or tumor is compressing the pancreatic and common bile ducts.

Hematogenous pancreatitis occurs in disseminated infections that embolize the pancreas and create cellulitis or abscesses. Therapy requires intensive and specific antibiotic therapy. *Staphylococcus aureus*, *E. coli*, *Cryptococcus neoformans*, group A streptococci, *Klebsiella*, and *Candida* species require intensive parenteral therapy and appropriate incision and drainage of the primary sites of infection. The patients need monitoring of blood sugars during and after infection for early diagnosis of diabetes mellitus.

Surgical drainage of pancreatic pseudocysts resulting from acute chronic pancreatitis is complicated by peritonitis and intra-abdominal abscess due to released enzymes and secondary infection, usually hospital acquired. Nosocomial strains of *Pseudomonas*, *Serratia*, *Acinetobacter*, and *Klebsiella* resist commonly used antibiotics. Piperacillin or imipenem combined with aminoglycoside provides specific therapy. It is essential to recognize recurrent peritoneal abscesses clinically and by CT. Prompt and repeated drainage by needle or laparotomy and smear and culture of exudate are necessary to sustain effective antibiotic therapy. Suppressant therapy using ciprofloxacin orally, ceftriaxone, or other third-generation cephalosporins intramuscularly is continued for several weeks after fever abates to prevent recurrent localized intraperitoneal infections.

Liver Abscess

When acute or chronic febrile illness occurs following cholecystectomy, an extra- or intrahepatic abscess should be suspect, as well as cholangitis. Drainage is necessary if CT or liver-spleen scan confirms the presence of an abscess. An abscess if often accessible to needle aspiration under CT guidance. Percutaneous needle aspiration should be done under antibiotic coverage, such as piperacillin alone or combined with an aminoglycoside, since the bacteria causing the complication are most likely resistant to the previously employed antibiotics. The initial aspirate of the abscess provides excellent material for microbiologic study. Adequate drainage options are by CT-guided pigtail catheter emplacement or open surgery. Surgical drainage is preferred to needle aspiration when multiple macroabscesses are demonstrated within the liver. Ciprofloxacin, ampicillin, and chloramphenicol are effective orally as single antibiotics if the bacteria isolated are sensitive and adequate drainage is assured.

The liver is in jeopardy of infection from bacteremia in addition to that from pyogenic cholangitis or post-cholecystectomy infection. Systemic infection with *S. aureus*, β-hemolytic streptococci, yeasts, or fungi may gain access by the hepatic artery and occasionally retrograde from hepatic vein thrombophlebitis. Intra-abdominal infections such as ruptured appendix, diverticulitis, or pericolic abscess may result in multiple abscesses from portal vein thrombophlebitis (pylephlebitis). Amebic liver abscess occurs in persons with asymptomatic colon infections with *Entamoeba histolytica*. Localized bacterial infections in the liver may follow accidents resulting in liver trauma and subsequent cryptogenic bacteremia. The diagnosis of liver abscess is suggested by acute or chronic febrile illness, anorexia, weight loss, and tender, enlarged liver. A chest roentgenogram revealing elevation of the anterior portion of the right diaphragm with or without infiltration in the lower lobe occasionally suggests the diagnosis. Abdominal ultrasonographic liver-spleen scan using technetium-sulfur colloid and gallium scan are diagnostic. CT is more prompt and precise in defining size and location of abscesses.

Management

Therapy of pyogenic abscess within or adjacent to the liver consists of determining etiology of systemic infection and administration of specific antibiotics against bacteria, protozoa, or fungi. Aggressive drainage, surgically or by percutaneous needle aspiration under CT guidance, is necessary to confirm etiology.

E. histolytica liver abscess is suspect in a patient with an illness several weeks in duration and consisting of low-grade fever, night sweats, anorexia, and weight loss. Physical findings include tender, enlarged liver, right anterior subcostal pain on deep breathing, and right-sided inspiratory lag. Leukocytosis with left shift, high level of serum alkaline phosphatase, and moderately increased AST are usually present. If liver-spleen scan and CT suggest a large intrahepatic abscess and CT-guided needle aspiration produces red-brown opaque material having no odor and no microorganisms by wet or stained preparations or culture, the syndrome is characteristic of an amebic abscess. A pig-tailed catheter with side holes should be inserted immediately and the abscess emptied. Further drainage is usually unnecessary. Metronidazole intravenously or orally should be given perioperatively while results of bacterial smear and culture and serologic test results against antigens of *E. histolytica* are awaited. In contrast, if the aspirate is malodorous, has an "anchovy sauce" appearance, and contains coccal and rod-shaped bacteria, the primary etiology may be *E. histolytica* associated with enteric anaerobes. Metronidazole should be given, but in combination with piperacillin, ampicillin, chloramphenicol, or clindamycin. Piperacillin or chloramphenicol with metronidazole is our preferred regimen. *E. histolytica* abscess may be treated also with chloroquine, 1 g orally daily for 2 days then 500 mg for 20 days. Emetine, up to 60 mg per day intramuscularly for 14 days, is effective but is cardiotoxic and the patient should be at bed rest. It is used only if chloroquine is not tolerated. Initial aspiration of nonputrid abscess and continued metronidazole therapy is followed by rapid convalescence. Neither surgical nor indwelling tube drainage is necessary. Metronidazole, 2 g per day orally, is continued for 3 weeks. When anaerobes are present, tube drainage and antibiotics should be continued until odor and bacteria disappear. Metronidazole should be continued for 3 weeks or longer. The patient is followed until the abscess has resolved by CT, usually for 3 to 4 months.

Patients who are immunocompromised may have multiple abscesses, too small and numerous to drain mechanically. These are the result of disseminated disease due to candidiasis, yeast phase of other fungi, *Mycobacteria tuberculosis*, or atypical mycobacteria. Disseminated mycoses and tuberculosis causing miliary granulomata may occur as primary disease in persons without evidence of deficient cellular or humoral immunity. However, miliary abscesses rather than granulomas constitute the pathology in most persons with AIDS. Remittant fever, leukopenia, or rarely leukocytosis, and abnormal levels of liver transaminases are indications for liver biopsy, cytopathology, and staining and culture for fungi, acid-fast bacilli, and other bacteria. The results of liver biopsy studies provide specific diagnoses much earlier than do findings from studies of bronchial washings, spinal fluid, and urine or lung roentgenograms of miliary densities or infiltrates.

Yeast and fungal dissemination demand intensive intravenous therapy using amphotericin B in single daily infusions given over 2 to 3 hours. The dosage is based on the minimal inhibitory concentration as determined in vitro. Daily infusions are necessary until fever abates. Thereafter, alternative-day therapy at no longer than 36- to 40-hour intervals are continued for 6 to 12 weeks, depending on the clinical response. *Candida* species are usually most sensitive (less than 0.8 μg per milliliter) and respond to 20 mg in 250 ml of 5 percent dextrose in water intravenously per day within 3 weeks. Histoplasmosis, blastomycosis, cryptococcosis, and sporotrichosis require 30 to 35 mg in 500 mg dextrose in water 5 percent per day, but 2 to 3 months' therapy is necessary. Coccidioidomycosis and mucormycosis require 50 to 75 mg per day, as tolerated. Most patients tolerate amphotericin B best if the therapeutic dose is attained slowly over 3 to 5 days. Those with severe acute and progressive illness, having received an initial 1-mg dose without hypotension, must receive increased dosage at 6- to 12-hour intervals until the therapeutic dose is attained. When fever, hypotension, and nausea follow a given increment in dose, the drug should be repeated within 6 hours with premedication, using first 25 to 50 mg up to 100 mg hydrocortisone by intravenous bolus. This reduces adverse effects and usually permits progression of amphotericin B to the desired daily dosage. Meperidine, antihistamines, or hydrocortisone should not be mixed with the amphotericin B but given as premedication. (See also *Antifungal Chemotherapy*.)

Combined isoniazid (INH) 300 mg per day, rifampin 600 mg per day orally, and streptomycin 500 mg twice daily intramuscularly are effective against most isolates of *M. tuberculosis* and *M. kansasii*. However atypical mycobacteria, particularly the *M. avium* complex (MAC), resist the first- and most second-line antituberculosis agents. It is impossible to differentiate the resistant atypical strains from sensitive *M. tuberculosis* by morphology alone. For this reason acutely ill persons with acid-fast organisms in liver biopsy should receive INH and rifampin orally plus amikacin intravenously or, if resistance to these drugs is suspected, with ansamycin and INH plus ciprofloxacin until identification has been accomplished. (See discussions of disseminated mycobacterial infections elsewhere in this volume.)

Acute or subacute hepatitis or hepatocellular infection occurs with systemic viral infections in children and adults. Often anorexia, nausea, abdominal pain, and jaundice occur for several days as part of an acute febrile illness with or without an exanthem. Enlarged cervical nodes and hepatosplenomegaly are associated with increased liver enzymes and bilirubin in the liver. Diagnosis is made clinically for the most part, since identifying a virus as the etiologic agent is expensive and is usually not essential. Currently available are acyclovir, gancyclovir, and ribavirin, which are specific against herpesvirus types 1 and 2, cytomegalovirus, and respiratory syncytial virus, respectively (see chapter on viral diseases). The availability of antiviral agents provides a greater incentive to identify the etiologic virus by serologic and/or isolation procedures or the presence of gene protein fragments in tissue. At present only supportive measures are indicated for patients with hepatitis as part of a viral syndrome. However if herpesvirus is identified and disease is progressive, acyclovir intravenously should be initiated (see also *Antiviral Chemotherapy* and *Acquired Immunodeficiency Syndrome*.)

Acknowledgment. The authors wish to thank Walker A. Long, M.D., for editing and Ms. Carolyn T. Sellars for word processing the manuscript.

SUGGESTED READING

Kevin H, Jones RB, Chowdhury L, Kabins S. Acalculous cholecystitis and cytomegalovirus infection in acquired immunodeficiency syndrome. Ann Intern Med 1986; 104:53–54.

Sackmann M, Delius M, Sauerbruch T, et al. Shock-wave lithotripsy of gallbladder stones. N Engl J Med 1988; 318:393–397.

Schiff L, Schiff ER, eds. Diseases of the liver. 6th ed. Particularly sections 42 (Warren K, Williams CI, Tan E); 11 (Zimmon DS); 12 (Pereiras R); and 1 (Rappaport AM). Philadelphia: JB Lippincott, 1987.

Schneiderman D, Cello JP, Laing FC. Papillary stenosis and sclerosing cholangitis in acquired immunodeficiency syndrome. Ann Intern Med 1987; 106:546–549.

Spies JB, Rosen RJ, Lebowitz AS. Antibiotic prophylaxis in vascular and interventional radiology: a rational approach. Radiology 1988; 166:381–387.

Stewart L, Smith AL, Pellegrini C, Matson RW, Way LW. Pigment gallstones form as a composite of bacterial microcolonies and pigment solids. Ann Surg 1987; 206:242–249.

Winkler AP, Gleich S. Acute acalculous cholecystitis caused by *Salmonella typhi* in an 11-year old. Pediatr Infect Dis 1988; 7:125–128.

Young LS, Berlin CG, Inderlied CB. Activity of ciprofloxacin and other fluorinated quinolones against mycobacteria. Am J Med 1987; 82: (Suppl 4A):23.

Young LS, Inderlied CB, Berlin CG, Gottlieb MS. Mycobacterial infections in AIDS patients with an emphasis on the *Mycobacterium avium* complex. Rev Infect Dis 1986; 8:1024.

VIRAL HEPATITIS

DAVID J. GOCKE, M.D.

DIFFERENTIAL DIAGNOSIS

When faced with a patient with jaundice and/or hepatic enzyme abnormalities, one needs first to decide whether the patient has one of the classic forms of viral hepatitis or is suffering from liver injury due to some other cause. Hepatic injury of an acute nature (i.e., evolving over days rather than weeks or months) can be caused by nonviral as well as viral agents. Chief among the nonviral causes is acute alcoholic hepatitis, which is common and usually accompanied by evidence of intoxication or binge drinking. Chemically induced hepatic injury is also fairly frequent and should be revealed by a careful medication and environmental history. Other nonviral etiologies such as biliary obstruction or metastatic carcinoma may occasionally present rather acutely, but the diagnosis is usually suggested by other accompanying features.

Among viral causes of acute hepatic injury, one must consider in the differential diagnosis the occasional case of severe infectious mononucleosis due to the Epstein-Barr virus, which may cause enzyme elevations and, rarely, jaundice. Almost invariably such patients have florid disease with fever, lymphadenopathy, and splenomegaly, which makes the diagnosis obvious. A mononucleosis-like illness with a negative mononucleosis test is due to cytomegalovirus infection and can also be associated with hepatic injury. This may be more confusing because the serologic test is negative, but again, the hepatic manifesta-

tions are usually minor compared with the systemic features. Other viruses (and, for that matter, other infectious agents) cause liver injury so rarely as to be negligible in the scope of this discussion.

Having considered the above possible causes of acute hepatic injury and concluded that one of the hepatitis viruses is the most likely etiology, the next step is to differentiate one type of viral hepatitis from another. This is not just an academic exercise because knowledge of the particular hepatitis virus responsible for the illness has important epidemiologic and therapeutic implications in management of the patient. Clinical and epidemiologic features of the illness may suggest that one or another of the hepatitis viruses is responsible. Some of these features are summarized in Table 1. However, there is considerable variation and overlap with regard to these features and, in the individual case, one must depend on serology to make a specific diagnosis.

In the past 20 years, the discovery of specific viral antigens and antibodies associated with type A and type B hepatitis viruses and development of reliable, widely available tests for these markers now permit specific differentiation of these two infections. In addition, clinical application of these tests has led, by a process of exclusion, to the recognition of so-called non-A, non-B (NANB) hepatitis, a serious form of hepatitis previously unappreciated. Even more recently, the discovery of the Delta hepatitis agent has revealed another new and important facet of viral hepatitis. Figure 1 illustrates the process involved in the serologic differentiation of acute viral hepatitis. The results of these sensitive, specific, and reliable assays for antibody to the hepatitis A virus (anti-HAV) and to the hepatitis B markers (HBsAg, anti-HBs, and anti-HBc) are usually available within 48 to 72 hours.

TABLE 1   Clinical and Epidemiologic Features in Viral Hepatitis

Type	Source	Risk Factors or Settings	Significance
Hepatitis A	Ingestion of contaminated food or water	Shellfish Day-care centers Institutions for retarded Prisons Male homosexuality Foreign travel	Often anicteric Usually self-limited Rarely fatal ($< 1\%$) No carrier state No chronic infection Requires public health intervention
Hepatitis B	Parenteral inoculation of contaiminated blood or blood products; sexual contact	Transfusion of blood or blood products Drug abuse Male homosexuality Sexual contact Health care professions Institutions for retarded Prisons	Often icteric High morbidity May be fulminant (1%–2%) 6%–10% become carriers and/or develop chronic hepatitis Hepatoma
Non-A, Non-B hepatitis	As for hepatitis B	As for hepatitis B	May be icteric May be fulminant 20%–60% become carriers and/or develop chronic hepatitis
Delta hepatitis	As for hepatitis B (Delta infection requires "help" from HBV, always occurs in patient concomitantly infected with HBV)	Transfusion of blood or blood products Drug abuse	Requires coinfection with HBV Increases severity of liver damage → fulminant hepatitis → death (10%–20%) → progressive chronic active hepatitis

As with most infectious diseases, the finding of viral antigen in the patient's serum usually indicates acute infection with the agent. Thus, the finding of a positive test for HBsAg in the serum of a patient with acute hepatic injury very likely signifies acute hepatitis B infection. One caveat to this is the occasional HBsAg-positive patient with what appears to be an acute process who is actually having an acute exacerbation of an underlying, previously unrecognized chronic form of hepatitis B. This exception may not become apparent without long-term follow-up of the patient and/or liver biopsy, but does not alter management for the acute episode. The presence of antibody to the infectious agent may represent either recent infection or prior exposure to the agent that is unrelated to the current illness. Differentiation of IgM and IgG components of the antibody response helps to distinguish recent from remote exposure. Thus, a positive test for anti-HAV predominantly of the IgM type is strongly suggestive of current HAV infection, whereas an IgG or mixed IgG/IgM response probably represents only prior exposure. Of the tests for hepatitis B virus (HBV) markers, detection of a positive anti-HBc in the presence of a negative anti-HBs is often useful in differentiating hepatitis B in the acute phase because the anti-HBc response appears earlier during the acute illness than the anti-HBs response, which may not be seen until the patient has recovered. When both the anti-HBc and anti-HBs are positive, this finding is compatible with either remote exposure to HBV unrelated to the current illness or with the late convalescent phase of an acute HBV infection. Thus, these tests always need to be interpreted in terms of the point in the patient's course when the blood was tested. Of course, documentation of recent seroconversion from negative to positive for any of the antibody tests is also strong evidence of recent infection. Finally, the tests for hepatitis Be antigen (HBeAg) and antibody (anti-HBe) are usually reserved for evaluation of patients with chronic forms of hepatitis B (see below).

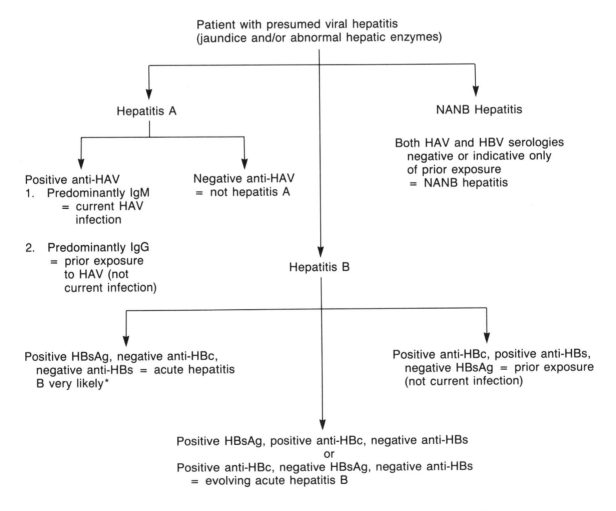

* Occasionally (~5%–10%) patients presenting with apparent acute hepatitis B are acutally having an acute exacerbation of an underlying chronic hepatitis B (see text).

Figure 1 Schema for serologic differentiation of acute viral hepatitis.

The significance of making a specific diagnosis of hepatitis A is that one can be assured the patient will almost always recover without serious sequelae. Chronic forms of hepatitis and the carrier state are essentially unheard of with this disease, and fulminant hepatitis is rare. However, this diagnosis should prompt epidemiologic investigation for the source of infection and institution of appropriate control measures (as discussed below). A diagnosis of hepatitis B, on the other hand, has more serious implications. The patient is more likely to be hospitalized or incapacitated for an extended time and has a significant chance of developing a major complication of HBV infection (fulminant disease, chronic hepatitis, the carrier state, hepatoma). These problems demand careful follow-up and proper management. Also, identification of contacts and immunization procedures need to be considered, as outlined below.

If a diagnosis of neither hepatitis A or B can be established after applying the above criteria, then one has arrived at a diagnosis of NANB hepatitis by exclusion. Obviously, this is not a specific way to make a diagnosis, but lacking tests for specific markers of the NANB agents, it is the best we can do at present. Occasionally, a case may be misdiagnosed in this manner, but this exclusion process is probably accurate at least 90 percent of the time. Clearly, NANB hepatitis is a real entity. At least two types of NANB agents have been demonstrated by epidemiologic and transmission studies, but these are not usually differentiated in the clinical setting at present. The major significance of establishing a diagnosis of NANB hepatitis is that it alerts the physician to the development of chronic disease, which occurs with disturbing frequency (20% to 60% of patients in various studies) and which requires appropriate follow-up and management.

Delta hepatitis is a newly discovered form of hepatitis caused by a defective or incomplete RNA virus that cannot produce infection by itself. This agent has an absolute requirement for coinfection with HBV, which provides essential help for replication of the Delta agent. Delta infection always occurs in a person who is concomitantly infected with HBV, either chronically or acutely. Delta "superinfection" may make an acute hepatitis much more severe (leading to fulminant hepatitis) or may exacerbate chronic hepatitis B (leading to early cirrhosis and hepatic insufficiency). Tests for Delta antigen and antibody are not yet widely available, but may appear in the next year or two.

MANAGEMENT

General Recommendations

When first seen, the course of the patient with presumed viral hepatitis is still unpredictable. Many recover uneventfully. Others develop serious, life-threatening complications that cannot be predicted at the outset. There is no specific antiviral therapy at present, but good management involves much more than benign neglect.

Early Recognition of Impending Hepatic Insufficiency. The syndrome of fulminant hepatitis leading to hepatic insufficiency, coma, and death is the least common but most dreaded complication of viral hepatitis. It occurs in less than 1 percent of patients with hepatitis A, in 1 to 2 percent of patients with hepatitis B or NANB hepatitis, and in 10 to 20 percent of hepatitis B patients superinfected with the Delta agent. Once coma occurs, the survival rate is only 30 to 40 percent in experienced centers, even with optimal care. The key to successful management is early recognition—before coma supervenes. The best predictor of impending hepatic insufficiency is the prothrombin time, which should be ordered along with the bilirubin, hepatic enzymes, and viral markers as a part of the initial evaluation. The levels of bilirubin, hepatic enzymes, and blood ammonia are not reliable guides, but if the prothrombin time is increased, especially if more than 20 seconds, the possibility that the patient will progress to full-blown hepatic insufficiency and coma is great. Deterioration can occur in a few hours, so close observation is required. The aim should be to start anticholemic measures (consult standard texts for details) before coma develops, rather than after.

When to Hospitalize the Patient with Hepatitis. There are only two indications for hospitalization of a patient with acute viral hepatitis. One is an elevated prothrombin time, as discussed above. The other is the patient with severe nausea and vomiting who is unable to maintain fluid balance or who is so weak and incapacitated as to be unable to care for himself at home. Most patients with acute hepatitis can and should be cared for at home in order to avoid unnecessary exposure of hospital staff and utilization of expensive hospital beds.

Isolation? All forms of viral hepatitis are capable of person-to-person transmission and certainly represent a hazard. In the hospital setting, both stool and needle/syringe precautions should be employed until the type and stage of hepatitis is defined (usually within 72 hours) and then modified along the following lines. Type A hepatitis is essentially never viremic in the acute phase (so serum precautions are not needed), and virus disappears from the stool very early in the acute phase (so even stool precautions are not needed in the convalescent phase). Types B and NANB require only needle/syringe precautions (not stool), but it is especially important that specimens sent to the laboratory and contaminated waste material be double-bagged and flagged to protect hospital personnel. A private room in the hospital is usually not necessary, unless the patient is a perambulatory child, has a bleeding diathesis, or is incontinent of stool or urine.

In the home setting, knowledge of the type and stage of hepatitis is also a guide. For hepatitis A, the patient should practice careful hand washing and good personal hygiene and avoid preparation of food for other family members. Decontamination of clothing, linen, and dishes can be satisfactorily achieved with conventional washing machines and dishwashers. Bear in mind that by the time the patient presents to a physician and a diagnosis is established, the virus has usually disappeared from the stool. Once the bilirubin and enzymes begin to decline in hepatitis A, isolation is no longer necessary. With hepatitis B and NANB, however, viremia may persist for weeks, months, or years, even though the bilirubin and enzymes are improving. Such patients may transmit disease. With hepatitis B, as long as the patient's blood contains HBsAg, he must be regarded as potentially infectious. In HBV infection, the presence of HBeAg in the serum is known to be associated with a high degree of infectivity, whereas patients with anti-HBe are much less infective, but this is only relative. For NANB hepatitis, since there is no antigenic marker to follow, one can be guided only by persistent enzyme elevations. The primary hazards for transmission of both type B and NANB disease in the home setting are close personal contact (usually sexual) and the sharing of toothbrushes, razors, and other articles that may be blood contaminated. Thus, it is the spouse or sexual partner who is at greatest risk of acquiring the infection and should be evaluated for evidence of infection and immunized if not already infected. Other members of the household are at much lower risk, except in special situations (a home dialysis patient, communal intravenous drug abuse, open wounds). Recommendations on immunization for hepatitis B are given below.

Diet. During the acute anorectic phase of viral hepatitis, the primary concern should be maintenance of caloric intake and fluid and electrolyte balance, orally, if possible, or with intravenous supplements, if necessary. Otherwise, the patient need only be instructed to eat and drink what appeals to him. As nausea subsides and appetite returns, most patients resume an adequate intake. The old idea of urging high-carbohydrate, high-calorie diets on an anorectic patient is counterproductive and has never been shown to hasten hepatic recovery. As noted above, if impending hepatic coma is suspected, protein restriction (20 g per day) or elimination (a no-protein diet) may be indicated.

Alcohol and Other Drugs. Alcohol is a direct hepatic toxin and acts in an additive fashion with viral hepatic injury. Alcohol should be strictly prohibited, not only in the acute phase but until the enzymes have returned to normal. Also, remember that the half-life of medications metabolized in the liver may be prolonged. Sedatives and tranquilizers should especially be avoided.

Activity. There is no evidence that strict bed rest speeds recovery in the average patient. However, most patients with hepatitis do not feel like doing much. Thus, limited activity around the home is advisable, but confinement to bed is unnecessary. The patient should be cautioned to resume normal activity only gradually and as tolerated. In some cases, the patient may not recover his usual stamina and well-being for 3 to 6 months.

Steroids. Corticosteroids are not indicated in the management of acute hepatitis of any type. Although steroids make the patient feel better transiently, they do not alter the ultimate course of the disease, may prolong full recovery, and are often associated with serious rebound hepatitis when discontinued.

Problems to Look for. Early recognition and treatment of impending hepatic insufficiency has been discussed above. As the acute phase passes and improvement begins, the next question is whether the patient will develop persistent infection, either in the form of an asymptomatic carrier state or some form of chronic hepatitis. As noted previously, this is rare with hepatitis A, but 6 to 10 percent of patients with hepatitis B and 20 to 60 percent with NANB develop some form of persistent infection. Thus, periodic follow-up (every 2 to 4 weeks) is indicated until it can be documented that the hepatic enzymes have returned to normal and stay normal and, in the case of hepatitis B, that HBs antigenemia has cleared. In some cases, this requires several months, during which time the comments made above about potential infectivity, alcohol prohibition, and activity still apply. An error commonly made in patients whose enzymes are still abnormal after 2 to 3 months is the unwarranted institution of steroid therapy. After 6 months, however, if the enzymes are still abnormal, liver biopsy is indicated. The management of chronic forms of hepatitis is beyond the scope of this discussion. Suffice it to say here that this is a difficult and controversial area that should be handled by an experienced hepatologist.

Specific Recommendations on Immunization

Guidelines for hepatitis immunization are given in Table 2.

Hepatitis. There is no hepatitis A vaccine available at present (although a candidate vaccine is currently in clinical trials and may be available in 1 to 2 years). Pools of normal human serum globulin (NSG) contain significant antibody to HAV and will prevent or ameliorate HAV infection if given within 2 weeks of exposure. Postexposure prophylaxis for close contacts of patients with hepatitis A and for individuals exposed in common-source outbreaks of hepatitis A is clearly indicated. The definition of ''close contact'' should be limited to members of the same household, not to entire schools, offices, neighborhoods, or social contacts. Preexposure prophylaxis of hepatitis A is indicated for travelers to areas of the world highly endemic for hepatitis A (basically, all the underdeveloped countries). The recommended dose of NSG is 0.04 ml per kilogram. In the event of continuing exposure, as with prolonged travel in endemic areas, this dose should be repeated every 3 to 4 months.

Hepatitis B. A safe, highly effective hepatitis B vaccine is now widely available. It is clearly indicated in persons at high risk of developing hepatitis B, i.e., those with exposure to contaminated blood and blood products. This includes susceptible health care workers (including surgeons, dentists, pathologists, and clinical laboratory workers), male homosexuals, and household contacts of hepatitis B patients. Regarding household contacts, if the patient is a chronic hepatitis B carrier (so that exposure may be prolonged), both active immunization with the hepatitis B vaccine and passive immunization with hepatitis B immune globulin (HBIG) are indicated for the susceptible contacts. This combination of passive/active immunization confers immediate protection from the

TABLE 2   Summary of Hepatitis Immunization Recommendations

	Vaccine		Immune Globulin	
	Setting	Dose	Setting	Dose
Hepatitis A	(vaccine not currently available)		Postexposure: household contacts common-source outbreaks	0.04 ml IG/kg IM
			Preexposure: travel to endemic area	0.04 ml IG/kg IM every 4-6 months
Hepatitis B	Postexposure: sexual contact* neonatal* Preexposure: risk of blood contact	} 3 doses† 20 µg each IM at 0, 1, and 6 months	Postexposure: needle stick sexual contact* neonatal Preexposure: not indicated (use vaccine)	0.06 ml HBIG/kg IM
Non-A, Non-B hepatitis	(Vaccine not currently available)		Postexposure: ? needle stick ? neonatal Preexposure: not indicated	0.04 ml IG/kg IM (controversial!)

Note: Abbreviations. IG = normal serum globulin: HBIG = hepatitis-B immune globulin.
*Use combined active/passive immunization with both HB vaccine and HBIG.
†Dose in children < 12 years old = 10 µg each injection.

HBIG pending later development of active immunity from the vaccine. This is especially important for sexual contacts of the infected carrier. This passive/active immunization against hepatitis B is also now the recommended approach for neonates born to HBsAg-positive mothers. To determine the susceptibility of contacts, and to rule out ongoing HBV infection, these individuals should be tested for anti-HBc, HBsAg, and hepatic enzyme levels. The presence of HBsAg and/or abnormal enzymes indicates current infection, whereas the presence of anti-HBc with negative HBsAg and normal enzymes indicates immunity. However, in any postexposure situation, early protection is important and administration of vaccine and HBIG to an individual already infected is not dangerous, so immunization should not be excessively delayed while waiting for test results. The hepatitis B vaccine must be given in three intramuscular injections (20 µg each) at 0, 1, and 6 months for optimal response. Children younger than 12 years require only half doses (10 µg each), and

immunocompromised hosts (i.e., dialysis patients) require larger doses (40 µg each). Finally, the usual dose of HBIG is 0.06 ml per kilogram.

For prophylaxis in the case of limited or one-time exposures—as in medical personnel with contaminated needle sticks, after limited sexual contact, or where the patient has promptly reverted to HBsAG-negative—adequate protection may be achieved with HBIG alone in the doses noted. In such cases, a second dose of HBIG should be given 1 month later.

Non-A, Non-B Hepatitis. There is no vaccine or hyperimmune globulin for NANB hepatitis. Whether normal serum globulin (IG) preparations contain enough antibody against NANB agents to be helpful is a controversial issue. However, since ordinary IG is inexpensive and harmless, many authorities would administer IG in high-risk situations, such as for contaminated needle sticks or the infant born of a mother with NANB hepatitis.

INFECTION CAUSED BY INTESTINAL HELMINTHS

MARTIN S. WOLFE, M.D.

Three major types of helminths occur in humans: nematodes (roundworms); cestodes (tapeworms); and trematodes (flukes). Intestinal helminths are the cause of some of the major disease problems worldwide. They are ubiquitous and must always be considered in dealing with populations in both the developing and developed world. In this chapter, the emphasis is on the therapy of infections as they occur in the United States. A broad definition of intestinal helminths is used here to cover certain parasites not discussed elsewhere that primarily localize to other organ systems such as the liver, lungs, skin, brain, or bladder.

With rare exceptions, helminths do not multiply within the human host. The majority of infected individuals, particularly in developed countries, harbor a low worm burden and have asymptomatic infections. Symptoms, when present, are usually related to the site of infection, but distant or systemic manifestations may occur with some species.

The clinical presentation and a careful geographic and travel history are the necessary first steps in consideration of helminthic infection. Intestinal helminths are generally diagnosed by examination of stools for eggs, larvae, or tapeworm segments; multiple examinations or special procedures or concentration tests may be required to confirm light infections.

For tissue-invasive flukes or tapeworms, scanning or serologic procedures may be necessary. In contrast to protozoal infections, helminths frequently cause a peripheral eosinophilia. This may be normal or mildly elevated in intestinal infections but can reach high levels in migrating or tissue-invasive stages of infection of certain species.

Most of the drugs described herein are commercially available in the United States. Some are not licensed for all indications discussed. A few drugs are not licensed in the United States but may be obtained from the Parasitic Disease Drug Service, Centers for Disease Control, Atlanta, Georgia (404–639–3670).

Summaries of oral drug therapies for these helminthic infections are given in Table 1. Relatively common adverse effects are listed in Table 2. Table 3 lists consensus safety of anthelmintic drugs in pregnancy and in younger children.

NEMATODE INFECTIONS

Ascaris lumbricoides (Roundworm)

Roundworm infection is not restricted to developing areas of the world and is present in certain areas of the southern United States. A number of safe and effective drugs are available for ascariasis. Mebendazole (Vermox) for 3 days is well tolerated and approximately 98 percent effective. This drug has not been sufficiently evaluated in children younger than age 2 years or in pregnant women for it to be recom-

mended in these situations. Pyrantel pamoate (Antiminth) in a single dose is a highly effective alternative, but adverse effects may be more common. Piperazine citrate (Antepar) in a 2-day course is a third choice. When *Ascaris* is present with another intestinal helminth, it should preferably be treated first; some drugs can cause *Ascaris* worms to migrate to unusual locations.

Hookworm Infections

The two common human species are *Necator americanus* and *Ancylostoma duodenale*, but clinical implications and therapy are similar for both. In the developing world heavy infections are commonly associated with iron deficiency anemia and with hypoproteinemia, particularly in malnourished young children. In temperate, developed areas, a distinction must be made between the less common hookworm disease with anemia and the more usual hookworm infection. Hookworm infection may be treated with anthelmintic drugs alone, while hookworm disease with anemia must also be treated with iron supplements, and in severe anemia, with transfusions. The drug of choice is mebendazole for 3 days. Pyrantel pamoate is an alternative.

Trichuris trichiura (Whipworm)

This is perhaps the commonest intestinal helminthic infection in the United States and is often associated with *Ascaris*, since both are acquired orally. Infection is usually light and asymptomatic. In the developing world, heavy whipworm infection may lead to dysentery, anemia, or rectal prolapse. Treatment is with mebendazole. Cure rates for trichuriasis are about 70 percent, but there is a 98 percent reduction in egg burden.

Anisakis Species (Anisakiasis)

Infection is from larvae ingested by eating certain species of raw, uncooked, pickled or salted fish. These larvae may cause infiltrative or mass lesions in the intestinal tract. Diagnosis is by direct observation of the characteristic tissue lesion at endoscopy and biopsy demonstrating larvae or eosinophilic granulomata. The preferred treatment is surgery. Thiabendazole (Mintezol) is considered an investigational drug that has been proven effective only in animal models.

Enterobius vermicularis (Pinworm)

This is a cosmopolitan infection, found more commonly in middle-class children in the United States than in children in developing countries. Adults, particularly parents of infected children, can also be infected. Unlike other intestinal helminths, pinworm eggs are not usually found by examination of stool specimens, but rather by obtaining specimens from the anal region. A number of simple, safe, and highly effective drugs are available for treatment, but reinfection commonly occurs. Single doses of mebendazole or pyrantel pamoate are initial choices. Pyrvinium pamoate, a cyanine dye, colors stools red and can stain clothes.

TABLE 1 Drug Therapy of Intestinal Helminths

Parasite	Drug	Adult Dose*	Pediatric Dose*	Availability
Ascaris lumbricoides	Mebendazole	100 mg b.i.d. × 3 days	Same as adult dose (>2 yr)	Vermox (Janssen) (tablets)
	or			
	Pyrantel pamoate	11 mg/kg single dose (max 1 g)	Same as adult dose (max 1 g)	Antiminth (Pfipharmics) (suspension)
	or			
	Piperazine citrate	75 mg/kg/day (max 3.5 g) × 2 days	Same as adult dose (max 3.5 g)	Antepar (Burroughs Wellcome) (syrup)
Trichuris trichiura	Mebendazole	As per Ascaris	As per Ascaris	
Hookworm	Mebendazole			
Necator americanus	or	As per Ascaris	As per Ascaris	
Ancylostoma duodenale	Pyrantel pamoate†	As per Ascaris	As per Ascaris	
Enterobius vermicularis	Mebendazole	100 mg single dose; repeat in 2 wk	Same as adult dose	
	or			
	Pyrantel pamoate	11 mg/kg single dose; repeat in 2 wk	Same as adult dose	
	or			
	Pyrvinium pamoate	5 mg/kg single dose; repeat in 2 wk	Same as adult dose (max 250 mg)	Povan (filmseals)
Strongyloides stercoralis	Thiabendazole	25 mg/kg b.i.d. × 2 days (max 3 g/day)	Same as adult dose	Mintezol (Merck, Sharp and Dohme) (suspension)
	or			
	Mebendazole†	As per Ascaris	As per Ascaris	
	or			
	Pyrvinium pamoate†	5 mg/kg once daily × 7 days (max 250 mg/day)	Same as adult dose	
Trichostrongylus species	Thiabendazole†	As per Strongyloides	As per Strongyloides	
	or			
	Pyrantel pamoate†	As per Ascaris	As per Ascaris	
	or			
	Mebendazole†	As per Ascaris	As per Ascaris	
Tapeworms				
Taenia saginata	Niclosamide	Single dose/4 tabs (2 g) chewed thoroughly	11–34 kg: single dose/2 tabs (1 g) >34 kg: single dose/3 tabs (1.5 g)	Niclocide (Miles) (tablets)
Taenia solium	or			
Diphyllobothrium latum and pacificum	Paromomycin†	1 gram q15min × 4 doses	11mg/kg q15min × 4 doses	Humatin (Parke-Davis) (capsules)
	or			
Dipylidium caninum	Praziquantel†	20 mg/kg once	Same as adult dose	Biltricide (Miles) (tablets)
Hymenolepis nana and diminuta	Niclosamide	Single 2 g/dose × 7 days	As above for other tapeworms, single dose daily × 7 days	
	or			
	Praziquantel†	25 mg/kg once	Same as adult dose	
Cerebral cysticercosis cellulosae (T. solim)	Praziquantel†	50 mg/kg/day in 3 divided doses × 14 days	Same as adult dose	
Schistosomiasis				
Schistosoma mansoni	Praziquantel†	60 mg/kg in 3 divided doses for 1 day	Same as adult dose	Biltricide (Miles) (tablets)
	or			
	Oxamniquine	Caribbean and S. American strains: 15 mg/kg single dose;	Same as adult dose	Vansil (Pfipharmics) (tablets)
		African strains: 15 mg/kg b.i.d. × 2 days	Same as adult dose	
Schistosoma japonicum	Praziquantel	As per S. mansoni	As per S. mansoni	
Schistosoma mekongi	Praziquantel	As per S. mansoni	As per S. mansoni	
Schistosoma intercalatum	Praziquantel	As per S. mansoni	As per S. mansoni	
Schistosoma haematobium	Praziquantel	As per S. mansoni	As per S. mansoni	

Table continues on the following page

TABLE 1 (*continued*)

Parasite	Drug	Adult Dose*	Pediatric Dose*	Availability
Intestinal flukes				
Fasciolopsis buski	Praziquantel[†]	25 mg/kg t.i.d.	Same as adult dose	
	or			
	Tetrachlorethylene	0.1 ml/kg single dose (max 5 ml)	Same as adult dose	Nema worm capsules Veterinary (Parke-Davis)
Heterophyes heterophyes	Praziquantel[†]	25 mg/kg t.i.d. for 1 day	Same as adult dose	
Metagonimus yokogawi	Praziquantel[†]	25 mg/kg t.i.d. for 1 day	Same as adult dose	
Liver and lung flukes				
Clonorchis sinensis *Opisthorchis viverrini*	Praziquantel[†]	25 mg/kg t.i.d. for 2 days	Same as adult dose	
Fasciola hepatica	Praziquantel[†] *or*	25 mg/kg t.i.d. for 3 to 5 days	Same as adult dose	
Paragonimus westermani	Bithionol[†] (Bitin) (capsule)	50 mg/kg on alternate days × 10 to 15 doses	Same as adult dose	Parasitic Disease Drug Service, CDC, Atlanta, Georgia

* All recommended drugs given by mouth.
† Considered an investigational drug for this purpose by the U.S. Food and Drug Administration.

It should be considered an alternative drug. It is acceptable practice to treat the entire family when at least one member is infected.

Strongyloides stercoralis (Strongyloidiasis)

This parasite can live for 30 to 40 years in an infected human host because of its unique autoinfection cycle, leading to self-perpetuating infection. The long-time presence of this often asymptomatic parasite poses a potential threat of lethal dissemination by hyperinfection if the infected individual becomes immunosuppresed or is treated with cancer chemotherapeutic drugs, radiation, or corticosteroids. It is therefore important to identify infected individuals and attempt to eradicate the infection. The current drug of choice in the United States is thiabendazole (Mintezol) given in a 2-day course. In disseminated strongyloidiasis, thiabendazole should be continued for at least 5 days.

Thiabendazole is a satisfactory but not always curative drug and is frequently not well tolerated, especially in adults. Adverse effects can include nausea, vomiting, dizziness, and, rarely, angioneurotic edema. Mebendazole is an alternative that is better tolerated but less effective. Another possible alternative that has had only little evaluation is pyrvinium pamoate. Albendazole, a new broad-spectrum anthelmintic (not yet available in the United States), has been effective

TABLE 2 Adverse Effects of Anthelmintic Drugs

Albendazole (Zentel)	Similar to mebendazole
Bithionol (Bitin)	Photosensitivity skin reactions, vomiting, diarrhea, abdominal pain, urticaria
Mebendazole (Vermox)	Occasional: diarrhea, abdominal pain
Niclosamide (Niclocide)	Occasional: nausea, abdominal pain
Oxamniquine (Vansil)	Occasional: headache, fever, dizziness, somnolence, nausea, diarrhea, rash, insomnia
Paromomycin (Humatin)	Gastrointestinal disturbance
Piperazine citrate (Antepar)	Occasional: dizziness, ataxia, urticaria, gastrointestinal disturbance
Praziquantel (Biltricide)	Sedation, dizziness, headache, abdominal discomfort
Pyrantel pamoate (Antiminth)	Gastrointestinal disturbances, headache, dizziness
Pyrvinium pamoate (Povan)	Red color to feces, staining of clothes, nausea, vomiting
Tetrachlorethylene (NEMA Worm Capsules, Veterinary)	Epigastric burning, dizziness, headache
Thiabendazole (Mintezol)	Nausea, vomiting, dizziness

TABLE 3 Safety of Anthelmintic Drugs in Pregnancy and in Young Children

Drug	Toxicity in Pregnancy	Recommendation in Pregnancy	Recommendation in Young Children
Bithionol	Experience not extensive enough to recommend in pregnancy	Caution*	Use with caution in children below age 8 yr
Mebendazole (Vermox)	Teratogenic and embryo toxic in rats	Caution*	Use with caution below age 2 yr
Niclosamide (Niclocide)	Not absorbed; no known toxicity in fetus	Probably safe	Limited experience; use with caution in children below age 2 yr
Oxamniquine (Vansil)	Embryocidal in animals	Caution*	No contraindication
Paromomycin (Humatin)	Poorly absorbed; toxicity	Probably safe	No contraindication
Piperazine citrate (Antepar)	Unknown	Best avoided at least in first trimester	No contraindication
Praziquantel (Biltricide)	Increased abortion rate in rats; no adequate studies in pregnant women	Caution*	Safety in children under age 4 yr has not been established; use caution
Pyrantel pamoate (Antiminth)	Absorbed in small amounts; no known toxicity in fetus	Probably safe	Not extensively studied in children
Pyrvinium pamoate	No studies done	Caution*	No contraindication
Tetrachlorethylene (NEMA capsules)	Caution is usually advised*	Caution*	No contraindication
Thiabendazole (Mintezol)	No well-controlled studies	Caution*	Safety and effectiveness not established in children weighing <15 kg

* Use only for strong clinical indication in absence of suitable alternative. Potential benefit should justify potential risk to fetus or young child.

against *S. stercoralis.* Ivermectin, a veterinary anthelmintic, has been highly effective against this parasite in investigational human studies.

Trichostrongylus Species (Trichostrongylosis)

This parasite is particularly common in Iran, Korea, and Indonesia, among other places. It can cause high eosinophilia and gastrointestinal symptoms in some of those infected. Thiabendazole, in doses used for strongyloidiasis, is the drug of choice. Pyrantel pamoate and mebendazole are alternative drugs. Trichostrongylosis is considered an investigational use for these drugs in the United States.

CESTODE INFECTIONS

Three of the most common intestinal cestodes (tapeworms), *Taenia saginata* (the beef tapeworm), *Diphyllobothrium latum* (the fish tapeworm), and the uncommon *Dipylidium caninum* (the dog tapeworm) are best treated with a single dose of niclosamide (Niclocide). *Hymenolepis nana* (the dwarf tapeworm) and the much less common *Hymenolepis diminuta* (the rat tapeworm) require a 7-day course of niclosamide. Niclosamide is best taken after a light breakfast. Alternatives for all the above tapeworms include praziquantel (Biltricide) and paromomycin (Humatin), but these are considered investigational drugs for these infections in the United States.

Tissue invasion of the brain or muscles with *Cysticercus cellulosa* of *T. solium* can now be treated nonsurgically with praziquantel on an investigational basis. Corticosteroids are usually given concomitantly to reduce any increase in cerebral pressure resulting from destruction of cysts. Praziquantel is not recommended for ocular cysticercosis.

Echinococcus granulosis (hydatid) cysts most frequently occur in the liver and less commonly in the lung and other organs. The treatment of choice remains surgery for resectable cysts. When surgery is contraindicated or cysts rupture spontaneously during surgery, mebendazole (experimental for this use in the United States) can be tried. Albendazole and flubendazole have also been tried investigationally with some success.

TREMATODE INFECTIONS

Schistosomiasis

The most common form of intestinal schistosomiasis seen in the United States is caused by *Schistosoma mansoni*, imported from such endemic areas as Africa, the Arabian peninsula, Brazil, and certain Caribbean islands. Rare cases of *Schistosoma japonicum* from East Asia, *Schistosoma mekongi* from Southeast Asia, and *Schistosoma intercalatum* from Central Africa may also be seen. *Schistosoma haematobium*, affecting the urinary system, is usually imported from Africa. The treatment of choice for all these species is praziquantel (Biltricide) in a single-day course. Praziquantel is highly effective and well tolerated, and all those with active schistosomiasis should be treated. Oxamniquine (Vansil) is an alternative drug for *S. mansoni* only. Somewhat higher doses of oxamniquine are required for the African versus the Caribbean and South American strains of *S. mansoni*.

Intestinal Flukes

Fasciolopsis buski, *Heterophyes heterophyes*, and *Metagonimus yokogawai* are rarely diagnosed. Frequently, infected individuals are asymptomatic. These parasites can be treated with praziquantel, which is presently an investigational drug in the United States for these indications.

Tetrachlorethylene is an alternative drug for *F. buski* infection only. Tetrachlorethylene is available only as a veterinary product (NEMA worm capsules); this should be taken on an empty stomach.

Liver Flukes

Clonorchis sinensis and *Opisthorchis viverrini* infections are not uncommon in residents of the Far East and Southeast Asia. *Fasciola hepatica* has a sporadic worldwide distribution. Praziquantel is the drug of choice for the former two parasites but is an investigational drug in the United States for these indications. Praziquantel has been successful in some but not all cases of infection due to *F. hepatica*. The definitive dose and duration of treatment with praziquantel for *F. hepatica* have not yet been determined. Bithionol (Bitin), an investigational drug in the United States, obtained from the Centers for Disease Control, is considered the drug of choice for *F. hepatica*.

Lung Fluke

Paragonimus westermani, the Asiatic lung fluke, usually presents with pulmonary lesions and clinical symptoms suggesting tuberculosis. Eggs of this parasite may be found in the stool, and rarely cerebral lesions can develop. Praziquantel is the drug of choice, with bithionol as an alternative; both of these drugs are investigational in the United States for this parasite.

TREATMENT OF PREGNANT WOMEN AND YOUNG CHILDREN

Information concerning the safety of most drugs during pregnancy and in early childhood is inadequate. Relatively few drugs have been studied in a sufficiently large population to assure complete safety. With some drugs, the only available toxicity studies have been done in animals, and the results are extrapolated for humans. Thus, recommendations for use of drugs during pregnancy and in early childhood are based on rather tenuous grounds, and the most conservative advice usually given is to avoid the drug unless the clinical indications are pressing. The greatest potential hazard is in the first trimester of pregnancy, so the later in pregnancy the drug is used, the better. Benefit versus potential hazard to the fetus must be weighed individually for each patient infected with a helminth. Fortunately, the great majority of these infections are light and cause few if any troublesome symptoms, and treatment can often be deferred until after delivery or until the child is at least 2 years of age.

Table 3 summarizes the best available information on safety of anthelmintic drugs during pregnancy and in early childhood.

SUGGESTED READING

Beaver PC, Jung RC, Cupp EW. Clinical parasitology. 9th ed. Philadelphia: Lea and Febiger, 1984.

Cline BL. Current drug regimens for the treatment of intestinal helminth infections. Med Clin North Am 1982; 66:721–742.

Davis A, Pawlowski ZS, Dixon H. Multicentre clinical trials of benzimidazolecarbamates in human echinococcosis. Bull WHO 1986; 64:383–388.

Mandell GL, Douglas RG, Bennett JE, eds. Principles and practice of infectious diseases. 2nd ed. New York: John Wiley, 1985.

Rudolph AM. Pediatrics. 18th ed. Norwalk, CT: Appleton and Lange, 1987.

Strickland GT. Hunter's tropical medicine. 7th ed. Philadelphia: WB Saunders, 1989.

CENTRAL NERVOUS SYSTEM INFECTIONS

BACTERIAL MENINGITIS IN CHILDREN

RONALD GOLD, M.D.

ETIOLOGY AND DIAGNOSIS

The majority of cases of bacterial meningitis occur in children less than 5 years of age. The age-specific attack rate peaks between 6 and 11 months of age. Between 2 months and 10 years of age, more than 95 percent of cases are caused by *Haemophilus influenzae* type b, *Neisseria meningitidis*, and *Streptococcus pneumoniae*. These pathogens account for approximately 70, 15, and 15 percent of cases, respectively, in North America. The relative proportions of meningococcal and pneumococcal meningitis vary from year to year because of cyclical changes in the incidence of meningococcal disease.

The pathogenesis of community-acquired bacterial meningitis in apparently normal children is almost always the result of hematogenous spread from the nasopharyngeal mucosa. Susceptibility to invasion of the bloodstream is determined primarily by the presence or absence of antibody directed against components on the bacterial surface, including the polysaccharide capsule, outer membrane proteins, and lipopolysaccharide.

Predisposing risk factors can be divided into three groups: (1) head trauma, neurosurgery, and congenital malformations of the central nervous system; (2) chronic ear and sinus disease; and (3) states with impaired host defenses (sickle cell disease, asplenia, agammaglobulinemia, malignancy and chemotherapy, and terminal complement component deficiencies). Meningitis following penetrating head injuries is caused by skin flora, especially *Staphylococcus aureus*, and/or by pathogens inoculated as the result of the injury. Meningitis associated with cerebrospinal fluid (CSF) rhinorrhea is most often caused by *S. pneumoniae*, whereas infections associated with dermal sinuses connected to the central nervous system (CNS) are usually due to *S. aureus*, *S. epidermidis*, or other bacteria colonizing the skin, depending on the site of the defect. More than 50 percent of episodes of meningitis in children with ventricular shunts are caused by *S. epidermidis*, with the remainder due to *S. aureus*, α-streptococci, enterococci, enteric bacteria, and *Haemophilus* species.

Meningitis in children with chronic middle ear disease is often caused by *Pseudomonas aeruginosa*, which frequently colonizes the external and middle ear in such patients. Infections of the CNS associated with acute or chronic sinusitis and chronic middle ear infection present more often as brain abscess or parameningeal infections than as meningitis.

Children with immunoglobulin deficiency and splenic dysfunction have a greatly increased incidence of meningitis due to the common childhood pathogens, especially *S. pneumoniae*. Children with deficiencies of the terminal components of complement have an increased risk of recurrent attacks of meningococcal meningitis. Children receiving cancer chemotherapy or immunosuppressive therapy may have meningitis caused by unusual organisms such as *Listeria monocytogenes*, *Candida albicans*, and *Cryptococcus neoformans*.

The diagnosis of bacterial meningitis must be considered in every acutely febrile child, especially in infants less than 2 years of age. Specific signs of meningeal irritation (nuchal rigidity, Brudzinki's and Kernig's sign) are often absent in young infants. The diagnosis should be suspected in any febrile infant with a significant alteration in consciousness (lethargy and/or irritability). The typical findings in the CSF consist of pleocytosis (1,000 or more white blood cells [WBCs] per cubic millimeter), glucose 2.0 mM or lower, and protein 0.4 g per liter or greater. However, the initial CSF will have less than 1,000 WBCs per cubic millimeter in one-third of cases, normal glucose in one-third, and normal protein in 20 percent. When performed optimally, the Gram stain is positive in more than 80 percent of cases of *H. influenzae* and pneumococcal meningitis and in two-thirds of meningococcal meningitis. Detection of capsular polysaccharide antigens in the CSF by means of latex agglutination or coagglutination correlate highly with results of Gram stains. They are particularly useful in the child who has already been treated with oral antibiotics prior to the lumbar puncture. Antigen detection methods are not reliable in detecting the antigen of group B meningococci and some pneumococcal serotypes.

Differentiation of viral from bacterial meningitis may be difficult as the clinical findings may be similar. Moreover, meningitis caused by enteroviruses characteristically produces a pleocytosis with an initial predominance of neutrophils. Repeating the lumbar puncture 8 to 12 hours after the initial tap has proven particularly useful in confirming an enteroviral etiology, as there is usually a switch from neutrophil to mononuclear cell predominance. Such a change does not occur in bacterial meningitis. Quantitative determination of C-reactive protein (CRP) in serum and CSF and also of lactic acid in the CSF has had variable success in differentiating bacterial from nonbacterial meningitis. The sensitivity and specificity of these assays have varied in different studies so that their use has not become routine.

Approximately one-third of children will have received oral antibiotics for 1 or more days before hospitalization as the result of having seen a physician for an acute febrile illness. The CSF cell count, glucose, and protein concentrations in children treated with usual oral antibiotics are not significantly different from those of untreated children. Moreover, most cases of *H. influenzae* type b meningitis will still have positive CSF cultures. However, partial treatment frequently leads to negative cultures and Gram stains of the CSF in meningococcal and pneumococcal meningitis. Antigen detection assays are particularly useful in such cases: both concentrated urine and CSF should be tested. If petechial or purpuric skin lesions occur, Gram-stained smears of skin scrapings should be performed; they will be positive in approximately 65 percent of cases of meningococcal disease.

THERAPY

Antibiotics

The initial antibiotic therapy of bacterial meningitis should utilize a regimen active against ampicillin-susceptible and -resistant *H. influenzae*, *N. meningitidis*, and *S. pneumoniae*. Although a rapid, specific diagnosis can often be made with Gram stain and/or antigen detection assays, the initial therapy must be broad enough to cover the three major pathogens. Specific therapy should be introduced after culture and antibiotic susceptibility results are known.

There are now a variety of equally effective regimens available for initial therapy including ampicillin plus chloramphenicol, cefotaxime, and ceftriaxone (Tables 1 and 2). These regimens have been utilized because of the 24 to 40 percent frequency of ampicillin resistance among isolates of *H. influenzae* and a slowly increasing prevalence of strains of pneumococci relatively resistant to penicillin, as well as occasional strains resistant to chloramphenicol.

Ampicillin plus chloramphenicol has been the standard regimen for more than 15 years. However, because of concern over the bone marrow toxicity of chloramphenicol and the need to measure serum concentrations in order to ensure safe and effective blood concentrations, ceftriaxone has become the drug of choice at The Hospital for Sick Children (Toronto). Cefuroxime is no longer used for initial therapy of meningitis because of reports of delayed sterilization of the CSF and of increased incidence of deafness in children with *H. influenzae* meningitis. Ceftriaxone can be given every 12 hours rather than every 6 hours, as with ampicillin plus chloramphenicol, saving pharmacy preparation and nursing time and effort.

As soon as the responsible pathogen is identified by culture, specific antibiotic therapy should be started. Because of the high cost of the cephalosporins, therapy should be changed to penicillin G for meningococcal or pneumococ-

TABLE 1 Choice of Antibiotics in Bacterial Meningitis

Bacteria	First Choice	Alternatives
H. influenzae, ampicillin-susceptible	Ampicillin	Cefotaxime Ceftriaxone Chloramphenicol
H. influenzae, ampicillin-resistant	Ceftriaxone	Cefotaxime Chloramphenicol
N. meningitidis	Penicillin G	Chloramphenicol Listed cephalosporin
S. pneumoniae	Penicillin G	Chloramphenicol Listed cephalosporin
Enteric gram-negative	Cefotaxime *or* ceftazidime	Ceftriaxone Ampicillin plus an aminoglycoside
Group B *Streptococcus*	Ampicillin	Listed cephalosporin
Enterococcus	Ampicillin *plus* gentamicin	Vancomycin plus gentamicin
S. aureus	Cloxacillin	Vancomycin
S. epidermidis	Cloxacillin	Vancomycin
L. monocytogenes	Ampicillin	Chloramphenicol

cal meningitis and to ampicillin for *H. influenzae* disease caused by susceptible strains. Ceftriaxone is continued if the isolate is ampicillin resistant.

Therapy should be by the intravenous route, although intramuscular administration is acceptable if intravenous access is so difficult as to require cut-downs or central lines. The minimal duration of therapy is 7 days for *H. influenzae*, meningococcal, and pneumococcal meningitis. This duration is shorter than those recommended in most standard texts. However, 7 days of therapy has been the standard regimen at The Hospital for Sick Children for more than 25 years. Repeated analysis of mortality and long-term morbidity shows no difference from results using regimens of 10 to 14 days. Moreover, two recent trials have compared 7 to 10 days of therapy and found no significant differences in outcomes.

Repeat lumbar punctures after 24 to 48 hours or at the end of therapy are not indicated routinely. The CSF findings do not help in management, except in children who fail

TABLE 2 Doses of Antibiotics in Bacterial Meningitis

Antibiotic	Dosage (mg/kg/day)*	Dosing Interval (hours)
Amikacin	15–22.5	8
Ampicillin	200–300	6
Cefotaxime	150	6
Ceftriaxone	100	12
Chloramphenicol	75–100	6
Cloxacillin	200	6
Gentamicin	7.5	8
Penicillin G	250,000 U	6
Vancomycin	20–40	6

* Ranges are standard so that a reasonable dose can be calculated for each child.

to respond clinically. Lumbar punctures should be repeated in the child who fails to respond to therapy as expected.

Therapy of the less common causes of bacterial meningitis will be determined by the results of cultures and susceptibility tests. CSF shunt infections are becoming increasingly difficult to treat because of the increasing prevalence of methicillin-resistance among *S. epidermidis*. The role of intraventricular therapy in such infections remains controversial. Gram-negative enteric meningitis is best treated with one of the new, third-generation cephalosporins such as—in order of preference—cefotaxime, ceftazidime, or ceftriaxone. These agents produce very high bactericidal levels in the CSF and usually eliminate the need for intraventricular therapy. Because of its activity against *P. aeruginosa*, ceftazidime is the drug of choice for pseudomonal meningitis.

Supportive Care

Fluid and electrolyte disturbances may occur in children with bacterial meningitis as the result of fever, vomiting, reduced intake, and inappropriate secretion of antidiuretic hormone (ADH). Fever should be controlled with antipyretics in order to reduce metabolic demands of the brain in the face of impaired cerebral blood flow. Fluid deficits should be corrected, with care taken to avoid overhydration. Inappropriate ADH secretion is present in almost all children with bacterial meningitis. Fluid intake should therefore be restricted to approximately two-thirds to three-fourths of daily maintenance requirements for the first 48 to 72 hours. Fluid and electrolyte balance can best be monitored by serum and urine osmolality determinations. Intake can be liberalized when serum sodium concentrations are normal and stable and urine output and specific gravity are normal.

Seizures occur in approximately 25 percent of children with bacterial meningitis, most often during the first 24 hours. Seizures should be controlled promptly in order to minimize metabolic demands on the brain, which is already compromised by impairment of cerebral blood flow. Most seizures are limited to the first day or two of the illness, and prolonged anticonvulsant therapy is unnecessary.

Increased intracranial pressure resulting from a combination of impaired resorption of CSF, cerebral edema, impaired cerebral blood flow, and vasculitis of cerebral vessels is the major cause of brain damage and death in children with bacterial meningitis. Children with significant impairment of the level of consciousness and other signs of increased intracranial pressure should be managed in an intensive care unit. The most rapid means of reducing cerebral pressure is by means of artificial mechanical hyperventilation. Rapid reduction of $PaCO_2$ by hyperventilation causes reduction of cerebral blood flow and of intracranial pressure. Oxygenation of the brain is maintained by the use of increased inspiratory fraction of oxygen. Muscle paralysis is usually required except for children in coma. Blood gases should be monitored with the aim of achieving a $PaCO_2$ of 25 to 27 torr and a PaO_2 of 85 to 95 torr.

Additional therapy with osmotic diuretics such as mannitol may be necessary to stabilize intracranial pressure initially. Rebound increases in intracranial pressure may occur 2 to 12 hours after administration of mannitol if controlled hyperventilation is not employed. Moreover repeated doses of mannitol are often associated with fluid and electrolyte disturbances.

The role of intracranial pressure monitoring with subarachnoid screws or bolts or with intraventricular catheters remains investigational. The benefit and risks of pressure monitoring in bacterial meningitis are still unclear.

The effectiveness of dexamethasone in prevention of deafness following bacterial meningitis has recently been reinvestigated. Four days of therapy with a dose of 0.6 mg per kilogram per day was shown in a placebo-controlled randomized trial to result in a significant reduction in the incidence of severe and profound deafness. However, before routine use can be recommended, the results must be confirmed in other populations. Previous studies of the use of corticosteroids in bacterial meningitis failed to show any benefit on mortality or morbidity.

MANAGEMENT OF COMPLICATIONS

Intracranial complications of meningitis occurring during the acute illness, in addition to those mentioned above, include cerebritis, ischemic infarction, communicating hydrocephalus, and subdural effusions. Such lesions should be suspected in any child who develops significant alteration in consciousness, prolonged or recurrent fever not otherwise explained, hemiparesis, prolonged seizures, or other focal neurologic signs. Computed tomography (CT) is indicated to evaluate children who develop signs of intracranial pathology.

Management of subdural effusions includes daily measurement of head circumference and transillumination in order to detect effusions. Subdural paracentesis should be performed only if focal neurologic signs or evidence of increased intracranial pressure develops or if a significant midline shift is detected on CT. Surgical drainage is rarely required.

Persistent (lasting more than 7 days) and recurrent fevers are the most common complication of bacterial meningitis in children, occurring in 10 to 15 percent of cases. Sources of such fevers include drug fever (especially with β-lactam antibiotics), thrombophlebitis at an IV site, intercurrent viral respiratory infection, focal bacterial infection (pneumonia, septic arthritis, otitis media, sinusitis, subdural empyema, and very rarely brain abscess or pericarditis), reactive vasculitis resulting in reactive (sterile) arthritis and/or skin rash, and subdural effusion. The cause of most persistent and recurrent fevers often is never discovered. If the child is clinically well and no source of fever is determined, antibiotics can safely be discontinued.

Survivors of bacterial meningitis should be followed for a minimum of 1 year or until 2 years of age, with careful developmental and neurologic assessment. Significant sequelae are most frequent following pneumococcal meningitis (40 to 50 percent), least frequent after meningococcal meningitis (5 to 10 percent), and intermediate with *Haemophilus* disease (20 to 30 percent).

Hearing should be tested at 4 to 6 weeks and 1 year after discharge in order to detect hearing impairment, the single most common neurologic sequela of bacterial meningitis.

ANTIBIOTIC PROPHYLAXIS

There is a significantly increased incidence of disease in household contacts of cases of meningococcal disease, regardless of the age of the contacts. There is also an increased incidence of invasive *Haemophilus* disease in household contacts less than 4 years of age. The purpose of antibiotic prophylaxis is to eradicate asymptomatic carriage. Therefore, all contacts should be treated promptly and simultaneously in order to interrupt further transmission within the household, thereby preventing infection of susceptible contacts. Because many secondary cases occur within a few days of onset of the index cases, prophylaxis should be administered immediately upon identification of the index case. Throat cultures to identify carriers are of no benefit and are not recommended.

For meningococcal prophylaxis, rifampin should be administered to all household contacts. Four doses are given every 12 hours. The unit dose is 10 mg per kilogram per dose (maximum, 600 mg per dose). Some authorities recommend a unit dose of 5 mg per kilogram for infants less than 1 year of age. Gastrointestinal side effects (nausea, vomiting, epigastric pain) appear to be less frequent when rifampin is administered every 12 hours.

There is a significantly increased risk of secondary cases of invasive *H. influenzae* disease among household contacts less than 4 years of age. Antibiotic prophylaxis should be given to all members of the contact household, regardless of age, if it contains children less than 4 years of age. The schedule is a single daily dose of 20 mg per kilogram per dose (maximum, 600 mg per dose) for 4 consecutive days. In addition, the index case should be treated with rifampin before discharge if there are contacts less than 4 years of age at home.

Rifampin is not commercially available as a liquid formulation. However, a 1 percent suspension in simple syrup can be readily prepared from the capsules and is stable for the 4 days required for prophylaxis. Antibiotic prophylaxis of day care center contacts of *Haemophilus* disease remains controversial because of conflicting results of studies of the secondary attack rates in day care centers. The controversy centers on whether prophylaxis should be given after a single case in a day care center or after two cases have occurred within an interval of 1 month. If there is an increased risk of disease, it appears to be limited to contacts less than 2 years of age. If prophylaxis is used in day care outbreaks, arrangements should be made to have all contacts treated at the day care center since interruption of transmission requires simultaneous treatment of all contacts.

Regardless of whether or not prophylaxis is used, parents should be informed of the risks of secondary disease and of the need to have all febrile illnesses seen promptly by a physician.

SUGGESTED READING

Jadavji T, Biggar WD, Gold R, et al. Sequelae of acute bacterial meningitis in children treated for seven days. Pediatrics 1985; 78:21–25.

Kaplan SL. Recent advances in bacterial meningitis. Adv Pediatr Infect Dis 1989; 4:83–110.

Lebel MH, Freiz BJ, Syriogiannopolous GA. Dexamethasone therapy for bacterial meningitis: results of two double-blind, placebo-controlled trials. N Engl J Med 1988; 319:964–971.

Lebel MH, McCracken GH. Delayed cerebrospinal fluid sterilization and adverse outcome of bacterial meningitis in infants and children. Pediatrics 1989; 83:161–167.

Lin TY, Chrane DF, Nelson JD, et al. Seven days of ceftriaxone therapy is as effective as ten days' treatment for bacterial meningitis. JAMA 1985; 253:3559–3563.

BACTERIAL MENINGITIS IN ADULTS

THOMAS R. BEAM, Jr., M.D.

Bacterial meningitis in adults is a disease that remains incompletely described. There is no formal reporting system of meningitis as a disease process other than that caused by meningococci. Thus, the incidence among adults is unknown. Large series of cases have been published, but the etiology often reflects the type of patients seen at a particular medical center and not necessarily the population at large. Meningitis is a reportable disease in New York City, but it is not clear whether the high numbers of cases caused by gram-negative bacilli and *Listeria monocytogenes* reflect the true nature of adult meningitis in other areas of the United States.

The treatment of meningitis in adults is also poorly studied. Rates of meningitis are too low for any single medical center to conduct a controlled clinical trial. Collaborative studies comparing various therapies have never been performed. As a result, data obtained from clinical trials conducted among neonates or children, or from epidemics of disease, are usually extrapolated to adults with sporadic disease. This approach may or may not be able to accurately define optimal chemotherapy.

Given these facts, the clinician should remain wary of bacterial meningitis in adults. Because the disease is almost always fatal when untreated, its presence should always be suspected and a diagnostic spinal tap performed even though many yield negative results. If the clinical circumstances are consistent with a diagnosis of bacterial meningitis, spinal tap should be performed promptly and antimicrobial therapy instituted as soon as possible following the spinal tap. If there is an epidemic of meningitis in the community, the first dose of antibiotic may be given prior to obtaining cerebrospinal fluid for analysis, if any delay in performing the spinal tap is anticipated.

Adults residing in a household that contains a case of meningitis caused by *Neisseria meningitidis* or *Haemophilus influenzae* are at increased risk for acquiring meningitis. Both pathogens spread to vulnerable household contacts with equal efficiency. Rifampin prophylaxis, 600 mg by mouth twice a day for 2 days, should be prescribed. Obtaining nasopharyngeal cultures and/or waiting until culture results become available are inappropriate in this setting. Should the adult develop signs or symptoms of meningitis, treatment with penicillin (meningococci), ampicillin (susceptible *H. influenzae*), or a third-generation cephalosporin such as ceftriaxone (isolate unknown or *H. influenzae*, susceptibility unknown) should be instituted.

Community-acquired adult meningitis is most often identified with a contiguous site of infection or concurrent infection, particularly pneumonia, which seeds the meninges by bacteremic spread. The most common organism isolated from such patients is *Streptococcus pneumoniae*. Penicillin G remains the drug of choice. However, all pneumococci should be tested for penicillin susceptibility, because a small minority of strains will be relatively resistant to penicillin G (minimal inhibitory concentration 0.2 μg per milliliter or more). Susceptibility screening is best done using an oxacillin disc. Chloramphenicol or third-generation cephalosporins may be used as alternative agents if resistance is known to be a problem within the local community, if the patient fails to respond to therapy, or if resistance is documented.

EPIDEMIOLOGIC CONSIDERATIONS AS A GUIDE TO THERAPY

Therapy for adult meningitis should be guided by epidemiologic considerations until a pathogen has been defined (Table 1). Sporadic disease among young adults is distinctly uncommon and most often caused by meningococci. The incidence is 0.6 cases per 100,000 population per year. Type B disease is usually responsible. Armed forces personnel are provided with vaccine against meningococci including types A, C, W135, and Y. These individuals remain vulnerable to type B disease in either sporadic or epidemic form. Pneumococci also occasionally cause meningitis in young adults. Therefore, the drug of choice for treatment is penicillin G.

Recent evidence suggests that the elderly are also susceptible to meningitis. Rough estimates of incidence suggest that the rate may be similar to that seen in young children.

Although pneumococci are the most common cause of meningitis among community-residing elderly individuals, *Escherichia coli*, *Klebsiella pneumoniae*, and *Listeria monocytogenes* are common enough to warrant coverage when empiric therapy is being prescribed. A combination of ampicillin and a third-generation cephalosporin (ceftriaxone, cefotaxime, or ceftizoxime) is preferred.

Certain adults with cutaneous infections caused by *Staphylococcus aureus* may become bacteremic and develop meningitis, particularly if the infection has been present for an extended period. A likely circumstance is the parenteral drug abuser who develops endocarditis and secondarily contaminates the central nervous system by bacteremic spread. Nafcillin is the drug of choice, unless methicillin-resistant staphylococci have been identified or are known to exist in the community at large. Vancomycin should be employed in these latter circumstances.

Adults with trauma to the head should be divided into several different groups. The first is trauma from neurosurgery, which then should be subdivided into procedures

TABLE 1 Likely Pathogens Responsible for Bacterial Meningitis in Adults

Clinical Parameters	Pathogens
No predisposing cause, sporadic	
Young adults	N. meningitidis, S. pneumoniae
Elderly (age ≥ 60 years)	S. pneumoniae, Enterobacteriaceae, L. monocytogenes
No predisposing cause, epidemic	N. meningitidis
Index case in household	N. meningitidis, H. influenzae
Predisposing factors:	
Contiguous or comcomitant infection	
Sinusitis, otitis, pneumonia	S. pneumoniae
Cutaneous infections	S. aureus
Endocarditis	S. aureus
Trauma	
Neurosurgery	
Without shunt	Enterobacteriaceae, S. aureus
With shunt or intracranial pressure monitor	Staphylococci, Enterobacteriaceae
Frontal fracture with CSF leak	S. pneumoniae
CSF leak plus antibiotics	Enterobacteriaceae, S. aureus
Skull fracture	S. aureus, Enterobacteriaceae
Immune compromise	
Splenic dysfunction, splenectomy	S. pneumoniae, N. meningitidis
Alcoholism	S. pneumoniae, L. monocytogenes
Hypogammaglobulinemia	S. pneumoniae
Immunosuppressive medications	L. monocytogenes, Enterobacteriaceae, S. pneumoniae
Complement deficiency (late components)	N. meningitidis

involving placement of a shunt or other device versus procedures with no placement of a foreign body. The foreign body strongly enhances the pathogenicity of coagulase-negative staphylococci. *S. aureus* and Enterobacteriaceae also warrant consideration. Vancomycin plus a third-generation cephalosporin, or trimethoprim-sulfamethoxazole as single-agent therapy, should be considered until Gram stain and/or culture information results are available (drugs are listed in order of preference).

Head trauma resulting in a leak of cerebrospinal fluid (CSF) predisposes the individual to pneumococcal meningitis. If the leak persists, recurrent episodes may ensue. If the patient is placed on prophylactic antibiotics to avoid meningitis, which is not advocated, Enterobacteriaceae and *S. aureus* become common pathogens. Treatment should be the same as that advocated for neurosurgical shunt complications.

If there is a skull fracture without rhinorrhea, antibiotic treatment should also be directed against these same pathogens.

The final group of adults vulnerable to bacterial meningitis have various forms of immunologic compromise. Each host-defense–, disease-, or medication-induced defect increases risk of infection caused by certain bacterial pathogens (see Table 1). Presumptive therapy should be directed toward those organisms most likely to be responsible.

DIAGNOSTIC CONSIDERATIONS AS A GUIDE TO THERAPY

In the majority of cases of bacterial meningitis among adults, therapy can be guided by rapidly available diagnostic test results. Following the considerations given to the patient's epidemiologic circumstances, certain clinical features of meningitis should be sought (Fig. 1). Fever, headache, photophobia, nausea and vomiting, and altered level of consciousness are the most important findings. If focal neurologic deficits are elicited on physical examination, a mass lesion must be ruled out before lumbar puncture is performed. In the absence of focal neurologic signs, a diagnostic spinal tap should be done immediately. If lumbar puncture is done without delay, one should await results before starting therapy. If lumbar puncture is delayed because of need for CT scan, time is a critical variable. A 1-hour delay is tolerable; a 6-hour delay is not. In the latter circumstance one dose of ampicillin plus ceftriaxone should be given. Gram stain, culture, glucose and protein levels, and white blood cell and differential counts should be requested. Counterimmunoelectrophoresis (CIE) or latex agglutination studies should be ordered and are particularly useful for diagnosis of bacterial meningitis when the patient has received prior antimicrobial therapy. *S. pneumoniae*, *N. meningitidis*, *H. influenzae*, and *E. coli* can be detected by these techniques. Group B streptococci, pathogens of importance for neonates, rarely cause adult meningitis but can also be detected. Assays take 30 to 45 minutes to perform

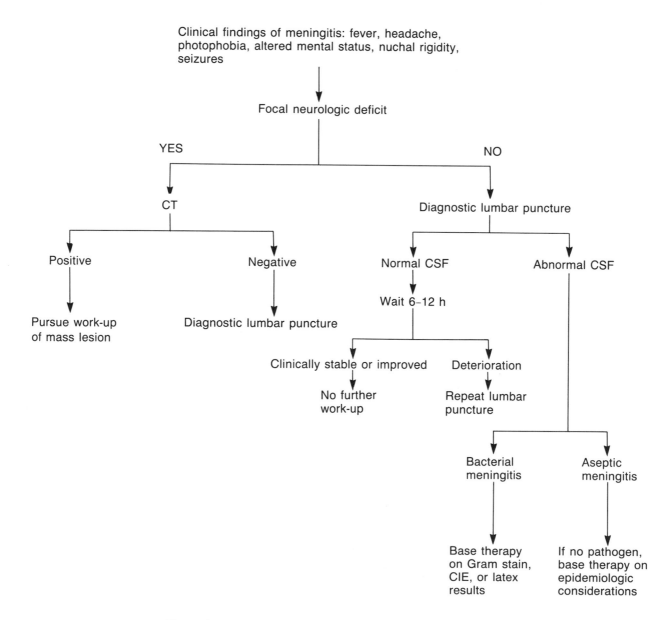

Figure 1 Diagnosing bacterial meningitis in adults.

and report to the clinician. Thus if available, they can be used to confirm or supplement Gram stain information.

If the Gram stain, CIE, and latex agglutination studies do not identify a presumptive pathogen but there is a CSF leukocytosis with polymorphonuclear predominance, hypoglycorrhachia, and elevated protein, empiric therapy should be started based on epidemiologic considerations, as previously described.

ANTIMICROBIAL THERAPY OF BACTERIAL MENINGITIS

As previously noted, therapy should be instituted as rapidly as possible once diagnostic material has been obtained. In addition to CSF, culture of blood, sputum (if available), and urine; complete blood count and differential; and urine for CIE are essential. A summary of recommendations is provided in Table 2.

The choice of antibiotic is based on several factors. It should be bactericidal. It should effectively penetrate into the central nervous system, achieving concentrations that are severalfold in excess of the minimum bactericidal concentration (MBC). Rarely, the nature of the infecting organism and the lack of penetrability of the chemotherapeutic agent may require a route other than parenteral to be chosen. Because of CSF flow dynamics, the optimal site for drug delivery is the cerebral ventricle. Neurosurgical consultation should be called to place a device such as an Ommaya reservoir if interference is anticipated with exchange of CSF from the choroid plexus to other areas.

The issue of bactericidal antibiotics requires clarification. Chloramphenicol is bactericidal for *S. pneumoniae, N. meningitidis*, and *H. influenzae* in concentrations achieved in the central nervous system during parenteral therapy. It is bacteriostatic for organisms such as *E. coli* and thus should not be used for meningitis caused by Enterobacteriaceae even when these organisms are reported to susceptible by in vitro testing.

Combining bactericidal antibiotics can be advantageous. Ampicillin plus chloramphenicol are prescribed because of the potential resistance of *H. influenzae* to either agent alone. One or the other may be discontinued upon determination of the organism's susceptibility pattern. However, combination of a bactericidal and bacteriostatic agent, such as penicillin plus tetracycline, can result in a substantially worse outcome than prescription of penicillin alone for treatment of meningitis caused by *S. pneumoniae*.

The development of third-generation cephalosporins has addressed the problem of inadequate therapeutic options available to treat meningitis caused by Enterobacteriaceae. Uncontrolled collections of cases have suggested that morbidity and mortality have been significantly reduced. However, prospective, randomized comparative trials conducted in neonates and children have failed to demonstrate appreciable benefit. This observation was made despite truly remarkable bactericidal activity achieved in CSF.

Although lumbar, cisternal, and direct intraventricular injections of antibiotics have not usually proved helpful (and in certain circumstances they are harmful), there remains a need for local instillation of antibiotics. An organism such as *Pseudomonas aeruginosa* is best treated with a combination of a β-lactam agent (piperacillin or ceftazidime) plus an aminoglycoside (gentamicin, tobramycin, or amikacin) (drugs are listed in order of preference). The β-lactam agent may be delivered parenterally, but the aminoglycoside is rendered more effective by local injection. Preservative-free gen-

TABLE 2 Antibiotic Therapy for Adult Meningitis

Organism	Preferred Antibiotic	Total Daily Dose	Dosing Interval	Alternative	Total Daily Dose	Dosing Interval
S. pneumoniae	Aqueous penicillin G*	24×10^6 U	2 h	Chloramphenicol	4 g	6 h
S. pneumoniae, penicillin-resistant	Chloramphenicol	4 g	6 h	Vancomycin* Cefotaxime	30 mg/kg 12 g	12 h 4–6 h
S. aureus	Nafcillin	12 g	4–6 h	Vancomycin*	30 mg/kg	12 h
S. aureus, methicillin-resistant	Vancomycin*	30 mg/kg	12 h	Trimethoprim-sulfamethoxazole*	12 amps	6 h
N. meningitidis	Aqueous penicillin G*	24×10^6 U	2 h	Chloramphenicol Ceftriaxone Cefotaxime	4 g 4 g 12 g	6 h 12 h 4–6 h
Enterobacteriaceae	Ceftriaxone Cefotaxime	4 g 12 g	12 h 4–6 h	Trimethoprim-sulfamethoxazole*	12 amps	6 h
H. influenzae	Ceftriaxone Cefotaxime	4 g 12 g	12 h 6 h	Ampicillin* ± chloramphenicol	12 g 4 g	4 h 6 h
H. influenzae, ampicillin-resistant	Ceftriaxone Cefotaxime	4 g 12 g	12 h 6 h	Chloramphenicol	4 g	6 h
L. monocytogenes	Ampicillin*	12 g	4 h	Trimethoprim-sulfamethoxazole*	12 amps	6 h

P. aeruginosa	Piperacillin* +
	  tobramycin*
		18 g
		5.1 mg/kg
			4 h
			8 h
				Ceftazidime* +
				  tobramycin*
					6 g
					5.1 mg/kg
						8 h
						8 h

* Requires dose adjustment for elderly or persons with renal dysfunction.

tamicin, tobramycin, or amikacin should be delivered through a device such as an Ommaya reservoir. Most experience and FDA approval exist for gentamycin only. The key consideration is to use a preservative-free preparation for local injection. There are, however, no data to recommend one agent in preference to others based on in vitro susceptibility results and correlation to outcome. Gentamicin is administered intrathecally in a dose of 4 mg once per day. A simple alternative to the Ommaya reservoir is to mix gentamicin with CSF in the syringe through which it is administered (barbotage). It should be continued until cultures of CSF are sterile.

Adverse reactions to therapeutic agents employed for treatment of bacterial meningitis are generally those characteristic of the class of drugs to which the specific antibiotic belongs. However, because these agents are used at maximal daily dosing, care must be taken to adjust standard regimens in the presence of impaired renal clearance. The most common problem is β-lactam toxicity attributable to reduced renal function in an elderly patient whose serum creatinine is "normal." The adverse effects that result from accumulation of the drugs include diminished level of consciousness, confusion, and seizure disorder. These drug-related phenomena must be distinguished from the natural history of the disease or failure to respond to therapy.

Although a repeat lumbar puncture is routinely obtained for neonates, infants, and children with bacterial meningitis, this is infrequently done for adults. The only justification is verification that the chosen antibiotic(s) have sterilized the CSF. In neurosurgical cases with direct ventricular access, this evaluation can be performed. Otherwise, it is only required when the patient clinically deteriorates while receiving allegedly effective therapy. Lumbar puncture at the end of treatment yields no useful information for predicting relapse and therefore is unwarranted.

The complications of meningitis are primarily neurologic and include cranial nerve palsies, impaired mental capacity, hearing loss, and a variety of other sequelae. No study has been done to assess the impact of effective antimicrobial therapy on neurologic residua. It is assumed that prompt diagnosis and rapid institution of appropriate therapy play a favorable role in outcome. This appears to be true for postneurosurgical gram-negative bacillary meningitis when contrasted with community-acquired disease caused by the same organisms.

The duration of therapy for effective treatment of bacterial meningitis in adults has not been critically appraised. Thus, arbitrary limits have been established and are both patient- and organism-specific. Defervescence, disappearance of abnormalities in mental status, relief of symptoms such as headache, and normalization of white blood cell count are required. Several additional days of antibiotics are generally prescribed before therapy is stopped. There is no

advantage to continued hospitalization to monitor for relapse once antibiotic therapy is complete. In general, adult meningitis is treated for 14 to 21 days.

FUTURE DIRECTIONS: ADJUNCTS TO ANTIBIOTIC THERAPY

Because the development of new antibiotics has not significantly improved morbidity and mortality associated with bacterial meningitis, the role of adjunctive therapy is being explored. It was first noted at the turn of the century that immunoglobulins could treat meningococcal disease. This was verified in the 1930s for *H. influenzae* meningitis. The development of potentially effective antibiotics caused a loss of interest in passive immunotherapy. Interest has regenerated with the development of safer immunoglobulin preparations and the lack of an antibiotic panacea. Under consideration are nonspecific and highly specific (monoclonal) immunoglobulin preparations instilled into cerebrospinal fluid or administered intravenously.

A second area of exploration is reduction of the inflammatory reaction within the central nervous system. Certain neurologic sequelae may be attributed to increased intracranial pressure from impaired CSF flow dynamics due to leukocytes. Also, it has been proposed that leukocyte products may be toxic to nerve cells. Using corticosteroids or nonsteroidal anti-inflammatory agents, it may be possible to reduce the incidence of neurologic sequelae. Since effective antibiotics are available, and since leukocyte function in the central nervous system is impaired by lack of immunoglobulins and complement, an overall reduction in inflammation may be beneficial.

There is insufficient clinical evidence available to consider immunoglobulin therapy, corticosteroid therapy, or nonsteroidal anti-inflammatory drug therapy at this time. Antibiotics may have shortcomings but remain the treatment of choice.

SUGGESTED READING

Beam TR. Cephalosporins in adult meningitis. Bull NY Acad Med 1984; 60:380–393.

McGee ZA, Kaiser AB. Acute meningitis. In: Mandell GL, Douglas RG Jr, Bennett JE, eds. Principles and practice of infectious diseases. 2nd ed. New York: John Wiley and Sons, 1985:560.

Sande MA, Smith AL, Root RK, eds. Bacterial meningitis. Contemporary issues in infectious diseases. Vol 3. New York: Churchill Livingstone, 1985.

Tauber MG, Sande MA. Principles in the treatment of bacterial meningitis. Am J Med 1984; 76(5A):224–230.

ASEPTIC MENINGITIS SYNDROME

P. JOAN CHESNEY, M.D., C.M.

The aseptic meningitis syndrome (AMS) was first defined by Wallgren in 1925. It is a syndrome of multiple etiologies, all of which produce symptoms and signs of meningeal inflammation with no evidence of a pyogenic organism by Gram stain or routine culture of cerebrospinal fluid (CSF). Other characteristics of AMS include an acute or subacute onset, the absence of severe cerebral manifestations, and a self-limited and usually benign outcome, depending on the etiology and the presence of a nonpurulent CSF (Table 1). Although exceptions clearly occur, as a general rule the CSF has a total white blood cell (WBC) count of less than 500 cells per cubic millimeter, a total protein (TP) concentration of less than 100 mg per deciliter, and a glucose concentration that is normal or rarely less than 20 mg per deciliter. The CSF WBC differential depends on the etiology. Although polymorphonuclear cells (PMNs) may predominate in the first 24 hours of a viral infection, Feigin et al found a shift to a lymphocytic predominance in 87 percent of patients within 8 to 12 hours of the first lumbar puncture (LP). Such a rapid shift in cellular morphology does not occur with bacterial meningitis.

The important challenge of AMS is that of identifying, as early as possible, the potentially treatable causes of the syndrome, including unusual presentations of bacterial infections of the central nervous system. Therapeutic strategies, such as the potential use of acyclovir and azidothymidine for the management of some of the viral causes of AMS; the continued availability of amphotericin B, 5-fluorocytosine, and the new imidazoles for fungal causes; antituberculous therapy for acid-fast organisms; and aggressive surgery and therapy for neural neoplasms and parameningeal foci, have

created an urgency for establishing a rapid and accurate diagnosis.

In general the term AMS is used to apply to syndromes in which the sole or predominant component is due to meningeal irritation, with other nonneurologic clinical features being less prominent or nonspecific. Thus, once the clinical and diagnostic evaluation establishes the presence of a specific entity such as Kawasaki disease or Rocky Mountain spotted fever, despite the presence of meningeal findings, these entities would no longer be called AMS.

The labels of meningoencephalitis and viral meningitis should be avoided when patients with AMS are initially evaluated. As opposed to the clinical findings of AMS, encephalitis connotes an acute, severe, persistent disturbance of cerebral function. Likewise, early use of the diagnosis of viral meningitis implies a known etiology, which may preclude continued evaluation for the many other, often treatable, causes of this syndrome (Table 2).

Although careful evaluation of body fluids, including the CSF, will provide the answer on occasion (Table 3), most

TABLE 1 Clinical and Laboratory Definition of the Aseptic Meningitis Syndrome

Symptoms and signs
  Fever and chills
  Headache
  Vomiting
  Nuchal rigidity
  Malaise
  Fatigue/anorexia
  Absence of severe cerebral disturbance
  Absence of readily diagnosed systemic syndrome

CSF evaluation
  WBC $\leq$ 500 cells/mm³ (rarely may be several thousand/mm³)
  WBC differential: either neutrophilic or lymphocytic predominance
  Total protein concentration $\leq$ 100 mg/dl
  Glucose concentration $\geq$ 20 mg/dl and usually normal
  Negative Gram stain
  Negative routine bacterial cultures

TABLE 2 Differential Diagnosis of the Infectious Etiologies of the Aseptic Meningitis Syndrome

INFECTIOUS ETIOLOGIES
  Viruses
    Enteroviruses (echo, coxsackie, polio, and others)
    Human immunodeficiency virus
    Lymphocytic choriomeningitis virus
    Varicella-zoster virus
    Epstein-Barr virus
    Arboviruses (eastern, western and Venezuelan equine; St. Louis, Powassan, California, and Colorado tick fever in the United States; others in other areas of the world)
    Mumps virus
    Herpes simplex type 2 virus
    Adenovirus
    Others (encephalomyocarditis virus; cytomegalovirus; measles virus; rubella virus; rhinovirus; coronavirus; parainfluenza virus; influenza A and B virus; rotavirus; variola virus)

  Bacteria
    Partially treated purulent meningitis
    Spirochetes
      Treponema pallidum (syphilis)
      Borrelia recurrentis (relapsing fever)
      Borrelia burgdorferi (lyme disease)
      Spirillum minor (rat bite fever)
      Leptospira species (leptospirosis)
    Mycobacterium tuberculosis (tuberculosis)
    Nocardia species (nocardiosis)
    Suppurative parameningeal focus
      Brain abscess
      Sinusitis, mastoiditis, middle ear infection
      Epidural abscess of cranium or spine
      Endocarditis or lung abscess with meningeal embolization
      Cranial osteomyelitis: subdural empyema or suppurative intracranial phlebitis

  Mycoplasmas
    Mycoplasma pneumoniae
    Mycoplasma hominis

  Rickettsia
    Rickettsia rickettsii (Rocky Mountain spotted fever)
    Rickettsia prowazeki (typhus)

Table continues on the following page

TABLE 2 *(continued)*

Fungi
  Blastomyces dermatitidis (blastomycosis)
  Coccidioides immitis (coccidioidomycosis
  Cryptococcus neoformans (cryptococcosis)
  Histoplasma capsulatum (histoplasmosis)
  Candida species
  Other (aspergillosis; mucormycosis)

Protozoa
  Amebas
    Naegleria fowleri (primary acute amebic menin-
      goencephalitis)
    Entamoeba histolytica (cerebral amebiasis,
      secondary)
    Acanthamoeba species (primary subacute or
      chronic amebic meningoencephalitis)
  Trypanosoma species (sleeping sickness)
  Plasmodium species (malaria)
  Toxoplasma gondii (toxoplasmosis)

Nematodes
  Strongyloides stercoralis (strongyloidiasis)
  Trichinella spiralis (trichinosis)
  Angiostrongylis cantonensis (eosinophilic
    meningitis)

NONINFECTIOUS ETIOLOGIES
Heavy-metal poisoning (lead, arsenic)
Postvaccination: measles, vaccinia, polio,
  rabies
Malignancy: leukemia, meningeal or
  parameningeal neoplasm
Unknown etiology:
  Behçet syndrome; lupus erythemato-
    sus; serum sickness; sarcoidosis;
    Kawasaki syndrome; Mollaret's
    recurrent meningitis; cat scratch
    disease; Vogt-Koyanagi-Hanada
    syndrome
Miscellaneous:
  Foreign bodies in the CNS: intra-
    thecal injections (procaine, soaps,
    or disinfectants)
  Drug associated (especially non-
    steroidal anti-inflammatory drugs):
    dermoid/epidermoid cysts adjacent
    to subarachnoid space

---

often the diagnosis used to initiate therapy of AMS will be based on the history, a careful review of possible epidemiologic factors, and physical examination.

ETIOLOGY AND EPIDEMIOLOGY

In prospective studies of AMS in which vigorous attempts were made to identify the etiology, a virus was identified in 70 percent of cases. Of those, the enteroviruses accounted for 85 percent of cases, with coxsackievirus B_5 and the echoviruses 4, 6, 9, and 11 as the most common enteroviruses. Arboviruses account for about 5 percent of AMS cases in North America, St Louis encephalitis virus and the California encephalitis virus being the most common. Although mumps used to be a common cause, it has become rare since the advent of the vaccine.

Since 1980, the human immunodeficiency virus (HIV) has become an important cause of virus-associated neuro-logic syndromes. HIV-linked AMS is most often associated with the initial mononucleosis-like acute infection. Clarification of potential host risk factors and of the patient's acute and convalescent enzyme-linked immunosorbent assay (ELISA) and western blot tests and HIV P_{24} antigen status should establish the diagnosis. Ongoing studies will determine whether antiviral therapy of this self-limited stage of the illness will modify the subsequent course.

Epidemiologic factors are important in establishing a tentative etiology for AMS. During the months of July to October, the presence of unexplained fever, rashes, pleurodynia, or pharyngitis in the community suggests the existence of an enteroviral outbreak.

For other agents (see Table 2) the history should include attention to recent travel, recreation, and residence at the time of onset, e.g., southwestern United States (cryptococcosis), southeastern United States (histoplasmosis), or Lacrosse, Wisconsin (California encephalitis virus). Environmental exposures, such as exposure in the woods to animals, insects, or mosquitoes (Lyme disease, relapsing fever, or rickettsial disease); to a beaver pond (blastomycosis); or to a freshwater pond or swimming pool (*Naegleria fowleri*) should be determined. Personal life style should be determined, particularly with respect to drug abuse and sexual activity (syphilis, HIV). Illness in other family members or pets may provide important diagnostic information. Underlying illnesses in the patient, such as those suggesting a recent or current sinusitis or middle ear infection or illness requiring a blood transfusion, dental work, antibiotics, or immunosuppressive agents or placement of intravascular or intracranial foreign bodies, should be determined. Other manifestations of the acute illness, such as a characteristic rash, pharyngitis, cough, adenopathy, conjunctival injection, jaundice, oral or genital ulcers or discharge, or previous episodes of meningeal inflammation, are also important in establishing an etiology.

Initial examination of the CSF will establish the presence of AMS in patients with obvious aberrations, e.g., TP of more than 200 mg per deciliter will immediately indicate further diagnostic tests. Hypoglycorrhachia in AMS suggests either mumps, lymphocytic choriomeningitis, or (in infants) enteroviral infection, the presence of a parameningeal focus, partially treated meningitis, brain tumor, CNS leukemic infiltration, or mycoplasmal, fungal, or acid-fast bacillus infection. Other diagnostic tests that may be utilized for the initial or subsequent CSF examinations are listed in Table 3.

Bacterial cultures of CSF and blood and of any other potentially infected site (urine, skin, catheter) should always be obtained first. If a viral diagnostic laboratory is available, viral cultures of CSF, throat, and stool, particularly during the summer and fall, may prove to be valuable in the management of problematic cases. The enteroviruses that grow in culture will give obvious cytopathogenic changes within 2 to 5 days. The stool culture has the greatest probability of being positive during enteroviral AMS, but CSF culture also has a high yield, with a positive culture 70 percent of the time. Thus, several studies have documented that, based on a positive viral culture result within 5 days of admission, the management of as many as 50 percent of patients with AMS will be changed. Problematic patients with AMS, such as infants or toxic-appearing or partially treated

TABLE 3 Additional Diagnostic Tests That May Assist in Establishing the Diagnosis of Aseptic Meningitis Syndrome

CSF
  Antigen detection*:   for pyogenic bacteria, *Cryptococcus neoformans* and HIV P_{24}

  Wet mount or hanging drop†:   amebas
  Cytology*:   may demonstrate smudge cells of Mollaret's or malignant cells

  Acid-fast stain of sediment*   positive in >80% of cases of
    (10 ml CSF):   tuberculous meningitis
  India ink*:   cryptococci and amebas
  Limulus lysate‡:   positive result indicates presence of endotoxin

  Chloride‡:   <110 mEq/L suggests TB if pyogenic meningitis ruled out

  Cultures*
    Bacterial: *Listeria* may take several days to grow, mycobacteria take several weeks, leptospires grow on special media

    Viral: positive in 70–80% of enteroviral AMS; growth of other viruses from CSF rare

    Fungal: need to culture large volumes of CSF as organisms present at low concentrations and generally take >10 days to grow

  Nonspecific tests: lactic   tend to be higher in bacterial
    acid, C-reactive protein‡:   meningitis
  CSF antibody†:   Antibody to viruses and *Treponema pallidum* may appear earlier and eventually in higher titer in CSF than in serum

  Darkfield examination†:   spirochetes may be seen

Blood
  Antigen detection†:   HIV P_{24}
  Acute/convalescent sera*:   obtained ≥3 weeks apart may establish diagnosis in retrospect: ELISA and western blot may be positive with acute HIV infection: viral specific IgM present in 83% of sera by day 3 for Lacrosse strain California encephalitis virus

  Culture* (bacterial fungal):   may yield agent when CSF cultures negative

  Heavy-metal levels†:   if indicated
  Serum/urine electrolytes*:   inappropriate ADH secretion (SIADH) definition

Other body fluids
  Stool viral cultures*:   positive for most enteroviral meningitis: growth in 2–5 days: allows specific serology for coxsackie A viruses

  Sputum and bone marrow   TB/fungi
    cultures†:
  Urine culture and antigen   positive for some viruses (CMV
    detection*:   and mumps), TB, and *Candida*: antigen detection for pyogenic bacteria)

Other tests
  Skull and sinus   sinusitis or cranial osteomyelitis
    roentgenograms†:
  CT or brain scan†:   sinus or intracranial abscess or inflammation

  EEG†:   diffuse or focal involvement
  PPD*:   TB

* Tests routinely performed on every patient with AMS.
† Tests to be performed if a particular agent or diagnosis is strongly suspected.
‡ Tests described in the literature but seldom of diagnostic help.

patients initially started on antibiotics, could have the medication stopped or changed on the basis of the positive viral culture.

"Partially treated meningitis" is the most puzzling initial diagnostic and management dilemma posed by patients with AMS, since 25 to 50 percent of patients will already have received antimicrobial therapy at the time of diagnosis. Recent studies have suggested that the only CSF findings altered significantly by prior intramuscular or oral therapy are the Gram stain and culture. Thus, several days of appropriate intravenous therapy are required to decrease the initial high percentage of PMNs and the elevated protein level and to increase the low glucose concentration of the CSF in bacterial meningitis. However, an early or atypical presentation of partially treated bacterial meningitis may initially mimic viral meningitis. In this case, a repeat LP demonstrating a predominance of lymphocytes within 8 to 12 hours, before starting antibiotics, may be justified and useful. Likewise, the CSF TP will not be significantly higher nor the CSF glucose concentration lower. Thus, if the initial physical evaluation and CSF examination strongly suggest either early AMS with a predominance of PMNs or partially treated probable viral AMS, physicians may choose to observe and monitor the patient closely without antimicrobial treatment and to repeat the LP after 8 to 12 hours.

MANAGEMENT

The specific management of the patient with AMS will be determined by the result of the initial evaluation (see Tables 1 to 3). The more general issues of management include the indications for hospitalization, initial cultures and tests to be obtained, isolation procedures, symptomatic therapy, careful fluid management, the need for possible surgical intervention (parameningeal infectious foci or neoplasms), and ongoing diagnostic evaluations including a repeat LP within 8 to 12 hours (Table 4). As with viral culture, the greatest advantage of repeating the LP prior to starting an antibiotic is that of shortening the duration of hospitalization.

Most patients with AMS will be admitted to the hospital with more specific indications for admission, listed in Table 4. Tests to be performed on the initial blood and CSF specimens (see Table 3) will be determined by the epidemiologic factors noted in the history and the possible suspected diagnoses (see Table 2).

Isolation precautions, fluid and electrolyte management, and symptomatic therapy comprise the initial therapy. Careful thought should be given to the administration of antimicrobial agents since, once started, they are seldom discontinued before 10 days, thus committing the patient to a potentially unnecessary and expensive hospitalization. Suggested indications for initiating antimicrobial therapy are listed in Table 4. Because of the frequent paucity of clinical manifestations, aberrant CSF findings, and rapid progression of bacterial meningitis in infants and immunocompromised hosts, antimicrobial agents should be started promptly in most of these patients. Likewise, antimicrobial agents should be

TABLE 4   Management of Patients with Aseptic Meningitis Syndrome

Indications for hospitalization
  Toxic-appearing with rapidly progressing symptoms
  High likelihood of treatable cause
  Age <12 mo
  CSF parameters suggesting bacterial etiology despite negative Gram stain
  Positive bacterial antigen test in blood/urine/CSF
  Dehydration or electrolyte imbalance
  Serious underlying disease

Isolation procedures
  Blood, respiratory, and secretion precautions until discharge or etiology clarified; enteroviruses may persist in stool despite clinical improvement

Aggressive and continued diagnostic attempts
  Repeat LPs if indicated
  Repeat bacterial, viral, and fungal cultures and antigen testing if disease progresses
  More complete serologic testing if indicated, i.e., for Epstein-Barr virus, *Mycoplasma* species, Rocky Mountain spotted fever, etc.

Antimicrobial therapy on admission
  Toxic-appearing with progressing symptoms and signs
  No switch to lymphocytic predominance in CSF on repeat 8–12-h LP
  Infant with suspected early or atypical bacterial meningitis or partially treated meningitis
  Immunocompromised individual with possible atypical CSF responses
  Demonstrated parameningeal focus of suspected bacterial etiology
  Selected viral infections

Surgical management
  Parameningeal focus requiring drainage
  CNS shunt manipulation
  Malignancy when indicated

Fluid and electrolyte management
  Intravenous fluid and electrolytes with fluid restriction and ongoing evaluation of serum and urine sodium and specific gravity for evaluation of presence of inappropriate ADH secretion (SIADH)

Symptomatic therapy
  Analgesics for headache, myalgias
  Decreased light, noise, and visitors for photophobia, hyperesthesia
  Antipyretics and antiemetics if indicated

started in patients who are toxic-appearing, who are strongly suspected of having a parameningeal infection, or who show rapid signs of clinical progression in the hospital. Selected patients with viral causes of AMS may benefit from antiviral drugs. The details of antimicrobial and antiviral therapy are discussed in the chapters devoted to each agent.

The outcome of AMS depends on the etiology. The course of enteroviral meningitis is usually benign and self-limited, with 3 to 5 days of fever and 1 to 2 weeks of neurologic dysfunction. Some patients continue to experience fatigue, irritability and decreased concentration, myalgias, incoordination, and muscle weakness and spasm for several weeks after the acute episode. Infants infected before 3 months of age may experience neurologic sequelae.

The patient with AMS presents a real challenge to the diagnostic and management skills of the physician. Antimicrobial therapy should be initiated soon after admission if the organism is identified or for the indications listed in Table 4. The more difficult and ultimately rewarding path of withholding antimicrobial agents and frequently reevaluating and reassessing the patient, if the etiology is unclear and the patient is stable, may result in a more accurate diagnosis and therapy, shorter hospitalizations, and thus fewer nosocomial infections.

SUGGESTED READING

Cherry JD. Aseptic meningitis and viral meningitis. In: Feigin RD, Cherry JD, eds. Central nervous system infections in pediatric infectious diseases. Philadelphia: WB Saunders, 1987.

Feigin RD, Shackelford PF. Value of repeat lumbar puncture in the differential diagnosis of meningitis. N Engl J Med 1973; 289:571.

Johnson RT, McArthur JC, Narayan O. The neurobiology of human immunodeficiency virus infections. FASEB J 1988; 2:2970–2981.

McGee ZA, Kaiser AB. Acute meningitis. In: Mandell GB, Douglas RG Jr, Bennett JE, eds. Principles and practice of infectious disease. New York: John Wiley, 1985.

Wallgren A. Une nouvelle maladie infectieuse du systeme nerveuse central? Acta Paediatr Scand 1925; 4(Suppl): 158–182.

LOCALIZED INFECTION OF THE CENTRAL NERVOUS SYSTEM

THOMAS M. KERKERING, M.D.

Localized infections of the central nervous system do not occur as frequently as bacterial or viral meningitis or encephalitis. Nevertheless, localized infections receive special attention because of the difficulty of accurate diagnosis, the controversy surrounding their management, and their often serious outcome.

The finding of a lesion has been made easier with the widespread use of computed tomography (CT) and the introduction of magnetic resonance imaging (MRI). Advances in neurosurgical procedures and the advent of newer antibiotics have altered the therapeutic approach, but mortality and neurologic sequelae remain unacceptably high. The optimal management of these infections requires the coordinated efforts of radiologist, neurosurgeon, and infectious disease specialist. This chapter discusses brain abscesses, subdural empyemas, epidural empyemas, spinal epidural abscesses, and mycotic aneurysms. Critical to the management of these infections is an understanding of the etiology, pathogenesis, clinical features, and laboratory and diagnostic modalities currently available. Because each of these infections presents a unique situation, each is discussed separately.

BRAIN ABSCESS

Etiology

Brain abscesses are the result of a contiguous spread of infection from a parameningeal focus, metastatic spread from distant sites, or the direct result of trauma or neurosurgical procedures. Approximately 75 percent of brain abscesses are single lesions, whereas 25 percent are multiple in nature. Of the latter, 50 percent are the result of metastatic spread from distant foci.

Despite therapy the mortality rate is 33 percent, and of the survivors, at least 58 percent have some neurologic sequelae ranging from mild to severe. Seizures are a common outcome of brain abscesses.

With few exceptions, the foci of infection leading to brain abscesses have changed little over the years, and in approximately 15 to 20 percent of cases a source is never found. The most common sources of infection are parameningeal, pulmonary, and then a miscellaneous grouping.

Parameningeal foci include the sinuses, ears, and mouth. Sinusitis accounts for approximately 20 percent of brain abscesses. Of the sinuses, the maxillary is the most frequently involved, leading usually to a temporal lobe lesion. Frontal and ethmoid sinusitis causes frontal lobe lesions, whereas infection of the sphenoid may result in frontal or temporal lobe lesions or even intrasellar processes.

Brain abscesses of otogenic origin are the result of chronic (not acute) otitis media and/or mastoiditis and account for 16 percent of brain abscesses. Lesions are most often found in the temporal lobes. However, when an abscess is found in the cerebellum it is almost always otogenic in origin.

Odontogenic infections cause about 13 percent of brain abscesses. Caries, periodontitis, and procedures such as extractions and root canals may all contribute to these infections.

Pulmonary infections are responsible for 16 percent of brain abscesses, and the most common focus is an anaerobic lung abscess. Other causes include pneumonia, bronchiectasis, and cystic fibrosis.

In the age of advanced life support, ventriculostomies and intracranial pressure devices account for 4 percent of brain abscesses. Congenital cyanotic heart disease is rarely a factor.

Sixteen percent of brain abscesses have miscellaneous causes, including endocarditis, abdominal and pelvic abscesses, head trauma, and a variety of procedures such as esophageal sclerotherapy.

Microbiology

Approximately 50 percent of brain abscesses are due to one organism, 25 percent to two organisms, and 25 percent to three or more organisms.

Aerobic organisms are responsible for 36 percent of brain abscesses, anaerobic organisms account for 41 percent, and microaerophilic streptococci cause 22 percent. The tiny remainder are caused by fungi and parasites.

Of the aerobic organisms, most are gram-positive cocci, and of these most are *Streptococcus* species, either unspecified or group D organisms. *Staphylococcus aureus* usually causes brain abscesses in the settings of endocarditis or head trauma. Infections due to gram-negative aerobes such as *Klebsiella*, *Escherichia*, *Pseudomonas*, and *Proteus* species are usually the result of otogenic infections, neurosurgical procedures, or head trauma. *Citrobacter* has a predilection for causing brain abscesses in neonates.

Anaerobic bacteria are the most common pathogens; streptococci, peptostreptococci, *Bacteroides*, and *Fusobacterium* are the most prevalent. These are usually sinus or odontogenic in origin.

Other organisms to consider are *Norcardia asteroides*, often seen with pulmonary disease, and most often, but not necessarily, in the immunosuppressed individual. As a consequence of human immunodeficiency virus infection, brain lesions due to *Toxoplasma* are becoming more common and must be considered in the differential diagnosis. Fungi are an uncommon cause of brain abscesses, but in the immunosuppressed host, disease due to *Aspergillus* or *Candida* may be present. In otherwise normal individuals abscesses due to *Blastomyces dermatitidis*, *Coccidioides immitis*, and the dematiaceous fungi have been reported. Cryptococcomas are usually associated with cryptococcal meningitis.

Clinical Features

Brain abscesses are more common in men in the second and third decades of life. Symptoms may have been present for hours to weeks and include headache (72 percent), fever (42 percent), seizures (35 percent), nausea and vomiting (35 percent), altered sensorium (26 percent), and visual or motor disturbances (40 percent).

Signs include mental status changes (75 percent), fever (60 percent), localizing neurologic signs (43 percent), and nuchal rigidity (35 percent). Papilledema is uncommon and seen in approximately 4 percent of patients.

Physical examination should also include an optimal ear, nose, and throat examination as well as pulmonary and cardiac examinations. Fever is not universally present in patients with brain abscesses.

Diagnosis

On the basis of the above signs and symptoms, the diagnosis should be suspected. CT of the head (with contrast) must be done promptly. If CT does not reveal a space-occupying lesion a lumbar puncture must then be

TABLE 1 Staging of Brain Abscess by Computed Tomography

Stage of Brain Abscess	Precontrast Scan	Pattern of Contrast Enhancement (10 min)	Delayed-Contrast Scan (30–60 min)
Early cerebritis	Irregular area of low density	May or may not show contrast enhancement; enhancement may be nodular, patchy, or ring-like	No significant decrease in contrast enhancement if present; further difference of contrast often occurs
Late cerebritis	Larger area of low density	Typical ring enhancement; ring is often diffuse and thick; however, it may be thin; if lesion is small, it will appear as a solid nodule; if lesion is larger, a lucent center remains	No significant decrease in contrast enhancement; further diffusion of contrast often occurs
Early capsule	Developing capsule delineated as a possible faint ring surrounding a lower-density necrotic center; area of low density (edema) surrounds developing capsule	Ring enchancement; may be thinner or ventricular or medial surface	Decay in contrast enhancement
Late capsule	Capsule visualized as a faint ring	Thin to moderately thick dense ring of contrast enhancement	Decay in contrast enhancement
Healed abscess	Collagen capsule commonly isodense with surrounding brain	May appear as nodular contrast enhancement for antibiotic treatment; no contrast enhancement	4 to 10 weeks after completion if cured

Adapted from Britt RH, Enzmann DR. Clinical stages of human abscesses on serial CT scans after contrast infusion. J Neurosurg 1983; 59:972–989.

performed to rule out acute bacterial meningitis. In the presence of a brain abscess, lumbar puncture increases the mortality but rarely gives a clue to the causative organism. On the other hand, spinal tap often gives a clue to the presence of a brain abscess because of pleocytosis and elevated protein and lack of organisms recovered on culture. Conversely, the cerebrospinal fluid may be normal in the presence of a brain abscess. It is the judgment of the physician whether the spinal tap can wait until after the CT scan. However, if lumbar puncture is delayed when bacterial meningitis is suspected, antibiotic therapy should be initiated before CT is performed.

As of this writing, CT with contrast is the most effective method of making the diagnosis. MRI may prove to be as or more useful, but the data are unavailable. Table 1 lists the stages of brain abscesses as seen before and after contrast in a CT scan. These classifications are useful in deciding upon surgical intervention and for following therapy. Obviously, the radiologist must be involved; the differential also includes hematomas and tumors. If present, ependymal or meningeal enhancement usually indicates infection, but these findings are not always seen with infection.

Management

In the stages of cerebritis (early infection of the brain parenchyma), some clinicians favor treating with antibiotics against the most likely organisms and following the CT without getting diagnostic material. In the latter stages, with capsule formation, drainage is usually needed. However, in patients in whom this procedure is too risky or the underlying medical condition does not allow for the procedure, empiric antibiotics alone have at times been successful.

The most prudent approach is to make an etiologic diagnosis. Here the neurosurgeon must be called on to determine the risks and possible consequences of aspiration of the abscess. However, CT or sterotactic guided-needle aspiration of the lesion is now commonplace and usually safe.

The single most important diagnostic procedure involving the aspirated material is Gram staining. This gives immediate information as to the causative agents and allows for an appropriate choice of antibiotics. The Gram stain is more important than the culture because many of the organisms are fastidious and may not grow, or, more likely, the patient may already have received antibiotics, making growth difficult. KOH and acid-fast stains should also be performed. Cultures should be performed for aerobic and anaerobic bacteria, fungi, and mycobacteria. If possible, histopathology should also be done if the aspirated material contains tissue.

Antibiotic therapy depends on the examination of the Gram stain. If this is not done, empiric therapy must cover anaerobes, streptococci, and gram-negative aerobes. In the past penicillin G was the preferred drug (12 to 24 million units per day intravenously), combined with chloramphenicol (1 g every 6 hours intravenously). However, many anaerobes are relatively penicillin-resistant, and many gram-negative aerobic bacilli are resistant to chloramphenicol. A newer combination that appears to be equally efficacious is any third-generation cephalosporin; ceftriaxone (2 g per day) is preferred, or ceftazidime (2 g every 8 hours intravenously) combined with metronidazole (500 mg every 6 hours intravenously) may be used. If staphylococci are suspected (endocarditis, head trauma) then nafcillin (12 g per day intravenously) should replace the cephalosporin.

If only gram-positive cocci in chains are noted in the smear, penicillin (12 to 24 million units per day) is the drug of choice. If mixtures of anaerobic organisms are seen, penicillin and metronidazole in the above doses are used. If gram-negative bacilli are seen, the third-generation cephalosporin replaces the penicillin until culture and sensitivities are known. For staphylococci in the penicillin-allergic patient, vancomycin (1 g every 12 hours intravenously) is used.

Steroids hinder the penetration of antibiotics into the abscess. Thus dexamethasone should be used only to reduce the surrounding edema. Dexamethasone (4 mg every 6 hours) tapered over 10 days to 2 weeks is usually sufficient.

Anticonvulsants (dilantin 300 mg daily) are indicated if the patient is having seizures.

Antibiotics are continued for 4 to 6 weeks, and CT is performed at regular intervals to note the decrease in edema, size, and contrast enhancement, as noted in Table 1. It may take 5 to 6 months for the CT to reach this stage.

SUBDURAL EMPYEMA

A subdural empyema is a collection of pus in the space between the cranial dura and arachnoid membranes.

Etiology

The majority of cases of subdural empyema (70 percent) are the result of acute sinusitis. The second most common underlying condition (25 percent) is a relatively new otogenic infection, as opposed to chronic otitis, which precedes brain abscesses. The remaining cases are secondary to bacterial meningitis (in children), osteomyelitis of the skull, and trauma. Infection of the subdural space is accomplished by direct extension of the infection (as in osteomyelitis) or by drainage of purulent material from the paranasal sinuses or ears via emissary veins, which frequently become thrombophlebitic. Hematogenous seeding from distant foci of infection occurs rarely if at all.

Microbiology

The causative bacteria are much the same as in cerebral brain abscesses. Anaerobes, microaerophilic streptococci, streptococci, and gram-negative aerobic bacilli (otogenic) are the usual organisms. Staphylococci are slightly more frequent secondary to osteomyelitis, trauma, or neurosurgical procedures. In children with

Haemophilus influenzae meningitis there may be direct extension of the organisms into a subdural effusion, giving rise to empyema.

Clinical Features

Signs and symptoms are related to three areas: those due to increased intracranial pressure, those associated with the focal site of infection, and those caused by meningeal irritation.

Headache and fever are prominent. Initially, the headache may be localized to the area of the infected sinus or ear, but later it becomes generalized. Nausea and vomiting are common, and other signs of increased intracranial pressure such as bradycardia and progressive obtundation may be evident. Papilledema is found in less than 50 percent of patients, while nuchal rigidity is seen in as many as 80 percent.

Focal neurologic signs such as hemiparesis or hemiplegia are frequent, as are either focal or generalized seizures. In some cases cranial nerve palsies may be evident.

Evidence of sinusitis or otitis is usually found.

Diagnosis

The diagnosis is made by CT of the head. Usually an elliptical hypodense region is seen directly next to the cranium or in the region of the falx cerebri. There is compression of the ipsilateral lateral ventricle. Evidence of sinusitis or mastoiditis may also be found with the scan.

If a subdural empyema is suspected, a lumbar puncture should not be done.

Management

Subdural empyema is a neurosurgical emergency. The pus must be drained to alleviate intracranial pressure and to help in clearing the infection. Controversy exists as to the use of multiple burr holes with irrigation or the use of craniotomy as the procedure of choice. I favor craniotomy for two reasons: It allows more space than burr holes for the brain to expand, and it allows for better drainage of thick, loculated pus. In infants with bulging fontanels, the pus may be drained by needle aspiration.

Numerous case studies have shown that drainage itself is not sufficient to effect a cure and that systemic antibiotics must be given for at least 3 weeks. Irrigation of the space with antibiotics has never been shown to affect the outcome.

A Gram stain of the pus is critical in determining antibiotic coverage. Treatment of gram-positive cocci in chains (streptococci) is penicillin. The adult dosage is 12 to 24 million units per day (1 to 2 million units every 2 hours). If the pus is foul smelling or the Gram stain shows a mixture of organisms, better anaerobic coverage should be added; metronidazole (500 mg every 6 hours) is preferred, or chloramphenicol (1 g every 6 hours) may be used. All drugs are given intravenously.

Gram-negative aerobic bacilli can be treated with a third-generation cephalosporin such as ceftriaxone (2 g per day) or ceftazidime (2 g every 8 hours). The latter drug also gives adequate *Pseudomonas* coverage until the results of culture and sensitivity are known.

If gram-positive cocci in clumps or clusters are seen, staphylococci should be suspected. The drug of choice is nafcillin (2 g every 4 hours intravenously). For the penicillin-allergic patient, vancomycin (1 g every 12 hours) is adequate with normal renal function.

In children with infections due to *H. influenzae*, the combination of chloramphenicol plus ampicillin or the use of a third-generation cephalosporin is sufficient.

Anticonvulsants are usually necessary.

The single most important prognostic factor is the level of obtundation at the time of drainage. With appropriate medical and surgical management the mortality rate varies between 10 and 20 percent.

CRANIAL EPIDURAL EMPYEMA (ABSCESS)

A cranial epidural empyema or abscess is a collection of pus between the dura mater and skull. Often there is coexistent subdural empyema.

The pathogenesis of cranial epidural abscess is generally the same as that of subdural empyema, that is, spread from a contiguous sinusitis or otitis. Orbital infections more commonly result in cranial epidural abscesses, and neurosurgery or compound skull fracture more often precedes the development of this infection.

Because of the limited anatomic space, infection in this area expands slowly and does not produce the dramatic neurologic changes seen with subdural empyema. Frequently persistent headache and fever are the only clues.

The diagnosis is made by contrast-enhanced CT of the head. The management (both surgical and medical) is the same as for subdural empyemas. Because of the effect of previous neurosurgery or trauma as the inciting event, there is a higher likelihood that *S. aureus* will be the causative agent than is the case with subdural empyema.

SPINAL EPIDURAL ABSCESS

Spinal epidural abscess is an infection in that space bounded by the dura of the spinal cord on the inside and the bony vertebral canal on the outside. These infections are uncommon, having a rate of occurrence of approximately one per year in large acute-care hospitals.

Etiology

Infection is introduced into the spinal epidural space either by hematogenous spread from a remote site or by direct extension from vertebral osteomyelitis. Recent spinal surgery or epidural anesthesia may also result in a spinal epidural abscess. Intravenous drug abuse is being seen with increasing frequency as an underlying condition.

The most common distant infections leading to hematogenous seeding are skin and soft tissue infections. Other sources include respiratory, abdominal, and urinary tracts. In addition to vertebral osteomyelitis, direct extension can occur from psoas, retropharyngeal, and perinephric abscesses.

Microbiology

S. aureus is the most commonly recovered agent. When infections due to *Staphylococcus epidermidis* and streptococcal species are added to those caused by *S. aureus*, gram-positive cocci account for 78 percent of all spinal epidural abscesses.

Aerobic gram-negative bacilli are largely responsible for the remainder of infections. Other causative organisms have been *Mycobacterium tuberculosis*, *Blastomyces dermatitidis*, *Coccidioides immitis*, *Cryptococcus neoformans*, *Aspergillus* species, and *Brucella*.

Clinical Features

Initially, the signs and symptoms of a spinal abscess are nonspecific. Backache is present in 90 percent of individuals, and fever is seen in 57 percent. Patients may be overtly septic from the initial site of infection.

Signs and symptoms generally go through four stages, and the time involved ranges from only a few hours to several weeks. The first stage is spinal ache or back pain. Secondly, root pain develops, and, depending on the location of the abscess along the spinal cord, this pain may present as abdominal in origin, mimicking pancreatic or gallbladder disease. Lumbar abscesses may have sciatica as the root pain. The third stage is weakness, and this may include bowel or bladder dysfunction. The fourth and final stage is paralysis.

Diagnosis

The difficult part of the diagnosis is suspecting the possibility of a spinal epidural abscess during one of the first three stages before paralysis sets in. The possibility of spinal epidural abscess must be included in many differential diagnoses.

Plain films of the spine may show evidence of vertebral osteomyelitis if this is the source, but films are frequently normal and thus cannot be relied on for the diagnosis of spinal epidural abscess. Similarly, bone scans may have the same results. In one series of spinal epidural abscesses, the CT was negative in two-thirds of the cases.

At times lumbar punctures are done in the evaluation of the clinical symptoms. Pleocytosis and elevated protein with negative cultures are usually found.

The time-honored method of making the diagnosis, and the procedure that is positive in almost all cases, is myelography. MRI may hold promise but has not yet been compared with the myelogram.

Management

Once the diagnosis is made, decompressive laminectomy and drainage must be done. Pus or granulation tissue should be cultured for bacteria (aerobic and anaerobic), mycobacteria, and fungi. Gram and acid-fast stains should also be performed.

Initial antibiotic coverage should be directed against staphylococci and gram-negative bacilli. Nafcillin (2 g every 12 hours intravenously) combined with gentamicin (2.0 mg per kilogram loading dose, followed by 1.5 mg per kilogram every 8 hours for patients with normal renal function) is an appropriate regimen. Once culture and sensitivity results are known, the antibiotics should be adjusted accordingly. Antimicrobial agents should be continued for 3 to 4 weeks after drainage and for 6 to 8 weeks if osteomyelitis is present.

The level and duration of neurologic impairment (above stages) at the time of laminectomy are the major factors determining the outcome.

CEREBRAL MYCOTIC ANEURYSMS

Cerebral mycotic aneurysms result from embolization of infected material to the bifurcation of the cerebral arteries or the vasa vasorum of these arteries. This process results in infection of the wall of the artery and, combined with the resultant inflammatory process, leads to weakening of the wall and dilatation. The term *mycotic* means *inflammatory*, not *fungal*.

The underlying condition is almost always bacterial endocarditis, and cerebral aneurysms occur in 4 to 10 percent of cases. The aneurysms may range from asymptomatic to rupture causing massive intracranial hemorrhage and death. Between these extremes the patient may have headaches, neurologic findings (cranial nerve palsies), or subarachnoid bleeding.

The definitive management of cerebral mycotic aneurysms is not clear and should be handled on a case-by-case basis. Of paramount importance is treating the endocarditis with antibiotics and performing valve replacement if indicated. Most aneurysms will resolve on their own over time, even after completion of a successful course of antibiotics.

If a mycotic aneurysm is known to be present, it should be followed by use of serial angiography. Rapidly enlarging lesions, subarachnoid hemorrhage, and evidence of an intracranial hematoma are indications for considering surgery to obliterate or clip the aneurysm. Decisions regarding the surgery also depend upon the accessibility of the aneurysm.

SUGGESTED READING

Britt RH, Enzmann DR. Clinical stages of human brain abscesses on serial CT scans after contrast infusion. J Neurosurg 1983; 58:972–989.

Chun CH, Johnson JD, Hofstetter M, Roff MJ. Brain abscess: a study of 45 consecutive cases. Medicine 1986; 66:415–431.

Morawetz RB, Karp RB. Evolution of intracranial bacterial (mycotic) aneurysms. Neurosurgery 1984; 15:43–48.

Sarwar M, Falkoff G, Naseem M. Radiologic techniques in the diagnosis of CNS infections. Neurol Clin 1986; 4:41–68.

Silverberg AL, DiNubile MJ. Subdural empyema and cranial epidural abscess. Med Clin North Am 1985; 69:361–374.

Verner EE, Mushen DM. Spinal epidural abscess. Med Clin North Am 1985; 69:375–384.

VIRAL ENCEPHALITIS

MARTIN S. HIRSCH, M.D.
DAVID D. HO, M.D.

Encephalitis, defined as inflammation of the brain, is not a rare disease. Approximately 1,400 to 4,300 cases are reported annually in the United States to the Centers for Disease Control, although the actual numbers are certainly much higher. Patients with encephalitis frequently also have meningeal inflammation, perhaps making meningoencephalitis a more appropriate term.

Meningoencephalitis has diverse causes. Despite the wide variety of agents that can cause encephalitis in the United States, 50 to 75 percent of all cases remain etiologically undefined. Although viruses cause the majority of the remainder, nonviral disease can also present with an encephalitic picture (Table 1). Since the morbidity and mortality of certain forms of encephalitis are high (5 to 10 percent overall fatality rates, but 70 to 80 percent with herpes simplex and eastern equine encephalitis), early recognition is important. Because antiviral agents can reduce the mortality from herpes simplex encephalitis, accurate diagnosis and prompt therapy have become imperative. A systematic diagnostic approach is necessary when patients present with altered mental status, fever, and headache. Analysis of cerebrospinal fluid (CSF) and attempts to evaluate focal abnormalities by physical examination, electroencephalography (EEG), computed tomography (CT), or technetium brain scans are indicated. If focal abnormalities are found, brain biopsy is required to confirm the diagnosis.

This chapter concentrates on acute meningoencephalitides caused by herpes simplex virus and arboviruses and presents guidelines for the diagnosis and management of patients with these disorders.

HERPES SIMPLEX VIRUS, TYPE I (HSV-I)

Herpes simplex virus accounts for 10 percent of all reported cases of encephalitis, and estimates of its frequency in the United States range from several hundred to several thousand cases a year. Individuals of all ages are susceptible, though neonates are usually infected by HSV-II and others by HSV-I. Beyond the newborn period, herpes simplex encephalitis may result from either primary infection (30 percent) or reactivation (70 percent). HSV-I has a predilection for involvement of the temporal lobe, possibly related to retrograde spread by olfactory or trigeminal pathways.

Previously healthy individuals of both sexes are most often affected. Presentation may be abrupt or insidious, following a nonspecific prodrome. Fever, headache, nuchal rigidity, and obtundation are the common presenting features. Personality change occurs in 85 percent of patients, dysphasia in 76 percent, seizures in 67 percent, autonomic dysfunction in 60 percent, and ataxia in 40 percent. Focal findings (hemiparesis, cranial nerve deficits, localized seizures) are present in 85 percent of patients.

TABLE 1 Important Nonviral Causes of Encephalitis

Mycobacterium tuberculosis
Mycoplasma pneumoniae
Rickettsia rickettsii
Lyme disease
Leptospira interrogans
Treponema pallidum
Coccidioides immitis
Naegleria species
Toxoplasma gondii, Cryptococcus neoformans, Listeria monocytogenes in immunosuppressed patients
Atypical presentation of bacterial meningitis, brain abscess, parameningeal infection, infective endocarditis*
Collagen vascular disease

*In addition, it is important to recognize that many conditions may mimic encephalitis. These include metabolic and toxic encephalopathies, carcinomas, lymphomas, and cerebrovascular accidents.

CSF formulas can range from normal (3 percent) to markedly abnormal, with neutrophils early and lymphocytes later in illness. Erythrocytes may be present, protein levels are usually elevated, and glucose levels are usually normal. Cultures of CSF for HSV are negative in more than 95 percent of patients.

Among neurodiagnostic tests, the EEG is the most sensitive early in herpes encephalitis. The characteristic pattern is one of periodic temporal spike and slow waves and is found in the majority of cases. Magnetic resonance imaging (MRI) may also be a sensitive early diagnostic test. Focal findings on technetium scan (enhanced localized radionuclide uptake) or CT scan (edema, mass effect, low-density lesion with contrast enhancement, hemorrhage) are seen in approximately 50 percent of patients. None of these neurodiagnostic findings, however, is specific for herpes encephalitis.

Brain biopsy is the only certain way to confirm the diagnosis. The yield from an open biopsy is extremely high and morbidity is low (2 percent). If one relies on clinical impressions alone, the diagnosis of herpes encephalitis is incorrect approximately 50 percent of the time. Biopsy can not only confirm this impression, but it can also provide alternative, treatable diagnoses. Proper ways to process biopsy specimens are discussed below (Clinical Guidelines).

Randomized, double-blinded, placebo-controlled, multicenter studies have demonstrated efficacy for vidarabine (adenine arabinoside) in reducing mortality from herpes simplex encephalitis. Age and state of consciousness at onset are important variables influencing outcome. More recent controlled trials in the United States and in Sweden showed that intravenous acyclovir was more effective than vidarabine in improving survival. Thus, at present, acyclovir (30 mg per kilogram per day in three divided doses) is the treatment of choice for herpes encephalitis. Individuals who are younger than 30 years of age fare better than those who are older, and patients who are merely lethargic respond to treatment better than those who are comatose.

ARBOVIRUSES

Although no longer an official taxonomic term, arbovirus refers to a group of more than 250 enveloped RNA viruses transmitted by arthropods. Nearly all cases of arbovirus encephalitis in the United States are due to St. Louis encephalitis (SLE), eastern equine encephalitis (EEE), western equine encephalitis (WEE), and California encephalitis (CE). Together these arboviruses account for about 10 percent of all cases of reported encephalitis, but this figure can be as high as 50 percent during an epidemic year.

SLE is the commonest arboviral disease in the United States. The largest epidemic of SLE occurred in 1975, with nearly 2,000 cases reported from the East Coast to Arizona; the case fatality rate was 10 percent. In urban areas of the Midwest, SLE virus is transmitted by *Culex* mosquitoes, which breed in stagnant sewage water. In the West, the disease occurs primarily in irrigated rural areas, whereas in Florida, the mosquito vector and disease are prevalent in both urban and rural areas. Asymptomatic or mild infections are common, particularly in children. Severe disease is more likely to involve the aged. In addition to typical encephalitic findings, dysuria, pyuria, and inappropriate ADH secretion may occur. There are no unique CSF or EEG findings. As with all of the arboviruses causing encephalitis in the United States, viral isolation from CSF or blood is uncommon, although the agent can be isolated from affected brain tissue by inoculation of appropriate cell cultures or suckling mice. Serology, however, is the mainstay of arboviral diagnosis, and a variety of techniques are used to assay for both serum and CSF antibodies. No effective antiviral treatment is yet available for SLE or any of the other arbovirus encephalitides.

Eastern equine encephalitis occurs sporadically near freshwater marshes of the Atlantic and Gulf coasts. Although cases are generally limited in number, mortality rates often exceed 50 percent. Birds are the main reservoir, and the virus is transmitted by a mosquito that does not ordinarily bite humans. Disease in neither horse nor man plays a role in the subsequent spread of virus. Disease is most frequent in those younger than 10 or older than 55 years. Often, EEE has an abrupt onset and a fulminant course, with progressive loss of consciousness and seizures. Cranial nerve abnormalities and periorbital edema are occasionally seen. The CSF often contains fewer than 1,000 leukocytes per cubic millimeter, with a preponderance of neutrophils. Survivors are often left with significant neurologic sequelae, including mental retardation, seizure disorders, or emotional lability.

Western equine encephalitis occurs sporadically in irrigated rural areas in the western two-thirds of the United States. As in EEE and SLE, birds are the major reservoir for infection. Highest attack rates are in infants younger than 1 year or those older than 55 years. Mild and inapparent infections are frequent, and case fatality rates are low (2 to 3 percent). However, children under 2 years may develop mental retardation seizures, or spasticity after recovery.

California encephalitis has a wide geographic distribution, but is particularly common in the upper Mississippi Valley. Among 10 subtypes of CE virus, the LaCrosse strain is the most prevalent and virulent. The vector is a forest-dwelling mosquito, and the reservoirs are small rodents such as squirrels; this explains the predilection of the vector for woodland campers. Disease occurs primarily among children in the 5- to 9-year-old age group, with adults usually having mild or asymptomatic infections. Fatalities are rare, but persisting personality problems or recurrent seizures are seen in up to 15 percent of affected children.

OTHER VIRUSES

Central nervous system manifestations can complicate many other viral infections. Varicella encephalitis can present as acute cerebellar ataxia with nystagmus and dysarthria. This syndrome is associated with an excellent prognosis. However, varicella encephalitis can also begin with seizures and focal neurologic deficits, with a mortality rate as high as 35 percent. Herpes zoster encephalitis is rare and largely seen in elderly immunosuppressed patients; it is usually self-limited and has a low mortality.

Encephalitis due to Epstein-Barr virus (EBV) can be diffuse or localized to the temporal lobe or cerebellum. When seen in the setting of heterophile antibody–positive infectious mononucleosis, the diagnosis can be readily made. However, encephalitis may be the only manifestation of EBV infection, requiring determination of specific antibodies to viral capsid or early antigens.

Cytomegaloviral (CMV) encephalitis is exceedingly uncommon in previously healthy individuals, but may occur in the setting of immunodeficiency. Disorientation, obtundation, paresthesias, and psychotic behavior occur. A syndrome of subacute encephalitis once thought to be secondary to CMV has been observed in patients with acquired immunodeficiency syndrome (AIDS). This disorder is characterized by apathy, depression, and progressive dementia. Recent studies suggest that the encephalopathy of AIDS is actually a consequence of brain infection by the human immunodeficiency virus (HIV). Acute self-limited encephalitis may also characterize the primary HIV syndrome 6 to 12 weeks following infection.

Enteroviral encephalitis occurs primarily in children during summer months. Although enteroviruses cause 30 to 50 percent of all cases of viral meningitis, they account for only 2 percent of encephalitis cases. Outcomes are generally benign, except in newborns, in whom fulminant encephalitis may occur, and in children with agammaglobulinemia, who sometimes develop chronic encephalitis.

Rabies virus encephalitis following animal bites is discussed elsewhere in this text. Lymphocytic choriomeningitis is a rare cause of encephalitis and is suggested by very high CSF lymphocyte counts and/or high protein values in the setting of recent exposure to rodents such as mice or hamsters.

Parainfectious encephalitides may follow viral infections or vaccinations and are thought to result from immunopathologic mechanisms. Most cases of measles encephalitis are thought to be parainfectious. Varicella, mumps, rubella, or influenza virus infections, as well as ill-defined upper respiratory infections, may be followed in 4 to 14 days by encephalitis clinically indistinguishable from that caused by direct viral involvement. Permanent neurologic sequelae are infrequent except in the setting of measles.

CLINICAL GUIDELINES

Alteration in brain function distinguishes viral meningoencephalitis from viral aseptic meningitis (see Table 2). Once this differentiation is made, the physician must consider epidemiologic features for clues concerning season, geography, prodromal illness, and insect or animal exposure. A summer case of encephalitis occurring near freshwater marshes of Massachusetts results in a different list of diagnostic possibilities than a winter case in Nebraska. In addition, nonviral, often treatable illnesses that may mimic viral encephalitis must always be considered (Table 1). Searching for such clues may occasionally lead to a laboratory test, such as a mono spot test or heterophile antibody determination, that provides the diagnosis.

Clinical features alone cannot usually establish an etiologic diagnosis. However, hints of temporal lobe involvement (focal seizures, speech difficulties, olfactory hallucinations) should suggest the diagnosis of herpes simplex encephalitis. The temporal sequence of the disease may also be helpful. Encephalitis following a viral exanthem by 1 to 2 weeks is more likely to be parainfectious, whereas a rapid progressive clinical course without prodrome suggests herpes or EEE.

Examination of CSF is important and can usually be performed following early lumbar puncture. If there is concern about elevated intracranial pressure and possible herniation, a cisternal puncture can be performed. If the CSF shows a neutrophilic response, bacterial processes

are likely, although early viral infections of the central nervous system can demonstrate a similar picture. A normal CSF formula suggests a toxic or metabolic encephalopathy, but does not rule out an early viral encephalitis. If the clinical suspicion is high, a repeat lumbar puncture may be necessary. A lymphocytic pleocytosis in the CSF is most frequently found in viral encephalitis, although fungal and mycobacterial processes must be excluded. Appropriate cultures, stains, and antigen testing must be performed on individual specimens. Attempts should be made to determine whether the process is generalized or localized in the central nervous system. Electroencephalography, CT scanning, and radionuclide scanning can all provide useful information. Anatomic definition is also helpful in directing the approach of neurosurgeons in subsequent brain biopsies. The need for a biopsy should be evaluated for each case. However, if a frontotemporal lesion is defined, we favor open biopsy of the involved area.

The brain biopsy specimen should be immediately cultured for virus and processed for histopathology. Immunofluorescence for herpesvirus antigens can provide confirmatory data, often within hours of biopsy. However, culture of the biopsy material remains the sine qua non for diagnosis. In herpes encephalitis, viral cultures are often positive within 24 to 48 hours, and the great majority are positive by day 5. Compared with viral isolation, histopathologic changes, e.g., intranuclear inclusions, lack sensitivity (56 percent), but are reasonably specific (86 percent). Immunofluorescence is quite sensitive (70 percent) and specific (91 percent). Electron microscopy for herpesvirus particles is insensitive (45 percent), but highly specific (98 percent).

Serology may be useful in making a retrospective diagnosis of herpes encephalitis. CSF HSV-I antigen tests are under study. Measurement of specific HSV-I antibodies in CSF and comparison of serum to CSF antibody levels are not sufficiently sensitive (50 percent) during the first 10 days of illness to influence management decisions. Measurement of early antibody to arboviruses may be more useful. If the physician's index of suspicion for arboviral encephalitis is high, several state and federal laboratories can detect small amounts of serum or CSF antibodies to these viruses early in the course of disease.

Because the level of consciousness is a critical prognostic factor in the outcome of herpes encephalitis, therapeutic decisions must be made prior to definitive diagnosis, which follows biopsy. Therapy with acyclovir, 30 mg per kilogram per day infused intravenously in three divided doses, should be instituted immediately after biopsy or earlier if biopsy is delayed. If cultures of herpesvirus are positive, treatment is continued for 10 days. If all assays are negative by the fifth day, acyclovir should be discontinued.

Treatment for other forms of viral encephalitis remains supportive. Attention must be directed toward reducing cerebral edema, if present, by agents such as dexamethasone or mannitol. Seizures are managed with intravenous anticonvulsive agents. Respiratory support may be required, and care is needed to prevent or treat secondary bacterial infections.

TABLE 2 Management of Viral Encephalitis

Is encephalitis present?	Check for brain dysfunction
Are there epidemiologic clues?	Review information such as season, geography, animal or insect exposure, prodromal illness
Are there CSF or serum abnormalities?	Check CSF cell and differential counts, protein, glucose, and obtain cultures or antigen tests for bacteria, fungi, mycobacteria Obtain CSF and peripheral viral cultures and appropriate studies on serum (heterophile and viral antibodies)
Are there focal neurologic abnormalities?	Review physical examination and consider EEG, CT scan, MRI
Should the site of focal abnormality be biopsied?	Culture biopsy material for viruses and examine by histology and immunofluorescence
Should treatment be started?	Begin acyclovir (10 mg/kg q8h) IV Continue for 10 days if brain biopsy herpes cultures are positive; discontinue on day 5 if herpes studies are negative

Approaches to diagnosis and treatment of viral meningoencephalitis are still in their infancy. Nevertheless, important advances have been made over the past decade. With the development of sensitive antigen- and nucleic acid–detection techniques, as well as advances in antiviral therapy, even more significant strides should occur in the relatively near future.

This chapter was supported by the Mashud A. Mezerhane B. Fund.

SUGGESTED READING

Gabuzda DH, Hirsch MS. Neurologic manifestations of infection with human immunodeficiency virus—clinical features and pathogenesis. Ann Intern Med 1987; 107:383–391.

Lakeman FD, Koga J, Whitley RJ. Detection of antigen to herpes simplex virus in cerebrospinal fluid from patients with herpes simplex encephalitis. J Infect Dis 1987; 155:1172–1178.

Whitley RJ, Alford CA, Hirsch MS, et al. Vidarabine versus acyclovir therapy in herpes simplex encephalitis. N Engl J Med 1986; 314:144–149.

URINARY TRACT INFECTIONS AND SEXUALLY TRANSMITTED DISEASE

BACTERIURIA AND PYELONEPHRITIS

CLARE L. CHERNEY, M.D.
DONALD KAYE, M.D.

Bacteriuria is defined as bacteria in the urine. Bacteriuria is quantitated to ascertain the probability of a truly infected urinary tract. Significant bacteriuria has traditionally been defined as 10^5 or more colony-forming units (cfu) per milliliter of urine, but lesser numbers may have significance in certain situations.

Bacteriuria may be symptomatic or asymptomatic. The clinical syndrome of dysuria, urgency, and frequency—with or without suprapubic tenderness—is defined as cystitis or lower urinary tract infection (UTI). The clinical syndrome of flank pain and/or tenderness and fever, with or without cystitis symptoms, indicates involvement of the kidney in the infectious process (i.e., pyelonephritis). The cystitis syndrome alone in no way excludes upper tract infection and, in fact, kidney involvement is common.

When discussing UTIs, it is important to differentiate reinfection from relapse. A relapse occurs when the same organism persists in the urinary tract so that infection recurs soon after antimicrobial therapy is discontinued. A reinfection is a new infection caused by a different or the same organism.

DIAGNOSIS

Microscopic examination of the urine is a quick, simple office procedure that can yield much useful information. Pyuria is present in many patients with symptomatic and asymptomatic bacteriuria. Pyuria is best defined as more than 10 polymorphonuclear leukocytes per cubic millimeter in a counting chamber. A less accurate definition is more than five to 10 white blood cells (WBCs) per high-power field in a centrifuged (5 minutes at 2,000 rpm) clean-catch urine specimen. It should be emphasized that many patients with pyuria do not have infection and other diagnoses should be entertained.

Methylene blue or Gram staining of the urine can aid in the predictability of significant bacteriuria. One bacterium visualized in each oil-immersion field in an unspun, stained, midstream, clean-catch urine correlates with 10^5 or more cfu per milliliter. If the urine is centrifuged and stained, one visualized bacterium per oil-immersion field correlates with 10^4 or more cfu per milliliter.

Quantitative urine cultures have been used to differentiate true and reproducible bacteriuria from urine contaminated from the urethra or vagina. In the asymptomatic patient, two separate clean-catch specimens, each with 10^5 or more cfu per milliliter of the same organism, are highly predictive of true bacteriuria. Since men and catheterized patients have less chance of contamination, 10^4 or more cfu per milliliter is considered significant in these groups. In women with dysuria and pyuria, 10^2 or more Enterobacteriaceae per milliliter is predictive of infection. Any growth from a suprapubic puncture of the bladder is considered indicative of infection.

MANAGEMENT OF SYMPTOMATIC LOWER URINARY TRACT INFECTION

Since not all patients with dysuria syndromes have UTI, a prerequisite to management is making the correct diagnosis. Herpes, chlamydial, gonococcal, and ureaplasmal infections of the urethra and vaginal infections can all cause dysuria, but routine urine cultures will be negative.

The majority of adults with symptomatic UTIs are young, healthy women. Some of these patients have a predisposition for recurrent UTIs, but few of them have underlying anatomic or surgically correctable abnormalities. Sexual intercourse and use of a diaphragm both increase the frequency of infection in this group. The prognosis is excellent since there is no evidence that recurrent UTIs in nonpregnant women without urinary tract obstruction lead to renal damage.

The majority of UTIs are caused by Enterobacteriaceae, especially *Escherichia coli*. *Staphylococcus saprophyticus,* a coagulase-negative, novobiocin-resistant staphylococcus, is a common cause of infection in sexually active young women.

Single-dose therapeutic regimens cure 80 to 100 percent of lower tract infections in women. One problem with this approach is the difficulty in identifying patients with asymptomatic upper tract infection, in whom there is a high risk of relapse. Single-dose therapy is applicable only with agents that have a relatively long half-life in serum and therefore provide prolonged urinary levels. Rather than advocate single-dose therapy, we prefer the concept of short-course therapy. This means giving doses of an agent that will provide 1 to 3 days of antimicrobial activity in the urine. This can be achieved, for example, with a single double-strength tablet of trimethoprim-sulfamethoxazole (160 mg of TMP, 800 mg of SMZ) or with 250 mg of amoxicillin or cephalexin every 8 hours for 24 hours. Some authorities prefer to give short-course therapy for 3 days on the assumption that 3 days will cure some patients with asymptomatic upper tract infection. This approach is probably preferable.

Table 1 lists some of the single-dose regimens that have been demonstrated to be effective. Some standard dosing regimens that can be given for short courses (1 to 3 days of therapy) are also listed. Urine cultures are not essential prior to short-course therapy.

Some women with frequently recurring symptomatic UTIs that follow sexual intercourse can be effectively managed with pericoital prophylaxis using a single, low dose of an antimicrobial agent such as one single-strength TMP-SMZ tablet (80 mg, 400 mg) or 100 mg of nitrofurantoin. Women with frequent symptomatic reinfections and children with frequent symptomatic or asymptomatic reinfections with no identifiable precipitating event are candidates for low-dose, long-term prophylaxis, which has been shown to reduce the number of episodes of cystitis by more than 90 percent and is well tolerated in the majority of patients. TMP-SMZ (one-half of one single-strength tablet nightly) or nitrofurantoin (50 mg nightly) have proven to be effective for this purpose. We recommend a trial of 6 months of prophylaxis and then reevaluation.

If patients remain asymptomatic after therapy, follow-up cultures are necessary only in pregnant women and children in whom it is important to treat asymptomatic bacteriuria. For the majority of women, follow-up cultures are not cost effective or warranted. If symptoms persist through therapy, the patient either does not have a UTI or has a UTI with a resistant organism, and a urine culture is indicated for diagnosis and susceptibility patterns.

If a patient responds and then relapses with symptoms after short-course therapy, urine cultures should be obtained and a 14-day course of antimicrobial therapy should be given to treat a possible renal focus. If symptomatic relapse again occurs, evaluation should be obtained to rule out stones and/or obstruction. In the absence of anatomic abnormalities, 4–6 weeks of therapy should be considered. Asymptomatic relapses are probably of little importance except in children and pregnant women.

Any child with a urinary tract infection should have an anatomic evaluation. Vesicoureteral reflux and obstruction are common and important to rule out since progressive renal damage can occur with these abnormalities alone and be accelerated in the presence of bacteriuria. Ultrasonography and radionuclide voiding studies are noninvasive diagnostic techniques that can be used for screening in this situation. Short-course therapy has not been extensively evaluated in

TABLE 1 Some Regimens for Patients Not Seriously Ill

Condition	Therapy	
	Duration	Agent and Dose
Cystitis	Single-dose therapy for women	TMP 400 mg* TMP-SMZ 320–1,600 mg*† Nitrofurantoin 200 mg Amoxicillin 3 g Tetracycline 2 g‡ Sulfisoxazole 2 g†
	Short-course (1–3 days) therapy for women; 7 days for men; 4–6 wk for relapse	TMP 100 mg q12h* TMP-SMZ 160–800 mg q12h*† Nitrofurantoin 100 mg q6h Amoxicillin 250–500 mg q8h Amoxicillin–clavulanic acid 250–500 mg q8h Sulfisoxazole 500 mg q6h† Cephalexin ⎫ Cephradine ⎬ 250 mg q6–8h Cefaclor ⎭ Norfloxacin 400 mg q12h* Ciprofloxacin 500 mg q12h* Tetracycline 250 mg q6h‡
Prophylaxis for frequently recurring UTIs in female (all in single doses each day)		Nitrofurantoin 50–100 mg/ day; children 1–2 mg/ kg/day TMP-SMZ 40–200 mg/day or thrice weekly*†; children 2 mg/kg/day of TMP component Trimethoprim 50–100 mg/ day*; children 2 mg/ kg/day
Children's doses for cystitis	7 days of therapy; 4–6 wk for relapse	TMP 4 mg/kg q12h TMP-SMZ 4–20 mg/kg q12h† Nitrofurantoin 1–2 mg/kg q6h Amoxicillin 20 mg/kg/day up to 20 kg divided q8h Sulfisoxazole 38 mg/kg q6h not to exceed 6 g† Cephalexin 6–12 mg/kg q6h Cephradine 6–12 mg/kg q6h Cefaclor 20 mg/kg/day divided q8h

* Not advocated during pregnancy because of possible teratogenicity.
† Should not be used close to term or in the newborn because of risk of kernicterus.
‡ Not to be used during tooth development, i.e., from the second half of pregnancy through 8 years of age.

children, and we recommend 7-day courses of therapy. Table 1 outlines drugs and dosages for children.

For the child who relapses, 2 weeks of therapy are used, and if relapse occurs again, 4–6 weeks of therapy are indicated. For the child with recurrent reinfections but no surgically correctable abnormality, low-dose, long-term prophylaxis may be indicated. Although new renal scarring in children after the age of 5 years is uncommon, we favor therapy of asymptomatic bacteriuria until young adulthood.

Males with urinary tract infection should be evaluated for structural abnormalities. Urinary tract obstruction is common in males with bacteriuria and, with and without bacteriuria, can lead to progressive renal damage. An ultrasound study with or without a radionuclide bladder-emptying study, may be sufficient. In men, short-course therapy has not been adequately evaluated, and we favor a 7-day course of therapy for lower urinary tract infection. A symptomatic relapse, as with women and children, should be treated for 14 days to cover the possibility of an upper tract focus. A subsequent relapse suggests the possibility of chronic bacterial prostatitis (see the chapter *Prostatitis, Epididymitis, and Balanoposthitis*), obstruction, or calculus. If surgically correctable lesions have been ruled out, longer courses of therapy, such as 4–6 weeks, are indicated at this time. Asymptomatic recurrences in the absence of urinary tract obstruction do not need to be treated in adults.

MANAGEMENT OF SYMPTOMATIC UPPER TRACT INFECTION

Acute pyelonephritis is suspected when a patient presents with fever, flank pain, nausea, and vomiting, with or without abdominal tenderness. Processes such as renal infarct, stones, obstruction, hemorrhage, tumor, spinal or epidural abscesses, intra-abdominal processes, and thoracolumbar herpes zoster can cause similar syndromes. Gram-negative bacteremia complicating pyelonephritis should be suspected when the patient presents with shaking chills, high fever, hypotension, confusion, and/or lethargy.

Patients should be admitted to the hospital when they are seriously ill, elderly, immunocompromised, or unable to take oral medication, or when the diagnosis is not certain. Both blood and urine cultures should be obtained, and the urine should be examined for the presence of pyuria and gram-negative or gram-positive organisms.

Table 2 lists commonly used drugs and dosages, depending on the clinical situation and urine Gram stain. There are many effective options. In the seriously ill patient, when bacteremia is suspected, we favor therapy with a third-generation cephalosporin until results of cultures are known. Patients can be switched to oral therapy when they are afebrile and doing well (see dosages in Table 1). Therapy should be given for a total of 14 days.

In the less-severely ill patient with pyelonephritis an oral drug can be administered. Outpatient care is an option when the patient is well enough to take oral medication, the diagnosis is clear, and the patient is reliable enough for adequate follow-up. Oral TMP-SMZ or norfloxacin or ciprofloxacin, or daily intramuscular ceftriaxone or aminoglycoside all are potential outpatient regimens for the moderately ill outpatient. Oral cephalexin, cephradine, and amoxicillin (alone or with clavulanic acid) are other options. Again, therapy should be given for a total of 14 days.

When the patient does not defervesce while being adequately treated for the urine and/or blood isolates, an underlying collection of pus must be suspected. Obstruction with hydropyonephrosis, intraparenchymal renal abscesses, and perinephric abscesses are most important to rule out. Plain films and ultrasonography of the abdomen aid in diagnosis

TABLE 2 Some Regimens for Seriously Ill Adults

Condition	Therapy
Community-acquired gram-negative bacteria in urine	TMP-SMZ 5–25 mg/kg IV q12h or PO*†
	Nonpseudomonal extended-spectrum cephalosporin, e.g., ceftizoxime 2 g IV q8h, cefotaxime 2 g IV q6h, ceftriaxone 2 g IV or IM q24h
	Gentamicin or tobramycin 1.7 mg/kg IV or IM q8h adjusted for renal insufficiency
	Aztreonam 2 g IV q8h†
Nosocomially acquired gram-negative bacteria in urine	Ceftazidime 1–2 g IV q8h
	Gentamicin or tobramycin 1.7 mg/kg IV or IM q8h adjusted for renal insufficiency
	Aztreonam 1–2 g IV q8h†
	Ciprofloxacin 500–750 mg PO q12h†
Community or nosocomially acquired gram-positive bacteria in urine	
Streptococci	Ampicillin 2 g IV q4h plus gentamicin
Staphylococci	Cefazolin 1–2 g IV or IM q8h
	Nafcillin 2 g IV q4h
	or
	Vancomycin 1 g IV q12h adjusted for renal insufficiency if methicillin-resistant†

* Should not be used close to term or in the newborn infant since it can cause kernicterus.
† Not advocated during pregnancy because of possible teratogenicity.

of stones, abnormal gas/fluid patterns, and hydronephrosis, but computed tomography (CT) is the imaging modality of choice to rule out intra-abdominal abscesses.

Intraparenchymal or corticomedullary renal abscesses have been increasingly recognized as more sensitive imaging techniques have been used. In many cases these abscesses represent infected foci that have not yet formed well-encapsulated abscesses. In general, they should be aggressively treated with parenteral antimicrobial agents, and only if no response is noted in 7 days or the patient is doing poorly should percutaneous or surgical drainage be attempted.

Perinephric abscesses probably occur after rupture of a corticomedullary abscess into the space between Gerota's fascia and the kidney. They usually have an insidious onset and are often unsuspected at the time of presentation. As opposed to corticomedullary collections, it is imperative to drain perinephric abscesses.

When upper tract infection is complicated by abscesses, more prolonged therapy is indicated. All patients with pyelonephritis should have at least an ultrasonic study to seek obstruction and/or stones. Follow-up urine cultures are mandatory 2 weeks after therapy is complete in pregnant women and children. In nonpregnant adults without symptoms, follow-up cultures are optional. Symptomatic relapses warrant prolonged antimicrobial therapy (e.g., 4–6 weeks) while anatomic evaluation of the urinary tract is ongoing. In the male, if there are no surgically correctable abnormalities, chronic bacterial prostatitis should be suspected and evaluated and treated as detailed in the chapter on prostatitis. Asymptomatic recurrences need be treated only in pregnant patients, children, and patients with uncorrectable obstructive uropathy.

MANAGEMENT OF ASYMPTOMATIC BACTERIURIA

Asymptomatic bacteriuria is a common finding that increases in frequency with age. Approximately 5 percent of middle-aged women are bacteriuric at any time. In the elderly population, at least 20 percent of women and 10 percent of men have bacteriuria on survey. Excluding pregnant women, patients with obstruction, and young children, the significance of asymptomatic bacteriuria is controversial and unclear. Asymptomatic bacteriuria has been associated with an increased risk of mortality in some community studies but not in others. It is not clear whether the increased mortality (if real) is secondary to bacteriuria itself or secondary to underlying diseases that predispose to bacteriuria. If it were established that bacteriuria definitely increased mortality, it would still be necessary to demonstrate that elimination of bacteriuria lengthened survival before therapy could be advocated in all cases.

With the following exceptions, we favor no therapy for asymptomatic bacteriuria at this time. In the pregnant patient, asymptomatic bacteriuria should be sought and treated (see Management of Bacteriuria During Pregnancy, below). In the presence of obstruction, urinary tract infection probably accelerates destruction of renal tissue and should be treated even if asymptomatic. In children, especially those younger that 5 years, vesicoureteral reflux is common, and in its presence urinary tract infection is likely to lead to renal damage and should be treated. Asymptomatic bacteriuria of lower urinary tract origin can usually be cured with short-course therapy (see Table 1). Asymptomatic bacteriuria of probable upper tract origin, as determined by relapse after short-course therapy, should be treated for 14 days when indicated.

MANAGEMENT OF BACTERIURIA DURING PREGNANCY

Bacteriuria during pregnancy is common (4 to 7 percent) and often asymptomatic. It is well documented that acute pyelonephritis leads to the premature onset of labor and grave risks to the fetus. Since 20 percent of pregnant patients with untreated bacteriuria subsequently develop acute pyelonephritis, asymptomatic bacteriuria during pregnancy should be sought and treated.

Pregnant women are the only group in whom screening for asymptomatic bacteriuria is advocated. Since 75 percent of women who develop bacteriuria during pregnancy are bacteriuric at the first prenatal visit, we recommend a screening urine culture at that time. If positive, a second culture with 10^5 or more cfu per milliliter confirms the diagnosis. In pregnant women, short-course therapy is generally effective (see Table 1). Follow-up cultures about 1 week after therapy are always necessary because of the need to assure eradication of bacteriuria and the consequent risk to the fetus, outlined above.

Table 1 outlines drugs and dosages. Most drugs given to pregnant women carry some risk for the fetus; therefore careful selection of drugs is mandatory. Drugs generally considered safe during pregnancy include ampicillin, amoxicillin, cephalosporins, nitrofurantoin, and sulfonamides. Sulfonamides should not be used near term because of increased risk of kernicterus. Norfloxacin and ciprofloxacin are not approved for use in pregnancy and childhood because of the theoretical risk of teratogenicity and malformations of cartilage.

Patients whose bacteriuria recurs after a short-course of therapy should be treated for 14 days. If a patient relapses after this, more prolonged therapy along with an ultrasound to evaluate for obstruction and/or stones is indicated. Following cure, monthly cultures are indicated for the duration of the pregnancy to detect reinfections.

MANAGEMENT OF CATHETER-RELATED BACTERIURIA

The incidence of bacteriuria in the catheterized patient with a closed, sterile-system indwelling catheter is 5 to 10 percent per day, and virtually everyone with a catheter for more than 30 days becomes bacteriuric. Catheter-induced bacteriuria increases the risk of morbidity and mortality secondary to bacteremia (2 to 4 percent of catheterized patients) (also see the chapter *Catheter-Associated Urinary Infection*). Since bacteriuria in the long-term catheterized patient is unavoidable and treatment of asymptomatic infection only predisposes to colonization with resistant organisms, treatment of asymptomatic bacteriuria in the catheterized patient is not advocated.

The most important preventative maneuvers are to not insert a catheter unless absolutely indicated and to remove the catheter as soon as possible. When this is not feasible, condom catheters for the unobstructed male and intermittent "in and out" catheterization of patients with neurogenic bladders are alternatives that carry definite but lower risks of infection. Prophylactic antibiotics, whether given systemically or placed topically around the catheter, do not decrease the acquisition of bacteriuria in the long-term catheterized patient and should not be used. Closed, sterile, nondisconnectable catheter systems should be used. Indwelling catheters should be changed whenever the flow of urine becomes obstructed.

When the catheterized patient becomes febrile or shows other signs of infection, sources other than the urinary tract should be considered. Obstruction of the catheter should also be ruled out. If the source of infection is likely to be the urinary tract, the infection should be treated with the full realization that relapse and/or reinfection is inevitable.

SUGGESTED READING

Boscia J, Kaye D. Asymptomatic bacteriuria in the elderly. Infect Dis Clin North Am 1987; 1:893–905.

Durbin W, Peter G. Management of urinary tract infections in infants and children. Pediatr Infect Dis 1984; 3:564–574.

Patterson T, Andriole V. Bacteriuria in pregnancy. Infect Dis Clin North Am 1987; 1:807–822.

Sobel J, Kaye D. Urinary tract infections. In:Mandell GL, Douglas RG Jr, Bennett JE, eds. Principles and practice of infectious diseases. New York: John Wiley and Sons, 1985.

Stamey T. Recurrent urinary tract infections in female patients: an overview. Rev Infect Dis 1987; 9(Suppl 2):S195–S210.

Warren J. Catheter-associated urinary tract infections. Infect Dis Clin North Am 1987; 1:823–854.

ACUTE DYSURIA IN WOMEN AND URETHRITIS IN MEN

WALTER E. STAMM, M.D.

ACUTE DYSURIA IN WOMEN

Acute dysuria occurs commonly in adult women and usually reflects the presence of lower genitourinary tract infection: cystitis (generally due to *Escherichia coli* or *Staphylococcus saprophyticus*), vulvovaginitis (due to *Candida albicans, Trichomonas vaginalis*, or bacterial vaginosis), or urethritis (due to *Chlamydia trachomatis, Neisseria gonorrhoeae*, or herpes simplex virus). The relative proportion of cases due to each of these agents depends on the age and sexual activity of a given patient population. Symptoms produced by these various infections overlap to such a degree that accurate diagnosis depends on the physical examination and simple laboratory tests. Of particular importance are the vaginal speculum examination, microscopic examination of vaginal secretions, and urinalysis. Recent studies clarifying the etiology of acute dysuria in women have demonstrated that, in acutely symptomatic women with *E. coli* infections and with pyuria, bacterial counts in midstream urine may often be in the range of 10^2 to 10^4 CFU per milliliter. Determination of a specific etiologic diagnosis is a necessity for optimal treatment.

Initially, women with dysuria should be evaluated to determine if their symptoms are attributable to vulvovaginitis, urinary infection, or urethritis (Fig. 1). Women with vulvovaginitis often characterize dysuria as external (that is, occurring as the urine contacts the inflamed labial tissue). Additional symptoms of vaginal discharge, pruritus, and vaginal odor suggest the presence of vulvovaginitis, which can be readily confirmed by pelvic examination. Complaints of suprapubic pain, hematuria, and urgency are infrequent with vulvovaginitis and should direct the evaluation to other etiologies.

The absence of symptoms and signs of vulvovaginitis necessitates an assessment of the dysuric patient for urinary tract infection and urethritis. The presence of pyuria in a midstream urine specimen is a sensitive indicator of probable infection but does not discriminate between the site or type of infection. Fever, flank pain, and costovertebral angle tenderness strongly suggest the presence of pyelonephritis. On the basis of clinical presentation alone, distinction between cystitis and urethritis can often be difficult. A history of previous urinary tract infections or current diaphragm use and complaints of either gross hematuria or suprapubic pain suggest cystitis. Infection with *N. gonorrhoeae* or *C. trachomatis* should be suspected in young, sexually active women who have had a recent change in sex partners or a history of previous sexually transmitted disease (Fig. 1).

The presence of one or more bacteria per oil immersion field on microscopic analysis of a Gram-stained, uncentrifuged urine specimen correlates with more than 10^5 organisms per milliliter in a urine culture and is helpful in the diagnosis of urinary infection when positive. To confirm the result of Gram stain, or in the absence of this finding, quantitative culture of a midstream urine specimen remains the preferred means to evaluate patients for urinary infection. The presence of lower quantitative counts (10^2 to 10^4 per milliliter of urine) of coliforms (e.g., *E. coli, Klebsiella*) in cultures of urine from dysuric women—particularly if the patient has concomitant pyuria—usually indicates acute urinary infection with these organisms.

Women with dysuria and pyuria in whom urinary infection is not confirmed by Gram stain (or culture if Gram stain is negative) or women whose illness suggests the presence of chlamydial or gonococcal infection should have a pelvic examination (Fig. 1). Findings consistent with mucopurulent cervicitis should be carefully sought in these women, and cultures for *N. gonorrhoeae* and cultures or antigen tests for *C. trachomatis* should be performed. If chlamydial tests are not available, the presence of a negative urine culture, pyuria, and a negative clinical and microbiologic evaluation for gonorrhea in a sexually active woman suggest infection with *C. trachomatis*. Examination of the patient's sexual partner may be useful in establishing a diagnosis as well.

Treatment of dysuric women should be directed against the specific etiologic agent identified. Urinary infections due to coliforms and *S. saprophyticus* are treated effectively by several antimicrobial agents including trimethoprim-sulfamethoxazole (TMP/SMZ), trimethoprim, nitrofurantoin, or quinolones such as norfloxacin or ciprofloxacin. Recent studies suggest that single-dose therapy for acute lower urinary tract infections is less effective than conventional 7- to 10-day regimens. However, the latter have unacceptably high rates of adverse reactions—especially rash and vulvovaginitis. Three-day treatment regimens appear to provide the increased efficacy associated with 7- to 10-day regimens

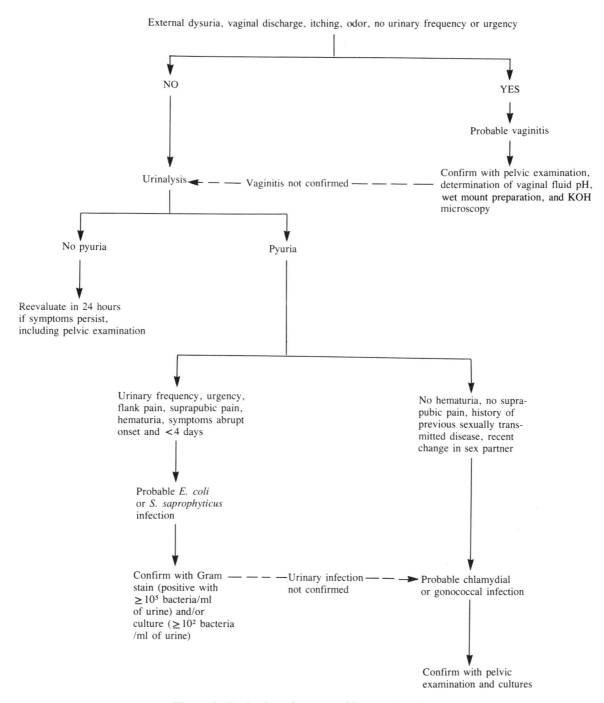

Figure 1   Evaluation of women with acute dysuria.

but have fewer adverse effects and lower cost. Currently recommended treatment regimens for acute cystitis thus include three consecutive daily doses of TMP (200 mg twice daily), TMP-SMZ (160/800 twice daily), nitrofurantoin (100 mg four times daily), norfloxacin (400 mg twice daily), or ciprofloxacin (250 mg twice daily). Patients with recurrent or persistent infection following single-dose therapy should receive 7 days of therapy as well as careful post-therapy evaluation to ensure eradication of infection.

Management of chlamydial, gonococcal, and other sexually transmitted infections should include evaluation and therapy of the sexual partner(s). For specific details regarding treatment of these infections, the reader is referred to the appropriate chapters in this volume. Women with acute dysuria without pyuria should be treated with pyridium (one tablet four times daily) to relieve symptoms and asked to return for reevaluation if symptoms persist. In most instances, symptoms will resolve spontaneously, and no further therapy is necessary.

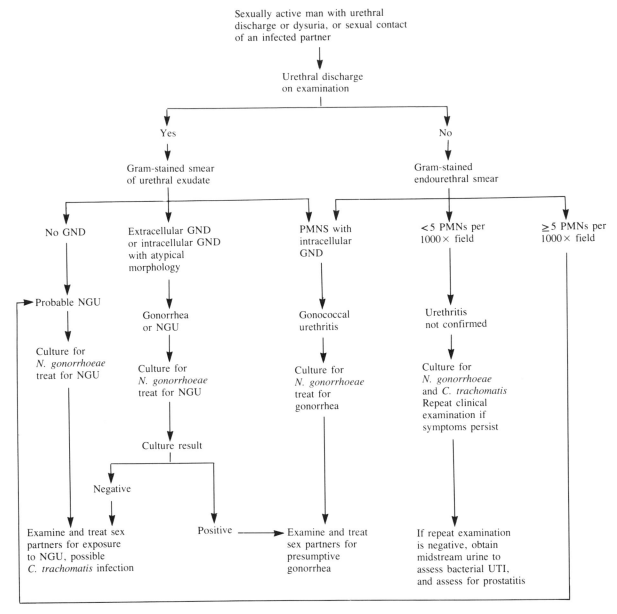

Figure 2 Management of a male with possible urethritis.

INITIAL MANAGEMENT OF
URETHRITIS IN MEN

Urethritis is the most frequent sexually transmitted disease (STD) syndrome seen in men. Customarily, clinicians categorize urethritis into gonococcal and nongonococcal etiologies. The relative frequency of nongonococcal urethritis (NGU) and gonococcal urethritis in a given clinic depends upon the racial and socioeconomic characteristics of the population served. *C. trachomatis* causes approximately 40 percent of cases of NGU, and *Ureaplasma urealyticum* may cause an additional 10 to 20 percent of cases. The remaining cases probably result from sexually transmitted pathogens, but their precise etiology remains unclear. Occasionally, urethritis results from infection with *T. vaginalis* or herpes sim-

plex virus. Most patients with urethritis due to genital herpes infection have obvious herpetic penile lesions, and many with urethritis due to *T. vaginalis* have sex partners with vaginitis.

The diagnostic approach to men with urethritis begins by distinguishing those patients who have urethral discharge on examination from those who do not (Fig. 2). Patients with a demonstrable discharge should be treated for NGU or gonococcal urethritis based upon the results of Gram stain of urethral secretions. Either a positive Gram stain showing intracellular gram-negative diplococci (98 percent sensitive and specific as compared with culture) or a positive culture confirms the diagnosis of gonococcal urethritis. Men with a urethral discharge on examination—but negative smears and cultures for *N. gonorrhoeae*—have, by definition, NGU. The Gram stain in patients with NGU usually shows five or more polymorphonuclear leukocytes (PMNs) per 1000 × field. It is generally unnecessary to make a specific etiologic diagnosis (i.e., perform chlamydial or ureaplasmal cultures) in men with NGU.

Patients without a demonstrable urethral discharge upon examination but with urethral symptoms or a history of an infected partner should also have urethral Gram stains done. Patients whose smears show PMNs with intracellular gram-negative diplococci should be treated for gonorrhea. In patients whose smears are not diagnostic of gonococcal urethritis, the number of PMNs per 1000 × microscopic field should be determined. Patients with fewer than five PMNs per 1000 × microscopic field, no history of recent contact with a known infected partner, and no symptoms should be advised that their examination results are normal and that they should return for reexamination only if symptoms arise or persist. Patients with fewer than five PMNs per 1000 × microscopic field but with history of contact with an infected partner should be treated epidemiologically in an appropriate manner. Patients having symptoms of urethritis and five or more PMNs per 1000 × microscopic field should be treated for NGU, and contacts of these patients should be examined and treated epidemiologically. Asymptomatic patients without demonstrable discharge and with no exposure history but with more than five PMNs per 1000 × microscopic field should be asked to return for reexamination in 7 days—or sooner if symptoms arise. If five or more PMNs per 1000 x microscopic field are still present, if discharge is now present, or if the *C. trachomatis* culture is positive, the patient and his contacts should be treated for NGU.

Men with NGU should be treated with tetracycline, 500 mg orally four times per day for 7 days, or doxycycline, 100 mg orally twice a day for 7 days. Alternatively, erythromycin, 500 mg orally four times per day for 7 days, can be used. The latter regimen should also be used in men with NGU who fail to respond to tetracycline therapy. Heterosexual men with gonococcal urethritis should be treated with 250 mg of ceftriaxone intramuscularly followed by tetracycline or doxycycline for 7 days to treat the concomitant chlamydial infection present in 25 percent of patients. Alternatively amoxicillin, 3.0 g plus 1.0 g probenecid, as a single oral dose, followed by tetracycline or doxycycline for 7 days can be used where PPNG strains are not prevalent. In homosexual men with gonococcal urethritis, 250 mg of ceftriaxone intramuscularly should be used; subsequent tetracycline therapy is unnecessary because of the lesser prevalence of concomitant *C. trachomatis* infection in this population.

It should be emphasized that clinical features alone do not reliably distinguish between gonococcal and nongonococcal urethritis. For this reason, a microscopic examination of the urethral smear and appropriate cultures must be undertaken to distinguish the two disorders. Further, heterosexual men seen in high-risk settings, such as an STD clinic, who have no history or signs of urethral symptoms and no history of contact with an infected partner should also have a urethral Gram stain and cultures or antigen detection tests for *Chlamydia* and *N. gonorrhoeae*. Some of these men will have asymptomatic gonorrhea or NGU, as evidenced by persistent urethral leukocytosis and/or a positive *C. trachomatis* culture. Since homosexual men are at less risk than heterosexual men of developing NGU or chlamydial infection, and since asymptomatic urethral gonorrhea is rare in this population, routine screening by urethral smear or chlamydial culture is not necessary for asymptomatic homosexual men who have no known infected partners.

SUGGESTED READING

Bowie WR. Urethritis in males. In: Holmes KK, Mardh PA, Sparling PF, Wiesner PJ, eds. Sexually transmitted diseases. 2nd ed. New York: McGraw-Hill, 1989.

Hooton TM, Stamm WE. Urethritis. In: Hurst J-W, ed. Medicine for the practicing physician. Stoneham, MA: Butterworth, 1988.

Johnson JR, Stamm WE. Diagnosis and treatment of acute urinary tract infections. Infect Dis Clin North Am 1987; 1:733–791.

Komaroff AL. Acute dysuria in women. N Engl J Med 1984; 310:368.

VULVOVAGINITIS, CERVICITIS, AND PELVIC INFLAMMATORY DISEASE

GARY E. GARBER, M.D., FRCPC
ANTHONY W. CHOW, M.D., FRCPC, FACP

GENERAL CONSIDERATIONS

Lower genitourinary symptoms are common complaints among adult women in primary care settings as well as in specialty clinics for sexually transmitted diseases. Among such women, vaginal symptoms are more than five times as common as urinary symptoms. Genital and urinary infections may often coexist, and their clinical distinction is not always clearcut. Furthermore, symptoms or signs of an abnormal vaginal discharge may be caused by a diverse variety of conditions or their combination (Table 1). Lack of uniformity in the clinical definition of these conditions, and of a consistent approach to laboratory confirmation also contributes to the diagnostic uncertainties and refractory response to therapy in many instances. Not surprisingly, considerable difficulty is also encountered clinically in differentiating true inflammatory conditions of the female genital tract from physiologic, functional, or psychosomatic causes of symptoms. For these reasons, a systematic approach to the diagnosis and management of urogenital infections is essential. Special emphasis should be given to the following considerations: (1) the history and physical examination should focus primarily on the epidemiology and anatomic localization of the likely sites of infection or inflammation; (2) specific etiologic diagnosis will require additional office or laboratory tests since the clinical diagnosis is imprecise and often misleading; (3) concomitant infection with multiple pathogens at different sites is common; (4) the presence of potentially serious but asymptomatic infection (e.g., cervicitis) should be excluded; (5) an important therapeutic goal should include prevention of upper genital tract infection and its sequelae in addition to eradication of lower genital symptoms and epidemiologic control of major sexually transmitted infections. A critical initial step in the evaluation of all lower genital symptoms, therefore, should be directed to detection and effective treatment of cervicitis or coexisting salpingitis.

An algorithm approach to the management of adult women with lower genital complaints is summarized in Figure 1.

TABLE 1 Conditions Associated with Vaginal Discharge

Infectious	*Noninfectious*

Vulvovaginitis
  Bacterial vaginosis
  Candidiasis
  Trichomoniasis
	Excessive mucorrhea and physiologic discharge

	Atrophic vaginitis

Cervicitis
  Chlamydial infection
  Gonorrhea
  Genital herpes
	Desquamative inflammatory vaginitis

Salpingitis	Foreign body, trauma, irradiation, hypersensitivity, or chemical irritation
Other sexually transmitted diseases	Endometriosis, neoplasms cysts, or polyps
Toxic shock syndrome	Others
Miscellaneous vulvovaginal pyogenic infections	

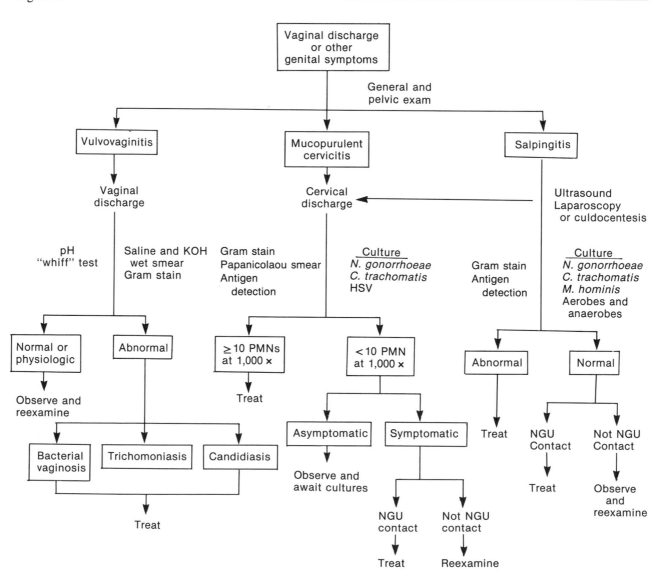

Figure 1 Approach to genital symptoms in premenopausal women.

SYSTEMATIC APPROACH TO DIAGNOSIS

History

Historical features are relatively nonspecific, but are useful for defining the epidemiology and natural history of specific infections. Inflammation of the cervix and vagina often produce similar symptoms, such as external dysuria, introital dyspareunia, and increased amount or altered quality of vaginal discharge. Patients with cervicitis often complain of intermenstrual or postcoital spotting. Abdominal pain or systemic complaints are uncommon with vulvovaginitis or uncomplicated cervicitis and should prompt a diligent search for accompanying pelvic inflammatory disease. Presence of fever may suggest acute salpingitis or primary genital herpes. Fever and multisystem involvement beginning during a menstrual period should raise the possibility of toxic shock syndrome.

The color and amount of discharge as perceived by the patient has little value in differential diagnosis. Although trichomoniasis and candidiasis can cause marked vaginal irritation, their clinical presentation can vary greatly from individual to individual. Vaginal odor may be the only symptom in bacterial vaginosis, a condition often associated with little vaginal irritation. The complaint of vaginal discharge does not in itself indicate a pathologic process. Physiologic discharge (mucorrhea) may be heavy enough to stain underwear, but it is not usually associated with external dysuria, vulvar irritation, or odor. The amount of discharge may vary with the phase of the menstrual cycle and may be increased by oral contraceptive use or pregnancy. Because the onset of physiologic discharge often coincides with the onset of sexual activity, women who feel anxious or guilty about their sexual activity may attach inordinate importance to small changes in normal vaginal discharge.

A complete and detailed sexual history is particularly important, since exposure to a new sexual partner increases the likelihood of sexually transmitted disease. The sexual history should include the number of recent new partners, patterns of sexual behavior, previous sexually transmitted diseases, and partner's sexual history. This line of questioning is often disconcerting for both the physician and patient. The patient is far more likely to discuss intimate sexual details freely if the impression projected is that of a routine but necessary and confidential procedure. This skill is acquired only with practice.

General Physical Examination

Particular attention should be directed to the skin, palms, soles, eyes, mouth, pharynx, anorectum, pubic hair, lymph nodes, and joints. Examination of the abdomen should include careful listening for diminished bowel sounds and evidence of peritoneal, suprapubic, or perihepatic inflammation. The pubic region should be inspected for lice and other pediculosis. The inguinal and femoral regions should be palpated for adenopathy. An anorectal examination by proctoscopy and digital palpation should be routinely performed.

The Pelvic Examination

The labia and the perineum should be examined for erythema, excoriation, and discrete lesions. Diffuse perineal erythema or edema may accompany trichomoniasis, candidiasis, or early toxic shock syndrome. Examination of extravaginal surfaces may reveal lesions of genital herpes, syphilis, chancroid, condylomata acuminata, molluscum contagiosum, or scabies. Vulvovaginal pyogenic infections such as abscesses involving Bartholin's and Skene's glands, infected labial inclusion cysts, furunculosis, and suppurative hidradenitis are readily apparent.

Next, the urethral meatus is examined and gently stripped with a finger placed inside the introitus. If urethral discharge is expressed, such material should be examined microscopically and cultured. A vaginal speculum, moistened with warm water and without lubricant, is then gently inserted. In the presence of severe genital herpes, or occasionally trichomoniasis, insertion of the speculum may be impossible due to intense discomfort. In such cases, a preliminary etiologic diagnosis is sometimes made from material recovered on a cotton swab gently inserted into the vagina.

After insertion of the speculum, the cervix is first examined, since cervicitis is a serious condition and is often asymptomatic. The cervix should be wiped clean and cotton-tipped swabs of endocervical secretions obtained through the cervical os. Mucoid material is normally observed at the cervical os and is present in increased amounts in women taking oral contraceptives. Normal cervical discharge is usually clear or white and is nonhomogeneous and viscous. Purulent or mucopurulent cervical discharge is associated with infective cervicitis and is readily recognized by the appearance of yellow or green exudate on the white cotton-tipped swab. The cervix should also be observed for erosions, friability, or easy bleeding. Mucopurulent cervicitis is most commonly caused by *Chlamydia trachomatis*, *Neisseria gonorrhoeae*, or both, and must be differentiated from cervicitis caused by herpes simplex virus (HSV), from vaginitis, and from simple cervical ectopy without inflammation. Cervical ectopy represents the presence of columnar endocervical epithelium in an exposed portion of the ectocervix and appears redder than the surrounding stratified vaginal epithelium. Ectopy, when not associated with visible or microscopic endocervical mucopus or with colposcopic epithelial abnormalities, is a normal finding and requires no therapy. Its prevalence is increased at the onset of menarche, by oral contraceptive use, and by pregnancy but gradually declines through later adolescence. Hypertrophic cervicitis manifests as intensely red, congested areas that appear to project from the surface of the cervix. It can be distinguished from ectopy in that it is usually asymmetrical and irregular around the cervical os, is rather friable and bleeds easily, and is usually accompanied by a mucopurulent cervical discharge. Presence of hypertrophic cervicitis is highly suggestive of chlamydial cervicitis, but it is an uncommon clinical finding. Similarly, findings of a "strawberry cervix" in association with increased purulent discharge is highly suggestive of trichomoniasis, but this observation was only 45 percent sensitive by colposcopy, although 99 percent specific.

Endocervical scrapings, swabs, or secretions should be collected for Gram stain, for antigen detection, or for culture (or other testing, depending on availability) of *N. gonorrhoeae*, *C. trachomatis*, and HSV. A Papanicolaou smear may identify trichomonads or cytologic findings characteristic of HSV infection.

After establishing the presence or absence of cervicitis, efforts should then be directed to establishing the presence or absence of vaginal infection. Not infrequently, cervicitis coexists with vaginal infection, particularly with bacterial vaginosis or trichomonal vaginitis. The amount, consistency, color, odor, and location of the discharge within the vagina should be noted. The character of vaginal discharge is relatively nonspecific. A yellow or green discharge is suggestive of trichomoniasis, but this occurs in less than one-fifth of infected women. Similarly, a frothy discharge is seen in only one-tenth of women with trichomoniasis, is nonspecific, and is equally suggestive of bacterial vaginosis. The amount of discharge in vulvovaginal candidiasis is highly variable, and one does not always see the classic curdy discharge. The vaginal wall should also be inspected for erythema, edema, and ulceration. Vaginal ulcers tend to occur in the right vaginal fornix, are chronic, and are associated with the use of tampons in some patients. A sample of discharge should be removed with a swab from the vaginal wall, avoiding contamination with cervical mucus. The vaginal pH should be determined directly by rolling the swab containing the specimen onto pH indicator paper. An additional specimen should be removed with a swab and mixed first with a drop of saline, then with a drop of 10 percent potassium hydroxide (KOH) on a microscope slide. The odor released after mixing the specimen with KOH is noted, and separate cover slips are placed on the saline and KOH wet mounts for microscopic examination to detect the presence and quantity of normal epithelial cells, clue cells, polymorphonuclear leukocytes (PMNs), motile trichomonads, or fungal elements.

Finally, the bimanual examination is performed to determine adnexal or cervical motion tenderness, and to exclude the presence of palpable adnexal or cul-de-sac masses. Adnexal tenderness is uncommon with local vaginal infections and suggests salpingitis; palpation of an abnormal adnexal or cul-de-sac mass may indicate tubo-ovarian abscess, ectopic pregnancy, or malignancy that requires prompt gynecologic or surgical consultation.

In most patients, the constellation of symptoms and signs together with the microscopic findings in vaginal secretions will allow a preliminary etiologic diagnosis of vulvovaginitis, and further studies are unnecessary (Table 2). However, it is prudent to request that the patient remain undressed in the examination room in case microscopic examination of the wet smear is unrevealing and further microbiologic studies are indicated. Patients generally do not mind waiting for 2 to 3 minutes for the results of the wet mount before the examination is continued. Depending on the clinical findings, these further studies may include culture for *Candida albicans* and *Trichomonas vaginalis* or Gram stain of vaginal fluid to differentiate between normal flora and the flora characteristic of bacterial vaginosis. In women with prominent vaginal complaints but no abnormal findings, each of these additional microbiologic tests may be indicated to differentiate vaginal infection from functional complaints and other causes of vaginal symptoms.

Routine Office and Laboratory Investigations

A number of bedside and office evaluations of clinical specimens are invaluable in the etiologic diagnosis of vulvovaginitis and cervicitis. These include vaginal pH, KOH "whiff" test, and microscopic examination of wet smears and Gram stains of vaginal and cervical specimens. Cervical and vaginal cultures should be obtained only for specific and selected pathogens and should be interpreted with caution.

Vaginal pH. The pH of vaginal discharge can be estimated at the bedside by use of pH indicators such as nitrazine paper, when the pH is between 4.5 and 7.0. A vaginal pH of 4.5 or less is most consistent with physiologic discharge or with vulvovaginal candidiasis. Vaginal pH greater than 4.5 is seen in patients with trichomoniasis or bacterial vaginosis.

KOH Whiff Test. Vaginal secretions from patients with bacterial vaginosis, when added to several drops of 10 percent KOH on a microscope slide will elicit a pungent fishy, amine-like odor. A positive whiff test can be expected in more than 90 percent of women with bacterial vaginosis and an undefined proportion of patients with trichomoniasis but is absent in women with vulvovaginal candidiasis or physiologic discharge.

Microscopic Examination of Vaginal Specimens. The wet mount of vaginal discharge is the single most useful technique in making an initial etiologic diagnosis of vulvovaginitis (Table 2). The following specific information is sought: (1) the nature of the vaginal epithelial cells and the presence of clue cells; (2) the presence and number of PMNs; (3) the presence of specific and readily identifiable pathogens such as motile trichomonads, budding yeasts, or pseudohyphae. Normal vaginal epithelial cells are flat and clean looking. The edges are sharply defined, and the nuclei, easily visible. Clue cells, which strongly suggest bacterial vaginosis, are squamous epithelial cells covered with coccobacilli, giving them a granular appearance with indistinct cell edges and nucleus. Presence of large numbers of PMNs may be either cervical or vaginal in origin. The number of PMNs is usually normal in bacterial vaginosis (i.e., one would not see an intense inflammatory response) and may be normal or increased in candidal vulvovaginitis or trichomoniasis. The presence of excessive PMNs should prompt further search for an inflammatory genital focus, but the absence of excessive PMNs does not rule out notable infection. The composition and normality of the bacterial vaginal flora is effectively assessed by Gram stain of vaginal fluid. Normal vaginal secretions contain predominantly gram-positive rods resembling lactobacilli, with or without gram-variable coccobacilli resembling *Gardnerella vaginalis*. In bacterial vaginosis, vaginal fluid contains few or no lactobacilli with a predominance of *G. vaginalis* plus other organisms resembling anaerobic gram-negative *Bacteroides* species, gram-positive cocci, or curved rods.

TABLE 2 Diagnostic Features of Vaginitis in Premenopausal Adults

	Normal or Physiologic Discharge	Bacterial Vaginosis	Candidal Vulvovaginitis	Trichomonal Vaginitis
Etiology	Uninfected; *Lactobacillus* predominant	*G. vaginalis* and various anaerobic bacteria	*C. albicans* and other yeasts	*T. vaginalis*
Predominant symptoms	None	Malodorous discharge	Vulvar itching and/or irritation; increased discharge	Profuse discharge, often malodorous
Vulvitis	None	Rare	Usual	Occasional
Inflammation of vaginal epithelium	None	None	Erythema	Erythema; occasional petechiae
Discharge				
Amount	Variable, but usually scant	Moderate	Scant to moderate	Profuse
Color	Clear or white	White or grey	White	Yellow
Consistency	Nonhomogeneous, flocular	Homogeneous, low viscosity, uniformly coating vaginal walls; occasionally frothy	Clumped, adherent plaques	Homogeneous, low viscosity; often frothy
Usual vaginal pH	<4.5	≥4.5	<4.5	≥5.0
Amine odor with 10% KOH ("whiff test")	None	Positive	None	Often positive
Microscopy (saline or KOH wet smears, Gram stain)	Normal epithelial cells; lactobacilli predominate	Clue cells; few PMNs; lacto-bacilli outnumbered by profuse mixed flora nearly always including *G. vaginalis* plus anaerobes	PMNs, epithelial cells; yeast or pseudo-hyphae in up to 80%	PMNs, motile tricho-monads in 80–90%

Modified with permission from Holmes KK. Lower genital tract infections in women:cystitis/urethritis, vulvovaginitis, and cervicitis. In: Holmes KK, Mordh P-A, Sparling PF, Wiesner PI, eds. Sexually transmitted diseases. New York: McGraw-Hill, 1984:583.

Microscopic Examination of Cervical Specimens. The Gram stain of endocervical secretions examined at 1,000× is the most useful and practical tool for the etiologic diagnosis of symptomatic or asymptomatic cervicitis. Visualization of yellow, mucopurulent endocervical secretions on a white swab or presence of 10 or more PMNs per 1,000× field are positively correlated with cervical *C. trachomatis* infection. Neither *N. gonorrhoeae* nor HSV infection is significantly associated with endocervical PMN leukocyte concentration or presence of macroscopic mucopus. On the other hand, demonstration of intracellular gram-negative diplococci in the Gram stain of endocervical secretions has a sensitivity of 60 percent and specificity close to 100 percent for the diagnosis of gonococcal infection. This compares favorably to isolation of *N. gonorrhoeae* from a single endocervical culture, which has a sensitivity of 80 to 90 percent. Giemsa-stained smears of endocervical scrapings are of less value for the diagnosis of chlamydial cervicitis since chlamydial inclusions can be identified in only a minority of infected women. Multinucleated giant cells and Cowdry type A intranuclear inclusions suggest HSV cervicitis; but in the presence of extensive tissue necrosis, the cellular architecture is distorted, and the typical cytologic findings are seen in less than one-third of infected patients. Similarly, the typical cytologic findings of HSV infection in Papanicolaou smears are reliable indicators of disease only when observed, but the sensitivity of this technique has been questioned.

Cultures. Prevalence is sufficient to recommend that endocervical, urethral, and anorectal cultures be obtained routinely for confirmation of gonorrhea and for detection of beta-lactamase production by *N. gonorrhoeae* isolates. Although endocervical cultures for *C. trachomatis* and HSV are desirable, they are not readily available in many centers. Routine aerobic and anaerobic vaginal cultures are not recommended, and results should be interpreted with great caution since the vagina is normally colonized by a wide variety of microorganisms. As an example, isolation of *G. vaginalis* from the vagina, even in high concentration, is not specific for the diagnosis of bacterial vaginosis.

Special Diagnostic Procedures

It is important to note that routine office and laboratory investigations are helpful in confirming an etiologic diagnosis of genitourinary infections in only 30 to 60 percent of symptomatic women. Nonroutine and more specialized and comprehensive microbiologic investigations are required to improve the diagnostic yield. Cultural procedures for the isolation of *C. trachomatis* are extremely expensive and labor intensive and may not be readily available. Two immunodiagnostic methods for detection of *C. trachomatis* antigen from cervical specimens, a direct immunofluorescence assay (DFA) and an enzyme immunoassay (EIA), have become widely available. Comparisons of these antigen detection methods in high-prevalence as well as low-prevalence populations have generally supported their usefulness (70 percent as sensitive as culture), although both false-positive and false-negative results can occur. The presence of ectocervical lesions suggestive of HSV infection should warrant laboratory confirmation by viral isolation and differentiation of HSV-1 and HSV-2 serotypes by use of type-specific monoclonal antibodies. Cytologic and immunofluorescent antigen detection techniques for genital herpes are 50 percent and 70 percent, respectively, as sensitive as viral isolation. DNA hybridization has been used to demonstrate human papillomavirus (HPV) in tissue. DNA hybridization is highly specific for demonstrating HPV and has the unique advantage of giving information on the virus serotype. It is much superior to antigen detection for HPV, which has poor sensitivity.

Cultures for *Ureaplasma urealyticum* and *Mycoplasma hominis* from cervical and urethral secretions may be useful for the diagnosis of nongonococcal and nonchlamydial cervicitis, endometritis, or salpingitis. These organisms have been implicated particularly in instances of postpartum fever or recurrent pregnancy loss. A variety of selective media are available for isolation of *T. vaginalis* from vaginal secretions, and culture is the most sensitive method for diagnosis of vaginal trichomoniasis. Vaginal cultures for yeast and *T. vaginalis* are particularly useful when symptoms or signs are suggestive of one or the other, but neither can be demonstrated by direct microscopy of wet smears.

Gas-liquid chromatography of vaginal fluid from women with bacterial vaginosis may show a characteristic pattern of organic acid metabolites: the concentration of lactate, the major metabolite of lactobacilli, is reduced, while succinate, acetate, propionate, butyrate, and other organic acids produced by the abnormal flora are increased. Toxin-producing *Staphylococcus aureus* may be isolated in high concentration from vaginal cultures of women with symptoms and signs suggestive of toxic shock syndrome (TSS). Toxic shock syndrome toxin-1, the major staphylococcal exotoxin implicated in TSS, can be detected in vaginal washings of some patients by solid-phase enzyme-linked immunosorbent assay during the acute illness; serum antitoxin antibodies in such patients are typically low in titer.

Colposcopy is increasingly used to evaluate women with abnormal cytologic smears consistent with cervical intraepithelial neoplasia. Colposcopic examination with magnification of the mucosal surface contour is invaluable for the detection of subclinical HPV infection and for cervicitis. Following application of 3 to 5 percent acetic acid during this procedure, papillomavirus-infected lesions typically appear white and shiny ("acetowhite") with irregular but distinct borders. Asperities (multiple, short, pointed surface projections) and reverse punctation (diffuse pattern of minimally raised white dots against the pink background of the vaginal epithelium) are often seen. If vascular abnormalities are also present, a biopsy should be obtained to exclude the possibility of intraepithelial neoplasia. Laparoscopy is invaluable for the visual diagnosis of salpingitis and is particularly helpful for microbiologic sampling and specific etiologic diagnosis of salpingitis and other pelvic conditions. Ultrasonography, radionuclide scanning, and computed tomography are particularly useful for detection and localization of tubo-ovarian and adnexal inflammatory masses.

MANAGEMENT OF SPECIFIC SYNDROMES

Vulvovaginitis

Vulvovaginitis may be the most frequent cause of genital symptoms in women. The cardinal manifestations are increased yellow or green discharge; vulvar itching, irritation or burning; external dysuria; introital dyspareunia; and malodor that is often increased following sexual intercourse. Treatment should be based on specific etiologic diagnosis that can usually be made at the time of initial clinical evaluation (see Table 2). The commonest cause of all vaginal discharge is bacterial vaginosis, which is also known as nonspecific vaginitis, followed in frequency by vulvovaginal candidiasis and trichomoniasis. Multiple and concomitant vaginal infections are not infrequent, especially trichomoniasis coexisting with *G. vaginalis*-associated bacterial vaginosis. Cervicitis may also present as vaginal discharge and must first be ruled out. Other causes of abnormal vaginal discharge, such as atrophic vaginitis, desquamative inflammatory vaginitis, and vaginal fistula or ulcers, are rare. In a patient with persistent vaginitis for which a specific pathogen cannot be identified, examination of the sexual partner may often provide the answer.

Common pitfalls that lead to misdiagnosis and treatment failure in the management of vulvovaginitis include (1) diagnosis based exclusively on macroscopic appearance of discharge, with failure to perform a wet smear; (2) "telephone" diagnosis and treatment; (3) broad-spectrum, "shotgun" remedies; (4) failure to use appropriate antimicrobial agents; and (5) failure to treat the sexual partner. Recommended therapeutic regimens for the most frequent causes of vulvovaginitis and cervicitis are summarized in Table 3. Adjunctive measures, such as warm tub baths to ease pain and reduce edema, careful attention to personal hygiene, and abstinence from sexual intercourse, are also important. Patients whose symptoms respond promptly to specific therapy should be seen about 1 week after completion of therapy for repeat clinical and microscopic evaluation. Women with physiologic discharge should be given a careful explanation of the condition. Persistence of worrisome symptoms in a woman in whom thorough and repeated evaluation has failed to reveal genital pathology may indicate psychosexual problems; such patients may well benefit from counseling provided by a trained therapist.

Bacterial Vaginosis or Nonspecific Vaginitis

Current evidence indicates that *G. vaginalis* (formerly known as *Hemophilus vaginalis* or *Corynebacterium vaginale*) in conjunction with high vaginal concentrations of anaerobic bacteria (particularly *Bacteroides* species, *Peptostreptococcus* species, and motile curved rods known as *Mobiluncus* species) is the primary cause of this condition. It is characterized clinically by symptoms of slightly increased, malodorous, watery vaginal discharge, with little pain or itching. The malodor may increase postcoitally (possibly due to release of amines by semen, which is alkaline). Examination often reveals a nonviscous, homogeneous, gray-white, uniformly adherent vaginal discharge, without gross inflammation of the vaginal mucosa. Bacterial vaginosis should be suspected in the presence of three of four of the following findings: (1) characteristic vaginal discharge; (2) vaginal pH above 4.5; (3) positive whiff test; (4) presence of clue cells. Symptoms alone are not reliable for diagnosis since many patients are asymptomatic. The diagnosis is readily confirmed by the characteristic changes in vaginal flora observed on

TABLE 3 Recommended Regimens for Treatment of Vulvovaginitis, Cervicitis, and Acute Salpingitis

Infection	Choice	Alternative
Vulvovaginitis		
Bacterial vaginosis	Metronidazole (500 mg PO b.i.d.) for 7 days	Ampicillin (500 mg PO q.i.d.) for 7 days
Candidiasis	Miconazole or clotrimazole vaginal cream (100 mg HS) for 7 days	Nystatin vaginal cream (100,000 units b.i.d.) for 7–14 days *or* Boric acid capsules (600 mg intravaginally HS) for 14 days
Trichomoniasis (sexual partner treated)	Metronidazole or tinidazole (2 g PO) single dose	Clotrimazole vaginal cream (100 mg HS) for 7 days
(sexual partner not treated)	Metronidazole or tinidazole (250 mg PO t.i.d.) for 7–10 days	Clotrimazole vaginal cream (100 mg HS) for 7 days
Cervicitis		
Chlamydial or mucopurulent	Tetracycline (500 mg PO q.i.d.) for 7 days *or* Doxycycline (100 mg PO b.i.d.) for 7 days	Erythromycin (500 mg PO q.i.d.) for 7 days *or* Sulfisoxazole (500 mg PO q.i.d.) for 10 days
Gonococcal		
PPNG not suspected	Ampicillin (3.5 g PO), amoxicillin (3 g PO), or APPG (4.8 mu IM), each with probenecid (1 g PO) and followed by tetracycline (500 mg PO q.i.d.) for 7 days	Tetracycline (500 mg PO q.i.d.) for 5 days
PPNG suspected	Spectinomycin (2 g IM) or ceftriaxone (250 mg IM), each followed by tetracycline (500 mg PO q.i.d.) for 7 days	Trimethoprim-sulfamethoxazole 80-mg/400-mg tablets (9 tablets PO OD) for 3 days
Genital herpes		
Primary or first episode	Acyclovir (5 mg/kg IV q8h or 200 mg PO q4–6h) for 5–7 days	Acyclovir cream topically to external genital lesions, 6 × daily for 7–14 days
Recurrent episodes	Acyclovir (200 mg PO q4–6h) for up to 6 mo for patients with frequent (>6 episodes per yr) and symptomatic recurrences (Routine therapy in immunocompetent hosts not recommended)	
Salpingitis		
Inpatient	Cefoxitin (2 g IV q6h) plus doxycycline (100 mg IV q12h) for 10–14 days	Metronidazole (500 mg IV q6h) plus doxycycline (100 mg IV q12h) for 10–14 days *or* Clindamycin (600 mg IV q6h) plus tobramycin (1.5 mg/kg IV q8h) for 10–14 days
Outpatient	Cefoxitin (2 g IM) plus probenecid (1 g PO), followed by doxycycline (100 mg PO b.i.d.) for 10–14 days	Ampicillin (3.5 g PO), amoxicillin (3 g PO) or APPG (4.8 mu IM), each with probenecid (1 g PO) and followed by doxycycline (100 mg PO b.i.d.) for 10–14 days *or* Trimethoprim-sulfamethoxazole 80-mg/400-mg tablets (2 tablets PO b.i.d.) plus clindamycin (300 mg PO t.i.d.) for 10–14 days

mu = million units.

Gram stain and by demonstration of a high ratio of succinate to lactate (greater than 0.4) or presence of specific amines (putrescine and cadaverine) in vaginal washings of affected patients. The latter two techniques may be useful if confirmation of diagnosis by the four findings above is difficult. The presence or absence of clue cells per se is not helpful since both false-positive (due to adherence by lactobacilli to desquamated vaginal epithelial cells) and false-negative (possibly due to presence of local IgA, which blocks bacterial attachment to vaginal cell surfaces) findings can occur. Culture of vaginal fluid is also not useful since isolation of *G. vaginalis*, even in high concentration, is not specific for bacterial vaginosis.

The recommended therapy of bacterial vaginosis is metronidazole, which appears to eradicate or suppress *G. vaginalis* and obligate anaerobes while promoting recolonization with lactobacilli (Table 3). Single-dose therapy, as used in the treatment of trichomoniasis, is associated with a high failure rate and is not recommended. Treatment with ampicillin is associated with success rates ranging from 33 to 100 percent. Erythromycin and doxycycline are ineffective, as are local measures such as triple-sulfa vaginal cream, or povidone-iodine vaginal tablets. Interestingly, treatment of the male sexual partner with metronidazole does not appear to prevent recurrence of bacterial vaginosis among women who had been treated with metronidazole.

Candidal Vulvovaginitis

This entity accounts for approximately one-third of all cases of vaginitis in office practice. Candidal vulvovaginitis is commoner during menstruation and in pregnancy and is associated with diabetes mellitus, immunosuppression, and use of broad-spectrum antibiotics, corticosteroids, or oral contraceptives. As many as 10 to 27 percent of male sexual partners of infected women may be found to have balanoposthitis. Clinically, candidal vulvovaginitis is characterized by symptoms of vulvar itching, burning, or other irritation, often associated with external dysuria and with scant, nonmalodorous discharge. Examination usually reveals reddened, inflamed vaginal mucosa with a thick, white, "cottage cheese" discharge. The vaginal pH is less than 4.5. Mixed infection with bacterial vaginosis or trichomoniasis is relatively uncommon. The diagnosis is confirmed by the presence of fungal elements either in saline or KOH smears or Gram stain of vaginal secretions. The KOH smear is considered the most sensitive noncultural method of diagnosis. Two drops of 10 percent KOH are mixed with the discharge on a glass slide under a cover slip and heated until boiling. This destroys the PMNs and epithelial cells and leaves intact the candidal budding and pseudohyphal forms. Cultures should be obtained if the clinical presentation is suggestive of vulvovaginal candidiasis but the wet smear is negative. Although *C. albicans* is the commonest isolate, other *Candida* species (e.g., *C. glabrata*) have also been implicated.

The recommended treatment for candidal vulvovaginitis is local application of antifungal imidazoles such as miconazole or clotrimazole nightly for 7 days and is associated with a cure rate of 90 percent over 6 to 8 weeks of follow-up (see Table 3). Three-day therapy with double strength clotrimazole has also been shown to be effective. Intravaginal nystatin cream can also be used, but requires twice-daily applications for 2 weeks and has a slightly lower cure rate of 70 percent. More recently, the use of 600 mg boric acid powder in gelatin capsules, inserted intravaginally each evening for 14 days, has been found to be as effective as nystatin but has the advantage of lower cost. Oral therapy with ketoconazole (200 mg twice daily for 5 days) does not provide added advantage in cure rate or prevention of recurrence and is not recommended except for patients with relapsing vulvovaginal candidiasis or for patients with chronic mucocutaneous candidiasis. The presence of *Candida* species per se in any asymptomatic woman does not require treatment. The need for treatment of the male sexual partner has not been determined.

Trichomonal Vaginitis

Symptoms associated with *T. vaginalis* vaginitis are highly variable and appear to correlate with the severity of the inflammatory response in a given host. *T. vaginalis* may also be associated with asymptomatic infection, which almost invariably leads to symptomatic disease eventually. In patients with minimal or no inflammatory response despite the presence of trichomonads, excessive vaginal discharge may be the only symptom. In more severe cases, the infection is characterized by a profuse, watery, foul-smelling vaginal discharge associated with burning, dysuria, and intermenstrual spotting. Examination shows a foamy, bubbly discharge adherent to an erythematous or often edematous vaginal mucosa with multiple petechiae. The vaginal pH is usually greater than 5.0. Numerous PMNs are seen in the wet smear. Diagnosis is confirmed by the presence of motile trichomonads in the saline preparation of vaginal discharge. In patients with minimal symptoms, the wet smear may not be sufficiently sensitive, and culture for *T. vaginalis* on selective medium (such as Diamond's medium) is highly recommended.

Systemic treatment with oral nitroimidazoles, such as metronidazole or tinidazole, are the only regimens consistently effective for *T. vaginalis* vaginitis (see Table 3). Simultaneous treatment of the male sexual partner is important for prevention of relapse or reinfection and is particularly important if the 2-g single-dose regimen is used. The presence of *T. vaginalis*, even in the absence of vaginal symptoms, should be treated since these women almost invariably develop symptomatic disease eventually. The commonest causes of recurrent *T. vaginalis* infection, or apparent treatment failure, are due to reinfection or patient noncompliance with therapy. Persistent infection despite good compliance and avoidance of reinfection should suggest the possibility of infection due to metronidazole-resistant *T. vaginalis*. Such patients may require 7- to 14-day retreatment regimens consisting of oral metronidazole, 2 to 3 g daily by mouth, together with a vaginal metronidazole tablet, 500 mg, inserted nightly each day until vaginal symptoms have completely subsided. Metronidazole remains the drug of choice for symptomatic trichomonal vaginitis during pregnancy; the dosage is the same as for a nonpregnant woman. Clotrimazole can be administered intravaginally as a topical trichomonicide, but it is clearly less effective than metronidazole.

Cervicitis

Infection of the cervix by sexually transmitted pathogens may lead to several potential complications, including endometritis and salpingitis leading to ectopic pregnancy or infertility; premature rupture of membranes, chorioamnionitis, and puerperal infection during pregnancy; and initiation or promotion of cervical neoplasia. Cervicitis can be difficult to diagnose because many women are asymptomatic, and infection is often discovered only after a sexual partner presents with urethritis. Alternatively, cervical infection may be misdiagnosed as vaginitis if a thorough pelvic examination is not performed. The typical finding of cervicitis is an inflamed cervix, with a mucopurulent exudate emanating from the os. The principal infectious causes are *C. trachomatis*, *N. gonorrhoeae*, and HSV. Although cervical infection with any of these pathogens is more likely to present with a mucopurulent endocervical discharge, only HSV is associated with characteristic ectocervical ulcerations, and only *C. trachomatis* is associated with the presence of mucopus or with 10 or more PMNs per high-power field in cervical mucus. *C. trachomatis* frequently coexists with *N. gonorrhoeae* in cervicitis; treatment for both gonococcal and nongonococcal cervicitis should, therefore, also be effective against *C. trachomatis*.

Mucopurulent or Chlamydial Cervicitis

Chlamydial infection should always be suspected in women with mucopurulent cervicitis whether or not gonorrhea is also found. Similar to the case of gonococcal urethritis in men, women with gonococcal infection treated with 4.8 million units of procaine penicillin G plus probenecid were associated with a significantly higher rate of posttreatment cervicitis and pelvic inflammatory disease as compared with similar women treated with agents effective against both *N. gonorrhoeae* and *C. trachomatis*. Tetracycline or doxycycline at equivalent doses for 7 days is currently the most effective regimen for mucopurulent cervicitis and eradication of *C. trachomatis* from the cervix (see Table 3). If coexisting gonococcal infection is found, additional therapy for gonorrhea should be provided in areas where tetracycline is no longer highly effective against *N. gonorrhoeae*. Erythromycin is recommended for women allergic to tetracycline or during pregnancy. Sulfisoxazole is another alternative for chlamydial cervicitis, but it should be avoided during pregnancy.

Gonococcal Cervicitis

Whenever endocervical gonorrhea is suspected, the urethra as well as paraurethral glands should also be carefully examined. Cultures should be obtained from multiple sites including the anorectum and the oropharynx. A confirmatory test for *C. trachomatis* is also desirable in women with cervicitis, even if gonococcal infection is found, since more than 40 percent of women with gonorrhea have coexisting chlamydial infection. Initial empiric therapy, therefore, should also be effective against *C. trachomatis* (see Table 3). Single-dose ampicillin or amoxicillin plus probenecid followed by 7 days of tetracycline is the regimen of choice for infections in which penicillinase-producing *N. gonorrhoeae* (PPNG) is not suspected. The combined regimen of ampicillin or amoxicillin followed by tetracycline will also eradicate pharyngeal gonococcal infection, for which ampicillin, amoxicillin and spectinomycin are not highly effective. Patients allergic to penicillin or in whom PPNG or pregnancy is suspected may be treated with spectinomycin or ceftriaxone. Trimethoprim-sulfamethoxazole is an alternative to ampicillin-tetracycline combination for dual endocervical infection with *N. gonorrhoeae* and *C. trachomatis*. However, this regimen is poorly tolerated and treatment failure has occurred with both organisms in 10 to 20 percent of cases. The new quinolones show some promise as effective therapy for dual infection with *N. gonorrhoeae* and *C. trachomatis*. Their activity against genital mycoplasmas is quite variable, however.

Herpes Simplex Cervicitis and Genital Infection

The first episode of genital herpes is frequently accompanied by systemic as well as local manifestations. Concomitant cervicitis occurs in the majority of cases (80 to 90 percent), in contrast to recurrent episodes (10 to 20 percent). Several anatomic sites besides the cervix may be involved, including the urethra, vulva, pharynx, and extragenital cutaneous regions. Primary HSV genital infection tends to be more severe in women, and complications occur more frequently than in men. The most prominent local symptoms include pain, dysuria, tender inguinal adenopathy, and neurologic complications such as sacral anesthesia, urinary retention, and constipation. The cervix may show diffuse friability with necrotic and ulcerative lesions of both the exocervix and endocervix. The presence of HSV is confirmed either by culture or direct immunofluorescent staining of scrapings from active lesions. Recurrent genital herpes is less severe and of shorter duration than primary or first episodes of infection. There is, however, considerable variability in the intensity and duration of symptoms and in the frequency of recurrence. Recurrent viral shedding from the cervix can also occur in the absence of symptoms or external genital lesions. This is of clinical importance particularly in late pregnancy because of concern of intrapartum transmission of HSV infection to the neonate. Pregnant women with a history of recurrent genital herpes should be closely monitored virologically or cytologically near term, usually starting between 32 and 36 weeks of gestation. Women with active external genital lesions or cervical viral shedding at the time of labor should be delivered by cesarean section. Women with two sequential negative viral cultures or cytologic studies performed 3 to 4 days apart and absent genital lesions at the time of labor may be delivered vaginally.

Acyclovir is effective in reducing some of the manifestations of primary genital HSV infection and in shortening the duration of viral shedding (see Table 3). Oral acyclovir is also effective in suppressing recurrent episodes among patients receiving continuous therapy and may be indicated in selected patients with severe underlying disease and immunosuppression. Topical acyclovir is useful for the treatment of external genital lesions in women during primary or first episodes of HSV infection. It is not approved for intravaginal use since the polyethylene glycol base is irritating and may cause vaginal erythema. Routine use of topical acyclovir in recurrent genital herpes is not recommended since it has no established role either in prophylaxis of recurrence or in prevention of acquisition of new infection.

Acute Salpingitis

Acute salpingitis, or pelvic inflammatory disease (PID), is believed to result from ascending infection, by contiguous spread of sexually transmitted pathogens and/or indigenous vaginal microflora, from the endocervix and endometrium. Major risk factors for salpingitis include an intrauterine device, previous gonococcal infection, previous episodes of PID, lower socioeconomic status, nulliparity, and number of sexual partners. Use of oral contraceptives appears to have a protective influence. The microbiology of acute PID is complex. Cultures obtained directly from inflamed fallopian tubes either at laparoscopy or laparotomy clearly indicate a polymicrobial etiology, including *N. gonorrhoeae*, *C. trachomatis*, *Mycoplasma hominis*, and mixed aerobes and anaerobes. Clinically, acute PID associated with endocervical gonorrhea tends to occur more frequently during the first 10 days of the menstrual cycle, and affected patients are more severely ill than those with nongonococcal

PID. On the other hand, patients with nongonococcal PID are more likely to have a history of previous PID and a less optimal response to conventional antimicrobial therapy, and are more likely to develop late sequelae such as recurrent PID, adnexal abscess, and infertility.

The clinical diagnosis of acute PID by history and physical findings alone is often inaccurate. The classic manifestations include fever, chills, malaise, and bilateral lower abdominal pain that is often aggravated by movement of the iliopsoas muscles. Pelvic examination reveals a mucopurulent cervical discharge, and exquisite tenderness on movement of the cervix. The adnexal regions are tender and thickened, and an adnexal or cul-de-sac mass may be palpable if infection is recurrent or chronic. Visual confirmation of tubal inflammation by colposcopy or laparoscopy can be very helpful and should be undertaken, particularly if the clinical diagnosis of acute PID is in doubt, or when the clinical presentation is atypical. Analyses of specimens obtained by culdocentesis for presence of PMNs and microorganisms by Gram stain and culture are helpful, but not very reliable for the diagnosis of chlamydial salpingitis. Cervical secretions should be routinely examined for PMNs as well as both *N. gonorrhoeae* and *C. trachomatis*. Since appropriate collection and microbiologic testing of specimens from the fallopian tubes are neither practical nor desirable in all cases of PID, treatment is often empiric, based on selection of antimicrobial agents active against the major recognized pathogens (see Table 3). Any IUD should be removed, and all sexual partners within 2 months prior to the patient's illness should be examined and empirically treated with a regimen effective against both *C. trachomatis* and *N. gonorrhoeae* before and irrespective of cultural results. Hospitalization should be considered for acutely ill patients, particularly if pelvic peritonitis is present, if the diagnosis of acute PID is in doubt and other surgical emergencies are possible, if an adnexal or cul-de-sac mass is palpable, or if the patient is pregnant.

It should be noted that none of the currently recommended regimens for acute salpingitis outlined in Table 3 are considered optimal therapy, and their relative efficacy remains to be established by controlled clinical trials. The cefoxitin-doxycycline regimen is theoretically most attractive, since cefoxitin has excellent activity against the anaerobes most frequently isolated in PID, as well as aerobic and microaerophilic streptococci, coliforms, and gonococci, whereas doxycycline is effective against *C. trachomatis* and *M. hominis*. The metronidazole-doxycycline combination is attractive since excellent tissue concentrations can be achieved by oral administration of these agents. However, this regimen may not be reliably effective against Enterobacteriaceae or against *N. gonorrhoeae* in areas where moderate tetracycline resistance is encountered. The clindamycin-aminoglycoside regimen is the least attractive since it does not provide optimal coverage for either *C. trachomatis* or *N. gonorrhoeae*. The combination of trimethoprim-sulfamethoxazole plus clindamycin for outpatient treatment of acute PID appears promising and deserves critical evaluation. Similarly, the combination of a new-generation quinolone plus either clindamycin or metronidazole may prove effective, but results from controlled clinical trials are not

yet available. Approximately 5 to 15 percent of women fail to respond to initial antimicrobial therapy, 20 percent have at least one recurrence, and 15 percent are left infertile. It is clear that a comprehensive assessment of any therapeutic regimen for PID must include evaluation for late sequelae such as recurrence, infertility, and ectopic pregnancy, as well as the immediate response to acute symptoms.

Vulvovaginal and Tubo-ovarian Abscess

Pyogenic Vulvovaginal Infections

These include abscess of Bartholin's and Skene's glands, infected labial inclusion cysts, labial abscesses, furunculosis, and hidradenitis. Mixed infection due to both aerobic and anaerobic vaginal bacteria is the general rule, and coliforms, *B. fragilis*, *B. bivius*, and anaerobic cocci are commonly involved. Coexisting *N. gonorrhoeae* should be excluded. Surgical drainage is the primary therapeutic modality, and antimicrobials are of secondary importance. In the absence of specific cultural and antibiotic susceptibility data, initial selection of drugs should include those effective against both aerobic and anaerobic bacteria of vaginal origin (Table 4). Subsequent modification of antimicrobial therapy should be guided by the clinical response and by microbiologic data based on specimens obtained by direct needle aspiration of lesions (avoiding contamination by normal vaginal flora).

Tubo-ovarian Abscess

Tubo-ovarian abscess (TOA) occurring in the absence of obstetric and postoperative infections is generally a consequence of acute or chronic PID. Unilateral presentation of TOA is not uncommon and is not uniquely associated with IUD usage. Tubo-ovarian abscesses are often polymicrobial, caused by mixed aerobes and anaerobes including *Escherichia coli*, *B. fragilis*, *B. bivius*, *Peptostreptococcus* species, and aerobic streptococci. The recommended antimicrobial regimens for initial empiric treatment of TOA are outlined in Table 4. The optimal duration of treatment has not been clearly established. The general recommendation is that antibiotic should be continued by oral administration for 6 to 8 weeks, until the adnexal mass is no longer palpable. Medical therapy with antimicrobial agents alone is successful in 40 to 70 percent of cases. Surgical intervention is indicated if rupture is suspected or imminent or if suboptimal clinical response is observed after 72 hours of initial antimicrobial therapy. Conservative initial management of TOA, particularly in young, nulliparous patients, is indicated in the majority of cases. Serial ultrasonography is particularly useful in assessing the therapeutic response and resolution of mass effect during follow-up.

Genital Warts

Genital warts are caused by specific serotypes of human HPV (types 6, 11, 16, 18, 31, 33, and 35). The association of HPV infection and cervical intraepithelial neoplasia is strong, and unique HPV serotypes are implicated. For ex-

TABLE 4 Recommended Regimens for Treatment of Vulvovaginal and Tubo-ovarian Abscess

Infection	Choice	Alternative
Vulvovaginal abscess		
Inpatient	Cefoxitin (1.5 g IV q8h) for 5–7 days	Metronidazole (500 mg IV q6h) or clindamycin (600 mg IV q8h) plus gentamicin or tobramycin (1.5 mg/kg IV q8h) for 5–7 days
Outpatient	Ampicillin (500 mg PO q.i.d.) plus metronidazole (500 mg q.i.d.) for 7–10 days	Trimethoprim-sulfamethoxazole 80-mg/400-mg (1 tablet PO b.i.d.) plus clindamycin (300 mg PO t.i.d.) for 7–10 days
Tubo-ovarian abscess		
Inpatient	Clindamycin (600 mg IV q8h) plus tobramycin (1.5 mg/kg IV q8h) for 10–14 days	Metronidazole (500 mg IV q6h) or cefoxitin (1.5 g IV q8h) or ticarcillin (3 g IV q4h), each plus gentamicin or tobramycin (1.5 mg/kg IV q8h) for 10–14 days *or* Cefotaxime (1.5 g IV q6h) ± gentamicin or tobramycin (depending on severity) (1.5 mg/kg IV q8h) for 10–14 days
Outpatient	Ampicillin (500 mg PO q.i.d.) plus metronidazole (500 mg PO q.i.d.) for 6–8 wk	Trimethoprim-sulfamethoxazole 80-mg/400-mg (2 tablets PO b.i.d.) plus clindamycin (300 mg PO t.i.d.) for 6–8 wk

Regimens are applicable after exclusion of endocervical or paraurethral *N. gonorrhoeae* or *C. trachomatis* infection.

ample, HPV type 16 or 18, which apparently causes only a small proportion of genital warts, is present in 70 percent of cervical cancers. Conversely, serotype 6, the most common cause of overt genital warts, is rarely found in genital cancer. Serotypes 10, 11, 31, 33, and 35 are also associated with cervical neoplasia but are found in a low percentage of cases.

HPV infection appears to be increasing rapidly in the general population and currently is among the three most common diseases diagnosed in patients attending STD clinics. Most genital warts are subclinical and may be detected only with colposcopy, cytology, biopsy, or DNA hybridization techniques. Infection may be overt, extensive, and symptomatic in immunocompromised individuals, such as in patients with the acquired immunodeficiency syndrome or following bone marrow or solid organ transplantation. Genital warts in women are generally more extensive than might be assumed from overt lesions. The posterior introitus is the most common location for overt warts (73 percent), followed by the vulva (30 percent), the vagina (15 percent), and the cervix (6 percent). However, over 50 percent of women with vulvar warts have colposcopic evidence of cervical HPV infection. As in men, anorectal involvement is not uncommon.

Therapy for HPV infection is primarily directed at symptomatic and overt lesions at present. It remains to be determined whether routine treatment of subclinical infection is warranted and is effective in preventing genital neoplasia. Weekly topical application with podophyllin has been widely used for clearing overt warts and is effective in 75 percent of cases, with an expected relapse rate of 65 to 78 percent within 3 to 12 months. Podophyllin is toxic if absorbed and can cause severe local reactions including ulceration and bleeding. It should be carefully applied under medical supervision, allowed to dry thoroughly, and washed off within 3 to 4 hours after the initial application. This interval may be extended as tolerated during subsequent treatments. Podophyllin should be avoided during pregnancy, and

its application to cervical lesions is not recommended. Cryotherapy with liquid nitrogen appears to be an effective alternative and is cost effective for initial therapy of nonextensive warts. Generally, 3 to 6 weekly applications are required. The main adverse effect is pain, but it appears to be better tolerated than electrical cautery. Laser ablation should be reserved for patients with extensive or refractory warts. Topical 5-fluorouracil (1 percent solution) may cause necrosis and sloughing of rapidly proliferating tissue, and its use is more limited. Finally, interferons, either topically, intralesionally, or systemically, have been used experimentally in the treatment of overt genital warts. The type of interferon preparations (leukocyte interferon, α- and β-interferons) and dose and treatment regimens have varied. The early results appear promising, but more careful evaluations are required before their role in the treatment of genital warts is established.

SUGGESTED READING

Berg AO, Heidrich FE, Fihn SD, et al. Establishing the cause of genitourinary symptoms in women in a family practice. JAMA 1984; 251:620–625.

Bruham RC, Paavonen J, Stevens CE, et al. Mucopurulent cervicitis. The ignored counterpart in women of urethritis in men. N Engl J Med 1984; 311:1–6.

Burnakis TG, Hildebrandt NB. Pelvic inflammatory disease. A review with emphasis on antimicrobial therapy. Rev Infect Dis 1986; 8:86–116.

Centers for Disease Control. 1985 STD treatment guidelines. MMWR 1985; 34:75s–108s.

Kirby P, Corey L. Genital human papillomavirus infections. Infect Dis Clin North Am 1987; 1:123–178.

Landers DV, Sweet RL. Current trends in the diagnosis and treatment of tubo-ovarian abscess. Am J Obstet Gynecol 1985; 151:1098–1110.

Noble MA, Kwong A, Barteluk RL, et al. Laboratory diagnosis of *Chlamydia trachomatis* using two immunodiagnostic methods. Am J Clin Pathol 1988; 90:205–210.

Paavonen J, Critchlow CW, DeRouen T, et al. Etiology of cervical inflammation. Am J Obstet Gynecol 1986; 154:556–564.

Paavonen J, Stamm WE. Lower genital tract infections in women. Infect Dis Clin North Am 1987; 1:179–198.

Sobel JD. Recurrent vulvovaginal candidiasis. A prospective study of the efficacy of maintenance ketoconazole therapy. N Engl J Med 1986; 315:1455–1458.

Sweet RL. Pelvic inflammatory disease and infertility in women. Infect Dis Clin North Am 1987; 1:199–215.

Wasserheit JN, Bell TA, Kiviat NB, et al. Microbial causes of proven pelvic inflammatory disease and efficacy of clindamycin and tobramycin. Ann Intern Med 1986; 104:187–193.

PROSTATITIS, EPIDIDYMITIS, AND BALANOPOSTHITIS

GERALD W. CHODAK, M.D.

PROSTATITIS

Current treatment of inflammatory diseases of the prostate still results in dissatisfied patients and frustrated physicians. Despite significant progress, there is a persistent difficulty in explaining why some patients respond so well to a short course of therapy and others have persistent or recurrent symptoms, even when prolonged therapy is employed. Nevertheless, a systematic approach to evaluation will enable the physician to localize the source of infection and determine whether it is likely to respond to antibiotic therapy.

Diagnostic Evaluation and Culture Techniques

In addition to the routine history and physical examination, information about the prostate can be obtained from microscopy and culture of the prostatic fluid. In order to localize the bacteria to the prostate, samples are taken from different parts of the voided urine as well as from fluid expressed by prostatic massage. At the time of evaluation, the patient should have a relatively full bladder. The urine is divided into the first 10 ml of voided urine (urethral sample) and the midstream urine (bladder sample). A digital examination is then performed, and fluid from the prostate is expressed into the urethra and collected (EPS). Another urine sample is then collected (VB3), which also contains prostatic fluid. The laboratory should be informed of the physician's interest in finding low densities of organisms. Evaluation of this test is difficult, but if pyuria is present, low counts of bacteria can be considered significant if no other diagnostic finding points to a differential diagnosis. The pathogens are usually the same as those causing urinary tract infections and include *Escherichia coli, Klebsiella, Enterobacter, Proteus,* and *Pseudomonas* species.

Microscopic Evaluation of Prostatic Fluid

Two criteria used to diagnose an inflammatory process in the prostate are the presence of leukocytes and lipid-laden macrophages (oval fat bodies) in the expressed prostatic fluid. The fluid must be compared with the first 10 ml of voided urine, which contains urethral contents. Normal prostatic fluid contains fewer than 10 white blood cells (WBC) per high-power field, and more than 15 or 20 WBC per high-power field are considered abnormal. Oval fat bodies are not typically found in the urethra, so that an increase in these cells in the prostatic fluid is also evidence for an inflammatory response.

Interpretation of Cultural Results

A bacterial infection in the prostate may not produce a count of more than 100,000 cfu per milliliter. Therefore, the diagnosis is made by comparing the prostatic cultures with those of the urethra and bladder. A prostatic infection is present when the urine from the bladder (VB2) contains fewer than 10,000 cfu/ml and the prostatic cultures (EPS and VB3) contain 10 times as many bacteria as does the urethral culture (VB1). In order to diagnose bacterial prostatitis when the bladder urine contains significant bacteria, the patient must first be treated for a few days with nitrofurantoin, which sterilizes the urine while not greatly affecting the prostate. Reculture at that time will permit the same comparison between the urethral sample and the VB3 and EPS cultures.

ACUTE BACTERIAL PROSTATITIS

Diagnosis

Patients with acute prostatitis present with fever, chills, and irritative voiding symptoms that include dysuria, frequency, and pain. Examination of the prostate reveals a tender prostate, and prostate massage is not recommended because of the possibility of producing a bacteremia. One underlying cause of this disorder is acute or chronic urinary retention, which is assessed by palpating an enlarged bladder. If significant residual urine is suspected following voiding, then the bladder is catheterized and an indwelling catheter is left in place when more than 100 ml is present.

Treatment

Hospitalization is usually advised for patients with high fever (greater than 101°F) and significant pain. Bed rest, hydration, and analgesics provide symptomatic relief. Antibiotic therapy is instituted with gentamicin (3 mg per kilogram intravenously in three divided doses) and ampicillin (2 g intravenously every 6 hours) until the cultures and sensitivities are available. When the fever has defervesced, the antibiotic can usually be changed to trimethoprim (160 mg) and sulfisoxazole (800 mg) orally twice a day. The usual course of therapy is 2 weeks. More recently, ciprofloxacin (250 to 500 mg twice a day for 7 to 10 days) may also be an excellent choice for treatment.

CHRONIC BACTERIAL PROSTATITIS

Diagnosis

Most men with chronic prostatitis complain of chronic irritative symptoms and pain in the pelvic area or in the penis following ejaculation. Patients may have recurrent urinary infections with the same organism and/or positive EPS or VB3 cultures.

Treatment

Optimal therapy requires obtaining high levels of antibiotic in prostatic secretions rather than in prostatic tissue (Fig. 1). The most effective treatment is trimethoprim (160 mg) and sulfamethoxazole (800 mg) orally taken in combination twice a day. Patients treated with short courses of therapy are more likely to have recurrences than those taking a longer course. The best approach is to initiate therapy for 2–4 weeks. Patients who develop recurrent symptoms after therapy is discontinued may improve following administration of low-dose daily therapy consisting of 80 mg of trimethoprim and 400 mg of sulfamethoxazole for another 1 to 3 months. An alternative therapy is carbenicillin indanyl sodium (382 mg, two tablets orally four times per day) for 4 weeks, which may be as effective, although it has a substantially higher cost. In some cases, patients fail to obtain prolonged relief of their symptoms, and these may warrant surgical intervention, which involves either transurethral prostatectomy or total prostatovesiculectomy. Although the transurethral procedure has far fewer adverse effects, the patient should be informed that his symptoms may not be to-

tally cured because some residual tissue will still remain. Urologists are generally reluctant to recommend surgery to treat this disorder.

NONBACTERIAL PROSTATITIS

Patients complain of the same symptoms found in bacterial prostatitis, and the prostatic fluid also contains more than 15 to 20 WBC per high-power field; however, the urine, EPS, and VB3 cultures are negative. There is no conclusive evidence that *Chlamydia* is a primary cause of this problem, and, yet, a trial of tetracycline, 500 mg orally every 6 hours for 10 to 14 days, may be warranted. If little or no response occurs, no additional antibiotics are warranted. Patients with negative cultures should not be placed on long-term antibiotic therapy. The optimal treatment is based on symptoms. Patients often feel better by taking hot sitz baths two or three times per day. Prostatic massage has no proven value in the management of this illness. Patients should be encouraged to maintain their normal sexual activity and physical exercise and should be informed that the problem is not serious but the symptoms are likely to persist for a variable period of time. Many patients notice that alcohol and caffeine worsen their symptoms, so that reducing these items from their diet may improve their symptoms.

ACUTE EPIDIDYMITIS

Acute epididymitis is a disorder characterized by an abrupt onset of pain and swelling in the tail of the epididymis and may be followed by diffuse swelling of the entire epididymis, ipsilateral testicle, and hemiscrotum (epididymo-orchitis). The causes may be either sexual or nonsexual; nonsexual causes are more likely to have an anatomic basis. Patients over 40 years of age who develop epididymitis usually have an associated urinary tract infection, which is due to some obstructive process such as a urethral stricture of benign prostatic hypertrophy.

Diagnosis

The initial diagnosis is made based on clinical findings, which include swelling and marked tenderness along the epididymis. As the disease progresses, epididymo-orchitis may develop as the testicle also becomes swollen and tender.

The cause of epididymitis in patients who have a history of sexual exposure may be determined by performing a Gram stain of a urethral smear obtained prior to voiding. If intracellular gram-negative diplococci are identified, then *Neisseria gonorrhoeae* is the cause. If no organisms are identified, then a culture must be performed to rule out gonococcal infection. In the absence of neisseriae, *Chlamydia trachomatis* is usually the responsible organism in this group.

For patients who develop epididymitis secondary to a urinary tract anomaly, a urine culture and sensitivity will identify the causative organism.

An important cause of epididymitis in the older population is urinary obstruction associated with an inability to empty the bladder. When the history or physical examina-

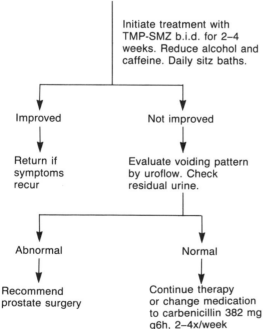

CHRONIC PROSTATITIS DIAGNOSED

Initiate treatment with TMP-SMZ b.i.d. for 2–4 weeks. Reduce alcohol and caffeine. Daily sitz baths.

Improved → Return if symptoms recur

Not improved → Evaluate voiding pattern by uroflow. Check residual urine.

Abnormal → Recommend prostate surgery

Normal → Continue therapy or change medication to carbenicillin 382 mg q6h, 2–4x/week

Figure 1   Treatment of chronic prostatitis.

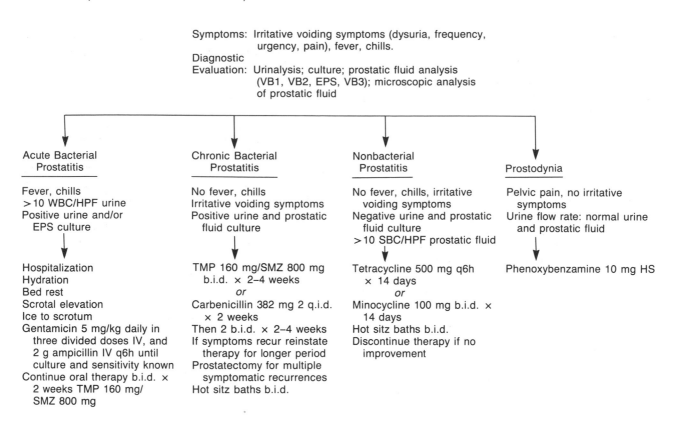

Figure 2 Diagnosis and treatment of prostatitis.

tion suggests a significant residual urine, a catheter is passed and left in place if more than 100 ml remains in the bladder following voiding.

Treatment

The optimal treatment of acute epididymitis depends on the underlying cause. Febrile patients with epididymitis secondary to bacteriuria are treated initially with ampicillin, 1 g intravenously every 6 hours, and tobramycin, 3.0 mg per kilogram intravenously in three divided doses, until the results of the urine culture and sensitivity are available. At that time either oral ampicillin, 500 mg orally every 6 hours for 10 days, or a first-generation cephalosporin may be substituted. Patients will usually benefit from symptomatic treatment, which includes hospitalization, bed rest, scrotal elevation, and ice packs to the scrotum to reduce swelling. If significant residual urine is detected, then a prostatectomy should be planned after the acute episode has resolved.

Men who develop acute epididymitis following sexual exposure are treated with ampicillin, 500 mg orally four times per day for 10 days, if *N. gonorrhoeae* has been cultured or found on Gram stain, or with tetracycline, 500 mg orally four times per day for 10 days, if there is no evidence for gonorrhea. In addition, symptomatic relief is provided by bed rest and scrotal elevation. When epididymitis has been caused by sexual transmission, sexual partners must also be treated.

BALANOPOSTHITIS

Infection of the glans penis and foreskin occurs almost exclusively in the uncircumcised male. Usually the foreskin cannot be retracted; this allows smegma and secretions to accumulate and provides a warm, moist culture medium that predisposes to infection. Balanitis and balanoposthitis are commonest in children and may be associated with impaired urination because of a tight phimosis. It also occurs following sexual contact with an infected partner.

Diagnosis

The initial diagnosis is made from physical examination. The foreskin may be difficult to retract over the glans. Inflammation and swelling of the glans and/or prepuce are present. A Gram stain of the material under the foreskin will determine the class of organisms present. Sexually active patients who develop balanoposthitis give a history of sexual contact within 6 to 24 hours prior to the onset of symptoms. These patients may have erosive soreness and ulceration of the glans penis. Microscopic examination should reveal the presence of *Candida*.

Treatment

Most cases of balanoposthitis in children can be treated with soap and water cleansing, provided that the foreskin can be retracted over the glans. Acutely, this may not be possible, and a dorsal slit procedure must be performed. This will allow improved hygiene, which helps to rapidly resolve the inflammation and swelling. Once this has resolved, the patient should undergo a circumcision. Antibiotics are usually not required.

Patients who develop balanoposthitis following sexual

DISSEMINATED GONOCOCCAL INFECTION

JONATHAN M. ZENILMAN, M.D.

Disseminated gonococcal infection (DGI) develops in approximately 0.5 to 1.0 percent of patients with gonorrhea, and is the most common cause of septic arthritis in persons under age 45 years. The manifestations of DGI are those of a febrile illness with prominent dermatologic and rheumatologic findings.

DGI has been clinically divided into two major syndromes: the dermatitis-tenosynovitis syndrome and the septic arthritis syndrome. Patients with the dermatitis-tenosynovitis syndrome usually present with chills, fever, polyarthralgias, and tenosynovitis and have three to 20 petechial, papular, pustular, hemorrhagic, or necrotic skin lesions, usually on the extensor surfaces of the distal extremities. The second common syndrome is septic arthritis, usually monoarticular, affecting large joints, most commonly the knee. Cultures of joint fluid are positive in about half the cases with effusion. Overlap between the two syndromes is not uncommon. A small proportion of DGI patients (approximately 1 percent) develop meningitis or endocarditis.

Blood cultures are positive in only half the patients with tenosynovitis dermatitis and in less than 20 percent of patients with septic arthritis. Often, patients with DGI have primary mucosal (either genital or pharyngeal) infection that may be mildly symptomatic or asymptomatic.

DGI should be suspected in sexually active patients with fever and rheumatologic or dermatologic symptoms. The differential diagnosis includes meningococcemia, acute rheumatic fever, Reiter's syndrome and other reactive arthritides, hepatitis B, endocarditis, viral illnesses such as Epstein-Barr or cytomegalovirus disease, and connective tissue diseases such as systemic lupus erythematosis, juvenile rheumatoid arthritis, and gout.

All patients with suspected DGI should have blood cultures performed by use of standard techniques and mucosal cultures at all sites of potential sexual exposure by use of selective medium (such as Thayer-Martin medium). Women should have cultures of the cervix, rectum, and pharynx. Men should have urethral and pharyngeal cultures, and rectal cultures should also be performed in homosexual men. If joint effusion is present, diagnostic arthrocentesis should

exposure to women with candidal vaginitis are treated with topical nystatin ointment, 100,000 units per gram, twice a day for 10 days. If phimosis is present and discharge is discovered under the glans, the sexual partner also receives the same treatment. Figure 2 provides a flow chart that summarizes the content of the discussion in this chapter.

be performed, with culture on nonselective media, such as chocolate agar. Gram stain and culture should be performed on aspirates of skin lesions; however, the sensitivity of these procedures is low. A confirmed diagnosis of DGI requires a positive culture from blood or synovial fluid; a probable case is defined as one with signs and symptoms of DGI with a positive mucosal site culture. In a small proportion of cases, all cultures may be negative (usually due to prior use of antibiotics). In these cases, the diagnosis is made by evaluating the signs and symptoms presented, ruling out other diseases in the differential diagnosis, and evaluating response to therapy.

CLINICAL AND EPIDEMIOLOGIC CONSIDERATIONS

Since all cases of DGI ultimately result from gonococcal bacteremia (whether or not blood cultures are positive), patients with this disorder must be closely monitored. All patients require daily cardiac evaluation for murmurs and evaluation of affected joints. Joint effusions typically resolve quickly with the institution of antimicrobial therapy. However, in some patients with septic arthritis, periodic arthrocentesis may be indicated, especially early in the course of the disease. Surgical intervention is rarely required.

The basic principle of therapy for DGI (Table 1) is that parenteral therapy is given until the patient defervesces and shows other signs of clinical improvement, including the resolution of joint symptoms and the lack of development of new dermatologic lesions. After the patient is afebrile for 24 hours, most authorities continue oral antibiotics for a total (parenteral plus oral antibiotics) therapy duration of one week.

TABLE 1 Principles of Management

Parenteral antibiotic therapy until defervescence or other measures of clinical improvement

Antimicrobial therapy for 1 week

Frequent (preferably daily) evaluation of cardiac and rheumatologic status

Arthrocentesis if indicated

Hospitalization if indicated (see Table 2)

Initial antibiotic therapy should be effective for treatment of antibiotic-resistant organisms

Clinical isolates should be tested for antimicrobial susceptibility and therapy adjusted accordingly

Most patients with DGI, even those with mild signs and symptoms, should ideally be hospitalized for evaluation and therapy (Table 2). Hospitalization is especially indicated for all patients with joint effusion or those with preexisting cardiac valvular disease or murmurs of uncertain etiology. Occasionally, reliable patients with uncomplicated disease who are not at high risk for complications can be managed with closely supervised daily parenteral outpatient therapy (see below).

Patients who are considered unreliable for compliance with regimens of outpatient therapy or follow-up should be hospitalized. Changes in the epidemiology of gonorrhea over the past 10 years have resulted in a larger proportion of gonorrhea patients from inner-city high-risk groups. Drug abuse, especially intravenous and use of "crack" cocaine, is extremely common in these groups. Clinical differentiation of DGI and bacterial endocarditis in these patients is extremely difficult, and they should be hospitalized.

ANTIMICROBIAL RESISTANCE

Over the past decade, the incidence of *Neisseria gonorrhoeae* isolates resistant to antibiotics has increased geometrically. Multiple types of antimicrobial resistance have emerged (Table 3) and include both plasmid-mediated and chromosomally mediated resistance determinants. As of this writing, most of the major metropolitan areas have had outbreaks of infection due to penicillinase-producing *Neisseria gonorrhoeae* (PPNG) and also have endemic chromosomally mediated resistance. Plasmid and chromosomally mediated tetracycline resistance is especially a problem, leading to recent recommendations that tetracycline not be used as sole therapy for any gonococcal infection. The Centers for Disease Control (CDC) expects the problem of antimicrobial resistance to get worse in coming years.

A commonly held notion among clinicians and in many textbooks is that the organisms causing DGI are "exquisitely" sensitive to penicillin and other antibiotics. Although true in the 1970s, this is no longer the case. In general, although antibiotic-sensitive isolates among DGI strains are apparently more frequent than those in the general population, antimicrobial resistance is by no means uncommon. PPNG and chromosomally mediated resistant strains causing DGI are occurring with increasing frequency. Additionally, PPNG occurs in DGI patients with approximately the same frequency as in the general population, which has important consequences in areas such as Florida, Detroit, Providence, Southern California, and New York City, where PPNG strains accounted for more than 10 percent of all *N. gonorrhoeae* isolates in 1988. Patients with antibiotic-resistant infection who are not treated appropriately are at risk for treatment failure and secondary complications.

Data on the prevalence of antibiotic-resistant gonorrhea are available from state and local health departments and may help to guide the choice of initial therapy. Unfortunately, in most areas, health department data reflect only the incidence of PPNG, because testing for susceptibility to other antibiotics is rarely performed. Thus, all isolates from patients with DGI should have β-lactamase assays and susceptibility determined to antibiotics that are candidates for therapy.

TABLE 2 Specific Indications for Hospitalization

Uncertain diagnosis

Presence of joint effusion

Unreliable or noncompliant patient

Preexisting cardiac valvular disease or presence of murmur

Altered immune status or complement deficiencies

Meningitis

INITIAL ANTIBIOTIC THERAPY

No large prospective studies on the antibiotic therapy of DGI have been performed since the mid-1970s. Therefore, the following therapy recommendations are based on experience of the author and other experts and the awareness of widespread resistance to antimicrobial agents among *N. gonorrhoeae*. Because of the potentially serious complications of treatment failure, initial therapy should be effective against PPNG and other antimicrobial-resistant strains. Unless isolates are documented to be sensitive to the penicillins, first-generation cephalosporins, or tetracyclines, these drugs should generally not be used as either initial or follow-up therapy in patients with DGI.

Parenteral therapy with third-generation cephalosporins (ceftriaxone, ceftizoxime, cefotaxime) is the cornerstone of initial DGI therapy (Table 4). The author prefers ceftriaxone because its half-life allows once-a-day dosing. In reliable patients with uncomplicated disease, daily supervised in-office intravenous or intramuscular therapy is a practical alternative to hospitalization. Alternatively, cefotaxime or ceftizoxime are equally effective in the appropriate doses. Generally, these drugs can be used in patients with a history of nonanaphylactic penicillin allergy because cross-reactivity is relatively infrequent. Patients with histories of severe allergic reactions to penicillin or anaphylaxis should be treated with spectinomycin.

Third-generation cephalosporins are preferred as initial therapy for several reasons. First, clinically important resistance of *N. gonorrhoeae* to third-generation cephalosporins has not been reported. Second, while second-generation cephalosporins (cefoxitin and cefotetan) are not commonly utilized for treatment of gonorrhea, recent sur-

TABLE 3 Antimicrobial Resistance in *N. gonorrhoeae*

Plasmid-mediated

Penicillin: penicillinase-producing
              N. gonorrhoeae (PPNG)

Tetracycline: High-level tetracycline-resistant
               N. gonorrhoeae (TRNG)

Chromosomally mediated

Penicillin
Tetracycline
Cefoxitin (cefotetan)
Spectinomycin (rare in the United States; seen primarily in Southeast Asia)

TABLE 4 Antibiotic Therapy for DGI

Parenteral-Inpatient	Oral-Outpatient
Ceftriaxone 1 g/d	Cefuroxime axetil 250 mg–500 mg b.i.d.
Ceftizoxime 1 g q6–8h	Ciprofloxacin 500 mg– 750 mg* b.i.d.
Cefotaxime 1 g q6–8h	Amoxicillin 500 mg + clavaulanic acid (Augmentin-500) 1 tab t.i.d.†
Cefoxitin 1 g q6h	
Cefotetan 1 g q12h	Amoxicillin 500 mg t.i.d.
Spectinomycin 2 g q12h	
Ampicillin 1 g q6h‡	

* Contraindicated in pregnancy.

† May be ineffective against organisms with chromosomally mediated resistance.

‡ Should be used only for infections due to organisms with documented sensitivity to penicillin; do not use for initial presumptive therapy except when local incidence of PPNG is less than 1 percent of all *N. gonorrhoeae* isolates.

veillance data from CDC indicate increasing chromosomal resistance to these agents. Last, although spectinomycin resistance is prevalent in Southeast Asia (although still rare in the United States) it is not commonly utilized in inpatients.

Initial therapy with ampicillin or amoxicillin is reasonable in patients with organisms documented to be sensitive to penicillin or in patients residing in geographic areas where resistant infection is rare (less than 1 percent of all gonorrhea, essentially eliminating most U.S. metropolitan areas).

Typically, most patients with DGI respond rapidly to initial therapy, with defervescence and resolution of joint symptoms within 24 to 48 hours. Cases without effusion or other complications can be discharged home to complete their 1-week course of antibiotics with an oral regimen.

In the past, the mainstays of oral therapy have been ampicillin and the tetracyclines. Because of the resistance problem, unless susceptibility data are known, these agents can no longer be recommended as oral therapy options. I recommend that outpatient therapy be completed with either cefuroxime axetil, ciprofloxacin, or amoxicillin–clavulanic acid. Amoxicillin–clavulanate is effective against PPNG. However, theoretically, the drug may be ineffective against chromosomally mediated resistant strains. Ciprofloxacin is

contraindicated in pregnant women; ciprofloxacin and other quinolones are also contraindicated in children and adolescents.

SPECIAL PROBLEMS

Pregnant Women

Pregnant women are the group at highest risk for developing DGI. All of the listed inpatient regimens are considered acceptable for use during pregnancy. Spectinomycin should be used only as a last resort because of the higher rates of pharyngeal infection, against which spectinomycin is less effective, in pregnant women. Of the outpatient regimens, only cefuroxime axetil and amoxicillin are considered safe to use in this group.

Public Health Issues

Persons with one sexually transmitted disease (STD) are at high risk for having another. Persons with DGI should also be evaluated for *Chlamydia* with either culture or standardized antigen detection tests, and treated appropriately if positive. Serologic testing for syphilis should be performed. Counseling and testing for human immunodeficiency virus should be strongly considered. Finally, sexual contacts of DGI patients should be treated for gonorrhea and evaluated for other STDs. This process is initiated by reporting of DGI cases to the local health authorities.

SUGGESTED READING

Centers for Disease Control. Disseminated gonorrhea caused by penicillinase-producing *Neisseria gonorrhoeae*—Wisconsin, Pennsylvania. MMWR 1987; 36:161–167.

Centers for Disease Control. 1989 sexually transmitted disease treatment guidelines. MMWR (in press).

Handsfield HH, Wiesner PJ, Holmes KK. Treatment of the gonococcal arthritis-dermatitis syndrome. Ann Intern Med 1976; 84:661–667.

Holmes KK, Counts GW, Beaty HN. Disseminated gonococcal infection. Ann Intern Med 1971; 74:979–993.

Masi AT, Eisenstein BI. Disseminated gonococcal infection and gonococcal arthritis. II. Clinical manifestations, diagnosis, complications, treatment, and prevention. Semin Arthritis Rheum 1981; 10:173–197.

O'Brien JP, Goldenberg DL, Rice PA. Disseminated gonococcal infection: a prospective analysis of 49 patients and a review of pathophysiology and immune mechanisms. Medicine 1983; 62:395–406.

Rompalo AM, Hook EW III, Roberts PL, et al. The acute arthritis-dermatitis syndrome: the changing importance of *Neisseria gonorrhoeae* and *Neisseria meningitidis*. Arch Intern Med 1987; 147:281–283.

SYPHILIS

HARRY C. NOTTEBART Jr., M.D., F.A.C.P.

The Great Pox, the great imitator, the great mimic: syphilis is all of that. There is hardly any medical specialty that does not encounter this disease. It affects and infects people from before birth to old age. Virtually any organ can

be involved. The outstanding clinicians of the past said that if one knew syphilis one knew medicine. Today many clinicians think of syphilis in a cookbook fashion: serologic tests and penicillin. The recipes for treatment are even published by the federal government, but, as with most things in the real world, the issues may not be so clear cut.

Syphilis in the past has been described as occurring in stages—primary, secondary, or tertiary. Some of these are so different from one another that they were once thought to be unrelated diseases.

In staging syphilis this way, I think there is the possibility of creating a false mental image of the progression of syphilis. One might think that in the primary stage syphilis is limited to the localized chancre. In secondary syphilis, the disease spreads to the skin and throughout the body. Finally, in tertiary syphilis, the disease is disseminated to deep organs and tissues such as the cardiovascular system or the central nervous system (CNS). This image is not correct.

Studies published 85 or more years ago and those published recently show that *Treponema pallidum* are disseminated by the blood throughout the body, including into the cerebrospinal fluid (CSF) in primary syphilis, and this occurs within minutes of infection. Does that help in understanding the progression and course of the disease?

It certainly could explain why some patients receiving "adequate" therapy have relapses. There are many reports in the literature of patients who have not been cured with "standard" therapy. It is too easy to attribute all of these relapses to reinfection. If the organism were sequestered in the CNS and the low blood levels of penicillin resulted in inadequate CSF levels of penicillin, the organism would not be affected. Afterward, the organism could diffuse back into the bloodstream and disseminate once again.

The fact that there are not more apparent relapses may be due to the functioning of a competent immune system. The severe course of neurosyphilis in human immunodeficiency virus (HIV) infections may then be explained on the basis that the immune system is not functioning appropriately. Perhaps the devastating course of neurosyphilis seen in HIV-infected patients is what would be seen in anyone whose immune system was not functioning properly.

On the same basis, then, the state of "serofast" syphilis may reflect a patient whose infecting organisms are walled off somewhere but still alive and well, much as occurs with the tubercle bacillus in tuberculin-positive individuals. One then might speculate whether high-dose, prolonged intravenous therapy might cure even the so-called serofast state.

It was first described when therapy was arsenicals and other heavy metals, which may not have been able to diffuse into various sites where the organisms were sequestered.

DIAGNOSIS

The consequences of missing the diagnosis and failing to treat this disease can be devastating not only to the patient and his or her family but also to future children, if the patient is a woman of childbearing age. Because of these dreadful consequences, it is important to diagnose this disease when present.

There are only three ways to diagnose syphilis: dark-field examination for spirochetes, special tissue stains of biopsy material for spirochetes, or serologic testing for antibodies. Routine culturing for the organism that causes syphilis, *T. pallidum*, has not yet been achieved.

The use of dark-field microscopy has been limited because of the lack of dark-field microscopes and of personnel trained to interpret such preparations. Many current clinicians have never seen a positive dark-field preparation. Also, there are treponemes indigenous to various parts of the body, which makes interpretation of the dark-field preparations not as easy as some would indicate.

Biopsy specimens other than those from tertiary gummas or autopsies are rarely obtained, and the special stains for spirochetes are not routinely used.

All of this results in the fact that serologic testing has been the most available and popular diagnostic test for syphilis for many years. Only a small sample of blood is needed, no special preparation of the patient is needed, and no special handling is necessary for the specimen. The physician receives a report that gives the answer in terms of positive or negative. If the result is positive, then most nontreponemal tests such as the VDRL or RPR will be titered so that the result may be reported as "positive, 1:8."

One needs to consider the result of a serologic test in the context of the individual patient's clinical setting since false-positive and false-negative results can occur. The following infectious diseases can give false positives: other spirochetal diseases, such as relapsing fever; parasitic diseases, such as malaria; viral diseases, such as measles and mumps (and their immunizations), and chicken pox; chronic infections, such as leprosy; autoimmune diseases, such as SLE. Even pregnancy is reported to cause false positives. The serologic test may be negative for any of the following reasons: no disease; syphilis acquired and incubating but serology not yet positive; syphilis treated intentionally or inadvertently with reversion of serology; false negative.

The serology may be positive for any of these reasons: current disease; serofast from disease in the past; rising titer reflecting recently acquired disease; falling titer reflecting disease responding to recent therapy—intentional or inadvertent; passively acquired antibody; false positive. It is obvious that the interpretation of positive or negative serologic results depends upon history and physical examination. It is a mistake to rely solely on the serology.

Tests should be used to confirm diagnoses and not to make them.

A positive serologic test in a patient who has a history of contact with a person with syphilis and has one or more physical findings that are compatible with primary or even secondary syphilis confirms the presumptive diagnosis of syphilis. However, a positive serologic test is more likely to be a false positive if the person has no history or physical findings indicative of syphilis. This is true for the nontreponemal tests, such as the VDRL and RPR, and also for the more specific treponemal tests, such as the FTA-ABS and MHA-TP. If there is an unexpected positive test, one needs to repeat the history and physical examination, asking specific questions about sexual contacts and illnesses and looking for chancres and other manifestations that might have been overlooked previously. At the same time serologic testing should be repeated using a treponemal test.

Sexual contacts of the patient should come in for a thorough history, physical, and serologic examination, if this is possible.

A small number of patients have false-positive nontreponemal tests and false-positive treponemal tests. At this point one can temporize by bringing the patient back in several weeks and repeating the history, physical, and serologic testing, or decide on clinical grounds that these test results are false-positives and do nothing more, or decide that the patient has syphilis and treat.

If the patient is pregnant, the nontreponemal test is reactive, and the treponemal test is nonreactive, no therapy is necessary. A repeat test in 4 weeks should show a negative test or constant or falling titers. If titers rise or there is anything in patient's history or physical examination compatible with syphilis, she should be treated. Of course, one should involve the patient so that whether treated or not the patient knows why and what the reasoning was behind such decision. This should be documented in the patient's chart.

From these problems it is obvious that doing serologic testing on unselected patients may result in additional work, more testing, and inconvenience to the patient and his or her sexual contacts for the few cases found.

Special problems arise in attempting to diagnose CNS syphilis. If there are physical signs that the CSF shows increased levels of white blood cells and protein and a VDRL test is positive, the patient should be treated for CNS syphilis. However, there are often no physical signs. One does not do CSF examinations routinely on asymptomatic patients, but sometimes one has CSF results on someone whose blood serology is positive. Then any abnormality in the CSF is a reason for presumptive treatment for CNS syphilis. Patients with completely normal CSF are usually not treated for CNS syphilis, although some studies have obtained organisms even from apparently negative CSF. These patients still need following.

If the patient has positive blood serology and any physical signs compatible with CNS syphilis, a lumbar puncture (LP) should be done for CSF examination. Again, any abnormality provides a reason for treating for CNS syphilis. However, with physical signs, even a completely normal CSF should be treated because 25 percent or more may be negative, even with CNS involvement.

Adequate follow-up for a minimum of 2 years is necessary for all of these patients.

TREATMENT

There is a tendency to believe that the Centers for Disease Control (CDC) recommendations give 100 percent cure rates. However, it has been recognized that not 100 percent of patients would be cured by such a regimen and that follow-up was absolutely necessary to assure that those patients who did not respond to standard therapy were identified and given longer courses with larger doses to effect a cure. In my opinion the importance of follow-up needs to be emphasized.

The dosage schedules publicized by the CDC are to be taken in this context. This is the public health approach in which one tries to cure the greatest number of patients with the shortest course since many patients will not return for multiple doses. In this context, one-dose therapy is ideal as long as it can cure a fairly large proportion of patients. The CDC recommended treatment does this. However, if you are treating patients who are highly motivated and will comply with multiple doses and a longer course, then higher initial cure rates may be obtained. One needs to remember that even healthy people have quite variable antibiotic blood (and CSF) levels after standard doses.

Differences in philosophy can be seen in the different recommendations for the treatment of various stages of syphilis (Table 1). It has long been recognized that the longer *T. pallidum* has had to become established in someone's body, the longer it takes to eradicate and the higher the doses required. This is based on animal experiments decades ago, clinical observations even before the use of penicillin and other potent antibiotics, and more recent observations on the time course of serologic response to therapy. This is reflected also in treatment schedules that recommend higher doses or longer courses or both as the stage of the disease progresses.

For example, in the epidemiologic treatment of possible incubating syphilis, one dose of 2.4 million units of benzathine penicillin intramuscularly (for those not allergic to penicillin) is good therapy. After contact, syphilis may incubate up to 3 months before presenting with a chancre, although on the average the incubation time is about 3 weeks. At this early stage even small doses of penicillin are very effective.

Of course, epidemiologic treatment is offered to contacts of known cases of syphilis, but probably only 50 percent of them would ever present with syphilis, so a fairly large percentage of possible patients will be treated even though they would not develop syphilis. In my opinion, the only appropriate use of benzathine penicillin in syphilis therapy is in incubating syphilis.

In comparing the treatment schedules there are several obvious points. First, there is a surprising amount of unanimity in spite of the fact that there are no long-term comparative studies and the guidelines are based on empirical experience and tradition.

The points of difference are particularly noteworthy. Notice that the Canadian guidelines for the treatment of neurosyphilis recommend only the use of intravenous aqueous crystalline penicillin G. In my opinion this is correct. Since intramuscular benzathine penicillin rarely yields detectable CSF levels, there is no place for the use of such a form of penicillin in the treatment of neurosyphilis. Aqueous procaine penicillin intramuscularly with probenecid four times daily usually yields adequate CSF levels of penicillin but requires a high degree of compliance, and, considering how devastating this disease can be if allowed to progress, this course should be chosen only for highly selected, well-motivated patients in whom there will be adequate follow-up.

The CDC recommendation in neurosyphilis to follow courses of aqueous crystalline penicillin intravenously and aqueous procaine penicillin intramuscularly with a course of benzathine penicillin intramuscularly has no data to justify it.

In congenital syphilis, also note that the Canadian recommendation is for crystalline penicillin intravenously alone. They recommend CSF examination before treatment to provide a baseline but recommend that all neonates be treated as if they had CNS involvement. This is certainly the most conservative approach to management of congenital syphilis.

The World Health Organization (WHO) recommendations are a few years older and rely heavily on aqueous procaine penicillin G in increasingly longer courses of therapy

TABLE 1 Guidelines for Treatment of Syphilis

Stage of Disease	CDC Guidelines*	Canadian Guidelines†	WHO Guidelines‡
Early	Benzathine penicillin G 2.4 x 10⁶U IM x 1	Benzathine penicillin G 50,000 U/kg (max 2.4 x 10⁶ IM x 1	Aqueous procaine penicillin G 600,000 U IM q.d. x 10 days *or* Benzathine penicillin G 2.4 x 10⁶ U IM x 1
If allergic to penicillin	Tetracycline 500 mg PO q.i.d. x 15 days Erythromycin 500 mg PO q.i.d. x 15 days	Tetracycline 500 mg PO q.i.d.; in children under 9 yr desensitization and use of penicillin is preferred *or* erythromycin 40mg/kg/day (max 500 mg) PO q.i.d. x 15 days	Tetracycline 500 mg PO q.i.d. x 15 days Erythromycin (not estolate) 500 mg PO q.i.d. x 15 days
Late§	Benzathine penicillin G 2.4 x 10⁶U IM once a week x 3 wk	Benzathine penicillin G 50,000 U/kg (max 2.4 x 10⁶) IM weekly for 3 wk	Aqueous procaine penicillin G 600,000 U IM q.d. x 15 days *or* Benzathine penicillin G 2.4 x 10⁶U IM weekly x 3 wk
If allergic to penicillin	Tetracycline 500 mg PO q.i.d. x 30 days Erythromycin 500 mg PO q.i.d. x 30 days (if compliance and serologic follow-up can be assured; otherwise manage in consultation with an expert)	Tetracycline 500 mg PO q.i.d. for 30 days; in children under 9 yr desensitization and use of penicillin is preferred *or* erythromycin 40mg/kg/day (max 500 mg) PO q.i.d. x 30 days	Tetracycline 500 mg PO q.i.d. x 30 days Erythromycin (not estolate) 500 mg PO q.i.d. x 30 days
Neurosyphilis	Aqueous crystalline penicillin G 12–24 x 10⁶U IV q.d. (2–4 x 10⁶U q4h) x 10 days followed by benzathine penicillin G 2.4 x 10⁶U IM q.w. x 3 *or* Aqueous procaine penicillin G 2.4 x 10⁶U IM q.d. and probenecid 500 mg PO q.i.d. both for 10 days followed by benzathine penicillin G 2.4 x 10⁶U IM q.w. x 3 *or* Benzathine penicillin G 2.4 x 10⁶U IM q.w. x 3	Crystalline penicillin G 2 to 4 x 10⁶U IV q4h (12–24 x 10⁶U per day) for at least 10 days	Benzathine penicillin should not be used. Aqueous procaine penicillin G 6 x 10⁵U IM q.d. x 20 days
If allergic to penicillin	Confirm allergy and manage in consultation with an expert	(Presumably the same as for late syphilis)	Tetracycline 500 mg. PO q.i.d. x 30 days Erythromycin (not estolate) 500 mg PO q.i.d. x 30 days
Syphilis during pregnancy			
Early	Same as for nonpregnant	Same as for nonpregnant	Same as for nonpregnant
Late	Same as for non-pregnant	Same as for nonpregnant	Same as for nonpregnant
If allergic to penicillin	Erythromycin as for stage of disease; infants then treated with penicillin	Desensitization and then use of penicillin are preferred Early: erythromycin 500 mg PO q.i.d. for 15 days Late: erythromycin 500 mg PO q.i.d. for 30 days Infants treated with penicillin early in neonatal period	Erythromycin (not estolate)

TABLE 1 *(continued)*

Stage of Disease	CDC Guidelines*	Canadian Guidelines†	WHO Guidelines‡
Congenital	Symptomatic or asymptomatic infants with abnormal CSF Aqueous crystalline penicillin G 5 x 10⁴U/kg IM or IV q.d. in 2 divided doses for at least 10 days *or* Aqueous procaine penicillin G 5 x 10⁴U/kg IM q.d. for at least 10 days Asymptomatic infants with normal CSF: no therapy if they can be followed; if no follow-up then many consultants would give benzathine penicillin G 5 x 10⁴U/kg IM	Crystalline penicillin G 5 x 10⁴U/kg/day divided q8–q12h for at least 10 days	Treat infants for congenital syphilis (a) if clinical or x-ray signs of syphilis (b) if serologic titers rise or persist at a high level (c) if mother's treatment was unknown, inadequate, or not penicillin Aqueous procaine penicillin G 5 × 10⁴U/kg IM q.d. for 10 days If follow-up unlikely, benzathine penicillin G IM, one dose Only penicillin for neonates; no tetracycline under 8 yr
Follow-Up Early and congenital	Repeat quantitative nontreponemal tests at least at 3, 6, and 12 mo after treatment	Repeat serologic testing at 1, 3, 6, 12, and 24 mo	Twice in 12 mo after therapy (every 3 mo if not treated with penicillin)
Late	Repeat serologic testing also at 24 mo after treatment	Repeat serologic testing at 1 and 12 mo	At 1, 3, 6, 12, 18, 24 mo, then annually as necessary
Neurosyphilis	Periodic serologic testing, clinical evluation at 6-mo intervals and repeat CSF examinations for at least 3 yr	Repeat serologic testing at 6, 12, and 24 mo and CSF examinations at 6 mo	CSF examinations until 2 yr at least 1 yr apart have normal protein and WBC count; serology may or may not return to normal

* Adapted from Centers for Disease Control 1985 STD Treatment Guidelines, MMWR 34:4S, October 18, 1985.
† Adapted from 1988 Canadian Guidelines for the Treatment of Sexually Transmitted Diseases in Neonates, Children, Adolescents and Adults, Canada Diseases Weekly Report 14S2, April 1988; 7–8 (kindly provided by Dr. G. Jessamine).
‡ Willcox RR. Treatment of syphilis. Bull WHO 1981; 59:655–663.
§ Defined as of greater than 1 year's duration by CDC and Canada; greater than 2 years' duration by WHO.

depending on the stage of syphilis. They also specifically recommend against the use of benzathine penicillin G in neurosyphilis.

I would follow the newer recommendations of the Canadian guidelines, although I would use benzathine penicillin intramuscularly only for epidemiologic treatment and use the procaine penicillin regimen for early and late syphilis (but not for neurosyphilis).

ALTERNATE THERAPY

The mainstay of therapy for syphilis is penicillin. No other drug has been studied so well and has such efficacy with so few adverse effects. Many people recommend a course of penicillin desensitization and then treat with penicillin in those patients who are allergic to penicillin. Alternatives to penicillin are oral tetracycline and oral erythromycin. These do not have studies substantiating their doses, course length, or efficacy. Also, tetracycline is not recommended in pregnant patients so one is left with oral erythromycin. Even erythromycin estolate is not recommended in spite of higher achievable blood levels, because there may be liver toxicity associated with its use in pregnancy.

Alternatives to penicillin should be used only when there is documented life-threatening allergy to penicillin and not as a matter of preference for oral or outpatient therapy.

Meticulous follow-up is even more important, if that were possible, when drugs other than penicillin are used to treat syphilis.

Some of the newer penicillins and cephalosporins should be effective in treating syphilis; however, there are few studies looking at their efficacy in syphilis.

Cephalothin, 1 g intramuscularly every 12 hours for 20 days, has been effective in primary syphilis, and the same dose for 25 days for secondary syphilis. Cephaloridine intramuscularly seemed to be effective when it was studied 20 years ago; it is no longer available. Cephalexin orally is also effective but does not add anything if the patient can take penicillin. A more recent cephalosporin, ceftriaxone, seems to be effective. Recent studies indicate that 250 mg intramuscularly every day for 10 days or 500 mg intramuscularly every other day for five doses (over 10 days) are effective in early syphilis. In another study, 2 g intramuscularly daily for 2 days or for 5 days were effective and even one dose of 3 g intramuscularly was effective in four of five patients. Future studies may clarify the use of this new agent in the therapy of early syphilis. Ceftriaxone can be used in patients allergic to penicillin who are not allergic to cephalosporins.

Ceftriaxone has even been used successfully in one patient with neurosyphilis who was allergic to penicillin. He was given 1 g intramuscularly daily for 14 days. Since this was done in a carefully controlled situation by a group of experienced venereologists, it cannot yet be recommended for routine use for neurosyphilis, but future studies may point the way to more alternatives in the treatment of syphilis. Another alternative that could be used when cost is not a major consideration is doxycycline.

In those situations in which tetracycline is recommended, there is now a possibility of using doxycycline 200 mg orally twice a day for 21 days. This has the advantage of a shorter course and fewer doses per day, which should yield better compliance and thus higher cure rates. This, however, has been studied in only a small group of patients, and the reported follow-up was not long enough to warrant its routine use.

JARISCH-HERXHEIMER REACTION

The Jarisch-Herxheimer reaction is a systemic response that may occur after the onset of treatment. It often occurs during the first 24 hours following start of therapy. The patient, as well as the physician, needs to be aware of this so that it is not confused with any sort of allergy to the treatment. There may be increases in temperature, pulse, blood pressure, and respiratory rate. This reaction usually begins 2 to 4 hours after the first dose, peaks about 8 hours after the first dose, and resolves by 24 hours after the first dose. No therapy is indicated for this reaction.

FOLLOW-UP

In all stages of syphilis, the mainstay of care for the patient is intensive, adequate follow-up. It is important to ensure that there are clinical improvement and decreasing quantitative serologic titers (or at least stable titers). Patients with early syphilis need to be followed for at least 1 year and patients with late syphilis, a minimum of 2 years. This may seem a great deal for a disease so readily treated, but it is necessary if relapses are to be eliminated and disease progression stopped.

During this follow-up period a quantitative serologic test should show about a fourfold decrease by 3 months after therapy and an eightfold decrease by 6 months. Those patients not falling within these guidelines are probably not responding to therapy, need to be followed carefully for possible relapse, and may need retreatment.

SUGGESTED READING

Nottebart HC Jr. Spirochetes from blood specimens. Spirochetes in CNS specimens. In: Dalton HP, Nottebart HC Jr, eds. Interpretive medical microbiology. New York: Churchill-Livingstone, 1986:132, 227.

Rein MF. General principles of syphilotherapy. In: Holmes KK, Mardh P-A, Sparling PF, Wiesner PJ, eds. Sexually transmitted diseases. New York: McGraw-Hill, 1984:374.

Stokes JH, Beerman H, Ingraham NR Jr. Modern clinical syphilology. 3rd ed. Philadelphia: WB Saunders, 1945.

CHANCROID, LYMPHOGRANULOMA VENEREUM, GRANULOMA INGUINALE, AND CONDYLOMA ACUMINATA

PETER JESSAMINE, M.D.
ALLAN R. RONALD, M.D.

Chancroid, lymphogranuloma venereum, and granuloma inguinale are infrequent diseases in North America and Europe. They are very common in some developing countries. Condyloma acuminata is prevalent in North America and Europe. Chancroid and possibly condyloma acuminata are important cofactors in the dissemination of human immunodeficiency virus.

CHANCROID

Chancroid is the most important cause of genital ulcer disease in developing countries. In North America and Europe, it occurs in sporadic outbreaks that have become frequent and widespread. The usual incubation period is 2 to 5 days but can be as long as 2 weeks. The initial lesion is a papule that erodes into a painful nonindurated ulcer. Lesions are most frequent on the genitalia. The ulcer has a base of friable granulation tissue that may be covered with a necrotic exudate. Inguinal adenopathy is frequently present, which may suppurate and rupture. Fistulas may drain for prolonged periods and leave sinus tracts.

The causative agent is *Haemophilus ducreyi*. The organism is fastidious, with a requirement for hemin and growing best under humid conditions, at 5 to 10 percent carbon dioxide and 33° C to 35° C. Two media should be used in order to ensure maximal yield. Our laboratory uses gonococcal agar base with bovine hemoglobin and Meuller-Hinton agar base with chocolatized horse blood. These are supplemented with coenzymes, vitamins, amino acids (CVA) enrichment and fetal calf serum, and made selective with vancomycin. Direct gram stain from the ulcer or bubo lacks sufficient sensitivity or specificity to be recommended.

Clinical differentiation of genital ulcers is unreliable, and possible occurrence of mixed infections makes laboratory evaluation essential. The culture of *H. ducreyi* is best done in combination with darkfield microscopy for syphilis. The darkfield should be done first and followed with the swab of the ulcer base of *H. ducreyi*. The media should be inoculated at the bedside as no transport medium exists.

Antimicrobial therapy at the time of presentation may be difficult because there is no rapid diagnostic test for chancroid and syphilis may be difficult to exclude. Specific therapy for chancroid may prevent the diagnosis of syphilis. Figure 1 illustrates treatment strategies. Fluctuant buboes should be aspirated with a large-bore needle, the needle passing through normal skin and then entering the bubo.

At present, the optimal regimen is ceftriaxone, 250 mg intramuscularly as a single dose. It provides the advantage of guaranteed compliance, with greater than 95 percent success. The disadvantages are important: it is ineffective for primary syphilis and may impair the Venereal Diseases Research Laboratory (VDRL) or rapid plasma reagin (RPR) tests.

Sulfamethoxazole-trimethoprim (SMZ-TMP) (800 mg SMZ and 160 mg TMP orally twice a day for 7 days) is more traditional therapy, but its effectiveness is decreasing because of the emergence of resistant strains. It has the advantage of not interfering with the diagnosis of primary syphi-

lis. Single-dose therapy with SMZ-TMP is much less effective than the 7-day regimen and is not recommended.

When an etiologic agent cannot be determined from clinical or epidemiologic data, SMZ-TMP is a reasonable choice. It permits the physician to provide relatively effective therapy for *H. ducreyi* infection and yet not impair the diagnosis of syphilis. If treatment failure occurs, laboratory data will provide the diagnosis, and definitive therapy may be given.

Ciprofloxacin, 500 mg orally twice a day for 3 days, has proved to be effective in treating chancroid with a greater than 95 percent cure rate. This may become the preferred therapy. Effectiveness for syphilis is undetermined.

The patient's sexual partners should be examined, cultured, and treated irrespective of symptoms. An asymptomatic endocervical state has been described.

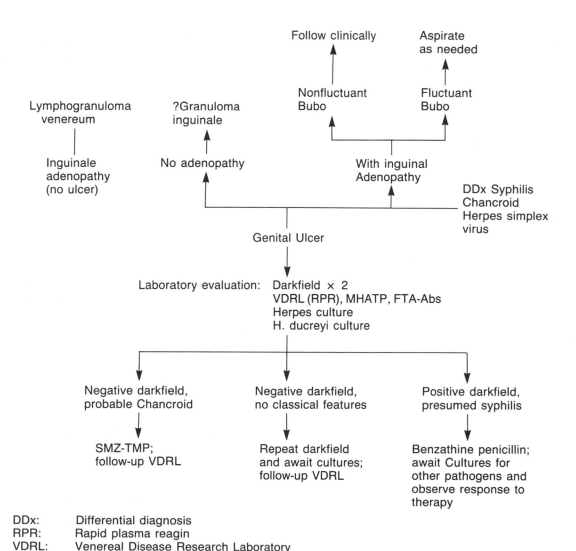

DDx: Differential diagnosis
RPR: Rapid plasma reagin
VDRL: Venereal Disease Research Laboratory
MHATP: Microhemagglutination treponemal antigen
FTA-Abs: Fluorescent treponemal antigen—absorbed

Figure 1 Genital ulcer adenopathy syndromes: management flow chart.

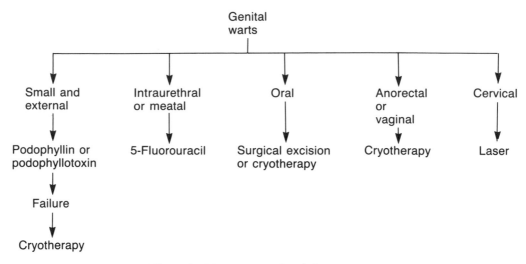

Figure 2 Management of genital warts.

LYMPHOGRANULOMA VENEREUM

This is a multisystem triphasic disease caused by *Chlamydia trachomatis*, serotypes L1, L2, and L3. It is endemic in tropical areas and occurs sporadically in North America and Europe. Cases occur in individuals who have had sexual contacts in endemic areas. The primary lesion is a painless papule that resolves without scarring and is often unnoticed. The site of the primary lesion determines the symptoms of subsequent phases.

Men most often develop an inguinal adenitis that may be unilateral or bilateral. Involvement of the corresponding femoral nodes results in the almost pathognomonic "groove sign." The adenitis is suppurative with a propensity to rupture and fistulae formation. In contrast to chancroid and syphilis, the adenitis is not temporally associated with a genital ulcer.

Women and homosexual men who have engaged in anal intercourse can develop a hemorrhagic proctitis. Fistulae may extend through the rectovaginal septum and into the ischiorectal area. Ultimately, fibrosis of the involved areas results in stricture and lymphatic obstruction.

Laboratory diagnosis of lymphogranuloma venereum is difficult. Isolation of the causative organism lacks sensitivity and is not routinely available. The complement fixation test is readily available but lacks specificity as the antigen is genus specific. A high titer (1:64 or greater) usually occurs with active disease. The microimmunofluorescent antibody test is more sensitive and specific, but it is technically demanding.

The unpredictable course of lymphogranuloma venereum makes assessment of uncontrolled clinical trials difficult. Traditional therapy has been with bubo aspiration and tetracycline (500 mg orally four times daily for 14 to 21 days). The former prevents rupture and fistula formation, while the latter treats constitutional symptoms. Buboes may not resolve with antimicrobial agents alone. Alternative antimicrobial regimens include erythromycin (500 mg orally four times daily) or doxycycline (100 mg orally twice daily) for the same duration.

Complications, such as sinus tract or stricture, may require surgery. Sexual partners should be examined and receive prophylactic therapy.

GRANULOMA INGUINALE

This disease is endemic in some tropical countries. It is rarely seen in North America or Europe. It begins as a painless subcutaneous nodule that erodes into a granulomatous ulcer. This is slowly progressive, extending to the fascia and into the groin and perineum. Subcutaneous tissue is primarily limited, and lymph nodes are seldom enlarged. Hematogenous spread to distal sites can occur through poorly understood processes.

The diagnosis is confirmed by examination of crush preparations of granulation tissue for Donovan bodies. The etiologic agent, *Calymmatobacterium granulomatis*, cannot be cultured. Biopsy specimens lack sensitivity. The presence of bipolar-staining bacilli in the cytosol of mononuclear cells establishes the diagnosis.

The traditional therapy has been tetracycline, 500 mg orally four times daily for 3 weeks. Lesions may heal within the treatment period, but this regimen should be completed to prevent recurrences. Alternative regimens include SMZ-TMP (800 mg SMZ and 160 TMP orally twice daily) or chloramphenicol (500 mg orally three times daily) for the same duration.

The disease has limited infectivity. Sexual partners should be examined and treated if lesions are present. In the absence of lesions prophylaxis is not indicated.

CONDYLOMA ACUMINATA

Genital and anal warts are collectively referred to as condyloma acuminata. They are among the commonest sexually transmitted diseases and are caused by specific human papillomaviruses (HPV). These viruses cannot be cultured, and typing is done by DNA hybridization. Twelve of the 45 serotypes are associated with anogenital tract lesions. The viral genome may be incorporated into the infected cell's genome or exist independently within the cell. The most frequent types causing genital infections are 6, 11, 16, 18, 31, 33, and 35.

The HPV lesions are polymorphic, usually multiple, and may coalesce into a larger mass. A subclinical infection was initially described for cervical warts but is now recognized to occur on the vulva, penis, and anus. The association of cervical neoplasia and HPV has been extensively studied. The HPV types most frequently associated with cervical dysplasia and neoplasia are 16 and 18. In several studies, 25 to 30 percent of asymptomatic pregnant women have been found to be infected with HPV, most being subclinical infections. There is increasing association of other genital and anorectal neoplasia with HPV. In addition, laryngeal papillomas occur in the infants of mothers with genital warts.

The diagnosis is usually established clinically but can be confirmed by biopsy. Subclinical infection can be detected by cytology or colposcopy. Cytology has excellent specificity but lacks sensitivity. Colposcopy has significant overlap with dysplasia, therefore necessitating biopsy. DNA hybridization can detect HPV genomes in tissue and cytologic preparations, therefore providing optimal sensitivity. The natural history of HPV infections and role in transformation are not established. The answers to these questions should provide guidelines for diagnosis and patient care.

Spontaneous regression of warts is to be expected, usually within 2 to 6 months. Recurrence is common. As a result, clinical studies must be placebo controlled with an adequate follow-up period. Few studies satisfy these criteria. Therapy should not be overly aggressive or costly.

Traditional therapy has been with podophyllin (10 to 25 percent) in a tincture of benzoin. This preparation is impure and has the potential for serious adverse effects. It should not be used on mucosal surfaces or in large quantities. It should be applied by the physician in small quantities to the lesion and washed off after 3 or 4 hours. Pregnancy contraindicates its use. It is applied at weekly intervals for 3 to 4 weeks and results in approximately a 30 percent cure rate at 3 months.

Podophyllotoxin is the active component of podophyllin. It is more efficacious and less toxic to normal tissue. It can be self-administered and will replace podophyllin when it becomes available.

Intraurethral warts should be treated with 5 percent 5-fluorouracil cream (2 ml) instilled twice per day into the urethra for 7 days. Surgery should be avoided, as stricture may result.

Vaginal, cervical, and anorectal warts should be treated with surgery or cryotherapy rather than podophyllin. Laser therapy has proved effective in cervical lesions and may develop wider applications. Consultation with a specialist should precede treatment of these lesions. Several controlled studies have evaluated the use of interferon either topically or systemically. It is definitely superior to placebo but requires further investigation to determine overall efficacy.

Although not clearly established, it would appear to be prudent to treat visible genital warts in pregnant women prior to delivery. Therapy should be with nontoxic ablative methods (e.g., cryotherapy). This strategy may prevent the development of laryngeal papillomas.

SUGGESTED READING

Eron LJ, Judson F, Tucker S, et al. Interferon therapy for condyloma acuminata. N Engl J Med 1986; 315:1059–1064.

Kirby P, Corey L. Genital papillomavirus infections. Infect Dis Clin North Am 1987; 1:123–143.

Krockta W, Barnes R. Genital ulceration with regional adenopathy. Infect Dis Clin North Am 1987; 1:217–233.

Meanwell CA, Blackledge G, Cox MF, et al. HPV 16 DNA in normal and malignant cervical epithelium: implications for the etiology and behavior of cervical neoplasia. Lancet 1:703–707.

Schmid GP, Sanders LL, Blount JH, Alexander R. Chancroid in the United States. reestablishment of an old disease. JAMA 1987; 258:3265–3268.

Taylor DN, Pitarang SI, Echeverria P, et al. Comparative study of ceftriaxone and trimethoprim-sulfamethoxazole for treatment of chancroid in Thailand. J Infect Dis 1985; 152:1002–1006.

SKIN AND SOFT TISSUE INFECTIONS

ACNE VULGARIS

PETER E. POCHI, M.D.

Acne vulgaris is among the commonest diseases of the skin for which patients seek treatment from dermatologists, pediatricians, and family physicians. Additionally, many other individuals with acne, particularly teenagers with mild forms of the disease, medicate themselves with over-the-counter acne products.

CAUSES OF ACNE

Acne is a multifactorial disease. One of the factors is bacteria; in fact, the main thrust of therapy for acne is antibacterial. In the last century, it was first appreciated that bacteria were important in this disease when histologic examination of acne lesions disclosed the presence of gram-positive diphtheroids within the follicles, the site of the acne lesions. It was thought that acne was an infection with these bacteria (*Propionibacterium acnes*), but when it was later discovered that the organisms could be cultured from the skin of individuals without acne, their causative role in acne fell into disrepute. Even decades later, it was believed that the only role of bacteria in acne was to infect acne lesions secondarily with pyogenic organisms such as staphylococci and streptococci. The occasional recovery of such pathogens in severe cases of acne supported this position and led to the use of sulfonamides and penicillin, with equivocal results.

The present view is that bacteria are indeed important for the induction of the inflammatory papules, pustules, and nodules ("cysts") in acne but are not the basic cause of the disease. The primary pathologic defect in acne is an abnormal differentiation of the follicular epithelium of specialized pilosebaceous follicles of the face and trunk. This altered epithelium permits the escape of low-molecular-weight peptides, elaborated by *P. acnes* organisms that reside in large numbers in these follicles. Polymorphonuclear leukocytes are attracted to the intrafollicular site where they ingest the *P. acnes* bacteria, with the resultant release of hydrolytic enzymes that rupture the follicular wall with the production of inflammation, both immunologically and nonimmunologically mediat-

ed. The inflammatory lesion heals in a period of 1 to 3 weeks, and the affected follicle apparently does not become inflamed again. The healing process is at times attended by the development of atrophic scars and, occasionally, hypertrophic scars, particularly on the trunk.

The sebaceous glands, which synthesize and secrete into the follicle a complex lipid substance called sebum, are also important in the acne process. Sebum is the substrate for *P. acnes*. The bacteria elaborate lipases that hydrolyze the triglyceride moiety of sebum to release irritant free fatty acids. It is believed, but has not been proved, that the initiating event in the acne lesion, i.e., the abnormal follicular differentiation, is the result of the action of sebum. From a therapeutic standpoint, any treatment that can substantially reduce the amount of sebum produced will also reduce acne.

THERAPEUTIC CONSIDERATIONS

Because acne is a disorder with a primary defect and several contributory endogenous pathogenic factors, best results are generally achieved by pluralistic therapy rather than monotherapy. Nonetheless, many cases, especially those of minimal severity, can be treated with a single agent. Approaches to treatment can be divided into four categories: antikeratinizing, antibacterial, sebostatic, and anti-inflammatory.

General Principles of Treatment

With the possible exception of oral isotretinoin, all treatments for acne do not alter the natural course of the disease, which may last from a few months to many years (the reason for the natural involution is unknown). Thus, any treatment that proves to be helpful needs to be maintained for an indefinite period of time. Most treatments do not accelerate healing of acne. The principal effect is the prevention of new lesions. For this reason it is important that topical medicaments be applied to the entire area of acne involvement and not just to individual lesions. The preventive effect of acne therapy is comparatively slow, taking at least 2 weeks for noticeable improvement and more often 3 to 6 weeks. During this time, the patient observes that few and smaller inflammatory lesions are erupting. Acne on the back and chest tends to respond less well than does facial disease, even with oral isotretinoin. This is particularly true for topical medications, which usually do not achieve any significant degree of control.

Specific Therapeutic Modalities

These embrace both topical and oral medication. Whenever possible, it is best to employ external therapy only. At times oral treatment may be required, particularly when there is resistance or incomplete response to topical treatment (this is more apt to be the situation in a patient with moderately severe or severe acne); where topical therapy cannot be tolerated by the patient because of sensitive skin, a circumstance not too uncommon, particularly in atopics; and when the disease affects the trunk. In actual practice, both oral and topical therapies are used in the patient who suffers from more than minimal-to-moderate disease.

Antikeratinizing Treatment

The goal is to reverse the abnormal differentiating follicular epithelium, the primary defect in the disease. The agent most effective in this regard is topical all-*trans* retinoic acid (tretinoin). Patients with comedonal acne, i.e., noninflammatory whiteheads and blackheads, benefit particularly, but the agent's comedolytic action eventually helps prevent the formation of inflammatory lesions.

Tretinoin is available as a gel (0.01 and 0.025 percent), as creams (0.025, 0.05, and 0.1 percent) and as a liquid (0.05 percent). While the gels contain, on the whole, lower concentrations of tretinoin, their efficacy is greater because of enhanced penetration into the follicle. On the other hand, gels are more irritating and are not well tolerated in cold climates or by persons with sensitive skin (the liquid is the most irritating of all and is generally best avoided). The creams are better tolerated but can still exert a primary irritant reaction, i.e., erythema, desquamation, pruritus, and so forth. The mildest but least effective form of topical tretinoin is the 0.025 percent cream; nonetheless, a relatively small sacrifice in efficacy is more than balanced by decreased irritation. For example, with 0.05 percent tretinoin cream, 25 percent of acne patients will experience some degree of irritation; with the 0.025 percent cream, this figure is reduced to 9 percent. This lower degree of irritation also permits the more ready use of a concomitant topical preparation. To reduce the potential irritant effect of tretinoin, it is preferable to have the patient apply it only every other night for 2 or 3 weeks, and then nightly; this procedure will allow the skin to accommodate to the irritancy (a few patients can tolerate twice-daily usage, but this is unusual). The irritant effect of tretinoin also makes the skin more vulnerable to the irritating effects of exposure to detergents, sunlight, and, as already mentioned, cold weather. A second disadvantage of tretinoin is the occasional worsening of the acne in the first month of therapy. This almost always subsides, but it is important that the patient be forewarned of this possible reaction and be informed that the reaction bears no relation to whether the acne will or will not ultimately respond satisfactorily.

A second comedolytic topical agent, less potent than isotretinoin, is salicylic acid, which has been used for many years for the purpose of unplugging obstructed pores at the skin surface. In actuality, the obstruction of the follicle is deep rather than superficial, so that a compound's having a keratolytic action, as do tretinoin and salicylic acid, does not ensure that it will be effective; follicular penetration is also necessary. Salicylic acid is commercially available in over-the-counter products, as saturated pads or as a lotion, and can be applied once or twice daily, as tolerated.

Antibacterial Treatment

This is the cornerstone of acne therapy. A substantial reduction of the *P. acnes* population, i.e., more than a two-log reduction, will ensure a beneficial response. The most frequently employed topical agent in this regard is benzoyl peroxide, in use for the treatment of acne for more than 20 years. Its presumed mechanism of action is the release of nascent oxygen, which inhibits the replication and proliferation of the facultatively anaerobic *P. acnes*. Formulations of benzoyl peroxide are available in a variety of concentrations (2.5 to 10 percent) and vehicles (gels, creams, lotions, cleansers, masks, and soaps). Most of the prescription benzoyl peroxide products are in the form of gels, but there are no experimental data indicating that these are more effective than nonprescription preparations, although one may assume that this is so because of the gel base. Also, there are no large-scale studies showing a dose response in the concentrations available, although one published study of a small number of subjects suggests that the lower concentrations (2.5 percent and 5 percent) are as effective as the highest concentration (10 percent). What is evident, however, is that cleansers and soaps containing benzoyl peroxide, while having been shown to be able to decrease *P. acnes* numbers in vivo, are less effective than products that are left on the skin rather than washed off. Benzoyl peroxide gels, lotions, or creams should be applied one or twice daily.

Advantages of benzoyl peroxide include a comparatively high degree of efficacy and no bacterial resistance. Disadvantages include irritation (although it is much less severe than with tretinoin), occasional contact sensitization, and bleaching of hair and colored fabrics. Another caution is that benzoyl peroxide should not be physically applied together with tretinoin, as the activity of the latter will be reduced by the oxidizing action of the peroxide. However, they can be used separately, i.e., one in the morning and one in the evening, with generally good to excellent results, as the comedolytic effect of tretinoin and the antibacterial effect of benzoyl peroxide result in a greater improvement of acne than occurs with either alone.

Topically applied antibiotics may be used instead of, or in addition to, benzoyl peroxide or tretinoin. All are prescription products and include clindamycin, erythromycin, meclocycline sulfosalicylate (a tetracycline derivative), and tetracycline itself. Their efficacy is variable, and they are probably not as beneficial overall as is benzoyl peroxide. They are available as liquids (clindamycin, erythromycin, tetracycline), gels (clindamycin, erythromycin), pads (erythromycin), a cream (meclocycline), and an ointment (erythromycin) and are usually applied once or twice daily. The advantage of topical antibiotics over benzoyl peroxide is that they are less irritating and essentially nonsensitizing. Those in liquid and pad forms are preferred by women for daytime use, as cosmetics are applied over them more readily then over gels or creams. Disadvantages include irritation in some patients (less severe with meclocycline cream and erythromycin ointment) and the development of bacterial resistance of *P. acnes* to the given antibiotic. This latter phenomenon, while not frequently a clinical problem, appears to be most common with erythromycin. As noted above, the effect of tretinoin can be vitiated by the concomitant presence of benzoyl peroxide. One antibacterial product contains both benzoyl peroxide (5 percent) and erythromycin (3 percent) in a gel base. Studies have indicated that the combination is more efficacious than either of the individual components and, moreover, that the primary irritant effect of the benzoyl peroxide is decreased with the combination. The product is unstable at room temperature, and it needs to be kept refrigerated.

The oral antibiotics used for the treatment of acne include tetracycline, erythromycin, and minocycline. All of these have been shown to inhibit *P. acnes* and in controlled clinical studies to be effective in treating patients with acne. The same has been demonstrated for trimethoprim-sulfamethoxazole and for clindamycin, but the risks of allergic sensitization from the former and pseudomembranous colitis from the latter limit their usefulness in acne, especially because of the necessity of the prolonged use of medications in acne. The antibiotic in longest use is tetracycline, administered initially in a dosage of 500 to 1,000 mg daily (250 mg or 500 mg twice a day) depending on the severity of the acne. Rarely, higher doses, up to 1.5 to 2.0 g, may be tried in severe cases, but alternative therapy to these doses is preferred. Once acne activity has diminished the dosage is decreased by 250 mg per day monthly to determine the optimal level of drug required for maintenance. Often, this can be as little as 250 mg per day or even 250 mg every other day. Adverse effects occurring in tetracycline-treated acne patients include gastrointestinal disturbances, yeast vaginitis (in 15 percent of cases), and phototoxicity, especially with higher doses. In most cases in which tetracycline or other oral antibiotics are employed, topical therapy is used as well, except in the unusual circumstance in which it cannot be tolerated. Concerns have been raised about the prolonged use of systemic tetracycline in treating acne patients. Among these concerns is the issue of bacterial resistance of the *P. acnes* but also of the emergence of resistance in other bacteria. Indeed, one such example is that of gram-negative rod folliculitis, an acne-like eruption occurring on the lower facial area that results from the infection of follicles with gram-negative organisms, including *Proteus mirabilis* and *Pseudomonas aeruginosa*. As a result of antibiotic treatment, gram-negative organisms establish residence in the nasal mucosa but produce no signs or symptoms of infection there. However, on gaining access to the skin surface, the organisms cause a folliculitis of the infranasal and perioral

areas, characterized by the appearance of occasionally pruritic (acne never itches), superficial pustules. The clinical appearance of this infection is characteristic to the experienced observer, but the diagnosis can be confirmed by bacterial cultures. The condition is eradicated or controlled by appropriate antibiotic therapy, usually with trimethoprim-sulfamethoxazole or ampicillin. No instance is known wherein the follicular gram-negative infection has become systemic.

If tetracycline is contraindicated, causes untoward effects, or proves ineffective, erythromycin treatment can be undertaken, in doses equivalent to those of tetracycline, and with essentially equal efficacy. Erythromycin can be taken with meals. Candidal infection is less a problem than it is with tetracycline, and phototoxity is absent. Some dermatologists are reluctant to prescribe the drug to patients who are allergic to penicillin in order to avoid the development of a resistance by penicillin-sensitive bacteria to erythromycin.

The third antibiotic used in acne is minocycline, a tetracycline, more effective than equivalent doses of tetracycline, presumably because of its increased gastrointestinal absorption, even if taken with food, and its highly lipophilic property allowing for greater concentrations in the pilosebaceous follicle. In terms of dosage, 50 mg of minocycline is approximately equivalent to 250 mg of tetracycline, so that the average starting dose is 100 to 200 mg daily (50 or 100 mg twice a day). This drug is used in the patient who requires oral antibiotic therapy but has not responded to oral tetracycline or erythromycin (if used). The advantage of minocycline is that it is the most effective of the acne-antibiotic drugs in general use, but this is offset by the occurrence of ototoxicity,—usually when doses exceed 100 mg daily, reversible pigmentary changes in the skin, and its cost.

Worthy of mention in discussion of the use of oral antibiotics for acne are two additional concerns. The first is the possible interaction of tetracyclines and oral contraceptive drugs that could result in lowered estrogen blood levels. This effect can be demonstrated in animals but has not been shown to occur in humans, and reports of the occurrence of pregnancy in women taking oral contraceptive drugs and tetracycline are rare. The putative interaction has probably been overexaggerated. A second issue, of only speculative concern, is the chronic suppression of *P. acnes* by oral antibiotics or by topical antibacterial substances. *P. acnes* is an immunoadjuvant in animal experiments. *P. acnes* occurs in large numbers in the acne-prone susceptible pilosebaceous follicles of the face and trunk. It has been suggested that these organisms serve an immunosurveillant function and that their chronic suppression might conceivably have adverse consequences. However, there is no clinical or epidemiologic evidence that such is the case.

Sebostatic Treatment

The sebaceous glands are androgen-dependent for their development and synthetic activity. Thus, approaches to inhibit androgenic stimulation of the glands would be of help. However, oral isotretinoin, the 13-*cis* isomer of tretinoin, is the most powerful sebostatic compound for acne, working not to affect androgens but to cause de-differentiation of the sebaceous gland and stop sebum production. Because the inhibition of sebum is so profound, the *P. acnes* organisms, which, as mentioned earlier, are dependent upon sebum for their growth and proliferation, are also reduced to even lower levels than result from administration of antibiotic. In addition, oral isotretinoin, like tretinoin, has an antikeratinizing action and an anti-inflammatory effect. Therefore, this oral retinoid is highly effective in acne, even in severe disease. Severe disease is the indication for the limited use of the drug in acne, because of the many adverse effects of this agent. Most of these are mucocutaneous and include cheilitis, xerosis, dermatitis, conjunctivitis, epistaxis, and hair loss. Systemically, musculoskeletal and arthritic symptoms, decreased night vision, and rarely, pseudotumor cerebri may occur. Minor elevations of liver enzyme concentrations and of lipids, particularly triglycerides, can be observed. Lipid abnormalities are rarely pronounced, but the triglyceride elevations can be of concern and, to avoid acute pancreatitis, should not exceed 500 mg per deciliter during isotretinoin treatment. All of the clinical and laboratory abnormalities revert to normal when the drug is stopped.

The most serious problem from the use of oral isotretinoin is its teratogenicity. If the drug is prescribed to women of reproductive capacity, pregnancy must be excluded by appropriate testing and prevented by strict contraception or abstinence. As oral isotretinoin has a relatively short half-life (terminal elimination half-life, 10 to 20 hours), pregnancy can occur safely 1 month after the drug is stopped. Isotretinoin is not mutagenic, so that future pregnancies are not affected.

The dosage of oral isotretinoin is 0.5 to 1.0 mg per kilogram per day for 16 to 20 weeks, depending on severity of the lesions. Laboratory tests should include liver enzyme and lipid tests and, in fertile women, a baseline pregnancy test. The tests should be repeated at 2-week intervals in the first month; if no significant changes are seen by the fourth week, no further testing is ordinarily required.

As already noted, isotretinoin is highly effective, even for very severe, treatment-recalcitrant cases of acne. Another aspect of treatment with this drug is that prolonged, sometimes permanent, remissions are induced. This is in contrast to all other acne treatments in which control is maintained only for as long as treatment is continued.

Inhibition of androgen to reduce sebaceous gland activity can be achieved only by systemic hormone administration, because none of the drugs in this category, even the antiandrogen spironolactone, can effect sebum inhibition by their topical application. Hormonal treatment, requiring systemic administration, has a further limitation in that its use is limited because of the feminizing effects that occur in males. In the adult woman who has had chronic acne and in whom standard acne therapy has proved unsatisfactory, estrogen, in the form of oral contraceptive drugs, can be given to suppress ovarian androgen production. Success from oral estrogen in controlling the acne, based on sebum studies, lies in the use of 50 μg of ethinyl estradiol or mestranol as the minimal level of benefit. Higher-estrogen-content pills increase the likelihood of improvement but bear nearly untenable risks. The lower doses of estrogen (i.e., 30 to 35 μg), now more commonly in use for oral contraception, are often ineffective in controlling acne.

In recent years, increased interest has centered on the treatment of acne in women (and men) with low-dose glucocorticoid (i.e., 5.0 to 7.5 mg of prednisone or 0.25 to 0.5 mg of dexamethasone) administered nightly to decrease adrenocortical androgen production. Much of the rationale for this treatment lies in the observation of increased levels of adrenal androgens, primarily dehydroepiandrosterone sulfate (DHEA-S) in 20 to 30 percent or more of women with acne, even without other signs of androgen excess. However, no controlled studies have been published to indicate to what extent these drugs are effective in treating patients with acne or whether there is a difference in response, depending upon baseline DHEA-S determinations. The same is true for estrogen; elevated testosterone levels but normal DHEA-S, which would suggest increased ovarian androgen activity, do not necessarily mean that the clinical response of the acne would be more predictable than if baseline testosterone levels were not increased.

The combination of estrogen and glucocorticoid has clearly been shown to reduce sebaceous gland activity and improve acne in women, even when severe disease is present. A 50-μg estrogen-containing oral contraceptive pill together with 5 mg of prednisone nightly has been shown to decrease sebum production, on average by 50 percent, a degree of suppression that results in significant clinical improvement. Adverse effects of such therapy are no more than those resulting from either alone, but as with most forms of therapy, the acne, if controlled, will remain so only if treatment is continued. In general, it is customary to treat patients for 6 months, and then to stop treatment to see if any degree of natural involution has taken place.

Another hormonal treatment, limited to women, is the use of spironolactone, which acts as a peripheral antiandrogen but has some central inhibiting effects as well. Dosages that cause a significant reduction in sebum secretion are from 100 to 200 mg per day, amounts higher than generally used to treat hirsutism and still higher than the dosages used for diuresis. Nonetheless, acne may respond well to spironolactone, although lower doses, i.e., 100 mg per day, are desirable, albeit less effective. The chief—and frequent—adverse effect is that of menstrual irregularity. For that reason, it is ideal if an oral contraceptive drug can be used together with spironolactone. If this is done, the incidence of menstrual irregularities, which at high doses can exceed 50 percent, is reducible to only 5 percent. Moreover, if a 50-μg estrogen-containing pill is chosen, it could increase the clinical benefit; however, this aspect of estrogen-spironolactone administration has received no study in acne patients. Nonetheless, it would seem both justified and desirable.

Anti-inflammatory

As noted earlier, most treatments for acne exert their effects by preventing the formation of new lesions.

However, inflammation itself, once present, can be ameliorated to shorten the duration of an existing lesion. The safest treatment, although not the most logistically feasible one, is the intralesional injection of corticosteroid (triamcinolone acetonide suspension 2.5 mg per milliliter) into individual lesions. This results in rapid resolution of the inflammation. The practicality of such treatment is that intralesional therapy is limited to the time of a patient's visit to the physician and does nothing to prevent the formation of new lesions. The use of systemic corticosteroids would have both effects, but their use in a chronic, asymptomatic disease of uncertain duration is generally contraindicated. If the person's history indicates the occasional problem of severe, periodic appearance of lesions, short courses of prednisone, in a dose of 30 mg daily for no more than 7 days, might prove necessary. The advent of isotretinoin has superseded this treatment.

Topically applied corticosteroids are ineffective in acne and are contraindicated for a variety of reasons, not the least of which is that the steroid, particularly if it is of the moderate or high-potency type, can cause follicular damage and an acne-like folliculitis ("steroid acne").

Nonsteroidal anti-inflammatory drugs have not been well studied in treatment for acne, but open, small clinical trials have shown that the majority of patients treated with 2.4 g of ibuprofen daily or 1.125 g of naproxen daily had a 60-percent decrease in inflammatory acne lesions. In one controlled study, the administration of ibuprofen, 2.4 g daily, was no more effective in patients with acne than oral tetracycline, 1.0 g daily, but combined administration was twice as effective, without an increase in adverse gastrointestinal effects.

SUGGESTED READING

Marks R, Plewig G. Acne and related disorders, Boca Raton: CRC Press, 1989.
Pochi PE. Management of refractory acne. Hosp Pract 1985; 20:73–82.
Pochi PE. Acne: androgens and microbiology. Drug Devel Res 1988; 13:157–168.
Strauss JS. Acne vulgaris. In: Fitzpatrick TB, et al, eds. Dermatology in general medicine. 3rd ed. New York: McGraw-Hill, 1987; 666–679.

ECTOPARASITIC INFECTION

HARLEY A. HAYNES, M.D.

Ectoparasites that affect humans include the following: (1) *Demodex folliculorum*; (2) sucking lice of the order Anoplura, including *Phthirus pubis* and *Pediculus humanis* (*P. humanis capitis, P. humanis corporis*); (3) mites of the suborder Sarcoptiformes, family Sarcoptidae, including *Sarcoptes scabiei* var. *hominis, Sarcoptes scabiei* var. *canis, Notoedres cati*, and *Knemidokoptes mutans* and *K. laevis*; and (4) Sarcoptiformes, family Psoroptidae. In addition, a variety of house mites, food mites, grain mites, harvest mites, and bird and rodent mites either bite or temporarily infest man or cause allergic reactions upon contact, but these are not truly parasitic in man.

DERMODICIDOSIS

Demodex folliculorum is a small mite that is an obligate parasite of the human pilosebaceous follicle but may not be the cause of any disease. Infestation involves nearly all people over the age of 5. The mite may be seen on scrapings of stratum corneum from time to time and is clearly increased in some cases of acne rosacea. However, treatment directed at the mite seems not to be required. Acne rosacea is usually treated with low doses of tetracycline (250-500 mg orally per day). Occasionally individuals, usually female, who never use soap and water on the face have large populations of *Demodex folliculorum*, which may contribute to inflammation. Cleansing with soap and water appears to be all that is required to restore the situation to normal.

PHTHIRIASIS PUBIS

Phthirus pubis is widespread and fairly common. Infestation is usually sexually transmitted but may be acquired from contact with clothing or towels or shed hairs on which adult lice or nits are attached. The clinical presentation is generally that of moderate to severe pruritus of infested areas. The pubic area is usually involved, but the body hair, such as on the axillae, eyebrows, and eyelashes, may be involved. The patient is often unaware of any infestation, but with good lighting the examiner should be able to spot the shiny white nits, which are the egg cases, attached to the hairs in the infested areas, and on closer inspection the adult lice, looking somewhat the color of freckles, will be seen on the surface of the skin, usually holding on to one or two hairs. Occasionally skin lesions representing a hypersensitivity reaction to the bite may be seen as blue-gray macules. Severe scratching and secondary infection are not common.

Treatment

The patient and sexual and household contacts should all be treated.

One percent gamma benzene hexachloride lotion (lindane, Kwell, Gammene) applied to the affected area (except eyelashes), washed off in no longer than 8 hours, and possibly as soon as 10 minutes, is usually effective in a single application. Retreatment in one week may be advised if indicated. This treatment is ovicidal, but the nits will remain attached to the hairs unless they are removed with a fine-tooth comb.

An over-the-counter treatment that is apparently as effective as gamma benzene hexachloride is a pyrethrum preparation, RID, which is available without prescription and includes a fine-tooth comb for nit removal.

Eyelash infestations are most easily treated by manual removal of nits and lice using forceps. Alternatively, an application of 0.025 percent physostigmine ophthalmic ointment will cause the lice to drop off. Smothering the lice with plain petrolatum jelly twice daily for 8 days also is effective.

Treatment of fomites is usually not necessary, but if desired, it can be accomplished by a spray of pyrethrum or gamma benzene hexachloride. Aerosol sprays should not be used for application on patients.

Consider obtaining cultures for gonorrhea and serologic testing for syphilis.

General facts about the life cycle of lice are important in the eduction and therapy of patients. The life cycle is similar for *Phthirus pubic* pediculosis and *Pediculosis humanis*; it is about 1 month, during which time the female lays 7 to 10 eggs each day. The eggs hatch in about 8 days, but may be delayed up to a month if away from body heat. The nits require an additional 8 days to reach maturity. A newly hatched louse must feed within 24 hours or die, and mature lice can survive no longer than 10 days without a blood meal. Even at the optimal temperature of 15 °C, they usually survive only 2 to 3 days away from the host. The eggs are attached to hairs near their exit point from the skin in the case of the pubic louse and the head louse. The length of time an infestation has been present may be estimated by how far out on the hairs nits can be seen. The poorly named body louse feeds on the host but lays the eggs on threads on the clothing in close contact with the skin, mostly on the inside seams. Nits may occasionally be attached to body hairs. All of these lice are about 3 to 4 mm long. The pediculi are longer than their width, the phthirus is wider than its length.

PEDICULOSIS CAPITIS

The head louse is seen worldwide and is fairly common in elementary school populations, even in affluent communities. Infestation is transmitted by very close contact and by shared hats, caps, brushes, and combs. The head louse is usually confined to the scalp but occasionally invades the beard. The number of nits greatly exceeds the number of adult lice, as patients have only 10 or fewer lice at any time. Pruritis is a major symptom, leading to scratching and frequent secondary infection. Occipital and cervical lymphadenopathy frequently develop and may be presenting signs.

Treatment

Identify and treat all affected individuals and, possibly, other close contacts as simultaneously as possible. Discontinue the sharing of hats, caps, towels, brushes, and combs.

The apparent first choice therapy for efficacy and some residual prophylaxis is permethrin 1 percent creme rinse (Nix, Burroughs Wellcome Company, Research Triangle Park, NC). This product is a synthetic pyrethroid. After shampooing with ordinary shampoo, rinsing, and drying, the permethrin creme rinse is applied to saturate hair and scalp. After remaining in place for 10 minutes, the product is rinsed off with plain water. A single treatment is usually sufficient but may be repeated in 10 days to 2 weeks without ill effect. Nits are not removed by this therapy, but most larvae are killed. Combing with a fine-tooth comb may be done for cosmetic effect, to reduce anxiety, and to help assess efficacy.

Natural pyrethrin preparations, synergized with piperonyl butoxide, are available without prescription and are only slightly less efficacious. Trade names are RID, A-200, and R and C Shampoo, among others. These generally involve contact times of 10 minutes and may be repeated as needed.

The standard therapy for the past 3 decades is 1 percent gamma benzene hexachloride shampoo. The shampoo is allowed to remain on the hair for 10 minutes before rinsing.

This may not be adequate contact time to kill the eggs; therefore, removal of as many nits as possible with a fine-tooth comb, or even clipping the hair to a shorter length in the case of an extremely long-lasting infestation, will reduce the possibility of viable eggs producing reinfection. A second shampoo treatment 10 days after the first is good insurance. Adverse side effects from gamma benzene hexachloride, particularly neurotoxicity, should not be a problem when it is used for public lice or head lice as described above, owing to the brief contact time and the small surface area treated.

If pyoderma is present, oral erythromycin or cloxacillin (in order of preference) and topical chlorhexidine (Hibiclens) washes are indicated.

PEDICULOSIS CORPORIS

Diagnosis of body lice usually requires finding nits in the seams of the inner garments, as examination of the skin surface generally shows nothing other than excoriations and possible secondary infection. Occasionally a nit or so may be found on body hair. Individuals with this infestation are generally exceedingly ill kempt. Differential diagnosis would include consideration of scabies—which should be sought by examining the skin for burrows and scraping the skin to see whether microscopic evidence of scabies can be found—and other metabolic causes of pruritus unrelated to infestation, such as liver or kidney dysfunction, lymphoma, polycythemia vera, and so on.

Treatment

Impound all infested clothing, place it in a plastic bag, spray with either gamma benzene hexachloride or pyrethrum, and close the bag tightly. Other effective pediculicides with which to treat the clothing are 1 percent malathion powder or 100 percent DDT powder. Alternatively, storing the clothes in the bag for 1 month without a chemical pediculicide will render them safe. Also, sending them to be cleaned and pressed or laundered and ironed is an effective way of killing the lice and their eggs.

If lice or nits are found on the skin or hair of the patient, treat with an overnight application of 1 percent gamma benzene hexachloride lotion, followed by bathing in soap and water.

SCABIES

The mite family *Sarcoptes* causes scabies in man and mange in other mammals. The mites are variants of a single species, *Sarcoptes scabiei*. While the host specificity is not complete, the mites survive for only a short period on another host. *Notoedres* is primarily responsible for infestation of cats and rabbits, but rarely of man. *Knemidokoptes* infests poultry but rarely man. Mites of the family *Psoroptidae* cause mange in many domestic animals and can be transmitted to man. *Sarcoptes scabiei* var. *hominis* is morphologically indistinguishable from the other races of this mite species. The female mite measures about 0.4 x 0.3 mm and when fertilized excavates a burrow in the stratum corneum. Each day she burrows an additional 2 mm or so and deposits 2 or 3 eggs to a total of 10 to 25 eggs and then dies in the burrow unless excoriation by the host removes her. The larvae emerge from the eggs after 3 to 4 days and migrate to the skin surface, where they reach maturity about 2 to 2-1/2 weeks after the eggs were laid. Copulation occurs on the skin surface; shortly thereafter the male dies and the impregnated female burrows into the stratum corneum to repeat the life cycle described above. The infestation may be spread by sexual contact or close personal contact. It is common for an entire household to become infested.

The mite tends to infest certain areas of the skin. The fingers, particularly the lateral aspects and the web spaces, and the flexor surfaces of the wrists are involved most frequently. In men the penis and scrotum and in women the region of the nipple are frequently involved. In children palms and soles are often infested. In a variation known as Norwegian scabies, there is massive infestation of the individual; erythema and scaling occur initially on the palms, soles, face, neck, scalp, and trunk and may become generalized. The diagnostic skin lesion is a burrow in the stratum corneum measuring about 0.5 mm in diameter and several millimeters in length. It has a wavy, linear shape. Upon close inspection using a hand lens, a grayish dot may be seen at the leading end of the burrow which is the location of the adult female mite. Burrows may be revealed by applying ink to the skin and then washing it off, staining the burrow track, but this is not usually necessary. The typical diagnostic burrows are produced only by *Sarcoptes scabiei* var. *hominis* and not by the animal mites. Microscopic identification of the mite, the larvae, or the fecal pellets is desirable before committing the patient and contacts to total cutaneous applications of gamma benzene hexachloride. The easiest technique is to take a #15 scalpel blade and shave off a whole burrow, place it upon a microscope slide, apply some 10 percent potassium hydroxide (but do not heat the slide), place a cover slip on top, and examine it directly under the microscope. Alternatively, scraping of the surface of the burrow may be done either dry or using a drop of mineral oil to collect the mite and ova and larvae. The whole droplet is then moved to the microscope slide and examined with a cover slip on top without the addition of KOH. A very pruritic patient will have many excoriations, and few typical lesions will be available for ready microscopic demonstration of the organism. Several tries to demonstrate the organism are desirable, but, if necessary, treatment on suspicion may be instituted.

Treatment

Treat all affected individuals and all close contacts as simultaneously as possible. Since the pruritus and most of the skin lesions seem to be hypersensitivity reactions occurring only after 3 to 4 weeks of infestation, it is not possible to rule out infestation because of lack of symptoms or easily visible signs. Great care must be used in treating premature infants, normal neonates, and pregnant women because of the concern about neurotoxicity from gama benzene hexachloride.

Apply 1 percent gamma benzene hexachloride lotion to the entire skin surface, giving special attention to web spaces and heavily infested areas. *Do not* recommend a hot bath or shower prior to the application. After 6 to 8 hours have the patient bathe thoroughly in soap and water. If this preparation is used on infants or pregnant women, the bathing is recommended after 4 hours. In general, a single such application will be effective, provided reinfestation from contacts does not occur. If necessary, preferably only if infestation can still be confirmed microscopically, retreatment in 10 to 14 days can be recommended.

Concomitant therapy for the hypersensitivity dermatitis is desirable in many cases. Anti-histamines, such as chlorpheniramine maleate, 4 to 12 mg every 4 to 6 hours as necessary and as tolerated, combined with a midpotency topical steroid such as triamcinolone cream 0.1 percent, and applications of 0.25 percent menthol lotion for itching as needed, to be continued for 2 weeks and extended as required are usually sufficient.

Patients should be warned about unnecessary overtreatment and retreatment with gamma benzene hexachloride, with emphasis on seizures as a major consequence. The physician should be prepared to encounter a certain amount of parasitophobia or other neurotic reaction to this infestation, which can result in pruritus and a belief that infestation is still active long after it has been objectively cleared.

Alternative therapies are either less efficacious or cosmetically unpleasant. The most reasonable alternative to gamma benzene hexachloride lotion is crotamiton cream or lotion (Eurax) applied once daily for 2 days. There are no reports of toxicity, but there have been no studies of its toxicity in infants and pregnant women. Six to 10 percent precipitated sulfur in a water-washable base or in petrolatum applied daily for 3 days is effective but messy. It is probably the safest treatment for infants and pregnant women. Another regimen that has been reported to be effective, but which I have never used, is 20 to 25 percent benzyl benzoate applied daily for 2 to 3 days, and

10 percent thiabendazole suspension applied twice daily for 5 days or taken orally in a dose of 25 mg per kilogram daily for 10 days. In the case of severe Norwegian scabies resistant to topical therapy, systemic methotrexate has been reported to be effective.

Treatment of fomites is not generally necessary, as fomite transmission is not as important as direct contact. Simple laundering of items is sufficient.

Consider obtaining cultures for gonorrhea and serologic tests for syphilis.

SUGGESTED READING

Meinking TO, et al. Comparative efficacy of treatment for pediculosis capitis infestations. Arch Dermatol 1986; 122:267–271.
Rasmussen JE, Lindane. A prudent approach. Arch Dermatol 1987; 123:1008–1010.
Taplin D, Meinking T. Infestations. In: Schachner, Hansen RC, eds. Pediatric dermatology. NY: Churchill-Livingstone, 1988:1465–1515.
Taplin D, et al. A comparative trial of three treatment schedules for the eradication of scabies. J Am Acad Dermatol 1983; 9:550–554.
Taplin D, et al. Eradication of scabies with a single treatment schedule. J Am Acad Dermatol 1983; 9:546–550.

CELLULITIS AND SOFT TISSUE INFECTION

DAVID SCHLOSSBERG, M.D., F.A.C.P.

Localized infection of the skin can be divided conveniently into two categories: localized purulent infection, or pyoderma, and cellulitis. Pyoderma is manifested by folliculitis, furunculitis, carbuncle, and impetigo. Cellulitis comprises various causes of cellulitis and the related entity of erysipelas.

In general, immediate clinical decisions regarding these infections must determine (1) the most appropriate empiric antimicrobial therapy, (2) the need for hospitalization and parenteral therapy, (3) the requirement for surgical intervention for diagnosis or therapy, and (4) the possible presence of a less common infecting organism, requiring therapy different from the usual.

PYODERMA

Folliculitis, furunculitis, and carbuncle are all aspects of the same process, i.e., infection around a hair follicle. Thus, these lesions tend to occur in characteristic areas of the body such as the head, neck, axilla, and groin. Infection of the follicle begins with a small pustule, which may later become crusted. At this stage, local treatment with warm compresses is usually sufficient. Extension of folliculitis results in a deeper nodule called a furuncle (boil). It may become fluctuant and drain spontaneously along the hair shaft.

Further and deeper extension of the furuncle produces a carbuncle. Whereas the furuncle has one site of drainage, a carbuncle usually has multiple drainage sites along many hair follicles and is more likely to be associated with systemic toxicity. As with folliculitis, most furuncles will resolve with application of moist heat. However, when a furuncle is associated with significant inflammation or systemic signs or if it is located on the face, treatment should include a systemic antibiotic and, if the lesion is large and fluctuant, incision and drainage. Similarly, carbuncles should be treated with an antibiotic and incision and drainage when indicated. Since most of these lesions are caused by *Staphylococcus aureus*, appropriate antibiotic therapy is oral dicloxacillin. (Antibiotic dosing regimens are provided in Table 1.) Alternative antibiotics include oral clindamycin and oral erythromycin.

Folliculitis caused by *Pseudomonas aeruginosa* has been described in patients with recreational water exposures such as hot tubs, whirlpools, and waterslides. This entity is self-limited and usually resolves without specific antimicrobial therapy.

Impetigo is characterized by eruption of vesicles, which become purulent and crusted, producing typical honey-colored crusts. They are superficial, grouped, painless lesions that occasionally have an inflammatory halo. Most cases involve the face or extremities. Group A streptococci are the most common cause, but staphylococci may also cause the lesion. Impetigo may be bullous; this form is seen more commonly in the newborn and is characterized by vesicles that become large bullae. These may rupture, the clear fluid producing thin brown crusts. This latter form of impetigo is more frequently caused by staphylococci. Impetigo is contagious and may be spread by direct contact to other patients or by the patient to other areas of the body. Antibiotic therapy should include an antistaphylococcal agent such as oral dicloxacillin, which treats both streptococci and staphylococci. Adjunctive therapeutic measures that may be helpful include gentle removal of crusts by soaking with soap and water. Additionally, patients (or their parents) should be warned about the ability to spread the infection.

ERYSIPELAS AND CELLULITIS

In contrast to the pyodermas discussed above, erysipelas and cellulitis involve large confluent areas of skin with an inflammatory erythema. Erysipelas is a superficial infection involving the dermis, with prominent lymphatic involvement. It most frequently involves the face and is seen particularly in patients with nephrotic syndrome, edema, or lymphatic obstruction. Erysipelas is characterized by an erythematous, indurated, advancing edge. It is usually associated with pain, fever, and toxicity and may be complicated by bacteremia. Recurrences are not unusual. Although usually caused by group A streptococci, other organisms such

TABLE 1 Antibiotic Regimens for Cellulitis and Soft Tissue Infection

Antibiotic	Children	Adults
Clavulanic acid + amoxicillin (Augmentin)	10 mg/kg q8h PO	0.5 g q8h PO
Cefoxitin	20 mg/kg q6h IV	2 g q6h IV
Cefuroxime	20 mg/kg q8h IV	0.75 g q8h IV
Clindamycin	4 mg/kg q6h, PO 8 mg/kg q8h IV	300 mg q6h PO 600 mg q8h IV
Clotrimazole	Topical 2x/day x 2 wk	Topical 2x/day x 2 wk
Dicloxacillin	25 mg/kg/day PO in 4 equal doses	0.5 g q6h PO
Erythromycin	50 mg/kg/day PO in 4 equal doses	0.5 g q6h PO 1.0 g q6h IV
Gentamicin	2 mg/kg q8h IV	4 mg/kg/day (divided q8h) IV
Nafcillin	30 mg/kg q4h–q6h PO	2 g q6h IV
Penicillin G	25,000 U/kg/day IV in 4 divided doses	2×10^6 U q6h IV
Penicillin V	50 mg/kg/day PO in 4 divided doses	500 mg q.i.d. PO
Piperacillin	50 mg/kg q4h IV	3 g q4h IV
Tetracycline	Not recommended	0.5 g q4h IV
Vancomycin	10 mg/kg q6h IV	1 g q12h IV

as group B streptococci, pneumococci, and, rarely, staphylococci may produce this syndrome. If the patient demonstrates significant toxicity or if the erysipelas involves the face, hospitalization is advised and treatment should be initiated with parenteral penicillin G. After clinical improvement, oral penicillin V-K may be employed to complete 10 days of therapy. The oral regimen may suffice for the entire course of therapy if the patient is not toxic, if the erysipelas is not extensive, and if the face is not involved. Alternative antibiotics include erythromycin and clindamycin, both intravenous and oral.

Cellulitis is an acute infection of the skin that extends deeper than erysipelas, to involve the subcutaneous tissue. Erythema (without a discrete advancing edge), pain, and fever are the usual manifestations. Secondary lymphangitis with characteristic red streaks may be seen, and bacteremia may ensue. Patients most prone to develop cellulitis are those with previous trauma or lesions allowing entry of microorganisms into the skin and patients with lymphedema or venous stasis for any reason. Thus, cellulitis may recur in patients who have had a mastectomy, coronary bypass (cellulitis frequently recurs in these patients at the vein-graft donor sites, particularly if tinea pedis is present), and in some women with lower extremity lymphedema (particularly postcoital, the "streptococcal sex syndrome").

The cause of cellulitis is usually *Staphylococcus* or *Streptococcus*, so that initial therapy is safely undertaken with an antistaphylococcal agent such as oral dicloxacillin. As with erysipelas, if the patient is toxic or if the infection is extensive or is in an area of the body where local spread or venous drainage could result in severe complications (e.g., the face or perineum), the patient should be hospitalized. Treatment

should then be undertaken with parenteral nafcillin. An oral antistaphylococcal agent like dicloxacillin may be used to complete 10 days of therapy after the patient improves. Alternative antibiotics include erythromycin and clindamycin.

Haemophilus influenzae may cause occasional cases of cellulitis, usually in association with bacteremic respiratory tract infection. The resultant cellulitis is sometimes blue-tinged. Most cases are in children and affect the face and arms. Treatment should include an agent active against staphylococci, streptococci, and *Haemophilus*, such as cefuroxime.

Several warnings must be mentioned regarding cellulitis. First, many clinical entities can mimic or complicate cellulitis (Table 2). Fasciitis and myositis, involving structures deeper than the subcutaneous tissues involved in cellulitis, require immediate surgical debridement as well as antibiotic therapy. This entity is frequently misdiagnosed as cellulitis, with disastrous results. The more invasive process should be suspected when a patient with apparent cellulitis has air in the soft tissues or symptoms out of proportion to

TABLE 2 Entities That May Mimic Cellulitis

Fasciitis/myositis
Mycotic aneurysm
Ruptured Baker's cyst
Thrombophlebitis
Osteomyelitis
Retro-orbital cellulitis/abscess
Herpetic whitlow

the observed inflammation, when blistering develops, or when the cellulitis spreads rapidly in spite of apparently appropriate therapy. An area of apparent cellulitis over the course of a major vessel, particularly in a patient with bacteremia, should raise suspicion of a mycotic aneurysm. Ruptured Baker's cyst and deep vein thrombophlebitis of the calf are often mistaken as cellulitis because of the overlying erythema and the pain and fever. Osteomyelitis involving the long bones may demonstrate an overlying erythema and pain and mislead the clinician to a diagnosis of a simple cellulitis. Herpetic whitlow, infection of the pulp of the finger, may resemble cellulitis with pulp abscess and lead to the unfortunate intervention of incision and attempted drainage. Retroorbital infection with or without abscess may be misdiagnosed as a simple periorbital cellulitis because of the preseptal inflammation. If there is any question about inflammatory involvement of retro-orbital structures, computed tomography should be performed because drainage might be required.

The other caveat regarding cellulitis is the need for concern for microbial etiologies other than the usual ones. These should be suspected when patients have particular underlying diseases or certain exposures. Although aspiration of cellulitis is not considered productive in most instances, subcutaneous aspiration for Gram stain and culture should always be attempted when an unusual etiology is suspected. An example of an underlying illness that predisposes to less common causes of cellulitis is diabetes mellitus, which may be associated with cellulitis due to *S. aureus*, streptococci, Enterobacteriaceae, and anaerobes.

Frequently, these infections have associated osteomyelitis and/or deep soft tissue extension requiring debridement. Such mixed infections, particularly when the treatment is supplemented by debridement, are usually treated successfully with a drug like cefoxitin, which eradicates the majority of the pathogens present. More extensive coverage in such patients, particularly if they are severely ill, includes a combination of clindamycin and an aminoglycoside.

TABLE 3 Less Common Etiologies of Cellulitis

Host Factors	Organisms(s)	Treatment (in order of preference)
Diabetes mellitus	*S. aureus*, streptococci, Enterobacteriaceae, anaerobes	Until cultures available (a) cefoxitin (b) if patient toxic or infection extensive, clindamycin and gentamicin
Intravenous drug abuse	*S. aureus*, coagulase-negative staphylococci, streptococci, Enterobacteriaceae, *Pseudomonas*, fungi (*Candida*)	Until cultures available: vancomycin and gentamicin
Compromised host	*S. aureus*, streptococci, Enterobacteriaceae, anaerobes, *Pseudomonas*, *Campylobacter fetus*, fungi (*Cryptococcus*)	Until cultures available: clindamycin and gentamicin *or* piperacillin and gentamicin
Burn patients	*S. aureus*, coagulase-negative staphylococci, Enterobacteriaceae, *Pseudomonas*, fungi	Vancomycin and gentamicin
Human bite	*S. aureus*, streptococci, anaerobes, *Eikenella corrodens*	Augmentin (ampicillin + clavulanic acid) Cefoxitin
Dog/cat bite	*S. aureus*, anaerobes, *Pasteurella multocida*, other gram-negative bacilli	Augmentin Cefoxitin
Freshwater exposure	*Aeromonas* *Pseudomonas*	Gentamicin, tetracycline Gentamicin
Saltwater exposure	*Vibrio* species	Gentamicin Tetracycline
Saltwater fish, shellfish, meat, hides	*Erysipelothrix*	Penicillin
Aquarium workers, veterinarians	Seal finger	Tetracycline
Diphtheria (unimmunized patients)	*C. diphtheriae*	Erythromycin
Tinea pedis (frequently seen in patients after vein grafts for coronary bypass)	Streptococci (various types), ? immunologic mechanisms	Penicillin (+ clotrimazole for the tinea)

Intravenous drug abusers may develop cellulitis due to unusual organisms or combinations of many organisms, including staphylococci, coagulase-negative staphylococci, streptococci, Enterobacteriaceae, *Pseudomonas*, and fungi, especially *Candida*. Empiric coverage for these patients includes vancomycin and an aminoglycoside until the results of tissue and blood cultures are available. The immunocompromised patient may develop cellulitis due to *Cryptococcus, Pseudomonas,* and *Campylobacter fetus* in addition to the more standard etiologies of cellulitis. Until cultures can be evaluated, initial empiric therapy could include a combination of clindamycin and gentamicin or piperacillin plus gentamicin. Finally, patients with burns may develop cellulitis complicated by infection with *Pseudomonas*, coagulase-negative staphylococci, and fungi in addition to the usual etiologies of cellulitis. Until cultures are available for such patients or if treatment is required prophylactically before manipulation of the wound, therapy would be best undertaken with a combination of vancomycin and gentamicin.

There are certain exposures and crucial points in a patient's history that may also suggest an unusual etiology of cellulitis (Table 3). As with routine etiologies, clinical judgment of severity and extent of infection will determine when hospitalization is necessary, if debridement should be considered, and if parenteral or oral therapy is required. Thus, cellulitis in a patient who has had exposure to fresh water suggests the possibility of infection with *Aeromonas* and is best treated with tetracycline or gentamicin. Exposure to saltwater, on the other hand, may result in severe necrotizing and blistering cellulitis caused by one of several species of vibrios. These patients are also treated with tetracycline or gentamicin. Saltwater fish, shellfish, meat, and hide exposure may result in the syndrome of erysipeloid, caused by *Erysipelothrix*. Penicillin is the treatment of choice for this infection. Aquarium workers and veterinarians who come in contact with seals may develop seal finger; the etiology of this cellulitis is not known but it may respond to treatment with oral tetracycline.

Infections associated with human bites are frequently caused by staphylococci and streptococci, but *Eikenella corrodens* is an important pathogen in this situation and will not be covered adequately by oral cephalosporin or antistaphylococcal antibiotics. Treatment for this form of cellulitis may be undertaken with ampicillin plus clavulanic acid (Augmentin). Similarly, infections from cat and dog bites, though frequently caused by staphylococci and other pathogens, may induce a cellulitis attributable to *Pasteurella multocida* which, like *Eikenella*, is not treated optimally by oral cephalosporins or antistaphylococcal agents. As with human bites, the safest approach to cellulitis resulting from a dog or cat bite is to use ampicillin plus clavulanic acid. Parenteral therapy for both human and dog and cat bites may be achieved with cefoxitin.

Tinea pedis is frequently seen in patients who have recurrent cellulitis of the legs, and the cellulitis stops recurring after the tinea is treated with topical antifungal agents such as clotrimazole. This syndrome is seen frequently in patients who have had coronary bypass and tends to occur at the vein-graft donor site on the legs.

Finally, one must not forget cutaneous diphtheria, which may produce soft tissue infection, particularly in the unimmunized. This syndrome may resemble cellulitis or impetigo and is documented by methylene blue stain and culture on special media. Both antitoxin and erythromycin constitute appropriate therapy.

Many of the unusual organisms just described show in vitro sensitivity to the quinolone class of antibiotics. At this writing, the role of the quinolones in the treatment of soft tissue infection is undefined, although their wide spectrum may ultimately prove helpful for treatment of both routine and uncommon etiologies of this group of infections.

SUGGESTED READING

Bisno AL. Cutaneous infections: microbiologic and epidemiologic considerations. Am J Med 1984; 76(5A):172–179.
Fitzpatrick TB, Eisen AZ, Wolff K, Freedberg EM, Austin KF. Dermatology in general medicine. New York: McGraw-Hill, 1979.
Hill MK, Sanders CV. Localized and systemic infections due to vibrio species. Infect Dis Clin North Am 1987; 1:687–707.
Mandell GL, Douglas RG Jr, Bennett JE. Principles and practice of infectious diseases. New York: John Wiley and Sons, 1985.

CREPITUS AND GANGRENE

E. PATCHEN DELLINGER, M.D.

Crepitus refers to the crackling sensation that is detected by the palpation of gas in tissue. However, roentgenography is more sensitive than palpation for detecting gas. Soft tissue gas is uncommon but always significant when found in conjunction with infection. Most facultative bacteria produce gas during anaerobic but not aerobic metabolism. The presence of gas with infection, therefore, indicates an anaerobic environment, incompatible with living human tissue, i.e., gangrenous infection. Gas may also be present in tissue as a result of trauma or surgery or as a result of a respiratory leak, either in association with severe obstructive pulmonary disease or positive pressure ventilation. In either case, the source of gas should be evident from the history, and the local signs of soft tissue infection should be absent.

The importance of recognizing dead tissue (gangrene) or the likelihood of dead tissue in conjunction with a soft tissue infection is that such an infection will not resolve without surgical intervention. Delay in intervention increases the risk of extensive tissue loss and death. Unfortunately, the literature that refers to these infections is complex and confusing, identifying many separate syndromes and specific gangrenous infections when, in fact, the great majority of them fall on a continuous spectrum of presenting signs and symptoms and relative severity. The most important distinction that should be made is between histotoxic clostridial myonecrosis and all other necrotizing soft tissue infections.

CLOSTRIDIAL INFECTIONS

Histotoxic clostridial myonecrosis, or gas gangrene, is the most feared form of clostridial infection. It is not the most common. Clostridia may be found in contaminated wounds that are not infected but merely need local care. These do not elicit a systemic response. Clostridia occasionally may be recovered with or without other bacteria in ordinary wound infections, which are adequately treated with simple incision and drainage. Clostridia commonly appear as part of a mixed flora in cases of necrotizing fasciitis (see below). Clostridial myonecrosis is the most serious, rapidly progressive, potentially fatal clostridial infection. Although there are some differences from the nonclostridial necrotizing infections in presentation and management, there are more similarities. These will be discussed in this chapter.

NONCLOSTRIDIAL INFECTIONS

Nonclostridial infections are much more common than clostridial infections but may also be life threatening and disfiguring. Different names have been applied to these infections depending on the responsible organism, the depth of tissue involvement, or the anatomic location of the infection, but the similarities in clinical presentation and management far outweigh these differences. Table 1 lists some specific terms for nonclostridial soft tissue infections that have been described as separate entities in the medical literature but that are more usefully regarded as different manifestations of the same basic infectious process. This process may be relatively superficial, in which case the most commonly applied term is necrotizing fasciitis. This label is not ideal, since in the majority of cases the fascia is not involved at all. The most common location of the infectious process is in the subcutaneous tissue, with relatively normal skin above and normal fascia below most of the affected area. If this process is caused by *Streptococcus pyogenes* alone it is termed hemolytic streptococcal gangrene. However, the clinical presentation and course are indistinguishable from cases caused by a polymicrobic flora of aerobes and anaerobes, gram-positive and gram-negative bacteria.

TABLE 1   Terms Used to Describe Nonclostridial Soft Tissue Infections

Necrotizing fasciitis
Necrotizing cellulitis
Nonclostridial crepitant cellulitis
Nonclostridial gas gangrene
Synergistic necrotizing cellulitis
Bacterial synergistic gangrene
Gangrenous erysipelas
Necrotizing erysipelas
Hemolytic streptococcal gangrene
Fournier's gangrene

When the infectious process involves tissues deep to the muscular fascia, it is sometimes called necrotizing cellulitis to distinguish it from necrotizing fasciitis. Individual muscle bundles may be infiltrated and in some cases rendered ischemic as the inflammatory process causes thrombosis of the blood supply. In most cases, however, the involved muscle is viable and contracts on stimulation. This contrasts with clostridial myonecrosis, in which muscle is killed by toxins in the presence of an intact blood supply. When necrotizing fasciitis begins on the penis, scrotum, or vulva it has been called Fournier's gangrene. There is nothing but the anatomic location to distinguish this from other examples of the same infectious process. Even the distinction between clostridial myonecrosis and other necrotizing soft tissue infections is less important than usually regarded in determining the clinician's initial response to infection. The most important step is to recognize gangrenous infection, whether or not clostridial. Subsequent steps in diagnosis and treatment will reveal the nature of the infection and allow the interested physician to make as precise a diagnosis as he or she wishes.

DIAGNOSIS

The most important initial step in approaching any soft tissue infection is to determine whether tissue necrosis is present. A simple subcutaneous abscess has a central necrotic portion but is distinguished from the infections discussed in this section by being localized. The gangrenous soft tissue infections are marked by the absence of localization or limitation. This accounts both for their severity and for many of the difficulties encountered in prompt recognition and treatment. In all cases the external evidence of infection and of gangrene is much less extensive than that found in deeper tissues. Both clostridial and nonclostridial infections appear rather ordinary when they begin. Table 2 highlights the similarities and differences between the clostridial and nonclostridial infections in presentation, diagnosis, and management.

Clostridial infections are marked by severe pain and some local swelling but little evidence of an inflammatory reaction. By contrast, the nonclostridial infections exhibit a more marked inflammatory response, with redness, swelling, and tenderness at the site of infection. In either case there is little or no initial evidence of tissue death. As the infection advances, clostridial myonecrosis will develop a bronze skin discoloration. Later hemorrhagic bullae may develop. Gram stain of the contents of these bullae may reveal gram-positive rods. Dermal gangrene and crepitus are signs of very advanced infection. Nonclostridial infections initially look no different than simple cellulitis without tissue necrosis. Rapid progression, a marked systemic hemodynamic response to infection, or failure to respond to conventional nonoperative therapy may be the earliest signs of the true nature of the process. Subtle bruising or ecchymoses almost invariably indicate underlying tissue necrosis. Bullae in an area of infection are also usually associated with this process. Dermal gangrene and/or crepitus, as in the case of clostridial myonecrosis, are very advanced signs and are unequivocal evidence of underlying necrosis that demands operative in-

TABLE 2   Similarities and Differences Between Clostridial and Nonclostridial Infections

	Clostridial Myonecrosis	Nonclostridial Necrotizing Infections
Erythema	Usually absent	Present, often mild
Swelling/edema	Mild to moderate	Moderate
Exudate	Thin	Dishwater
White blood cells	Usually absent	Present
Bacteria	GPR* ± others	Mixed ± GPR, may be GPC† alone
Advanced signs	Bronzing, hemorrhagic bullae, dermal gangrene, crepitus	Ecchymoses, bullae, dermal gangrene, crepitus
Deep involvement	Muscle >>>‡ skin	Subcutaneous tissue ± fascia ± muscle (uncommon) >>> skin
Histology	Muscle necrosis with little or no inflammation	Viable muscle with acute inflammation
Physiology	Tachycardia, hypotension, volume deficit ± intravascular hemolysis	Tachycardia, hypotension, volume deficit
Treatment		
General	Aggressive cardiopulmonary resuscitation	Aggressive cardiopulmonary resuscitation
Antibiotics	Penicillin G§	Cefotaxime + metronidazole‡
Hyperbaric O$_2$	If it does not delay other treatment	No
Surgery	Aggressive removal of infected tissue; amputation of extremity often required	Debridement and exposure; not much removal required; usually no amputation
Antitoxin	No	No

* GPR = gram-positive rods.
† GPC = gram-positive cocci.
‡ > > > = much more extensive than.
§ See text for doses and alternate choices.

tervention. Although nonclostridial gangrenous infections usually progress quite rapidly, some cases—alike in all other respects—spread slowly over many days with a correspondingly less severe systemic response.

In both cases the local exudate is initially unimpressive, being described as thin or like dishwater. In addition, the transition between the infected and the surrounding normal tissues is gradual, and no clear border or limit is evident by surface inspection of the intact skin. Gram stain of drainage usually reveals multiple organisms and morphologic forms in both clostridial and nonclostridial infections. Some cases of clostridial myonecrosis, however, have few organisms evident on Gram stain and may not produce positive cultures. Clostridial species do not form spores in soft tissue infections, and thus the absence of spores does not rule

out a *Clostridium* species as the infectious agent. White blood cells are usually absent from the histotoxic clostridial infections. This accounts for the thin nature of the exudate and the lack of external signs of an inflammatory reaction.

Culture of a clostridial infection may recover multiple species of clostridia and often includes other anaerobic and facultative bacteria, whereas nonclostridial infections usually show multiple species, except in cases where *Streptococcus pyogenes* is the sole pathogen. Conversely, clostridial organisms may be recovered from infections that are not classic gas gangrene (histotoxic clostridial myonecrosis). Clostridia occur more commonly in infections that are not myonecrosis, and so this diagnosis and the subsequent therapeutic decisions must be made on clinical grounds, operative findings, and response to therapy, not simply on the presence of gram-positive rods on stain or in culture.

When an infection occurs in an open wound, special care must be taken in obtaining specimens and interpreting culture results. An open wound often contains a great variety of organisms, many of which are contaminants and not true pathogens in the infectious process. The best cultures are obtained in the operating room through previously intact skin and at a distance from any open wounds. An alternative is needle aspiration of the tissues at a distance from the open wound. If sufficient material is obtained in this manner, then the sample is reliable. If no material is obtained, however, this is not valid evidence of the absence of a necrotizing infection. The location and extent of underlying involvement is unpredictable, and needle aspiration may be unproductive despite an overwhelming infection.

The most common soft tissue infections with crepitus and/or gangrene are not clostridial. They may involve subcutaneous tissue only, subcutaneous tissue and muscular fascia, or both and muscle. It is rare to see a deep infection that does not also involve subcutaneous tissue. The depth of tissue involvement is probably determined by the depth of the original wound of entry. The most common site of origin is an accidental wound or surgical incision. Wounds that have communicated with the bowel lumen or perineum are at higher risk, and any wound closed under tension is at higher risk. Necrotizing fasciitis of the abdominal wall often follows coeliotomy for intra-abdominal infection. If it occurs after bowel surgery it often indicates deeper intra-abdominal infection. Spontaneous episodes occur more commonly in the perineum and may be related to perirectal abscesses, Bartholin cysts, or unrecognized minor skin defects. These infections are usually polymicrobial, with several anaerobic and facultative species present. Cases can also occur after trivial scratches or insect bites. These are most commonly caused by *S. pyogenes*, which is the only organism that has been recorded with any frequency as the sole cause of this syndrome.

One of the difficulties presented by these infections is that they are neither rare nor common. Thus, nearly every primary care practitioner or infectious disease specialist will see several over a lifetime of practice, but most physicians see them seldom and have little experience in their diagnosis or treatment. The primary physician must suspect the diagnosis, and the consulting infectious disease specialist and surgeon must have the courage to act aggressively once the diagnosis has been suspected. When necrotizing soft tissue infection has been suspected, the clinician is obligated to move rapidly to confirm or refute the diagnosis and institute treatment. For practical purposes, this can only be done in the operating room, where the necrotic tissue can be exposed and its extent confirmed. Recently, some have suggested biopsy and frozen-section tissue stains to confirm the diagnosis. In fact, if the diagnosis is under serious enough consideration to warrant biopsy, the most important step has been taken. The incision that must be made to obtain biopsy material will allow the diagnosis to be made by direct inspection, and definitive therapy can be initiated at once.

TREATMENT

Significant fluid sequestration and a marked hemodynamic response are common with the gangrenous soft tissue infections. Among the nonclostridial infections, the range of responses is wide, from minimal response to profound septic shock. The responses parallel those seen with intra-abdominal infection. Clostridial myonecrosis is notable for a more rapid and more severe hemodynamic impairment. Profound cardiovascular collapse may occur with minimal evidence of infection. This constitutes the major difference between the histotoxic clostridial infections and all others. In every case, the potential for profound cardiovascular compromise exists, and careful cardiorespiratory evaluation, monitoring, and support are mandatory.

Empiric antibiotic selection must cover a wide range of potential pathogens—similar to those found in peritonitis and intra-abdominal abscess. A regimen of cefotaxime, 2 g intravenously every 8 hours, plus metronidazole, 500 mg intravenously every 8 hours, is a good initial choice. Another third-generation cephalosporin or an aminoglycoside can be substituted for cefotaxime. If an aminoglycoside is used, then penicillin should be added to ensure coverage against streptococcal species. Clindamycin, 900 mg intravenously every 8 hours, can be given as a substitute for metronidazole. Imipenem-cilastatin alone, 500 mg intravenously every 6 hours, is another reasonable alternative. If the initial Gram stain shows a predominance of gram-positive rods and few or no white blood cells, penicillin G, 20 million units per day, should be given. Since many cases of clostridial myonecrosis also involve other mixed bacterial flora, it is prudent to include cefotaxime and metronidazole as indicated above until the details of culture and clinical response are clear. For penicillin-allergic patients chloramphenicol, 1 g intravenously every 6 hours initially, then 500 mg intravenously every 6 hours, or cefotaxime and metronidazole are acceptable alternatives.

Hyperbaric oxygen prevents clostridial organisms from manufacturing new toxins but does not inactivate toxins already present in tissue. Hyperbaric oxygen often causes a transient improvement in the hemodynamic status of a patient with clostridial myonecrosis but is inadequate as a sole treatment. No adequate clinical trials of its use in this condition have been or are likely to be done. If a hyperbaric chamber is readily available, it is reasonable to add this treatment according to the protocol of the local chamber after adequate hemodynamic resuscitation, antibiotic administration, and operative treatment. It is contraindicated to transport a patient with clostridial myonecrosis for hyperbaric oxygen before the other measures have been instituted. Many medical centers with hyperbaric chambers provide excellent care for these patients since they have acquired an interest and a large experience generated by patient referrals. There is no accepted role for antitoxins in the treatment of clostridial myonecrosis.

The extent of surgical excision and debridement is determined by the gross findings during the procedure. In cases of clostridial myonecrosis, all infected tissue must be excised. All margins in muscle must contract on stimulation and bleed freely. In cases of infection of the extremities, amputation is often required. In cases of nonclostridial infection, less excision of tissue is required. All infected tissue must be exposed, and the challenge is to find all extensions of the process. Large areas of infection may communicate by narrow tracts. Once all areas have been exposed and debrided, the infection usually resolves. The extensive unroofing required by some infections may result in interruption of the blood supply to superficial tissues and loss for that reason. Careful planning and placement of incisions can minimize such tissue loss.

In all serious cases of either clostridial myonecrosis or nonclostridial gangrenous infections, at least two operative procedures are required. The infectious process infiltrates widely beneath skin, and an extension may be overlooked at the first procedure or not adequately debrided in hopes of saving tissue. The second procedure should be scheduled within 24 to 48 hours of the first. If significant amounts of infection are discovered at the second operation, a third must be scheduled and so on. Once no further infection is found on operative inspection, the surgical phase of treatment is completed.

The surgical management of these infections leaves large soft tissue defects in most cases. The management and closure of these wounds is a significant problem. Topical agents such as sulfamylon and other techniques used in the management of large open burn wounds are useful in these circumstances. Often a plastic surgery or burn service consultation will be helpful in resolving these problems and achieving expeditious wound closure.

SUGGESTED READING

Dellinger EP. Severe necrotizing soft tissue infections: multiple disease entities requiring a common approach. JAMA 1981; 246:1717–1721.

Kaiser RE, Cerra FB. Progressive necrotizing surgical infections—a unified approach. J Trauma 1981; 21:349–355.

Meleney FL. Hemolytic streptococcus gangrene. Arch Surg 1924; 9:317–364 (one of the earliest good clinical descriptions—a surgical/infectious diseases classic).

Pessa ME, Howard RJ. Necrotizing fasciitis. Surg Gynecol Obstet 1985; 161:357–361.

VanBeek A, Zook E, Yaw P, et al. Nonclostridial gas-forming infections. Arch Surg 1974; 108:552–557 (discusses the physiology of insoluble gas production by bacteria under anaerobic circumstances).

OCULAR AND PERIORBITAL INFECTIONS

ENDOPHTHALMITIS

ANN SULLIVAN BAKER, M.D.

Endophthalmitis is one of the catastrophic complications of ocular surgery, penetrating ocular trauma, and systemic infection. Until recently, infectious endophthalmitis was associated with an almost uniformly poor prognosis; in one large series between 1950 and 1977, 67 percent of patients with postoperative endophthalmitis lost all light perception. Both experimental and clinical evidence indicates that the expeditious use of intraocular antibiotics and therapeutic vitrectomy favorably alters the outcome of endophthalmitis.

Endophthalmitis is defined as inflammation of intraocular structures, typically severe in character and often associated with pain, decreased vision, inflammatory cells in the anterior or posterior chamber, hypopyon in many instances, lid swelling, chemosis, and loss of the red reflex. In infectious or bacterial endophthalmitis one or more microorganisms are recovered from vitreous or aqueous fluids on at least two culture media (see below).

Most cases of bacterial endophthalmitis follow cataract extractions, with onset typically in the immediate postoperative period. Others that occur more than 3 months after surgery are termed late postoperative infections; these are often infections of blebs raised for therapy of glaucoma. Endophthalmitis may rarely follow penetrating ocular trauma, after which multiple organisms may be found. Finally, endophthalmitis may follow bacteremic infections.

Symptoms of endophthalmitis include headache over the infected eye, eye pain, and decreased vision. Signs include swelling or chemosis of the conjunctiva and upper lid, hypopyon (or cells in the anterior chamber), and a decreased red reflex. Visual acuity may also be decreased.

Ultrasonographic examination of the orbit may be helpful in identifying a vitreous infiltrate as well as establishing the status of the retina.

To confirm the diagnosis of endophthalmitis, fluid should be aspirated from the anterior chamber and always from the vitreous, or the material from vitrectomy washings (which may be a total of more than 200 ml) should be collected on a 0.45-micron filter. The tiny drop of aspirate (or the filter paper) is then placed on *Brucella* agar and chocolate agar plates, anaerobic media, and a Sabouraud's slant. Because the specimen is so tiny, the drop should be placed in the center of the plate.

The criteria for infectious endophthalmitis include eyes from which organisms are cultured from a specimen of aqueous or vitreous fluid on at least two media. (The area of growth on the culture plate may be so small that growth is required on at least two media to rule out contamination.)

Organisms cultured from most postoperative cataract infections include coagulase-negative staphylococci, streptococci, and *Staphylococcus aureus*. In traumatic endophthalmitis, multiple organisms may be cultured; in these patients, the incidence of anaerobic (clostridia), gram-positive (*Bacillus*) and gram-negative infections is high.

Finally, endogenous or metastatic endophthalmitis secondary to a focus elsewhere may be due to streptococci, staphylococci, gram-negative, or anaerobic organisms.

TREATMENT

There are several tenets of therapy for endophthalmitis. Treatment within 24 hours of diagnosis improves the outcome considerably. A delay of more than 24 hours in the performance of therapeutic vitrectomy has been associated with a dismal outcome; 50 percent of patients with late vitrectomy had no light perception in one series. Vitreous sampling is crucial in establishing a bacteriologic diagnosis. Coagulase-negative *Staphylococcus* is the commonest pathogen in postoperative endophthalmitis. Visual outcome is poor in the late-onset (or more than 3 months' onset) endophthalmitis. It is also poor in the patient with gram-negative or anaerobic infection.

VITRECTOMY

Evidence is increasing for the need for a vitrectomy and/or intravitreal antibiotics versus medical therapy alone. It is our clinical impression that vitrectomy and intravitreal antibiotics improve the outcome of endophthalmitis. A vitrectomy includes removal of all or part of the 3.9 ml of material in the vitreous.

Advantages include drainage of the abscess; the vitreous is a tiny closed space, and drainage is imperative. The

**TABLE 1   Endophthalmitis: Intravitreal Doses
(Total Volume, 0.1 to 0.2 ml)***

Antibiotic	*Dosage*
Aminoglycosides	
Gentamicin	0.2 mg
Tobramycin	0.2 mg
Amikacin	0.2 mg
Penicillins	
Methicillin	2.0 mg
Oxacillin	0.5 mg
Ampicillin	5.0 mg
Carbenicillin	2.0 mg
Miscellaneous	
Cefazolin	1.0 mg
Erythromycin	0.5 mg
Clindamycin	1.0 mg
Vancomycin	1.0 mg
Chloramphenicol	2.0 mg
Antifungal antibiotic	
Amphotericin B	5–10 μg

Note: Choice of antibiotic is determined by the organism isolated.
* Adapted from Peyman GA. Surv Ophthalmol 1977; 21:332–346.

gel matrix of the vitreous is also removed so that diffusion for antibiotic delivery is better. Disadvantages include the risk of retinal tear or detachment and new fibrovascular ingrowths. The vitrectomy must be performed early to be of any value.

Indications for vitrectomy include gram-negative organisms on Gram stain or vitreous sample, fungal infection, or a gram-positive organism in a patient with visual acuity of 20/400 or less. In severe, progressive cases, repeat vitrectomy and reinstillation of antibiotics may be necessary.

ANTIBIOTIC THERAPY

There are four suggested approaches to antibiotic therapy in endophthalmitis:

Intravitreal Injection

Diffusion of the antibiotic occurs readily in the vitreous. Loss of the drug from the vitreous occurs through two routes; anteriorly to the posterior chamber and out through the aqueous drainage system (aminoglycosides); or by active transport across the retina (e.g., beta-lactam drugs or clindamycin). Competitive inhibitors such as probenicid inhibit this pump and may prolong the vitreous concentration of beta-lactams.

There is a concern about toxicity of intravitreal antibiotics, and thus several precautions should be taken. The intravitreal antibiotics should be given in the anterior part of the vitreous as a slow injection. A rapid-fire stream toward the back of the retina may tear the retina.

Suggested initial doses for endophthalmitis of unknown etiology include vancomycin (1 mg) and an aminoglycoside such as gentamicin (200 μg). Table 1 lists antibiotics and dosages used after the organism has been identified.

Subconjunctival Therapy

Subconjunctival therapy has been recommended (for one or two doses) if there are no bleeding or pressure complications. Doses of cefazolin (50 mg) and tobramycin (50 mg) result in good concentrations in the cornea that exceed the aqueous concentration by severalfold; the vitreous levels are usually less than 1 μg per milliliter, however. Thus, the usefulness of this approach in endophthalmitis is still debated.

Topical Therapy

Topical therapy should be combined with other modes of therapy especially in the patient with a draining wound. One to two drops of antibiotic every 1 to 4 hours are usually sufficient. Cefazolin, 33 mg per milliliter, vancomycin, 14 mg per milliliter, and gentamicin, 14 mg per milliliter, are useful initial antibiotics.

Systemic Therapy

Systemic intravenous administration of antibiotics results in poor penetration of the vitreous barriers. Peak levels in the vitreous are typically only 1 percent of the serum level; penetration of the aqueous is slightly better, i.e., 2 to 10 percent of the peak level.

Preferred intravenous antibiotics in order of choice are vancomycin, 1 to 2 g per day, or cefazolin 3 to 4.5 g per day. In patients from whom methicillin-resistant *Staphylococcus epidermidis* has been isolated, vancomycin may be substituted. The role of intravenous antibiotics remains to be defined and must await studies of vitreal levels obtained after intravenous administration. Specific antibiotic therapy is adjusted when cultural and sensitivity data become available. Most cases due to coagulase-negative staphylococci respond well to a 7- to 10-day course of parenteral antibiotics, vitrectomy, and topical therapy; complicated cases involving *S. aureus*, gram-negative bacteria, or fungal endophthalmitis require a longer (14-day or more) course of parenteral therapy until the vitreous clears. Traumatic endophthalmitis therapy should include vancomycin or clindamycin to cover anaerobic organisms. Fungal endophthalmitis generally clears with systemic amphotericin B alone; rarely, vitrectomy and vitreous instillation of 5 to 10 μg of amphotericin B is necessary.

Close follow-up is mandatory to detect posttreatment complications including glaucoma, retinal detachments, and sterile uveitis.

STEROIDS

Systemic steroids may be used in the severely inflamed and infected eye to decrease inflammation in this tight, small space. Prednisone, 60 mg a day tapered rapidly after 5 days, may be used.

DIFFERENTIAL DIAGNOSIS

The differential diagnosis of endophthalmitis following cataract extraction should include sterile inflammation as well as bacterial and fungal infection. Sterile uveitis has been reported to occur in 2 to 3 percent of patients following intraocular lens implantation. Like bacterial infections, sterile endophthalmitis generally develops during the first week following the lens implantation.

PSEUDOPHAKIC ENDOPHTHALMITIS

Bacterial pseudophakic endophthalmitis (intraocular lens) is a postoperative complication of intraocular lens implantation. The presentation is similar to postcataract endophthalmitis. Most commonly, the bacteria are coagulase-negative staphylococci, *Staphylococcus aureus*, *Propionibacterium acnes*, and streptococci, but a wide variety of gram- positive and gram-negative organisms have been isolated. The therapy should be similar to that for the patient with routine postoperative cataract endophthalmitis. Although it has been suggested that in cases of pseudophakic endophthalmitis the intraocular lens should be removed, this may be a difficult procedure with high morbidity. Most patients can be cured without removal of lens; in fact the removal may lead to a poorer visual outcome.

FUNGAL ENDOPHTHALMITIS

Fungal endophthalmitis may occur as an indolent infection, with the first symptoms often occurring days to weeks after the initial surgery. Pain in the involved eye, headache, and lid edema may be less pronounced than in bacterial infections. The commonest symptom is decreased vision. Fluffy exudates or nodules on examination frequently suggest fungal endophthalmitis. Intravitreal and systemic amphotericin B are the usual modes of therapy.

ANTIBIOTIC PROPHYLAXIS

For topical prophylaxis before cataract surgery we suggest polymyxin B sulfate and bacitracin ophthalmic ointment (Polysporin) on the evening before surgery and in the postoperative period.

Systemic antibiotics such as cefazolin might be given prophylactically for vitreal or retinal surgery. It is our impression that the patient with some type of immunosuppression such as steroid use or chemotherapy as well as patients with intraoperative complications such as vitreous loss during cataract surgery have a higher incidence of endophthalmitis than would be expected. Unplanned extracapsular extraction or vitreous loss had occurred in one-third of our reported cases of endophthalmitis. In the case of vitreous loss, one may speculate that the intact hyaloid face has some barrier function against intraocular penetration of microorganisms. Thus, a heightened index of suspicion for infectious endophthalmitis is warranted in cases of complicated cataract extraction. Subconjunctival and/or systemic antibiotics as well as topical antibiotics should be considered in the immunocompromised patient before cataract surgery.

Speed is of the essence in the evaluation and therapy of endophthalmitis. The goal should be to salvage vision rather than to perform enucleation, an all too common outcome of bacterial endophthalmitis.

SUGGESTED READING

Davey RT, Tauber WB. Post-traumatic endophthalmitis: The emerging role of *Bacillus cereus* infection. Rev Infect Dis 1987; 9:110–123.

Tabbara KF, Hyhdiuk RA. Infections of the eye. Boston: Little, Brown, 1986:563.

Talley AR, D'Amico D, Talamo J, Kenyon K. The role of vitrectomy in the treatment of post-operative bacterial endophthalmitis: An experimental study. Arch Ophthalmol 1987; 105:1699–1702.

Weber DJ, Hoffman KL, Thoft RA, Baker AS. Endophthalmitis following intraocular lens implantation: Report of 30 cases and review of the literature. Rev Infect Dis 1986; 8:12–20.

INFECTION OF THE CONJUNCTIVA, EYELIDS, AND LACRIMAL APPARATUS

MICHAEL D. WAGONER, M.D.
RHOADS E. STEVENS, M.D.

CONJUNCTIVITIS

Conjunctivitis denotes inflammation of the mucous membrane covering the eyelids and sclera. The broadest classification scheme of conjunctivitis differentiates between infectious and noninfectious etiologies of conjunctival inflammation. Regardless of the etiology, signs and symptoms of conjunctivitis may include hyperemia, lid swelling, irritation or foreign body sensation, mild photophobia, and intermittent foreign body sensation.

Conjunctival infections are the most commonly encountered eye disease. Because of its location, the conjunctiva is constantly exposed to microorganisms from the air, from skin of the eyelids, and from hand-to-eye contact. Nevertheless, the normal conjunctiva is remarkably resistant to infections, and except in rare cases such as trachoma, most conjunctival infections are self-limited.

Disorders primarily involving the conjunctiva that must be distinguished from infectious conjunctivitis include allergic conjunctivitis (prominent itching, "ropy" mucoid accumulations that may be mistaken for discharge), medications (especially epinephrine), contact lens irritation, cicatricial disorders such as Stevens-Johnson

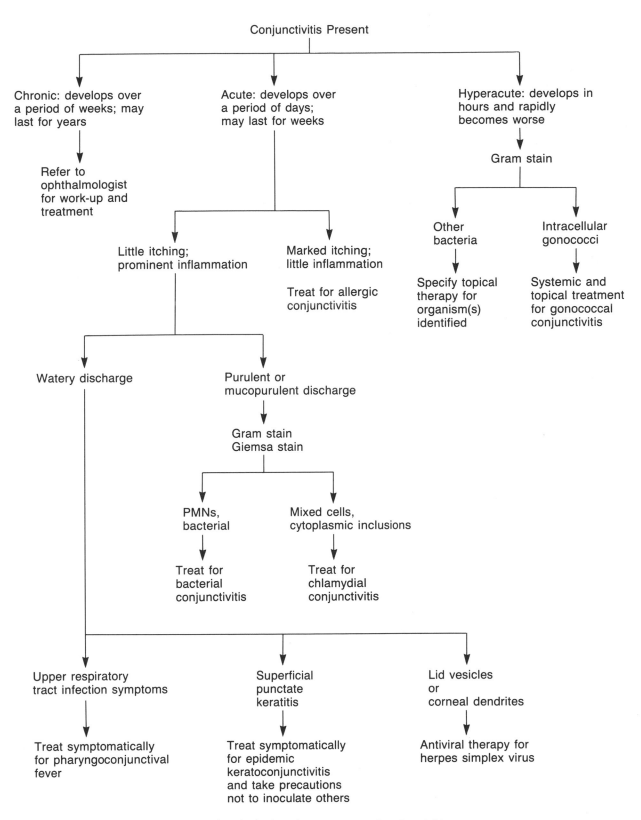

Figure 1 Diagnosis and management of conjunctivitis.

syndrome or pemphigoid (chronic injection, conjunctival shrinkage, and fibrosis), superior limbic keratoconjunctivitis (localized inflammation of the superior bulbar conjunctiva sometimes associated with thyroid disorders), lymphoid hyperplasia (localized salmon-pink elevation of the conjunctiva, usually in the fornices), and tumors such as pterygium, carcinoma-in-situ, and squamous cell carcinoma (usually interpalpebral fissure, elevated, well-circumscribed vascular lesions that may encroach upon the cornea). Disorders primarily affecting nonconjunctival sites but associated with reactive conjunctival hyperemia include episcleritis, scleritis, keratitis, uveitis, and angle-closure glaucoma. All of these disorders are characterized by a notable absence of discharge.

True discharge is the essential sign and symptom of infectious conjunctivitis. This may be watery, purulent, or mucopurulent. Although some crusting or mattering of the eyelids in the morning is normal, infectious conjunctivitis usually produces significant sticking together of the eyelids, especially upon awakening. A conjunctival reaction to infection may result in elevations of the tarsal conjunctiva, called follicles (predominantly lymphoid reaction) or papillae (predominantly vascular), which may aid in the differential diagnosis (see below). Lymphatic drainage from the conjunctival sac is to the submandibular and preauricular nodes, where reactive lymphadenopathy may occur. Infrequently, in severe cases, fibrin and inflammatory debris may collect on the conjunctival surface to form ''pseudomembranes.''

Acute conjunctivitis (developing over several days) is almost always a self-limited disease that can be diagnosed and managed on purely clinical findings. Appropriate bacteriologic diagnosis is indicated in all cases of hyperacute conjunctivitis (develops in a matter of hours and worsens), ophthalmia neonatorum (conjunctivitis in infants), and all cases of chronic (present longer than 3 weeks) or unresponsive conjunctivitis. The conjunctiva can be swabbed with a sterile calcium alginate swab that has been moistened with sterile saline prior to the instillation of antibiotics or topical anesthetics. This should be inoculated onto blood agar, chocolate agar (for *Neisseria* and *Haemophilus*), and thioglycolate broth (for anaerobes). Smears should be examined with both gram and Giemsa stains. Gram stain is particulary useful for identifying bacteria and cell morphology. Although nondiagnostic, polymophonuclear cells are seen in acute bacterial conjunctivitis, mononuclear cells in viral conjunctivitis, and eosinophils or basophils in allergic conjunctivitis. Giemsa stain is essential for the identification of basophilic paranuclear cytoplasmic inclusions within the epithelial cells in chlamydial disease. Smears of the conjunctiva can be examined by immunofluorescent staining with antichlamydial monoclonal antibody (Micro Trak).

Figure 1 provides a scheme for the diagnosis of hyperacute, acute, and chronic conjunctivitis.

Hyperacute Conjunctivitis

The most important task in the diagnosis and management of conjunctivitis is to properly identify all cases of hyperacute conjunctivitis due to *Neisseria* species. *Neisseria gonorrhoeae* is by far the most common cause of hyperacute conjunctivitis. It can be seen in adults of all ages and in neonates (see ophthalmia neonatorum). *Neisseria meningitidis* can produce an equally severe conjunctivitis, especially in young children, and must not be overlooked because it may be a prelude to meningococcemia or meningitis. Although other types of conjunctivitis may produce significant discomfort and occasionally become chronic with significant sequelae, ocular infection caused by *Neisseria* species may rapidly lead to an ulcerative keratitis and perforation of the globe if not promptly treated. In young children, *Haemophilus influenzae* may produce a hyperacute conjunctivitis (discussed elsewhere).

Hyperacute conjunctivitis has an explosive onset that occurs over a several-hour period and is associated with continued worsening. The patient is usually extremely uncomfortable, and the eye is tender to the touch. Often the lids are difficult to open owing to extensive swelling. Discharge is copious and tends to drain continuously from the eye. The conjunctival chemosis is severe. If it is due to *Neisseria* species, an invasion of the cornea through intact epithelium may occur, especially near the limbus. A rather prominent preauricular node may be present.

A laboratory work-up is mandatory in all cases of hyperacute conjunctivitis. Conjunctival scrapings, rather than smears of the ocular discharge, are preferred for Gram staining. The inflammatory cell response is overwhelmingly polymorphonuclear. Gram-negative diplococci are seen primarily within these cells, but may be seen extracellularly. Chocolate agar should be inoculated for culture. Appropriate studies should be performed to distinguish gonococcus from meningococcus.

Present recommendations by the Centers for Disease Control for the treatment of adult gonococcal ophthalmia depend on the prevalence of penicillinase-producing *N. gonorrhoeae* in a given community. Communities are defined as nonendemic, endemic, or hyperendemic depending on whether penicillinase-producing *N. gonorrhoeae* represent less than 1 percent, 1 to 3 percent, or more than 3 percent of all gonococcal isolates. In nonendemic areas, the recommended treatment is hospitalization and treatment with aqueous penicillin G, 10 million units intravenously daily, for 5 days. In endemic or hyperendemic areas, the recommended treatment is hospitalization and treatment with either 1 g of ceftriaxone (intravenous or intramuscular) or equivalent third-generation cephalosporin daily for 5 days. In both cases, topical antibiotics (aqueous penicillin drops, bacitracin, tetracycline, or tobramycin) should be administered every 2 hours. There is evidence that in the absence of corneal involvement, however, a single injection of 1 g of ceftriaxone, combined with conjunctival saline lavage, may be clinically and microbiologically curative of uncomplicated nonneonatal gonococcal conjunctivitis.

Acute Conjunctivitis

Acute conjunctivitis develops over a period of several days. The principal differential is between acute infectious conjunctivitis and acute allergic conjunctivitis. When itching, not discharge, is the most prominent symptom, allergy is by far the commonest cause. The history is usually positive for hay fever or multiple allergies. The onset may be sudden, with intense itching and severe conjunctival chemosis, or, more commonly, the onset is more insidious, with mild redness and itching. In the former case, the diagnosis is obvious. In the latter case, the patient is usually more symptomatic than the clinical appearance suggests. There are milky edema of the bulbar conjunctiva, mild conjunctival injection, a ropy mucoid discharge, and papilla on the upper tarsal conjunctiva. Treatment modalities include allergen avoidance, cool compresses, and, if necessary, an ocular astringent-decongestant-antihistamine drop (Vasocon A, Naphcon A), up to four times a day for a limited period of time. Cromolyn 4 percent can be used prophylactically in seasonally recurrent allergic conjunctivitis to reduce the reactivity of the conjunctiva to allergens.

Acute infectious conjunctivitis is classically divided into nonfollicular and follicular causes, as determined by the predominant morphologic changes in the tarsal conjunctiva. Acute nonfollicular conjunctivitis is classically of bacterial origin, while common causes of acute follicular conjunctivitis include adenovirus (pharyngoconjunctival fever, epidemic keratoconjunctivitis), herpes simplex virus (types 1 and 2), acute hemorrhagic conjunctivitis, and *Chlamydia* (inclusion conjunctivitis, trachoma). Generally, acute infectious conjunctivitis is a self-limited disorder. Delays in diagnosis of bacterial (*Moraxella, Staphylococcus aureus* blepharoconjunctivitis) or chlamydial disorders that can produce a chronic conjunctivitis will not adversely affect the ultimate prognosis. The most serious mistake that can be made in the empiric diagnosis and treatment of acute infectious conjunctivitis is the precipitation of corneal epithelial keratitis with unrecognized herpes simplex virus accompanying the use of topical steroids.

Acute bacterial conjunctivitis is most commonly caused by *S. aureus, Streptococcus pneumoniae, Haemophilus influenzae, Haemophilus aegyptius,* α- or β-hemolytic *Streptococcus,* or *Moraxella.* With the exception of the blepharoconjunctivitis associated with *S. aureus* or *Moraxella,* all are self-limited disorders that heal without complications. Acute bacterial conjunctivitis is characterized by a purulent or mucopurulent discharge with significant sticking together of the eyelids in the morning. Because these organisms are surface pathogens with low invasiveness, regional adenopathy is not seen. A prominent follicular reaction does not occur. In some cases, petechial conjunctival hemorrhages may be seen. The diagnosis is suspected by the history and physical findings and is confirmed by smears revealing a predominantly polymorphonuclear leukocyte response and the corresponding gram-stain and morphologic characteristics of the specific organism. Cultures may be helpful but are usually not necessary for appropriate treatment.

In the western world, *S. aureus* is the commonest cause of infection of the conjunctiva and lids. It causes conjunctivitis in all age groups and has no seasonal prevalence. Infection usually originates from the patient's own hands, face, or nares. In cases of acute inoculation, the conjunctivitis is self-limited and easily amenable to therapy with topical bacitracin or erythromycin ointment. In cases in which conjunctivitis and keratitis are secondary to chronic colonization of the lid margins, control and eradication are exceedingly difficult (see Chronic Conjunctivitis, below). *S. epidermidis* is part of the normal ocular flora in a majority of humans. If present in sufficient numbers, it can produce an acute conjunctivitis or chronic blepharoconjunctivitis.

S. pneumoniae is a common cause of bacterial conjunctivitis. It is seen most often in children, in northern latitudes, and in cold months. It may be found in the upper respiratory tract of healthy carriers, especially children. It produces a purulent conjunctivitis with patchy areas of subconjunctival hemorrhage. It is a self-limited infection but can be quickly eradicated with topical sulfacetamide drops or ointment, erythromycin ointment, or bacitracin ointment.

H. influenzae is a common cause of bacterial conjunctivitis in elderly, debilitated patients with chronic pulmonary disease and in children between the ages of 6 and 36 months in whom it produces a distinctive form of preseptal cellulitis in association with a moderately severe mucopurulent discharge. It is seen more commonly in warmer environments, especially in the summer months. The presentation may be hyperacute and must be differentiated from hyperacute conjunctivitis of *N. gonorrhoeae.* The infection is accompanied by systemic signs and symptoms of fever, irritability, and upper respiratory tract infection. Both the upper and lower lids may be edematous with well-demarcated areas of purple coloration. Leukocytosis is usually present. Appropriate work-up consists of conjunctival smears and cultures as well as blood cultures. Chloramphenicol drops should be administered four to six times daily. Systemic therapy with ampicillin is adequate in areas where ampicillin-resistant strains of *H. influenzae* are uncommon. If ampicillin-resistant strains are common in the area, systemic treatment with intravenous chloramphenicol has traditionally been used pending sensitivity testing. Recent evidence suggests that cefotaxime (150 mg per kilogram per day given in three divided intravenous doses) may be substituted for chloramphenicol and may eliminate the potential risk of aplastic anemia.

Numerous other bacteria may produce acute conjunctivitis. In general, all of these are self-limited, and they are important only if a concomitant bacterial keratitis is present. Therapy can be tailored on the basis of Gram-stain characteristics, with several suitable antibiotics available for both gram-positive (sodium sulfacetamide, erythromycin, bacitracin), gram-negative (gentamicin, tobramycin), and mixed or unidentified species (bacitracin-polymyxin B [Polysporin]). Combination antibiotic preparations that contain neomycin (e.g., neosporin) should be avoided because of the high incidence (10 percent) of ocular sensitivity to neomycin. Chloramphenicol drops should be reserved for infections with *H. influenzae* because of the rare reports of bone marrow toxicity from topical chloramphenicol therapy.

Adenovirus causes one of the more frequent and severe forms of follicular conjunctivitis. If the adenoviral infection is accompanied by pharyngitis and fever, it is called pharyngoconjunctival fever (PCF). Although adenovirus 3 is the most common cause of PCF, practically any of the adenoviral types can produce the syndrome. After an incubation period of 5 to 12 days, the patient experiences the onset of pharyngitis and fever, followed by the onset of conjunctivitis, usually unilateral, with preauricular adenopathy. The other eye frequently becomes involved, but to a lesser degree, several days later. The conjunctivitis runs a 7- to 16-day course, although some symptoms may linger for months. The discharge is usually watery, although there may be significant sticking of the lids upon awakening. There may be a mild keratitis, which will produce foreign body sensation and photophobia. The infectious contagious period is 10 to 14 days, but virus may be shed from the eye up to 30 days after the onset of the illness. Because of this, patients should be cautioned not to expose others to their ocular secretions. The treatment of PCF is entirely supportive. Antipyretics for fever, cool or warm compresses, and a bland antibiotic preparation such as erythromycin or bacitracin may provide comfort, especially for the associated keratitis.

Adenoviral infections may produce a particularly severe form of follicular conjunctivitis known as epidemic keratoconjunctivitis (EKC). Adenovirus type 8 is the commonest etiologic agent for EKC, but epidemics have also been reported from types 7, 19, and 37. Less than 5 percent of the general population has the antibody to adenovirus type 8, and the infection rate following exposure is high. Extensive contamination of patients by health care professionals can occur by hand-to-eye contact and instrument-to-eye contact (especially tonometers). After an incubation period of 5 to 7 days, there is an unusually uncomfortable follicular conjunctivitis with watery discharge, marked conjunctival chemosis, eyelid erythema and edema, and recurrent formation of "pseudomembranes" of the conjunctiva, which may form "casts" of the upper and lower tarsal conjunctiva. After approximately 1 week, numerous areas of superficial punctate keratitis (SPK) occur and produce foreign body sensation and photophobia. These symptoms persist for at least 1 more week, although the conjunctival symptoms may begin to ameliorate. Finally, all symptoms of conjunctival and corneal discomfort abate, but the numerous corneal subepithelial infiltrates may form and blur vision and produce might glare for weeks or months. The treatment of EKC is mostly supportive. As with PCF, the use of cool or warm compresses, combined with a bland antibiotic ointment such as erythromycin or bacitracin may produce some relief. Removal of pseudomembranes as they occur may reduce the duration and severity of the disease. Many ophthalmologists use weak topical steroids such as prednisolone acetate 0.125 percent several times daily early in the course of EKC to reduce inflammation and symptoms. There is some evidence that the use of steroids early in the course of the disease may suppress the later development of subepithelial infiltrates. Unfor-

tunately, these infiltrates may still occur or reappear when topical steroids are tapered or discontinued. Topical steroids may be required late in the course of EKC for the treatment of severe subepithelial infiltrates that significantly disturb visual acuity. Once again, tapering the steroids may be difficult, and it is preferable, if possible, to allow spontaneous resolution of the subepithelial infiltrates.

Although both forms of adenoviral conjunctivitis (PCF and EKC) are self-limited disorders, an occasional patient may end up with a chronically red and irritated eye that is poorly responsive to any form of therapy. There may be some residual glare and mildly decreased vision from persistent subepithelial infiltrates. Late canalicular obstruction may result in persistent epiphora (tearing).

Herpes simplex virus can produce a follicular conjunctivitis with or without associated vesicles on the eyelids from primary or recurrent infection. If the conjunctivitis is associated with lid vesicles, topical antiviral therapy with trifluorothymidine (Viroptic) drops every 2 hours or vidarabine ointment five times a day can be used for 5 to 10 days as prophylaxis against corneal involvement until the conjunctivitis and lid lesions resolve. More often, there are no associated lid vesicles and the clinical picture is identical to that of adenoviral conjunctivitis. Unfortunately, treatment with topical steroids in these cases will often precipitate the onset of herpetic epithelial keratitis. For this reason, it is best to try to avoid the use of topical steroids in all cases of suspected viral conjunctivitis, with the possible exception of severe epidemic keratoconjunctivitis (see above).

Acute hemorrhagic conjunctivitis (AHC) first appeared in West Africa in 1970. Since that time, many epidemics of AHC have occurred in densely populated areas of the world, including several recent outbreaks in Florida. Crowded populations with low socioeconomic status are more commonly affected. This infection by enterovirus type 70 is characterized by the sudden onset of ocular pain, itching, photophobia, eyelid edema, and watery discharge after a short incubation period (1 or 2 days). Both eyes soon become involved with a hemorrhagic, follicular conjunctivitis. Improvement in this self-limited disease occurs over a 2- to 4-day period and is virtually complete by 7 days.

In industrial countries, *Chlamydia* produces a non–self-limited form of acute follicular conjunctivitis called inclusion conjunctivitis. It affects both neonates (see Ophthalmia Neonatorum, below) and sexually active adults (see Chronic Conjunctivitis, below). In its early stages it is virtually indistinguishable from adenoviral follicular conjunctivitis. Failure to suspect and properly treat this condition leads to a persistent conjunctivitis, which rarely, if ever, is associated with the occurrence of permanent, adverse sequelae. Although rare in the United States, *Chlamydia* produces trachoma in endemic areas such as North Africa, the Middle East, and Southeast Asia. It is the most common ocular infection in the world, affecting 400 to 500 million people. Although it may produce an acute follicular conjunctivitis, its late sequelae of conjunctival and corneal scarring are responsible for its reputation as the world's leading cause of blindness.

Rare types of acute follicular conjunctivitis include Newcastle's disease, measles, mumps, vaccinia, influenza, herpes zoster, cytomegalovirus, lymphogranuloma venereum, *Rickettsia*, and psittacosis.

Chronic Conjunctivitis

Chronic conjunctivitis is defined as any conjunctivitis that has developed over a period of weeks or any acute conjunctivitis that has not responded to primary therapy. Like acute conjunctivitis, chronic conjunctivitis can be both infectious and noninfectious. Noninfectious etiologies must be seriously considered in any patient with conjunctival redness of greater than 3 weeks' duration, particularly in view of the potential seriousness of some of these conditions (e.g., cicatricial pemphigoid, chronic atopic keratoconjunctivitis, conjunctival and lid tumors). The diagnosis and management of these conditions require extensive work-up by an ophthalmologist.

Infectious causes of chronic conjunctivitis include *S. aureus*, or *S. epidermidis*, *Moraxella*, *Chlamydia trachomatis*, *Phthiris pubis*, *Molluscum contagiosum*, or Parinaud's syndrome (cat scratch disease, tularemia, or sporotrichosis). Chronic nasolacrimal obstruction may produce chronic, recurrent conjunctivitis (see below).

Blepharoconjunctivitis caused by chronic colonization of the lid margins with *S. aureus* or *S. epidermidis* is the commonest cause of chronic infectious conjunctivitis. Increased colonization of the lid margins with these organisms may be associated with aging, acne rosacea, keratoconjunctivitis sicca, atopy, ocular cicatricial pemphigoid, use of eyelid cosmetics and mascara, and immunodeficiency states. The history is of indolent conjunctivitis that is minimally responsive to topical antibiotic therapy but always recurs after cessation of therapy. Signs include crusting and greasy scaling of the lid margins, dilated meibomian gland openings, microchalazia, recurrent hordeolum, and thickened and telangiectatic lid margins. Symptoms include discharge and burning sensation that is particularly prevalent upon awakening and chronic conjunctival redness. Exotoxins produced by staphylococcal species may produce epithelial keratitis, peripheral corneal infiltration and ulceration, and angular blepharoconjunctivitis. The latter is characterized by dry, scaly flaking of the lateral canthus. Angular blepharitis can also be caused by *Moraxella*, but the scaling in this condition is classically wet and moist.

Treatment of chronic blepharoconjunctivitis is very difficult and frustrating to both the physician and patient. *Moraxella* is easier to eradicate. It is responsive to all topical antibiotic ointments and zinc. Because *Staphylococcus* species are part of the normal flora of the lid, the goal of treatment of staphylococcal blepharoconjunctivitis is to lower the bacterial cell counts below symptomatic levels and maintain them at that level. During acute exacerbations, application of bacitracin ointment to the lids two to four times a day, followed by rapid tapering, will help reduce the bacterial flora. This is further facilitated by meticulous scrubbing of the eyelashes at least twice daily with a warm, moist cloth. This regimen of lid hygiene must be continued indefinitely to reduce symptoms. Topical steroids may be required for treatment of corneal infiltrates related to staphylococcal exotoxins. Concomitant therapy includes the avoidance of eyelid makeup, use of tear substitutes for any associated keratoconjunctivitis sicca, and long-term oral tetracycline therapy if acne rosacea is present.

Inadequately treated acute chlamydial conjunctivitis (inclusion conjunctivitis) is a common cause of chronic conjunctivitis in sexually active adults. *Chlamydia trachomatis* is usually acquired from the urethral or vaginal discharge of infected sexual partners, although direct eye-to-eye transmission or contamination from nonchlorinated swimming pools is possible. Often there is a history of acute conjunctivitis that initially responded to topical therapy but never quite cleared up. The condition may be predominantly unilateral. Clinically, tarsal conjunctival follicles are prominent, especially inferiorly. There may be associated superior limbal pannus. In rare cases, there may be associated corneal involvement with superficial punctate keratitis and subepithelial infiltrates,which are indistinguishable from those of epidemic keratoconjunctivitis. A preauricular lymph node is often present. If untreated, the conjunctivitis may persist for more than 1 year. In women it may be associated with cervicitis, vaginitis, or salpingitis. In men it may produce nongonococcal urethritis. In any young, sexually active patient with conjunctivitis of greater than 3 weeks' duration, conjunctival epithelial cells should be examined with Giemsa stain for characteristic intracellular inclusions, although the incidence of false-negative results is quite high. Immunofluorescent studies with monoclonal antibodies (Micro Trak) will be positive in most cases. If the history is suggestive, the diagnosis should be considered, and treatment may be initiated even in the absence of abnormal cytology or immunofluorescent testing.

Topical therapy is inadequate in the treatment of inclusion conjunctivitis of adults. The preferred treatment is systemic tetracycline, 1 to 1.5 g orally daily in four divided doses for 3 to 4 weeks. The sexual partner should also be treated. If the patient is allergic to tetracycline, or the woman is pregnant, alternative therapy of erythromycin, 1.0 g orally daily in four divided doses, is indicated.

Trachoma, also caused by *Chlamydia trachomatis*, is the commonest ocular infection in the world but, fortunately, is rarely seen in the United States. It should be suspected in any patient who has visited or is from an endemic area and presents with chronic conjunctivitis with conjunctival and/or corneal scarring.

Phthiris pubis, the common pubic louse, can infect the eyelids and produce chronic, intensely pruritic conjunctivitis. It is easily diagnosed with the slit-lamp biomicroscope; large numbers of the transparent, blood-engorged lice can be seen attached to the lash follicles. Ocular therapy consists of mechanical removal of the lice followed by frequent treatment with any antibiotic ointment that eliminates the organisms via suffocation. Physostigmine 0.25 percent (Eserine), which was once the treatment of choice, is no longer readily available. Systemic therapy of other body hair with appropriate antilouse shampoo is indicated.

Molluscum contagiosum is a waxy, pearly white nodular lesion with an umbilicated center of viral etiology that may occur on the lid margin and produce a chronic, unilateral follicular conjunctivitis from continuous viral shedding onto the conjunctiva. The lesions may be single or multiple and are often overlooked. The patient presents with a history of chronic, unilateral redness and discharge. Findings include follicular hypertrophy of the tarsal conjunctiva, often with associated superior limbal pannus and keratitis. It may be indistinguishable from chlamydial inclusion conjunctivitis. Culture-negative cases of presumed inclusion conjunctivitis that are unresponsive to systemic tetracycline should prompt thorough reinspection of the lids and lashes for a molluscum lesion. Treatment by excision is completely curative. Topical medications are ineffective and unnecessary.

An unusual form of chronic conjunctivitis is Parinaud's syndrome. This produces a unilateral granulomatous conjunctivitis characterized by the presence of a single large conjunctival granuloma and a significantly large preauricular node. Although a variety of organisms may be associated with this syndrome, the most commonly encountered etiologies are cat scratch disease, tularemia, and sporotrichosis. Cat scratch conjunctivitis occurs 7 to 14 days after inoculation. The ocular syndrome is self-limited, with complete resolution in 2 to 3 months. This may be facilitated by excision of the conjunctival granuloma. Treatment of associated systemic symptoms and disease is the mainstay of therapy, particularly in tularemia or sporotrichosis.

Ophthalmia Neonatorum

Ophthalmia neonatorum is arbitrarily defined as inflammation of the conjunctiva in the first month of life. Passage through the birth canal exposes the neonate to all the organisms present there. In the absence of sexually transmitted disease or cervicitis, the normal endocervical canal has an average of more than five species on routine culture. Seven to 10 percent of pregnant women shed cytomegalovirus (CMV), and 12 percent are culture-positive for *Chlamydia* during the third trimester. The infection rate for CMV is fortunately low, but that of *Chlamydia* may be as high as 20 percent. Because of the severe ocular and systemic disease associated with gonococcus and herpes simplex type 2 (HSV-2), it is necessary to establish these diagnoses in pregnant women. All pregnant women should be cultured for gonococcus and, if positive, should be treated. Obstetric management of women with genital HSV infection is beyond the scope of this discussion.

Neonatal prophylaxis has significantly reduced the incidence of ophthalmia neonatorum. Chemical prophylaxis with silver nitrate has greatly reduced the incidence of neonatal gonococcal conjunctivitis, but it is ineffective against *Chlamydia*. In addition, chemical conjunctivitis may develop a few hours after instillation and lasts 24 to 36 hours. Prophylaxis with erythromycin or tetracycline ointment is used in some centers because of its additional efficacy against *Chlamydia*.

Neonatal conjunctivitis can present at any time. Although there is some correlation with the time of onset and the infectious pathogen, this should not be relied upon to establish the diagnosis. All cases of ophthalmia neonatorum should receive cytologic and microbiologic work-up.

Neonatal infection with HSV-2 is almost invariably secondary to direct exposure to an HSV-2–infected birth canal during the late prenatal period or during passage through an infected birth canal. The infant's transplacental antibodies do not seem to protect against major ocular disease, although they may prevent life-threatening visceral involvement. In almost every case, there is a vesicular eruption of the skin, which is an aid in rapid diagnosis. The skin lesions will resolve spontaneously without scarring. If there is associated conjunctivitis or the skin lesions are in close proximity to the eyes, treatment with topical trifluorothymidine drops (every 2 hours for 14 to 21 days) or vidarabine ointment (five times daily for 14 days) is indicated. The ultimate prognosis is dependent upon the presence of associated corneal, lenticular, or chorioretinal involvement. The diagnosis and management of these conditions are beyond the scope of this discussion.

N. gonorrhoeae bacterial infection produces the severest form of ophthalmia neonatorum and if untreated may result in corneal perforation. Despite a dramatic reduction with use of silver nitrate prophylaxis, its incidence is still 0.6 percent. Classically, it presents as a hyperacute conjunctivitis beginning 2 to 4 days after birth, with grossly purulent exudate, chemosis, and lid swelling. The diagnosis is established by Gram stain and appropriate cultures.

Because of the imminent threat to the integrity of the globe as well as the high rate of systemic involvement, admission to the hospital for both topical and parenteral therapy is indicated. The eye should be lavaged frequently with saline. Therapy with aqueous penicillin drops (20,000 units per milliliter), tobramycin drops or ointment, bacitracin ointment, or tetracycline ointment is equally effective but must be administered at least every 2 hours as prophylaxis against corneal invasion. If the cornea is already infiltrated at the time of diagnosis, more aggressive therapy is indicated. Parenteral therapy traditionally consists of intravenous penicillin G, 50,000 units per kilogram per day in two divided doses for 7 days. As is the case with uncomplicated adult gonococcal conjunctivitis, there is some evidence that single-dose therapy with 1 g of ceftriaxone may be curative in uncomplicated neonatal gonococcal conjunctivitis.

Chlamydia is currently the leading cause of ophthalmia neonatorum, with an incidence of 2 to 6 percent. The conjunctivitis may appear at any time within the first month, although it is most frequent between days 5 and 14. It usually presents with a mild unilateral or bilateral mucopurulent discharge. Unlike adults, neonates do not produce follicles in response to chlamydial infection. The presence of basophilic intracytoplasmic inclusions is much commoner on smear than in adults. Immunofluorescent detection of the organism with monoclonal antibodies confirms the diagnosis. Although this was once considered a benign, self-limited disorder, it is now apparent that both ocular (conjunctival scarring, pannus) and systemic (otitis media, pneumonitis) sequelae may occur in untreated or inadequately treated cases. Topical treatment is with sulfacetamide ointment or drops, tetracycline ointment, or erythromycin ointment four times daily for 3 to 4 weeks. Systemic therapy is with oral erythromycin syrup (50 mg per kilogram daily in four divided doses) for 21 days. The mother and her sexual partner should be treated as well.

Neonates are susceptible to the same entire spectrum of bacterial and viral causes of acute conjunctivitis as the adult. While *S. aureus* is the most frequent bacterial pathogen, involvement with *Pseudomonas aeruginosa*, *H. influenzae*, or other organisms is also seen. Because of the increased risk of septicemia in the neonate, all cases of presumed bacterial conjunctivitis should be cultured. Initial therapy for gram-positive organisms is erythromycin ointment four to six times daily until improvement is observed. For *H. influenzae*, erythromycin ointment or chloramphenicol drops may be used. For gram-negative organisms, gentamicin or tobramycin drops or ointments are the treatment of choice. For mixed infections or undiagnosed bacterial conjunctivitis, a combination antibiotic ointment such as polysporin (bacitracin/polymyxin) may be used. Systemic therapy is indicated for associated septicemia.

INFECTIONS OF THE EYELIDS

Infections of the eyelids may involve superficial dermis (impetigo), the subcutaneous tissue (preseptal cellulitis, erysipelas), or the meibomian or Zeis glands of the eyelid (hordeolum). Chronic staphylococcal or *Moraxella* blepharoconjunctivitis has been considered separately under Chronic Conjunctivitis.

Infections of the eyelids are their associated edema and swelling are prevented from spreading into the deeper tissues of the orbit by the presence of the orbital septum, unless its integrity has been disrupted by trauma. Spreading into the forehead or cheek is likewise contained by dense fibrous bands. The infectious process or its associated edema may spread to the other lid of the same eye and sometimes cross the bridge of the nose to involve the lids of the fellow eye.

Although infections of the preseptal structures are relatively benign, infections within the orbit (orbital cellulitis) potentially are both sight- and life-threatening. They are distinguished from preseptal infections by the presence of proptosis, restricted ocular motility, and pain on attempted extraocular movement. Furthermore, marked chemosis, reduced corneal sensation, and blurred vision may be present. The diagnosis and management of orbital cellulitis is discussed elsewhere.

Impetigo is a highly contagious, rapidly spreading, superficial primary pyoderma that is seen more commonly in children than adults and that may involve the eyelids. It begins as small red macules that rapidly progress to thin-walled vesicles that rupture, ooze, and crust. Peripheral spreading occurs, sometimes with satellite lesion formation. The conjunctiva and globe remain uninvolved. Lid swelling develops beneath the surface infection. Impetigo is caused by *S. aureus* and group A *Streptococcus pyogenes*, perhaps by mutually promoting each other's growth.

Laboratory work-up should include Gram stain and culture of the vesicle fluid. Treatment consists of oral dicloxacillin for 10 days and topical bacitracin ointment to the vesicular eruptions four times daily. Cephalexin can be substituted for dicloxacillin in penicillin-sensitive patients. Intravenous nafcillin therapy may be necessary in severely afflicted or in extremely young patients. See also the chapter *Cellulitis and Soft Tissue Infection*.

Erysipelas is a superficial form of streptococcal cellulitis that uncommonly affects the eyelids. The group A β-hemolytic streptococci gain access to the dermis via any break in the skin and incite a spreading, acute inflammatory response. The involved area is bright red, hot, tender, indurated, and well-defined. The overlying surface skin may exfoliate. Signs of systemic toxicity and orbital inflammation may be present. Microbiologic confirmation of the infection is often difficult. Needle aspiration of the lesion should not be attempted because the infection may be spread. Blood cultures may be positive for streptococci. Erysipelas of the eyelid is treated with intravenous penicillin G until there is clinical improvement, followed by oral penicillin VK for a total of 10 days.

Bacterial preseptal cellulitis usually results from trauma around the orbit. The preseptal cellulitis of *H. influenzae* is associated with acute conjunctivitis and is discussed in that section. *S. aureus* is the commonest cause of preseptal cellulitis, although any bacterial organism (aerobic or anaerobic) may be isolated. Preseptal cellulitis usually presents with tender inflammation of the eyelid with some degree of fluctuance. There may or may not be evidence of overt trauma or penetration of the skin. The patient does not appear extremely ill, nor is there any evidence of orbital cellulitis (unless the orbital septum has been penetrated).

Therapy of bacterial preseptal cellulitis includes incision and drainage (if a focal abscess exists), microbiologic work-up, and systemic antibiotics. The lid should be incised horizontally for 2 to 3 cm along the area of fluctuation and allowed to drain continuously. Depending on the severity of the infection, oral or intravenous therapy is initiated and modified on the basis of the microbiologic findings. Oral dicloxacillin or intravenous nafcillin is the mainstay of treatment for suspected *S. aureus* preseptal cellulitis. If other organisms are seen on Gram stain or are identified on culture, the appropriate antibiotics are used in full systemic dosage. If intravenous therapy is employed, oral antibiotics may be substituted when clinical improvement is sufficient. Treatment should be continued for a minimum of 7 days or until resolution of the purulent drainage. In cases of streptococcal preseptal cellulitis, 10 days of therapy are mandatory. Tetanus toxoid and tetanus immune globulin are administered if necessary.

Infections of the glands of Zeis or the meibomian glands result in a well-localized, tender, fluctuant swelling within the lid, called a hordeolum. This is usually secondary to stasis complicated by secondary infection with *S. aureus*. Depending upon the involved gland, the fluctuance may point externally (gland of Zeis) or internally (meibomian gland). Resolution may occur spontaneously or with frequent applications of warm compresses. Drainage through the tarsal conjunctiva or lid skin will result in resolution of the infection. Residual scarring of the skin or conjunctiva may result from drainage. Persistent inflammation of the meibomian or Zeis glands may result in persistence of localized, nontender granulomatous swelling (chalazion). Systemic therapy is not needed for a simple, localized hordeolum. Antibiotic prophylaxis of the conjunctiva with erythromycin or bacitracin ointment may prevent a secondary bacterial conjunctivitis.

INFECTIONS OF THE LACRIMAL SYSTEM

The lacrimal system consists of the main lacrimal gland in the upper temporal aspect of the orbit and the drainage system that permits tear flow from the conjunctival sac into the nose. The drainage system opens with the puncta,near the inner canthus of each lid, which are in communication with the canaliculi. The canaliculi course medially and join near the lacrimal sac to form a common canaliculus. The common canaliculus enters the lacrimal sac 3 to 4 mm below its domed fundus. Tears flow from the tear sac down the nasolacrimal duct to enter the nose beneath the inferior turbinate.

Dacryoadenitis is inflammation or infection of the lacrimal gland. Noninfectious causes of dacryoadenitis include Sjögren's syndrome, sarcoidosis, leukemia, lymphoma, amyloidosis, and eosinophilic granuloma. Infections of the lacrimal gland are usually viral in origin. Mumps is the most common virus causing dacryoadenitis, although measles and influenza are also seen. Treatment of viral dacryoadenitis is entirely supportive. Bacterial dacryoadenitis produces purulent swelling in the region of the lacrimal gland. Bacteria associated with dacryoadenitis include *N. gonorrhoeae*, *S. pneumoniae*, *S. aureus*, mycobacteria, and *Treponema*. If bacterial dacryoadenitis is suspected, the treatment includes incision and drainage, culture and smears of the drainage material, and appropriate systemic antibiotic therapy for the involved organism. In rare situations, parasitic infection of the lacrimal gland with *Onchocerca volvulus* may occur.

Infections of the lacrimal drainage system are almost always preceded by stasis due to obstruction within the canaliculi or lacrimal sac. There is often a chronic history of epiphora and chronic, recurrent conjunctivitis. Depending on the site of acute infection, there may be tender swelling of the canaliculi (canaliculitis) or lacrimal sac (dacryocystitis).

Isolated canaliculitis usually involves only one canaliculus. The involved canaliculus is usually swollen and tender, and the associated punctum may be swollen and enlarged ("pouting"). Most commonly it is due to *Actinomyces israelii*, an anaerobic, gram-positive, weakly acid-fast organism. The diagnosis is made by expressing the yellow-tinged concretions from the canaliculus, which on cytologic examination show gram-positive branching filaments. Treatment consists of emptying the canaliculus with external pressure on the surface of the lid with a chalazion clamp, dilatation and curettage of the canaliculus with a chalazion curette, or, rarely, with horizontal incision of the canaliculus, followed by topical sulfacetamide four times daily for 1 week. Recurrences are common, especially if evacuation of the canaliculus is incomplete. Other causes of canaliculitis are *Arachnia*

propionica (*Streptothrix*), *Streptomyces*, or fungi (*Nocardia*, *Candida albicans*, *Aspergillus niger*).

Dacryocystitis is almost always secondary to stasis and subsequent infection as a result of nasolacrimal duct obstruction. In the newborn, this obstruction may be due to membranous occlusion of the nasolacrimal duct. This results in chronic epiphora, recurrent conjunctivitis, and recurrent dacryocystitis. This can be managed supportively with warm compresses, massage of the lacrimal sac, and topical antibiotics for up to 9 months, since 70 to 90 percent of the time the nasolacrimal duct will open spontaneously, with complete relief of symptoms. If spontaneous resolution does not occur, simple nasolacrimal probing will provide a permanent cure in almost all cases.

In adults, chronic stasis may lead to chronic epiphora, followed by acute inflammation if occlusion occurs. Acute dacryocystitis presents with a red, tender, sometimes fluctuant swelling inferomedial to the eye. Reflux of mucus or pus from the puncta on massage of the sac is confirmatory evidence of dacryocystitis. Culture of this discharge most commonly reveals *S. pneumoniae* as the causative organism, although other streptococci, staphylococci, diphtheroids, *Klebsiella pneumoniae*, *H. influenzae*, *P. aeruginosa*, and *Actinomyces*, *Candida*, and other fungi have been cultured from patients with acute dacryocystitis. Treatment of acute dacryocystitis consists of oral dicloxacillin (1 g per day), topical antibiotic drops (e.g., sodium sulfacetamide four times daily) and warm compresses. This is continued until amelioration of symptoms occurs. Transcutaneous incision and drainage of the tear sac in acute dacryocystitis can temporarily improve the clinical picture. However, induced drainage produces scarring and is not curative. A permanent cure results only if normal nasolacrimal drainage is reestablished. In an initial case, probing and irrigation of the nasolacrimal system may occasionally be successful in reestablishing permanent patency. More commonly, a surgical correction of normal drainage, dacryocystorhinostomy, is required for permanent cure.

In chronically neglected cases, recurrent infections of the lacrimal sac may lead to spontaneous fistula formation between the lacrimal sac and skin. Cultures usually are positive for a variety of aerobic and anaerobic organisms. In such cases, dacryocystorhinostomy is the only procedure that affords the possibility of a permanent cure.

SUGGESTED READING

Darnell RW. Follicular conjunctivitis. In: Darnell DW, ed. Viral diseases of the eye. Philadelphia: Lea & Febiger, 1986:296.

Haimivici R, Roussel TJ. Treatment of gonococcal conjunctivitis with single dose intramuscular ceftriaxone. Am J Ophthalmol 1989; 107:511–513.

Jones DB. Microbial preseptal and orbital cellulitis. In Duane TD, ed. Clinical ophthalmology. Vol 4. Philadelphia: Harper & Row, 1982.

McCulley JP. Blepharoconjunctivitis. Int Ophthalmol Clin 1984; 24:65–77.

Sandstrom K, Bell TA, Chandler JW, et al. Microbial causes of neonatal conjunctivitis. J Pediatr 1984; 105:706.

Smolin G, Tabbara K, Whitcher J. Infectious disease of the eye. Baltimore: Williams & Wilkins, 1984.

Ullman S, Roussel TJ, Forster RK. Gonococcal keratoconjunctivitis. Surv Ophthalmol 1987; 32:199.

INFECTIOUS KERATITIS

JOHN F. STAMLER, M.D., Ph.D.
DEBORAH PAVAN LANGSTON, M.D.

The cornea is a unique tissue with the specialized functions of refraction, efficient transmission of light, and the formation of a physical barrier between the internal eye and the external environment. These functions necessitate a smooth curved surface and a structurally competent transparent tissue. Infectious keratitis, with its associated inflammation, disrupts the normal corneal architecture with scarring, thinning, vascularization, edema, cellular infiltrates, and epithelial defects, thereby threatening all three functions of the cornea. There are four main categories of infectious keratitis: bacterial, viral, fungal and protozoal (*Acanthamoeba*). A systematic and rapid approach to diagnosis and appropriate therapy is the key to preservation of vision.

DIAGNOSTIC LABORATORY INVESTIGATION

If the diagnosis of bacterial, fungal, or acanthamoebic keratitis is considered, scrapings for culture and staining must be taken prior to the institution of therapy (Table 1). Premature antibiotic treatment in the absence of adequate diagnostic tests may obviate later attempts to isolate the offending organism if initial therapy fails. Since these scrapings require an ophthalmologist, consultation early in such cases is advisable.

After topical administration of proparacaine or a similar anesthetic, with slit-lamp or loupe magnification, the edge and center of the ulcer are vigorously scraped with a Kimura spatula or Bard Parker number 15 blade. The material obtained by the scrapings is smeared onto microscope slides and placed directly onto culture media. The spatula or blade is sterilized by heat from an alcohol lamp after each scraping.

When bacterial pathogens are suspected, two slides are smeared with corneal scrapings and stained with Gram and Giemsa stains, and a third is prepared in the event more specialized stains are desired later. Although filaments and yeast may be seen on the Gram and Giemsa stains, slides for wet mount, potassium hydroxide, and/or methamine silver are prepared if fungus is suspected. Special stains for *Acanthamoeba* are calcofluor white and trichrome. The calcofluor white reacts only if the specimen is formalin-fixed. Acid-fast preparations are used if mycobacteria are suspected.

Often the clinical picture is sufficient to make the diagnosis of herpes zoster or adenoviral keratitis. A rapid diagnostic kit (Herpcheck, DuPont) for office diagnosis of herpes simplex is now available. The results of the smears are used to guide the initial therapy (Table 2).

After the smears are obtained, additional scrapings are streaked in successive rows of *C*s directly onto blood, chocolate, and Sabouraud's agar plates. Organisms are considered significant if they grow on a *C* and probable contaminants if they are located on another part of the plate. A sterile swab with either cotton or calcium alginate tip on a wooden handle is then wetted with sterile saline, rubbed on the ulcer, and then inserted to the bottom of a chopped meat broth or thioglycolate broth tube.

Blood agar will support growth by the most common gram-positive and gram-negative bacterial pathogens, and any hemolysis provides early clues for differentiation. Chocolate agar also supports most bacteria and enhances isolation of *Moraxella, Neisseria,* and *Haemophilus* species. Sabouraud agar will grow most fungi, filamentous or yeast, and may be supplemented with an antibiotic to inhibit bacterial overgrowth, but should not be supplemented with cycloheximide, which inhibits some pathogenic fungi. If Sabouraud agar is not available, a good alternative is blood agar incubated at room temperature. Cultures are taken for fungi, even when the diagnosis seems unlikely; the infiltrates in the early stages often have the clinical appearance of a bacterial ulcer. The meat broth or thioglycolate will support

TABLE 1 Initial Work-up of a Corneal Ulcer

Suspected Pathogen	Stains	Culture Media
Bacteria	Gram, Giemsa	Blood, chocolate, meat broth, thioglycolate
Neisseria	Gram, Giemsa	Thayer-Martin in high CO$_2$
Fungus	Wet mount, KOH, methamine-sliver	Sabouraud
Acanthamoeba	Calcofluor white, trichrome	*E. coli*-layered non-nutrient
Mycobacteria	Acid-fast	Lowenstein-Jensen
Herpes simplex	Herpcheck	Cell culture
Adenovirus	No diagnostic stain	Cell culture
Herpes zoster/ herpes varicella	Giemsa	Cell culture

TABLE 2 Initial Antibiotic Therapy for Infectious Keratitis

Smear Results	Antibiotic Drugs (in Order of Preference)
No organisms or gram-positive or -negative bacteria other than *Pseudomonas*	Cefazolin 133 mg/ml* q1h *and* tobramycin 14 mg/ml* q1h
Pseudomonas	Cefazolin 133 mg/ml q1h, tobramycin 14 mg/ml q1h, *and* ticarcillin 6 mg/ml q1h
Filamentous fungi	Natamycin 50 mg/ml q1h *or* miconazole 10 mg/ml q1h
Yeast	Flucytosine 1% q1h
Acanthamoeba	Propamidine 0.1%† q1h, miconazole 10 mg/ml q1h, neomycin-polymyxin B-gramicidin q1h
Infectious herpes (positive Herpcheck)	Trifluridine 1% 9 doses/day, vidarabine 3% ointment 5 doses/day

* Prepared by hospital pharmacy from systemic drug.
† Not FDA approved; available over the counter in England as Brolene.

anaerobic bacterial growth. *Acanthamoeba* is cultured on *Escherichia coli*–layered non-nutrient agar. The live trophozite produces tracks in the bacteria. A positive culture can then be confirmed with the appropriate stains. Herpes simplex, varicella, and adenovirus can be cultured if special cell culture facilities are available.

BACTERIAL KERATITIS

Clinical Findings

Bacterial keratitis is usually characterized by pain, photophobia, mucopurulent discharge, and decreased visual acuity. Accompanying signs are conjunctival injection, white stromal infiltration, epithelial defect (ulcer), anterior chamber inflammation, and in severe cases, hypopyon. Epithelial defects are most easily detected with rose bengal or fluorescein stain.

Bacterial keratitis often follows trauma, contact lens abuse, chronic steroid dosing, or chronic underlying disease such as corneal herpes. The site of infection is usually single and round with distinct edges, often with surrounding stromal edema. The signs and symptoms tend to progress rapidly over hours or days depending on the organism. Gram-negative bacteria such as *Pseudomonas* or *Neisseria* are known for rapid progression over hours, whereas gram-positive bacterial infections tend to progress more slowly over 1 to 2 days. The most frequent etiologic agents are the gram-positive *Staphylococcus* and *Streptococcus* and the gram-negative *Pseudomonas, Moraxella,* and *Proteus,* but virtually any organism may infect the cornea, hence the need for a broad variety of cultures.

Therapy

Antibiotics are initiated immediately after the examination of the smears. The choice of initial agents is guided by the smear results (Table 2). If no organisms or gram-positive bacteria are seen, the topical fortified antibiotics cefazolin (133 mg per milliliter) and tobramycin (14 mg per milliliter) are both given hourly, alternating on the half hour. If *Pseudomonas* is suspected, hourly ticarcillin (6 mg per milliliter) is added. This regimen usually necessitates hospitalization to ensure compliance. The clinical response or culture-sensitivity testing may lead to a change in antibiotics. The concentrations of other commonly used antibiotics are listed in Table 3. Topical fortified antibiotics deliver high drug levels to the cornea and have proved effective in experimental and clinical bacterial infections.

Subconjunctival injections can also provide high drug levels to the cornea and are recommended by some. However, subconjunctival injections also have the disadvantage of producing pain and anxiety in many patients. Furthermore, repeated injections scar the conjunctiva and risk intraocular infection. For these reasons, we limit the use of subconjunctival injections to those cases in which the administration of hourly drops is not feasible. Systemic antibacterial agents are not used because they do not supply significant additional drug to the cornea. Cycloplegia (e.g., 0.25 percent scopolamine twice daily) combats synechia formation and relieves the pain of ciliary spasm.

TABLE 3 Doses of Topical Fortified Antibiotics for Corneal Ulcers

Antibiotic	Topical Dose
Bacitracin	5,000 U/ml
Cefamandole	133 mg/ml
Cefazolin	133 mg/ml
Carbenicillin	4 mg/ml
Chloramphenicol	5 mg/ml
Gentamicin	14 mg/ml
Natamycin	50 mg/ml
Ticarcillin	6 mg/ml
Tobramycin	14 mg/ml
Vancomycin	25–50 mg/ml

The epithelial defect, infiltrate, and anterior chamber reaction are measured at least daily. If the ulcer improves during the first 48 hours, the antibiotic frequency is reduced to every 2 hours. If an organism is cultured, the least-sensitive antibiotic is discontinued. As the ulcer improves, the schedule is reduced by one-half each 24 to 48 hours until the dosage interval reaches every 6 hours. At this point the dose of cefazolin can be reduced to 33 mg per milliliter and tobramycin to 3 mg per milliliter (commercial drops) and continued until the cornea is fully healed.

If worsening or no improvement is noted at 48 hours and the cultures are negative, the ulcer is recultured and/or biopsied. Often fungal or acanthamoebic infections are misdiagnosed as bacterial ulcers and only correctly diagnosed later after failing to respond to antibiotic therapy.

The use of steroids in the treatment of bacterial ulcers is controversial. Topical steroids may decrease the inflammation and thus reduce corneal scarring. However, the inflammation may also help to eradicate the infection. Only when the ulcer is central, is associated with significant inflammation, and has received 4 to 5 days of intensive antibiotic treatment and showed clinical improvement do we consider adding a small amount of topical steroid (0.125 percent prednisolone once or twice daily). Pseudomonal ulcers are generally not treated with steroids because of possible persistence of live organisms even weeks after initiation of appropriate antibiotic therapy. If steroids are used, the cornea needs to be monitored closely for signs of thinning or recurrence of the infection. Persistent epithelial defects may remain after the ulcer is sterilized and are treated as discussed in the section on neurotrophic ulcers.

Intraocular surgery on an infected cornea carries the risk of endophthalmitis and a greater than normal risk of graft rejection. Visual rehabilitation may require corneal transplantation, but every effort is made to sterilize the cornea first. However, corneal perforation or progressive infection may require emergency penetrating keratoplasty to preserve the eye.

FUNGAL KERATITIS

Clinical Findings

Fungal corneal ulcers differ from bacterial ulcers in that they tend to be elevated and gray, have a feathery, less-discrete edge, and possibly have small separate satellite lesions. Fun-

TABLE 4 Antiviral Drugs and Dosages

Drug	Concentration	Frequency
Trifluridine	1.0%	q1–2h 9 times/day × 14 days
Idoxuridine ointment	0.5%	5 times/day × 14 days
Idoxuridine drops	0.1%	q1h days, q4h nights × 14 days
Vidarabine ointment	3.0%	5 times/day × 14 days

gal ulcers also tend to produce less purulent discharge than do bacterial ulcers. However, the distinction cannot be made on clinical grounds alone. All suspected fungal and bacterial ulcers are scraped and cultured for both.

Fungal keratitis is more common in southern and tropical areas than in northern climates, but is not as common as bacterial keratitis in any area. The most frequent pathogens are the nonpigmented filamentous fungi *Fusarium* and *Aspergillus*. Also seen are the brown-pigmented filamentous fungi such as *Curvularia* and yeasts such as *Candida albicans*.

Therapy

The three extensively used types of antifungals are the polyenes (amphotericin B, natamycin), imidazoles (miconazole, ketoconazole), and pyrimidines (flucytosine). The polyenes function by binding to ergosterol, the major sterol moiety in fungal cell membranes. They bridge the cell membrane and allow ionic fluxes, creating intracellular ionic imbalances and cell death. The imidazoles interfere with ergosterol synthesis and bind to cell membrane fatty acids. These effects cause the cell membrane to become leaky, thus destroying the organism. Flucytosine enters the fungal cell and is deaminated by a fungal enzyme to fluorouracil. This uracil analogue is incorporated into the fungal RNA, making it dysfunctional and causing inhibition of protein synthesis and cell death. The polyenes and imidazoles are relatively insoluble in water and thus have limited penetration into the cornea. Flucytosine is water soluble and penetrates well.

Amphotericin B has been the most used topical antifungal drug for corneal infections and is highly effective. However, natamycin (commonly pimaricin) is less irritating, has better penetration into the cornea and has a better spectrum of action against the most common fungal pathogens, particularly *Fusarium*. Topical natamycin is given hourly in a 50 mg per milliliter (5 percent) solution. Miconazole is also active against filamentous fungi, especially *Aspergillus*. Miconazole, in a 10 mg per milliliter (1 percent) solution is given topically every 1 to 2 hours or subconjunctivally in 10-mg doses. Flucytosine has the best antimicrobial action against yeast. It is given in a 1 percent solution topically, beginning with hourly doses, and can be given orally, although careful adjustment of serum concentrations is required. Therefore, our first choice for filamentous fungi is natamycin and flucytosine for yeast.

Other topical antifungal agents that can be used if the particular sensitivities or clinical picture (for example, if the

infection does not respond to treatment or if the patient is allergic to the initial therapy) dictate are hourly topical drops of amphotericin B 0.1 to 0.3 percent, nystatin 50,000 units per milliliter, and ketoconazole 10 to 20 mg per milliliter. As in bacterial keratitis, the infection is monitored closely and the therapy is tapered according to the clinical improvement and altered according to the cultures if the clinical response is not satisfactory. Cycloplegia is maintained by twice-daily drops of 0.25 percent scopolamine. Steroids tend to enhance the growth of fungi and thus are avoided if there is still viable fungus in the cornea.

Surgical intervention is the exception in cases of keratomycosis. However, a significant number of cases are too advanced at the start of treatment or have resistant organisms and medical therapy is inadequate. Penetrating keratoplasty is the surgical treatment of choice for these cases. Ideally, the surgery should excise all of the infected cornea, necessitating surgical intervention before the fungus spreads to the limbus.

VIRAL KERATITIS

Herpes Simplex Keratitis

Herpes simplex virus (HSV) is the most ubiquitous infectious virus in humans. It becomes latent primarily in neurons and can reactivate periodically, causing recurrent disease throughout the lifetime of an individual. Approximately 500,000 cases of HSV keratitis are reported in the United States annually, making HSV the leading infectious cause of blindness in the United States. The types of HSV keratitis can be divided into infectious epithelial, trophic ulceration, and immune stromal keratitis. These may occur separately or in any combination.

Infectious Epithelial Keratitis

Clinical Findings. The hallmark of infectious epithelial HSV keratitis is the dendritic ulcer. This branching epithelial defect stains with rose bengal or fluorescein and has a discrete edge. Occasionally, the dendrite becomes large and forms a geographic pattern. There is usually scant inflammation or discomfort at this stage; however, irritation, photophobia, tearing, and conjunctival injection are often present.

Therapy. Treatment usually begins with gentle debridement of the loosely attached infected cells with a cotton-tipped applicator. This may reduce the load of virus and reduce the antigen-induced inflammation. This is followed by topical antiviral therapy (Table 4).

There are several antiviral drugs that have demonstrated efficacy in the treatment of HSV keratitis. They include idoxuridine, vidarabine, trifluridine, and acyclovir. Trifluridine and idoxuridine are thymidine analogues that are incorporated into viral DNA and inhibit viral enzymes. Vidarabine inhibits DNA polymerase and is incorporated to some extent into viral DNA. Acyclovir is phosphorylated by a herpesvirus-specific thymidine kinase, but not by host cells. The phosphorylated drug is a potent inhibitor of viral DNA polymerase, but is relatively inactive against host enzymes. Topical acyclovir (3 percent ointment) appears to be as effective as idoxuridine or vidarabine. However, it is not yet commercially available in this country for topical ophthalmic use. Of the three available drugs, all are effective clinically; trifluridine is probably slightly superior and is our first choice. They are all moderately toxic to the corneal epithelium and cannot be used in high doses for long periods of time. Topical steroids promote HSV infections and are strictly contraindicated in infectious HSV keratitis.

Noninfectious (Trophic) Herpetic Epithelial Ulceration

Clinical Findings. The epithelium may not fully heal after a herpesvirus infection, or it may break down again once it has healed despite adequate antiviral therapy, thus producing a chronic sterile (trophic) ulceration. As opposed to infected dendrites, trophic ulcers are ovoid, have a smooth, rolled edge of epithelium, and are relatively stable in their configuration. Persistence of the epithelial defect can lead to bacterial infection and/or stromal melting.

Therapy. Therapy is aimed at promoting reepithelialization. Initial treatment is lubrication with antibiotic ointment and patching. Bandage soft contact lenses with frequent artificial tears and twice daily topical antibiotics help promote epithelial healing. Severe cases often respond to tissue adhesive cyanoacrylate glue (not FDA approved for ocular use) in the bed of the ulcer covered with a bandage lens. Topical medroxyprogesterone (1 percent Provera) (not FDA approved for ocular use) four times daily may also help reepithelialization by reducing underlying stromal inflammation without enhancing the danger of stromal thinning. Provera is used when trophic ulcers are accompanied by mild inflammation.

Lateral or medial tarsorrhaphy can help protect the ocular surface and promote epithelial healing. Conjunctival flap is a treatment held in use for eyes with ulcers that do not respond to medical treatment. Corneal transplantation is reserved for frank or impending corneal perforation if tissue adhesive has failed or is not available and to rehabilitate eyes that have had conjunctival flaps or significant scarring.

Stromal Immune Disciform, Interstitial Herpetic Keratitis, and Immune Rings

These forms of keratitis are the result of an immune reaction to the residual viral antigens that are left in the stroma after multiple active infections. This reaction is characterized by focal or diffuse areas of stromal edema with or without necrosis. Keratitic precipitates may be present on the endothelium. Severe cases have diffuse stromal and epithelial edema with Descemet's folds, neovascularization, dense white infiltrates, and iritis.

Immune HSV keratitis is usually responsive to topical steroid treatment. However, once started, it may be difficult to taper without a flare of inflammation. Therefore, steroids should be used only in severe cases or if the visual axis is threatened. If steroids such as 1 percent prednisolone are used more than once or twice daily, concomitant antiviral coverage should be used three (ointment) to five (drops) times daily. If the epithelium is not intact, topical steroids should be minimized or stopped and oral prednisone (20 to 30 mg daily for 7 to 10 days) may be used if needed to reduce significant intraocular inflammation (iritis). Topical antibiotics should be added when there is an epithelial defect as prophylaxis against bacterial superinfection. Cycloplegia (0.25 percent scopolamine twice daily) helps to reduce the iritis, prevent synechia, and reduce ciliary spasm. In some cases active viral dendrogeographic infection occurs during active disciform keratitis. If live virus is thought to be present, initiation of antiviral treatment should precede the use of steroids by 1 to 2 days.

Penetrating keratoplasty (corneal transplant) plays a role in the rehabilitation of eyes plagued by interstitial or disciform HSV keratitis. Penetrating keratoplasty has a high rate of success if the operation is performed on an uninflamed eye with sparse neovascularization and high-dose topical steroid treatment follows the surgery. Corneal transplantation not only can restore a clear cornea but will also reduce the antigenic load in the eye and thus decrease the frequency of inflammatory episodes.

Herpes Zoster (Varicella-Zoster Virus) Keratitis

Clinical Findings

The primary infection with herpes zoster virus (HZV) usually occurs during childhood as chickenpox. The virus, like HSV, gains access to the sensory ganglia and may remain latent within the ganglion during the life of the individual or may reactivate at any time. A reactivation, usually through the immunosuppression of age or disease, produces an active viral infection that travels along the nerve to the end organ. If the first division of the fifth cranial nerve is involved, any ocular structure may be affected. The corneal manifestations of HZV keratitis include punctate epithelial staining, pseudodendritic epithelial defects, stromal infiltrates, endotheliitis, disciform keratitis, and neurotrophic and exposure keratitis.

Therapy

A role for topical antiviral medication has not been established. Uncontrolled studies have suggested a possible benefit from the use of topical acyclovir, which is not commercially available in the United States. However, oral acyclovir (600 mg orally five times daily) does appear to speed resolution of the active infection and reduce the inflammation if started within 72 hours of disease onset.

Topical steroids are useful in suppressing the ocular inflammation of HZV keratitis. However, the patient who is started on topical steroids is committed to a long course. Late flare-ups are common and are treated by increasing the dose again. Therefore, tapering of the dose must be slow and gradual. Furthermore, steroids can promote stromal melting and inhibit epithelial growth. Since these eyes are also prone to neurotrophic ulcers and exposure, the lowest amount of topical steroid needed is the best amount to use.

Systemic steroids are used to help prevent postherpetic neuralgia. Oral prednisone 40 to 60 mg per day alternating within 10 to 14 days of disease onset and tapered over 4 weeks probably reduces the risk of postherpetic neuralgia (the lower dose and shorter course are used for elderly or small individuals). However, it may also increase the risk of disseminated zoster. Because of this risk, oral steroids are avoided in immunocompromised patients.

Cimetidine is a histamine-blocking drug used extensively to treat peptic ulcer disease. This drug appears to relieve the early symptoms of pain, itching, and erythema that accompany the vesicular skin eruptions of HZV. The dose is 300 mg orally four times daily for 4 to 6 days (duration depends on the symptoms) and probably needs to be started in the first 72 hours to have a significant effect.

Other medical therapy includes topical antibiotics for an epithelial defect, cycloplegia for iritis, and analgesics for neuralgia. Artificial tears and ointment may be used for lubrication if there is evidence of exposure. Amitriptyline, 40 to 80 mg orally daily is preferred, or Triavil, 2 to 10 mg orally four times daily, may provide symptomatic relief from postherpetic neuralgia. The neuralgia itself tends to self-resolve over a several-month period.

Lateral and/or medial tarsorrhaphy can be used to protect the cornea from exposure and to help prevent or heal neurotrophic ulcers in anesthetic eyes. Conjunctival flaps will help stabilize chronically inflamed, ulcerated eyes. Penetrating keratoplasty has a low rate of success in eyes scarred from HZV. The transplanted corneas are prone to ulceration, bacterial infection, rejection, and melting. Any anterior segment surgery, such as corneal transplantation or cataract extraction, is best postponed for at least 3 years after active inflammation has subsided.

Adenovirus

Clinical Findings

Adenovirus ocular infections generally present two clinical syndromes: epidemic keratoconjunctivitis (EKC) and pharyngeal conjunctival fever (PCF). EKC is most often caused by serotypes 8 and 19, but also 2 through 4, 7 through 11, 14, 16, and 29 have been reported. As the name implies, EKC is quite contagious and is generally spread by direct contact. Contaminated instruments and fingers of medical personnel are major fomites, as are person-to-person contact and swimming pool water.

EKC starts with a sudden onset of watery discharge, foreign body sensation, and variable photophobia. Enlarged and tender preauricular lymph nodes and a follicular conjunctival reaction are hallmarks of the syndrome. Punctate keratitis, conjunctival hemorrhages, and a mild iritis may be present. During the second or third week of symptoms, the typical subepithelial round infiltrates develop.

Therapy

Therapy is primarily symptomatic or aimed at preventing the spread of the disease. Hand washing and sterilization of instruments are vital preventative measures. Some symptomatic relief can be provided by cold compresses, analgesics, and artificial tears. Topical antibiotics and antiviral agents are of no value unless there is concomitant herpetic or bacterial infection. If the subepithelial infiltrates are in the visual axis and are symptomatic, topical steroids can

reduce their size and improve acuity. Therapy is started with 1 percent prednisolone four times daily and tapered to a minimal dose as dictated by the symptoms.

PCF is most frequently caused by adenovirus serotypes 3, 4, and 7. The syndrome consists of acute follicular conjunctivitis with injection, watery discharge, pharyngitis, fever, and regional lymphadenitis. It is spread by aerosolized water droplets or direct contact. The disease is self-limited and requires no specific treatment for the conjunctivitis. The fever and pharyngitis can be treated symptomatically with oral antipyretics and analgesics.

ACANTHAMOEBIC KERATITIS

Infectious keratitis from the protozoan *Acanthamoeba* is one of the most feared corneal infections. Medical cure has been reported, but is presently the exception rather than the rule. The frequency of recognized cases is increasing, but fortunately this infection is still uncommon.

Clinical Findings

Acanthamoeba causes an indolent keratitis that is typically unilateral and is associated with minor trauma, soft contact lens wear, and/or exposure to soil or standing water. Most infections can be traced to contaminated contact lens solutions, such as homemade saline solution. Early in the infection the epithelium may be irregular, but essentially intact, with dendritiform perineural infiltrates. Pain is usually more prominent than with other forms of infectious keratitis and is out of proportion to the degree of inflammation. Later in the disease, iritis, scleritis, epithelial erosion, and the characteristic ring infiltrate develop. The most reliable prevention is to use commercially prepared contact lens solutions, which are discarded after 2 weeks, and to heat and disinfect soft contact lenses daily.

Therapy

Most reported cases of acanthamoebic keratitis have come to penetrating keratoplasty. However, with earlier diagnosis and prompt institution of appropriate medical therapy, more medical cures should result. The antimicrobial agents that are amebecidal in vitro and are used clinically are neomycin, polymyxin B, natamycin, miconazole, and propamidine. Propamidine isethionate (Brolene) is not available in the United States but is available over the counter in England as a 0.1 percent solution, and dibromopropamidine, as a 0.15 percent ointment. Neomycin and polymyxin B are marketed in combination with gramicidin as Neosporin. Miconazole and natamycin are produced in 10 and 50 mg per milliliter solutions, respectively.

Treatment begins by the gentle removal of the infected epithelium with a Kimura spatula. This is thought to reduce the infectious and immunologic load of *Acanthamoeba* and allow better penetration of drugs into the stroma. After debridement, hourly propamidine 1 percent, miconazole 10 mg per milliliter, and Neosporin are initiated. The drugs are tapered according to the clinical response, but treatment generally lasts for at least a year, once- to twice-daily drops.

Additionally, cycloplegia (0.25 percent scopolamine twice daily) and topical steroids are used to control inflammation. Oral nonsteroidal antiinflammatory agents and codeine are used for pain relief. If medical treatment is unable to control the progressive ulceration or if stromal melting progresses, penetrating keratoplasty is indicated. A large graft is used to maximize the chances of encompassing all of the organisms. Medical treatment should be continued after surgery and tapered slowly.

SUGGESTED READING

Duane TD, ed. Clinical ophthalmology. Vol 4, chapters 7, 18, 19, 21, 26. Hagerstown, MD: Harper & Row, 1987.
Pavan-Langston D, ed. Manual of ocular diagnosis and therapy. 2nd ed. Boston: Little, Brown, 1985:65.
Smolin G, Thoft RA, eds. The cornea. In: Scientific foundations and clinical practice. Boston: Little, Brown, 1987:193.

TRACHOMA

MOHSEN ZIAI, M.D.

Trachoma is the leading cause of blindness throughout the world. It is estimated that 400 million individuals suffer from this disease. The overwhelming majority of affected persons live in endemic areas of Southeast Asia, the Middle East, and Africa, where environmental and personal standards of hygiene are suboptimal and where virtually every child under 2 years of age is affected.

The infection produces a chronic form of conjunctivitis with bacterial superinfections that lead to scarring if the cycle is not broken. These conjunctival scars result in trichiasis and entropion with consequent damage to the cornea causing ulcerations, opacity, and loss of vision.

The causative agent of trachoma is *Chlamydia trachomatis*, and in endemic areas the disease is associated with the serotypes A, B, and Ba, in contrast to other serotypes causing inclusion conjunctivitis and urethritis in nonendemic areas. The mode of transmission is eye-to-eye spread by contaminated hands or objects. In the uncomplicated form the disease has a relatively self-limited natural history and eventual recovery is expected. Initial symptoms consist of photophobia and lacrimation, with a clear or purulent discharge. The course of the disease is chronic, and even in the absence of reinfection there are frequently remissions and exacerbations.

In the early stages a chronic follicular conjunctivitis is observed, manifested by follicles on the upper tarsal plate and papillary hypertrophy as well as by inflammatory infiltration of the conjunctiva of varying degrees. Linear scars follow, and if they are severe they may lead to tear deficiency syndromes, dacryostenosis, and trichiasis with entropion which usually affects the upper lid, causing corneal ulceration and scarring. The vascular pannus (neovascularization) is superficial, more marked in the area of the superior limbus. Other forms of scars as well as inflammatory processes are found in chronic cases.

In the United States the disease is seen mainly in Mexican Americans and American Indians as well as some other minorities. Older individuals who have lived in the area known formerly as the Trachoma Belt of Oklahoma and Texas may manifest recurrences of the disease, with some active infection found in their children.

The diagnostic features of the disease are its insidious onset, the presence of upper tarsal follicles, limbal follicles, corneal infiltration, and scars. In addition, one can observe vascular pannus developing early over the cornea, where epithelial keratitis and marginal infiltrates are also seen. Laboratory diagnosis of trachoma in the initial stages can be made by direct immunofluorescence or Giemsa stain of conjunctival scrapings as well as by detection of tear micro-IF antibody or isolation of the organism in tissue culture.

Treatment of trachoma must be considered in the context of two separate objectives. First and foremost is the organization of campaigns for the control of the disease or at least prevention of blindness. Second is the treatment of individual patients with the best possible method, notwithstanding the usual obstacles encountered in campaigns and public health efforts directed at the masses.

In mass treatment campaigns systemic use of antimicrobials often results in serious complications. Sulfonamide drugs, although effective against trachoma, are associated with undesirable side effects, particularly allergic skin and systemic reactions. The use of tetracyclines is risky for children as well as pregnant or lactating women. The expense involved in the use of rifampin and certain serious side effects associated with the use of some forms of erythromycin are examples of difficulties that could be encountered with the use of systemic drugs in such campaigns. Therefore, the procedure of choice in these mass treatment campaigns is to emphasize the promotion of hygiene as well as prolonged use of topical antimicrobials in the form of ointments. For the latter purpose ointments of either 1 percent tetracycline or 1 percent erythromycin are reasonable choices. I recommend the intermittent administration of the drug topically for 5 consecutive days every month for 6 months or periodic community-wide treatment (5 days per week for 6 weeks). In case sensitivity or superinfection by resistant organisms develops, the drug should be discontinued. Effective vaccines against trachoma are not available.

As far as the treatment of individual patients is concerned, it must be remembered that systemic use of antimicrobials is preferable, as topical treatment will usually not eradicate the organism even though it may greatly improve the signs of infection. I recommend any of the three drugs: tetracyclines, 2 g per day in four divided doses for adults (this drug is not recommended for children); sulfonamides, for example, sulfisoxazole, 6 g per day in four divided doses for adults, 150 mg per kilogram per day for children in four divided doses; or erythromycin, for example erythromycin ethyl succinate, 30 mg per kilogram per day in four divided doses for children, 2 g per day in four divided doses for adults. Effective treatment of the disease and eradication of the organisms require 3 weeks of systemic drug administration. Clinical improvement may not become apparent for 2 weeks or more after the initiation of systemic therapy. The patient should be under supervision and the necessary precautions concerning the side effects should be kept in mind. In infants and young children erythromycin is probably preferable to sulfonamides.

Trichiasis and cicatricial entropion resulting from chronic trachoma can be treated surgically. Cryotherapy is useful in certain cases. When corneal damage is occurring, corrective therapy must be considered a matter of emergency.

SUGGESTED READING

Dawson CR, Schachter J. Strategies for treatment and control of blinding trachoma: cost effectiveness of topical vs. systemic antibiotics. Rev Infect Dis 1985; 7:768–773.

Maybey DCW, Robertson JN, Ward ME. Detection of chlamydial trachomatis by enzyme immunoassay in patients with trachoma. Lancet 1987; 2:1491–1492.

CARDIOVASCULAR AND RELATED INFECTIONS

INFECTIVE ENDOCARDITIS AND MYCOTIC ANEURYSM

C. FORDHAM VON REYN, M.D.

Optimal management of native valve infective endocarditis (IE) is a multistep process beginning with selection of an appropriate antimicrobial agent and continuing through posttreatment evaluation and counseling (Table 1). Most patients require 4 weeks of intravenous antibiotic therapy, and at least 2 of these weeks of treatment should be under observation in a hospital. Consultation with both an infectious disease specialist and a cardiologist is advisable, and reliable microbiologic support (in-house or reference laboratory) is essential. Patients with congestive heart failure complicating IE should be evaluated by a cardiac surgeon and are generally treated where valve replacement can be performed promptly if necessary. With proper management, overall mortality from infective endocarditis should be 15 percent or less.

SELECTION OF APPROPRIATE ANTIMICROBIAL AGENT(S)

General

The most common organisms causing infective endocarditis are viridans streptococci, enterococci, and *Staphylococcus aureus*. In most cases, antibiotic therapy will ultimately be directed against a specific organism isolated from blood cultures. However, the physician may be required to select an antibiotic before the diagnosis of IE is established, before the infecting organism is identified, or when blood cultures remain negative but IE is suspected. Treatment guidelines will first be offered for specific organisms and then for initial or empiric therapy.

Successful treatment of IE requires sustained serum levels of bactericidal antibiotics, generally 4 weeks of parenteral therapy. Single agents are used against some organisms, but if synergistic combinations are available, two drugs are often used for at least part of the course (Tables 2 to 5).

TABLE 1 Steps in the Management of Infective Endocarditis

Select appropriate antimicrobial agent(s)

Monitor antimicrobial efficacy
    Blood cultures
    Serum antibiotic level
    Serum bactericidal level

Monitor for development of complications
    Cardiac dysfunction requiring valve replacement
    Extracardiac suppurative foci requiring drainage

Monitor for antimicrobial adverse effects

Provide posttreatment evaluation and counseling

Such combinations are recommended for patients with organisms that are difficult to eradicate (e.g., nutritionally deficient viridans streptococci or penicillin-tolerant strains). Congestive heart failure or suppurative foci of infection (e.g., myocardial abscess, extracardiac visceral abscesses, mycotic aneurysms) also are best treated with a combination. More than 4 weeks of treatment may be necessary in patients who have suppurative complications and/or require cardiac surgery.

Except for β-hemolytic streptococci, minimum inhibitory concentrations (MICs) and/or minimum bactericidal concentrations (MBCs) should be determined for all organisms. Since antibiotic adverse effects often necessitate selection of an alternative drug, MICs should be determined for two or more drugs at the outset. The following antibiotics should be tested: (1) viridans streptococci—penicillin, vancomycin, cefazolin, ceftriaxone, and gentamicin; (2) enterococci—gentamicin and vancomycin; (3) *S. aureus*—penicillin, oxacillin, cefazolin and vancomycin; (4) gram-negative bacteria—ampicillin, gentamicin, ceftriaxone, and chloramphenicol.

Several regimens are effective in treating IE caused by penicillin-sensitive streptococci (Table 2). The most potent regimen is intravenous penicillin for 4 weeks plus gentamicin for the first 2 weeks (regimen A). This combination is standard for any patient with complicated IE and for most hospitalized patients. Since gentamicin is given for its synergistic effect, the dosing is lower than in serious gram-negative bacillary infection, and toxicity is less common. Nevertheless, gentamicin can be omitted for uncomplicated

254

TABLE 2 Antibiotic Treatment of IE Due to Penicillin-Sensitive Streptococci

Standard (4 wk) regimen

Most patients treated in the hospital should receive this regimen. It should always be used in those with complicating factors, including congestive heart failure, prolonged endocarditis (≥ 3 mo), mycotic aneurysm and other extracardiac foci of infection, nutritionally deficient viridans streptococci, penicillin-tolerant streptococci, or history of long-term penicillin prophylaxis

Penicillin G	4×10^6 U IV q4h $\times$ 4 wk
	and
Gentamicin	1 mg/kg IV q8h (first 2 wk)

Penicillin alone (4 wk) regimen

May be used in patients at special risk for gentamicin toxicity (age 65 yr, underlying renal insufficiency or 8th cranial nerve damage) who do not have complicating factors (see above).

Penicillin	4×10^6 U IV q4h

Penicillin allergic (4 wk) regimen

Convenient and suitable for completing IV treatment in a home setting. Vancomycin should be used if the patient has had an anaphylactic reaction to penicillin.

Ceftriaxone	2 g IV q12h
	or
Vancomycin	1 g IV q12h

Penicillin-sensitive streptococci include viridans streptococci (e.g., *S. sanguis, S. mitior, S. mutans*), β-hemolytic streptococci, *Streptococcus bovis*, and other streptococci with penicillin MIC of ≤ 0.1 μg/ml.

TABLE 4 Antibiotic Treatment of IE Due to Staphylococci

S. aureus (penicillin-sensitive)
  Penicillin G 4×10^6 U IV q4h $\times$ 4 wk*
    plus
  Gentamicin 1 mg/kg IV q8h (first week only)
S. aureus (methicillin-sensitive)
  Nafcillin 2 g IV q4h $\times$ 4 wk*
    plus
  Gentamicin 1 mg/kg IV q8h (first week only)
S. aureus (methicillin-resistant or patient penicillin-allergic)
  Vancomycin 1 g IV q12h $\times$ 4 wk*
S. epidermidis (4–6 wk)
  Vancomycin 1 g IV q12h
    plus
  Gentamicin 1 mg/kg IV q8h
    plus
  Rifampin 300 mg PO q8h

* 4 wk sufficient for patients who respond within 1 wk; 6 wk recommended if course is complicated by fever or bacteremia >1 wk, metastatic *S. aureus* infection, or need for valve replacement.

dose gentamicin during the first week is recommended for its synergistic activity against *S. aureus*. Patients with staphylococcal IE are particularly at risk for metastatic suppurative infections requiring surgical drainage and antibiotic treatment for up to 6 weeks. Even in the absence of documented complications, patients with delayed response to therapy (as evidenced by bacteremia or fever beyond 1 week) should also receive 6 or more weeks of antibiotic therapy. The management of prosthetic valve endocarditis due to coagulase-negative staphylococci is discussed elsewhere (see the chapter *Prosthetic Valve Endocarditis*).

Antibiotic regimens for treating other less common organisms should be based on the MIC for the isolate (Table 5). If MICs are not available (e.g., fastidious organism), an attempt should be made to determine a serum bactericidal level (see later). Therapy for these organisms should generally be continued for 4 weeks (see exceptions in footnotes to Table 5).

Initial Treatment and Treatment of Culture-Negative IE

Antibiotics often must be started on the basis of organism morphology, before final identification is available. When gram-positive cocci are reported, the combination of vancomycin, 1 g intravenously every 12 hours, and gentamicin, 1 mg per kilogram intravenously every 8 hours, will offer initial coverage for viridans streptococci, staphylococci, and enterococci. When gram-negative rods are reported, ampicillin, 2 g intravenously every 4 hours, and gentamicin, 1.5 mg per kilogram intravenously every 8 hours, will provide initial coverage for most organisms.

Antibiotics may sometimes need to be initiated as soon as blood cultures are obtained. Prompt empiric treatment is recommended when IE is suspected and the patient is toxic or is in frank septic shock or congestive heart failure. In these situations, vancomycin and gentamicin should be started to cover the three most common organisms (viridans streptococci, enterococci, and staphylococci).

cases in patients considered at significant risk for aminoglycoside toxicity; in this situation, penicillin is given alone (regimen B). Regimen C offers two alternatives for patients who are allergic to penicillin. These regimens may also be used to treat (or complete treatment) at home for patients with uncomplicated IE.

Enterococci (*Enterococcus faecalis* and *Enterococcus faecium* [formerly *Streptococcus faecalis* and *S. faecium*]) and penicillin-resistant streptococci (MIC >0.1 μg per milliliter) must be treated with a synergistic combination of two drugs for 4 weeks (Table 3). Penicillin has been chosen over ampicillin because of its reduced risk of hypersensitivity reactions, especially delayed maculopapular rashes.

The choice of antibiotics for IE due to staphylococci (*S. aureus, S. epidermidis*) is determined by the sensitivities of the infecting organism (Table 4). The addition of low-

TABLE 3 Antibiotic Treatment of IE Due to Enterococci and Penicillin-Resistant Streptococci

Regimen	Comments
Standard (4 wk)	
Penicillin 4×10^6 U IV q4h	
plus	Both drugs must be given for 4 wk
Gentamicin 1 mg/kg IV q8h	
Penicillin-allergic (4 wk)	
Vancomycin 1 g IV q12h	This combination may have an increased risk of nephrotoxicity; renal function should be monitored carefully.
plus	
Gentamicin 1 mg/kg IV q8h	

Penicillin MIC of >0.1 μg/ml.

TABLE 5   Antibiotic Treatment of IE: Other Organisms

Organism	Regimen
Haemophilus species	Ampicillin 2 g IV q4h *and* Gentamicin 1 mg/kg IV q8h
Actinobacillus *actinomycetemcomitans*	Ampicillin 2 g IV q4h *and* Gentamicin 1 mg/kg IV q8h
Cardiobacterium hominis	Ampicillin 2 g IV q4h *and* Gentamicin 1 mg/kg IV q8h
Eikenella corrodens	Ampicillin 2 g IV q4h *and* Gentamicin 1 mg/kg IV q8h
Kingella kingii	Ampicillin 2 g IV q4h *and* Gentamicin 1 mg/kg IV q8h
Brucella species	Doxycycline 100 mg PO b.i.d. *and* Gentamicin 1.5 mg/kg IV q8h
*Coxiella burnetii**	Doxycycline 100 mg PO b.i.d. *and* Trimethoprim 160 mg/sulfa- methoxazole 800 mg PO b.i.d.
Diphtheroids	Vancomycin 1 g IV q12h
E. coli	Cefazolin 1 g IV q8h *and* Gentamicin 1.5 mg/kg IV q8h
Serratia marcescens†	Amikacin 7.5 mg/kg IV q12h *and* Piperacillin 2 g IV q4h
Pseudomonas aeruginosa†	Tobramycin 1.5 mg/kg IV q8h *and* Piperacillin 2 g IV q4h
Bacteroides fragilis	Metronidazole 7.5 mg/kg IV q6h
Fungi	Amphotericin B 0.7 mg/kg IV qd *and* 5-flucytosine 35 mg/kg PO q6h

* Treatment may need to be continued for 1 yr; valve replacement may be required.
† Treatment requires ≥6 wk of therapy and valve replacement.

Culture-negative endocarditis (CNE) may be due to partial treatment of sensitive organisms such as viridans streptococci or fastidious gram-negative organisms such as the HACEK group (organisms 1 to 5 in Table 5). Combined treatment with ampicillin and gentamicin (as in Table 5) offers coverage of these possible etiologies. *S. aureus* is not covered with this regimen for CNE, so if antistaphylococcal coverage was given prior to blood cultures or if the history suggests a possible primary site of staphylococcal infection, nafcillin (or vancomycin) and gentamicin should be chosen (as in Table 4). Organisms 6 to 8 in Table 5 may also cause CNE and should be covered with the indicated regimen if the organism is suspected on the basis of epidemiology or serology.

MONITORING ANTIMICROBIAL EFFICACY

Since clinical expression of antibiotic failure may be insidious or delayed in recognition, an attempt should be made to determine whether the chosen antibiotic regimen and dose are producing bactericidal serum levels against the isolated organism. This is generally not necessary for evaluation of treatment of penicillin-sensitive streptococcal IE where standard regimens have a high success rate, but should be considered for all other organisms. Efficacy is determined by blood cultures while the patient is receiving treatment and by either comparing serum antibiotic levels to the MBC of the organism or determining a serum bactericidal titer (SBT).

Blood cultures should be repeated during the first few days after antibiotic treatment is instituted. Two blood samples should be obtained for culture at least 30 minutes apart at the expected trough antibiotic level. With penicillin-sensitive streptococcal IE, repeat blood cultures should be negative after 1 or 2 days of therapy. With *S. aureus* IE, blood cultures should become negative at approximately 1 week. With enterococcal IE and other organisms, blood cultures should become negative within a few days up to a week. Bacteremia that persists beyond the expected interval or fever that persists beyond 1 week suggests an inadequate antibiotic regimen, extensive infection of the valve ring, a metastatic focus of infection, or drug fever.

Bactericidal activity in serum should be assessed on the second day of treatment or on the second day after a significant change in dose or antibiotic. When the patient is receiving a single antibiotic and an MBC of the chosen antibiotic is available, bactericidal activity can be assessed by obtaining a peak serum level of the antibiotic. The peak serum level should be adjusted to a level four to eight times higher than the MBC (but not in excess of toxic levels, e.g., 10 to 12 μg per milliliter for gentamicin).

When a peak SBT is used to assess bactericidal activity, serum factors such as complement become part of the test system and enhance the apparent activity of the antibiotic. Thus, the SBT may provide a more biologic measure of antibacterial activity in vivo than the ratio of serum antibiotic level to MBC. The SBT will be the only feasible test of bactericidal activity when an MBC is unavailable and is the most practical test when multiple antibiotics are employed. A peak SBT of 1:8 or greater is advisable. The antibiotic dose should be raised or the drug(s) changed if the SBT is 1:8 or less and the patient is not responding clinically.

MONITORING FOR DEVELOPMENT OF COMPLICATIONS

Cardiac Dysfunction Requiring Valve Replacement

Approximately 20 to 30 percent of patients with active IE will require valve replacement (or debridement). All patients with IE should be seen by a cardiologist or a cardiac surgeon for a baseline evaluation. Indications for cardiac surgery in native valve IE are given in Table 6. Significant valvular incompetence in IE requires valve excision and replacement with a prosthesis. Obstruction from a vegetation requires debridement. Excision without replacement with a prosthesis may be successful when valvular complications occur in right-sided endocarditis. Bacteremia and fever that persist beyond a week and are not due to mycotic aneurysm or other extracardiac suppurative focus and can-

TABLE 6 Indications for Cardiac Surgery in IE

Congestive heart failure due to valvular insufficiency or obstruction

Persistent bacteremia

Myocardial abscess

Fungal endocarditis

Systemic emboli (see text)

not be eradicated with modification of the antibiotic regimen are other indications for valve replacement. Myocardial abscess cannot be confirmed without surgery but should be suspected in the patient with fever persisting beyond 1 week and/or with conduction defects; surgical drainage is required for cure. Fungal IE and some gram-negative bacillary IE requires valve excision for cure (see Table 5).

Indications for valve replacement in the face of systemic embolization are controversial. Surgery should be considered in the patient with two or more systemic emboli and a persistent vegetation by echocardiogram. The benefits and risks of surgery should be reviewed in patients with a single embolus.

Extracardiac Suppurative Foci Requiring Drainage

Embolization may result in extracardiac suppurative foci, including abscesses in brain, spleen, liver muscle, and soft tissue. Parenchymal abscesses are suggested by prolonged fever plus signs and symptoms in the affected organ and are usually documented by computed tomography. Surgical drainage is indicated if macroscopic abscesses fail to resolve on antibiotic therapy.

MONITORING FOR ANTIMICROBIAL SIDE EFFECTS

Prolonged parenteral antibiotic therapy is frequently complicated by drug hypersensitivity and other adverse effects. As a result, as many as 30 percent of patients will require a change in antibiotic during treatment for IE. Patients should be questioned and examined on a regular basis for evidence of antibiotic side effects. With some drugs, serum levels should be obtained to ensure that toxic concentrations are not exceeded. Standing orders are often advisable to follow for laboratory evidence of drug toxicity (Table 7).

POSTTREATMENT EVALUATION AND COUNSELING

After completion of therapy, the patient should be evaluated to confirm cure. Two blood cultures should be obtained 3 to 7 days after antibiotics have been discontinued. Positive cultures for the original organism confirm the need for retreatment, usually with valve replacement. Cardiac evaluation should assess whether complications such as valvular insufficiency require further intervention. Patients with *Streptococcus bovis* IE should have barium studies or endoscopy of the entire gastrointestinal tract to exclude underlying tumor or other bowel pathology. Finally, all patients should be con-

sidered at risk for subsequent episodes of IE and should be given the standard American Heart Association guidelines for antibiotic prophylaxis during potentially bacteremic procedures.

MYCOTIC ANEURYSM

Infection of an artery with associated aneurysmal dilation of the vessel is known as mycotic aneurysm (MA). In the preantibiotic era, most cases of MA were the result of emboli in patients with underlying infective endocarditis (embolomycotic aneurysm). In recent years, as many as 50 percent of cases have other causes. These include bacteremic seeding of preexisting aneurysms, infection of traumatic pseudoaneurysms, and spread of contiguous foci of infection.

Mycotic aneurysm complicates approximately 5 to 10 percent of cases of IE. MA may be responsible for persistent fever in IE and may rupture or cause symptoms from

TABLE 7 Monitoring for Adverse Effects of Antibiotics

Antibiotic	Major Side Effects	Standing Orders (frequency)
Penicillin Ampicillin	Neutropenia Hepatitis Interstitial nephritis	Complete blood count (2 ×/wk) Chemistry profile (1 ×/wk) Urinalysis (1 ×/wk)
Nafcillin	Phlebitis (see penicillin)	(see penicillin)
Piperacillin	(see penicillin)	(see penicillin)
Cefazolin Ceftriaxone	Neutropenia Interstitial nephritis Phlebitis	(see penicillin) (see penicillin)
Amikacin Gentamicin Tobramycin	Ototoxicity Nephrotoxicity	Peak and trough levels (1 ×/wk) Creatinine (3 ×/wk) Audiogram (1 ×/wk)
Vancomycin	Ototoxicity Nephrotoxicity	Peak and trough levels (1 ×/wk) Creatinine (3 ×/wk) Audiogram (1 ×/wk)
Erythromycin	Phlebitis Nausea/vomiting	None
Rifampin	Hepatitis	None*
Trimethoprim-sulfamethoxazole	Cytopenia Hemolytic anemia	Complete blood count (2 ×/wk)
Doxycycline	Gastrointestinal symptoms	None
Metronidazole	Antabuse effect Neurologic reactions	None
Amphotericin B	Renal insufficiency Hypokalemia	Creatinine (3 ×/wk) Potassium (1 ×/wk)
5-Fluorocytosine	Cytopenia	CBC (1 ×/wk)

Hypersensitivity and pseudomembranous colitis are possibilities for all drugs listed.

* Question for symptoms of hepatitis.

progressive enlargement. As many as 80 percent of MAs are multiple, and many are asymptomatic. A ruptured MA may be the presenting feature of IE, but the peak incidence is 2 to 3 weeks after diagnosis, and symptomatic lesions may develop as late as 6 months after treatment. Because of their frequency, multiplicity, and potential for serious consequences, MAs should be sought with angiography in patients with IE who have suggestive focal symptoms, persistent fever, or one or more clinically apparent emboli.

The site of MA in patients with IE is cerebral in 50 percent and extracerebral in 50 percent (especially extremities, but also visceral and ascending aorta). Infecting organisms have a distribution similiar to that for all cases of IE, with a slight increase in frequency of *S. aureus*.

In MA complicating IE, antibiotic treatment is the same as for the underlying IE, but treatment should be extended to at least 6 weeks for all organisms. As an embolic event, MA becomes a factor in the decision to proceed with valve replacement in active infective endocarditis (see above). Intracranial aneurysm requires surgery for expansion or hemorrhage. Surgical management of asymptomatic cranial MA depends on the size and location of the aneurysm since small lesions may resolve with antibiotic therapy alone. Symptomatic extracranial aneurysm should also be managed with surgical excision. When revascularization is necessary, an autogenous graft is preferred, but a prosthesis may be required (and should be placed in an extra-anatomic location). Early removal of peripheral emboli will help prevent the development of mycotic aneurysms. Anticoagulation is contraindicated in cerebral mycotic aneurysm and has no proven value in other sites.

Other MAs (those not associated with IE) occur in various settings. In men over age 50 years with underlying vascular disease, bacteremic seeding of the abdominal aorta occurs with *Salmonella* species and with *Escherichia coli*. Intravenous drug abusers develop brachial or femoral infected pseudoaneurysms due to *S. aureus* at injection sites. Other

types of trauma (e.g., penetrating injuries) and contiguous infection (e.g., cervical cellulitis, vertebral osteomyelitis) may cause MA with various organisms.

When MA occurs in the absence of IE, antibiotic therapy should be given for 6 weeks and should be based on sensitivity results. For *S. aureus*, treatment is with nafcillin (2 g intravenously every 4 hours). For *E. coli*, treatment should combine gentamicin (1.5 mg per kilogram intravenously every 8 hours) with either ampicillin (1 g intravenously every 4 hours) or cefazolin (1 g intravenously every 8 hours). For *Salmonella*, sensitive strains should be treated with ampicillin (1 to 2 g intravenously every 4 hours), chloramphenicol (12.5 mg per kilogram intravenously every 6 hours), or trimethoprim-sulfamethoxazole (3.5 mg of TMP per kilogram intravenously every 8 hours). Surgical excision is always indicated, following the same principles for revascularization as for MA with IE.

Acknowledgment. The author wishes to thank Robert Arbeit, M.D., for reviewing the manuscript and Pauline Carter for secretarial assistance.

SUGGESTED READING

Dean RH, Meacham PW, Weaver FA, et al. Mycotic embolism and embolomycotic aneurysms: neglected lessons of the past. Ann Surg 1986; 204:300–307.
Douglas A, Moore-Gillon J, Eykyn S. Fever during treatment of infective endocarditis. Lancet 1986; 1:1341–1343.
Enzler MJ, Rouse MS, Henry NK, Geraci JE, Wilson WR. In vitro and in vivo studies of streptomycin-resistant, penicillin-susceptible streptococci from patients with infective endocarditis. J Infect Dis 1987; 155:954–958.
Sande MA, Kaye D, Root RK, eds. Endocarditis. New York: Churchill Livingstone, 1984.
Tuazon CU, Gill V, Gill F. Streptococcal endocarditis: single vs. combination antibiotic therapy and role of various species. Rev Infect Dis 1986; 8:54–60.
Wilson SE, et al, eds. Vascular surgery: principles and practices. New York: McGraw-Hill, 1987.

PROSTHETIC VALVE ENDOCARDITIS

PHILLIP I. LERNER, M.D.

The burgeoning use of prosthetic heart valves over the past quarter century produced an important new disease of medical progress, prosthetic valve endocarditis (PVE), a devastating complication estimated to follow 1 to 4 percent of all such operations. The unique characteristics of PVE demand recognition if the incidence, morbidity, and mortality of this infection are to be controlled. At major medical centers with active cardiac surgical programs, PVE currently accounts for 15 to 30 percent of all cases of endocarditis. Mortality rates ranged from 50 to 60 percent during the period 1965 through 1975. Although more recent experiences offer some encouragement, overall case-fatality rates remain discouragingly high, particularly for certain organisms. During the past 15 years, both the risk of infection and the types of infecting organisms have changed consequent to improved surgical techniques and equipment, a better understanding and application of antibiotic prophylaxis, and increased use of bioprosthetic devices (combining cloth-covered supporting struts with homologous or heterologous tissue, especially porcine valves) as opposed to completely mechanical valves.

INCIDENCE

Early PVE originally designated infections beginning within 60 days of surgery; in *late PVE*, endocarditis developed more than 60 days after valve insertion. Sixty days was chosen arbitrarily in the hope of separating those infections related to the operation from those not related to surgery and/or the immediate postoperative period. A recent modification, proposed by investigators at the Massachusetts General Hospital, argues for 12 months as the preferred breakpoint for defining nosocomial (early onset) PVE because of the very high incidence of methicillin resistance among coagulase-negative staphylococci isolated from patients with PVE in the first 12 months after surgery (approximately 85 percent), when compared to an incidence of only 22 percent methicillin resistance among coagulase-negative staphylococcal strains causing PVE beyond the first postoperative year. The spectrum of infecting organisms was similar throughout the first 12 months after surgery (Table 1), an observation suggesting that these cases probably share a similar pathogenesis and that the methicillin-resistant coagulase-negative staphylococci (MRCNS) may be a marker for hospital acquisition of strains, and, thus, in turn, a marker for nosocomial infection. The attack rate of early PVE was considerably higher before 1969 (2.5 percent), compared with an average risk of 0.75 percent among reports published during 1969 through 1976. Before 1975 there were few good prospective studies of the risk of late PVE, which is now appreciated to be a time-related event, with a greater risk in the early months after surgery and a lower risk thereafter. Early estimates of the incidence of PVE overlooked the time-related nature of this infection and often failed to appreciate the importance of the comprehensiveness and duration of the follow-up.

Since 1975, prospective studies have provided a more detailed and accurate picture. A prospective analysis of 1,465 consecutive valve replacement survivors at the University of Alabama Medical Center (January 1975 through July 1979) found the cumulative actuarial risk per person to be 3.0 percent at 12 months and 4.1 percent at 48 months. The risk for PVE was greatest at 5 weeks but subsequently declined to a stable level 12 months after operation. Original surgery

for native valve endocarditis (NVE) resulted in a fivefold incremental risk for subsequent PVE, whether the NVE was active or inactive at the time of valve replacement. PVE following NVE usually became evident within the first 6 months after surgery; organisms causing PVE in patients operated on for NVE were often different from those that caused the NVE. Black race was a risk factor (fourfold increment), and male gender doubled the risk, the latter also being more important in the first few months after surgery. Patients with a mechanical prosthesis had a threefold higher risk of PVE, especially in the early months after operation, than did persons with bioprostheses. There was no higher risk of PVE associated with aortic valve prostheses compared with mitral valve replacements. Thirty-four (64 percent) of the 53 patients with PVE died; most deaths occurred within 3 months of the onset of PVE.

An equally detailed analysis of risk factors for the development of PVE among 2,642 patients undergoing initial valve replacement at the Massachusetts General Hospital from 1975 through 1982 confirmed many of the findings in the Alabama survey; PVE developed in 116 patients (4.4 percent), with an actuarial risk for PVE of 3.1 percent at 12 months and 5.7 percent at 60 months (mean length of follow-up, 39.8 months). These investigators also found no overall difference between infection rates in patients with aortic and mitral prostheses and confirmed the higher early risk of PVE in recipients of mechanical prostheses vs. porcine prostheses ($p = .02$) in the first 3 months after surgery, but they uncovered a higher risk for porcine valve recipients 12 months or more after surgery ($p = .04$), although there was no significant difference in the cumulative risk of PVE by 5 years of follow-up between mechanical and porcine valve recipients. The Boston study confirmed that older patients had a higher risk of late PVE after multiple ($p = .04$) or mitral ($p = .08$) valve replacement but not after aortic valve replacement. Recipients of multiple valves

TABLE 1 Bacteriology of Prosthetic Valve Endocarditis

| | Onset Following Surgery | | | |
| | Cases Prior to 1975* | | Cases 1975–1983† | |
	<2 months	>2 months	<12 months	>12 months
Coagulase-negative staphylococci‡	41	36	41	10
S. aureus	30	22	5	5
Gram-negative bacilli; coccobacilli§	30	19§	4§	8§
Streptococci (viridans and other nonenterococci)	9	41	1	11
Enterococci	6	14	2	4
Pneumococci	2	0	0	1
Diphtheroids	12	6	4	1
Fungi	18	9	4	1
Others and mixed#	—	—	5	1
Culture-negative	3	7	6	2
Total	151	154	72	44

* From Karchmer AW, Swartz MN. Infective endocarditis in patients with prosthetic heart valves. In: Kaplan EL, Taranta AV, eds. Infective endocarditis. American Heart Association Symposium monograph no. 52. Dallas: American Heart Association, 1977.

† Calderwood SB, Swinski LA, Karchmer AW, et al. Prosthetic valve endocarditis. J Thorac Cardiovasc Surg 1986; 92:776–783; with permission.

‡ Mostly *S. epidermidis*.

§ Includes fastidious gram-negative coccobacilli (HACEK; see text).

Includes two patients infected with coagulase-negative staphylococci plus a second organism.

had a higher risk of PVE than single valves ($p = .01$). Male gender was a risk factor for PVE on aortic prostheses in the 12 months after surgery ($p = .008$) but not thereafter, but gender did not influence the risk of infection on mitral valve prostheses.

MICROBIOLOGY

Microorganisms responsible for PVE differ considerably from those producing NVE, with clear-cut differences in the relative importance of certain pathogens in early and late PVE whether one uses the 2-month or the 12-month breakpoint for this designation (Table 1). *Staphylococcus epidermidis* is the single most common organism in both groups, accounting for 30 to 40 percent of all cases; in NVE, it is responsible only 1 to 3 percent of the time. Rarely, other coagulase-negative staphylococci are involved in PVE. *Staphylococcus aureus* is no longer a dominant organism, probably because of proper use of prophylactic antibiotics, but the case-fatality rate remains high. Streptococci currently cause few early infections. Gram-negative bacilli and fastidious gram-negative bacilli and coccobacilli, infrequent pathogens in NVE, account for 5 to 20 percent of early and 12 to 18 percent of late PVE cases. Case-fatality rates are high, especially in early PVE. The range of enteric and nonfermentative gram-negative bacilli associated with PVE is extensive and includes *Escherichia coli*, *Klebsiella* species, *Enterobacter* species, *Proteus* species, *Pseudomonas* species, *Serratia* species, and the *Mima/Herellea/Acinetobacter* complex. Increasingly, especially in late PVE, fastidious gram-negative coccobacilli, the so-called HACEK group (*Haemophilus* species, *Actinobacillus actinomycetemcomitans*, *Cardiobacterium hominis*, *Eikenella corrodens*, and *Kingella* species), are responsible, in addition to occasional anaerobic rods, such as *Bacteroides fragilis*.

Fungal PVE is not uncommon and is consistently associated with a poor prognosis. Early diagnosis may be difficult, due to minimal or nonspecific signs and symptoms; embolic events often herald the diagnosis and fungemia may be intermittent, with delayed growth in routine blood cultures not uncommon. *Candida* species are the most common isolates, followed by *Aspergillus* species, but *Histoplasma capsulatum*, *Cryptococcus neoformans*, *Mucorales*, and even saprophytes such as *Penicillium*, *Curvularia*, *Phialophora*, and *Paecilomyces* have been reported. *Trichosporon* species, normally strict cutaneous commensals or superficial pathogens, also on occasion attack prosthetic heart valves.

Contaminated gluteraldehyde-fixed porcine prostheses caused several cases of PVE with *Mycobacterium chelonei*. Other mycobacteria, *Corynebacterium diphtheriae*, *Listeria*, *Lactobacillus*, *Nocardia*, *Brucella*, *Neisseria*, *Rickettsia*, *Chlamydia*, and *Mycoplasma* have been implicated. Culture-negative cases account for 5 to 15 percent of cases in large series, particularly in patients recently exposed to antibiotics or in those with fungal PVE. The lysis centrifugation technique (DuPont Isolator system) may be more productive than conventional blood cultures (e.g., BACTEC system) for recovering fungi. Nutritionally variant (pyridoxal-dependent) streptococci may not grow in routine culture media. A deliberate search for *Legionella* species (*L. pneumophila* and *L. dumoffii*, nosocomially acquired) uncovered seven cases of late (3 to 19 months) PVE at Stanford University Medical Center since 1982; special culture methods directed at recovery of these organisms from blood cultures or valves at reoperation should not be neglected. *Legionella* species or other organisms with special growth requirements must be responsible for cases of unquestionable PVE with negative bacteriologic findings reported not uncommonly from a number of centers.

PATHOGENESIS AND DIAGNOSIS

It now seems evident that PVE developing in the first year after prosthetic valve surgery commonly derives from persistent and prolonged colonization with weakly pathogenic, perioperatively acquired organisms, probably suppressed by prophylactic and/or postoperative antibiotics. Small-colony variants, metabolically dormant and relatively immune to host defenses, may play a role in the prolonged, dormant course that often characterizes *S. epidermidis* PVE. Excluding *S. epidermidis* and the emerging occurrence of the HACEK group, the microbiology of late PVE beyond the first year increasingly resembles that seen in subacute NVE, with a predominance of streptococci, presumably from the transient bacteremias associated with dental, genitourinary, or gastrointestinal sources.

Cultures of valve prostheses and native cardiac tissues obtained during surgery often (70 percent) yield skin organisms (*S. epidermidis*, diphtheroids); the same bacteria may also be found in blood from the heart-lung machine and extracorporeal circulation and even from air in the operating room. Perioperative and postoperative sources of infection include arterial lines, intravenous catheters, cardiac pacing wires, chest tubes, urethral catheters, and endotracheal tubes—all vital but invasive elements in the intensive care setting. Pneumonia and/or an infected pleural space, sternal/mediastinal wound infections, phlebitis, urinary infections, and infected decubiti add to the risk of bacteremia in this vulnerable period.

The signs and symptoms of early PVE are neither sensitive nor specific, and the occurrence of fever and leukocytosis in the immediate postoperative period provokes a lengthy differential diagnosis. Splinter hemorrhages are of little diagnostic value in early PVE, as they occur commonly in uninfected patients following cardiopulmonary bypass. Pulmonary emboli and the postpericardiotomy syndrome readily mimic infectious complications. Some patients develop a febrile mononucleosis-like illness (postperfusion syndrome) 4 to 6 weeks after surgery, probably due to blood transfusions that transmit cytomegalovirus, or rarely Epstein-Barr virus.

Although bacteremia is its hallmark, fortunately not all early bacteremias in prosthetic valve recipients result in PVE. Some patients, in the early postoperative period, have obvious extracardiac sources of bacteremia without signs of endocarditis; provided that no such signs develop during treatment, such patients can be managed with short (2 to 3 weeks) courses of antibiotic therapy. Others have persistent bacteremia (often with gram-negative organisms) even after elimination of the extracardiac sources of infection. Bacteremia that persists for 24 or more hours suggests PVE when there is no proven extracardiac source or after extracardiac sources have been eliminated. Bacteremia associated with murmurs of prosthetic incompetence or stenosis, evidence of excessive or abnormal prosthetic motion, systemic embolization (particularly to large vessels), and new or progressive atrioventricular or bundle branch conduction disturbances usually poses no diagnostic problem.

Splenomegaly is often absent in early PVE, and 40 percent of patients may have a normal white blood cell count. Petechiae, particularly conjunctival, are the most common peripheral manifestations of PVE and occur in 30 to 60 percent of patients. Roth's spots, Osler nodes, and Janeway lesions, common peripheral stigmata of subacute NVE, are more likely to be found in late PVE than in early PVE. Anemia, microscopic hematuria, and an elevated erythrocyte sedimentation rate are useful findings, although obviously much less so in the early postoperative period; increased concentrations of circulating immune complexes may offer additional support to the diagnosis of PVE, regardless of the timing. Systemic emboli to the central nervous system, kidneys, spleen, and major peripheral vessels occur in 7 to 28 percent of patients, and splenomegaly occurs in approximately one-third of later cases.

Daily auscultation of the heart is essential to detect new or changing murmurs (particularly those of a regurgitant nature), changes in valve sounds in patients with a mechanical prosthesis, and the appearance of new sounds such as gallops or friction rubs. In contrast to NVE, where infection is usually confined primarily to the valve leaflet(s), PVE more commonly occurs at the interface of the sewing ring of the prosthesis and the valve annulus, with extension to adjacent cardiac tissues occurring in up to 60 percent of cases, and frank intraseptal aortic root or myocardial abscess, in almost 40 percent of cases. The murmurs of mitral and/or aortic insufficiency often indicate paravalvular leaks from dehiscence of the seat of the prosthesis from the periannular tissue. The absence of a regurgitant murmur unfortunately does not exclude the presence of a paravalvular leak. Infections primarily involving the central structures of the mechanical valve (i.e., the disk or ball) produce obstruction and thus muffle or obliterate the prosthetic heart sounds or cause other new or unusual murmurs.

Purulent pericarditis occurs in approximately 10 percent of autopsy cases (more commonly in staphylococcal infections); mycotic aneurysms and diffuse myocarditis are less common complications. In patients with aortic valve PVE, pulse pressure changes usually herald important developments; narrowing of the pulse pressure may accompany worsening heart failure or signal valve obstruction or thrombosis due to vegetations. Serial electrocardiograms may detect heart block or other arrhythmias, indicating conduction system involvement by an intraseptal abscess extending from paravalvular infection. New murmurs or congestive heart failure also can result purely from mechanical complications, such as tears along the annular suture line, without PVE. Beyond the first several months, the clinical and laboratory features of PVE more closely resemble the picture of NVE.

Late PVE caused by *S. epidermidis* may be indolent, with few classic signs. Valve dysfunction, arrhythmia, or a major embolus may be the first clue. Not all blood cultures yield the organism, and it may be difficult to differentiate infection from contamination. *S. epidermidis* PVE with annulus involvement or valve dehiscence or obstruction is more likely to involve a methicillin-resistant organism and will require surgery for cure. Uncomplicated cases more nearly resemble NVE with this organism: a higher percentage of methicillin-sensitive organisms and a 55 percent cure rate with antibiotics alone.

Early reports suggested that infection involving porcine bioprosthetic valves was usually confined to the central leaflets and was not notably invasive; subsequent experiences document invasion of paravalvular tissues in up to 50 percent of such cases, particularly when infection begins during the initial postoperative year, less so when porcine PVE begins more than a year after valve implantation. Occasionally, the tissue leaflets themselves are destroyed by the infection, producing significant valvular incompetence.

M-mode echocardiography is not always useful in the diagnosis of PVE, since intense echoes generated by mechanical prostheses can distort images and subtle changes indicative of a vegetation or abnormal valve motion. Two-dimensional studies are more helpful in detecting vegetations, documenting prosthetic dehiscence and paravalvular leaks and abscesses (aortic root, annular or intramyocardial), and assessing left ventricular function. Cinefluoroscopy may demonstrate abnormal rocking motion of the valve from disruption of the suture line, but unless a vegetation is demonstrated, it is difficult to distinguish infectious complications from purely mechanical difficulties. Finding decreased excursion of radiopaque elements of the prosthetic valve may suggest invasion by clot or vegetation, whereas excessive rocking motion may signal an aortic root or annular abscess. Cardiac catheterization and angiography have also been employed to assess prosthetic function and left ventricular performance, detect dysfunction of a second valve, examine the coronary circulation, and detect fistulae, aneurysms, and/or filling defects. Although there is some concern about dislodging thrombi and vegetations at the time of catheterization and angiography in patients with PVE, the risk is extremely small. Whether patients with PVE should have preoperative cardiac catheterization and angiography is a matter of some debate, despite its reported relative safety. Angiography is less sensitive than echocardiography for identifying vegetations. Currently, cross-sectional echocardiography provides an excellent method for visualizing intracardiac masses and vegetations, assessing valvular and myocardial status, and even detecting sinus of Valsalva aneurysms, fistulae, and aortic ring abscesses, although it is less helpful in detecting a myocardial abscess. Intraoperative (epicardial) echocardiography, performed just prior to cardiopulmonary bypass, may offer yet a further dimension to this technique in the preoperative assessment of PVE patients.

ANTIMICROBIAL THERAPY

The same principles guiding successful antimicrobial treatment of NVE pertain, including the use of parenteral bactericidal antibiotics, singly or in combination, given over extended periods. Precise in vitro susceptibility testing of the infecting organism (including studies for possible synergy) and assessment of the in vivo effectiveness of the antibiotics selected (serum bactericidal levels) are, with a few exceptions, essential. Most patients with PVE receive at least 6 weeks of antibiotic therapy, but infection with more virulent or resistant organisms occasionally extends treatment to 8 weeks.

Withholding antimicrobial therapy pending isolation and identification of an etiologic agent in a suspected case of PVE can pose a therapeutic dilemma. The clinical status of the patient will dictate the degree of urgency regarding the initiation of therapy, but since the range of pathogens is so great in the presence of an intravascular foreign body, every effort must be made to recover and identify the infecting organism before initiating therapy to insure optimal antimicrobial treatment and monitoring. When signs and symptoms suggest acute PVE, especially in the early postoperative period, empiric therapy (as described below for culture-negative PVE) should be instituted immediately after a series of blood samples is drawn. Likewise, when the patient is critically ill with congestive heart failure secondary to a recent onset of valvular insufficiency or a paravalvular leak with suspected valve ring abscesses, immediate empiric antimicrobial therapy is necessary. When the history suggests a more indolent process without evidence of hemodynamic deterioration, antibiotics may be withheld for 24 to 48 hours, either pending recovery of an organism from the blood cultures or simply to provide a longer antibiotic-free interval to obtain multiple blood samples for subsequent incubation. In the early postoperative period, when prophylactic or other antibiotics (employed for the treatment of specific extracardiac infections) are being used, blood samples should also be inoculated into culture media containing antibiotic-binding resins. Organisms normally considered contaminants, such as S. epidermidis, Micrococcus, and diphtheroids, should raise one's suspicion for PVE and always prompt the drawing of multiple additional samples for culture. Diphtheroids and other fastidious bacteria often do not provoke a high-grade bacteremia; consequently not all blood cultures will be positive, and many days may elapse before a blood culture is recognized as positive.

A combination of vancomycin, gentamicin, and ampicillin usually initiates presumptive treatment for suspected or culture-negative PVE. Ampicillin (2 g intravenously every 4 hours) is included because of the increasingly prominent role of fastidious gram-negative coccobacilli (HACEK group). Doses for vancomycin and gentamicin are similar to those given for proven S. aureus PVE (see below). Blood cultures are often negative (or delayed in turning positive) in fungal endocarditis, especially those not due to candida species (e.g., Aspergillus), and this possibility must be carefully considered when undertaking antibiotic therapy for "culture-negative" PVE. In selected patients with negative blood cultures, careful bacteriologic and histologic study of surgically extracted peripheral arterial emboli may yield an etiologic diagnosis. A search for Legionella species should also not be neglected.

Antibiotic therapy is usually initiated with two bactericidal antibiotics potentially synergistic for the suspected or proven pathogen (a penicillin or cephalosporin plus an aminoglycoside). A trough serum bactericidal level of 1:8

should be the minimum goal of therapy in these patients. In experimental animal models of endocarditis, antibiotics exhibiting in vitro synergy (checkerboard technique) sterilize vegetations more rapidly than do single-drug regimens. While the in vivo benefits of this phenomenon remain controversial in the treatment of NVE, most investigators generally employ such combinations when treating PVE.

In all cases of suspected or proven PVE due to S. aureus, therapy should be initiated with a penicillinase-resistant penicillin, provided that the patient has no history of penicillin allergy. Parenteral nafcillin or oxacillin (2 g every 4 hours) given for at least 6 weeks is generally recommended. High-dose penicillin G therapy, in the range of 20 to 30 million units per day, can be substituted if the MIC of the organism is less than 0.1 μg per milliliter. Gentamicin or tobramycin (1.5 mg per kilogram every 8 hours) is usually combined with the penicillinase-resistant penicillin or penicillin G in the treatment of S. aureus PVE, at least for the first 2 to 4 weeks of therapy, with careful renal functional monitoring. In patients with a history of penicillin allergy, either a first-generation cephalosporin (e.g., cefazolin 1 g every 8 hours) or vancomycin alone (1 g every 12 hours) can be substituted. In patients with PVE caused by methicillin-resistant strains of S. aureus, vancomycin is the antibiotic of choice; an aminoglycoside (gentamicin preferred or tobramycin) is added only with extreme caution if the response is incomplete or the blood culture remains positive. Vancomycin or a combination of nafcillin (or oxacillin) plus gentamicin (or tobramycin) has been advocated for patients whose S. aureus isolate is determined to be "tolerant" in vitro (as indicated by serum bactericidal studies). For patients failing conventional therapy, or in those where bacteremia persists, adding rifampin (300 mg orally every 8 hours in adults; 18 mg per kilogram per day in three divided doses in children) may produce a striking clinical and laboratory response.

The literature suggests that the prognosis for HACEK PVE is reasonably good for both clinical and bacteriologic cure; 80 percent of cases are cured by antibiotics (penicillin or ampicillin with or without an aminoglycoside) alone without the need for valve replacement; β-lactamase-producing strains of Haemophilus influenzae would require use of a β-lactamase-resistant cephalosporin, such as cefuroxime, ceftazidime, or ceftriaxone, until susceptibility test results are available.

Antimicrobial therapy for S. epidermidis and diphtheroid PVE requires a more detailed discussion. To treat S. epidermidis PVE properly, methicillin-resistant strains, which are very common, must not be overlooked. The microbiology laboratory can easily and mistakenly designate S. epidermidis strains methicillin-susceptible when they are actually methicillin-resistant, since only a small portion of the total bacterial population (one resistant cell in 10^5 to 10^7 susceptible cells) expresses resistance in the absence of exposure to that antibiotic. While every cell in the methicillin-resistant subpopulation is genetically capable of expressing resistance, only a small number do so under nonselective growth conditions (i.e., absence of methicillin). When exposed to methicillin, the resistant subpopulation declares phenotypic resistance, but takes 48 to 72 hours to do so. Therefore, standard antibiotic susceptibility test systems employing low inocula (10^5 colony-forming units per milliliter), such as agar dilution or microtiter broth or tube dilution, automated turbidimetric systems or those requiring rapid confluent growth around a paper disk (agar diffusion), usually fail to detect the cryptic, slow-growing, resistant subpopulation.

Methicillin-resistance is most reliably identified (Table 2) by testing higher inocula (10^7 colony-forming units per milliliter) incubated for 72 hours, easily performed by the properly alerted laboratory. Kirby-Bauer plates containing a methicillin disk incubated for 24 hours at 30°C may isolate resistant colonies in the clear zone around the disk, but the preferred method is described in Table 2. For clinical purposes, strains resistant to methicillin are considered resistant to all β-lactam antibiotics but are susceptible to vancomycin and usually to rifampin and gentamicin.

A prospective, randomized multicenter trial compared two 6-week regimens: (1) vancomycin, 7.5 mg per kilogram intravenously every 6 hours, plus rifampin, 300 mg orally every 8 hours; or (2) vancomycin and rifampin, as noted, plus gentamicin, 1 mg per kilogram intravenously every 8 hours during the initial 2 weeks of therapy. There was a 75 to 80 percent cure rate with either regimen (combined with surgical intervention in 64 percent of cases), but rifampin-resistant *S. epidermidis* strains were isolated from surgical specimens or blood cultures at the time of relapse in 40 percent of patients receiving the first regimen, whereas none were recovered from the group that received 2 weeks of gentamicin therapy. Therefore, the three-drug regimen, which minimizes the risk of nephrotoxicity by utilizing only 2 weeks of gentamicin, appears to be the current regimen of choice. When PVE is due to a methicillin-susceptible strain of coagulase-negative staphylococcus (*S. epidermidis* or otherwise), a semisynthetic penicillin or a first-generation cephalosporin is appropriate therapy; many investigators add either gentamicin and/or rifampin as second or third drugs. The addition of a second or third drug must always be monitored by in vitro studies documenting enhanced serum bactericidal activity, since not all such additions are enhancing.

Determining appropriate antimicrobial therapy for diphtheroid PVE may pose a problem, as these fastidious gram-positive coccobacilli may be difficult to isolate and maintain in culture and the microbiology laboratory may have difficulty performing MICs, MBCs, and serum bactericidal studies. When the isolate is sensitive to penicillin, a combination of penicillin G (4 million units every 4 hours) plus gentamicin (1.5 mg per kilogram every 8 hours) is administered for 6 weeks, because 90 percent of diphtheroid strains from PVE patients are synergistically killed by this combination. Isolates with MICs for penicillin as high as 256 μg per milliliter will yield to the synergistic influence of gentamicin, so long as the isolate is susceptible to gentamicin. Others recommend vancomycin in this situation. For patients allergic to penicillin or for those whose diphtheroid isolates are resistant to gentamicin, vancomycin, 7.5 mg per kilogram every 6 hours for 6 weeks, is recommended, alone or with the addition of gentamicin and rifampin. Renal function must be monitored closely.

Fungal PVE always requires combined medical and early surgical treatment. For candidal endocarditis, intravenous amphotericin B (up to 1 mg per kilogram per day) is combined with oral flucytosine (5-fluorocytosine; 200 mg per kilogram in four divided doses for as long as amphotericin B is given), with the dose adjusted for renal function, which is closely monitored. A total dose of 2 g of amphotericin B is usually the goal of postvalve replacement therapy. Oral imidazole compounds under current investigation (e.g., fluconazole, itraconazole) may offer future alternative approaches to the current need for long-term therapy with intravenous amphotericin B; ketoconazole has no current role in therapy of fungal PVE.

Prolonged parenteral therapy is the optimal way to treat PVE. Oral therapy has little or no role here, certainly not during the early stages of treatment. The average duration of treatment is 5 weeks, but patients infected with staphylococci or enteric and nonfermentative gram-negative bacilli or fungi often receive 6 or 8 weeks of therapy, respectively, because of the severe consequences of relapse in these patients. Serial (weekly) monitoring of C-reactive protein levels and the erythrocyte sedimentation rate may help determine how long a time antibiotic therapy must be continued; measurement of circulating immune complexes is probably just a more expensive way of accomplishing the same goal. Streptococcal infections (particularly those occurring after the first year) often respond to shorter courses of therapy (4 weeks), with intravenous penicillin (18 to 30 million units per day in six divided doses), with (my preference) or without the addition of gentamicin (1 mg per kilogram every 8 hours for the first 2 weeks, at least). Patients cured with antibiotic therapy alone are usually those developing PVE a year or more after surgery who are infected with relatively avirulent organisms highly susceptible to antibiotics: streptococci, fastidious gram-negative coccobacilli (HACEK), and methicillin-susceptible *S. epidermidis*. Such patients are usually hemodynamically stable with no evidence of an invasive infection.

Although more in vitro data and many more human studies remain to be done, teichoplanin, an experimental glycopeptide antibiotic structurally related to vancomycin and bactericidal for most gram-positive bacteria (except enterococci), has a much longer serum half-life than vancomycin (up to 40 or more hours), permitting once-daily injections

TABLE 2 *Staphylococcus epidermidis*: Tests for Methicillin Susceptibility

Pick four or five colonies of strain and grow overnight in brain heart infusion broth (organisms = 5×10^8 cfu/ml)

Inoculate with 0.1 ml (5×10^7 cfu) by spreading on surface:
Mueller-Hinton agar with 20 μg methicillin/ml
Mueller-Hinton agar with 12.5 μg methicillin/ml

Incubate agar plates 72 hours at 37°C

Read:
Colonies on agar with 20 μg methicillin/ml
= methicillin-resistant strain
No colonies on agar with 20 μg or 12.5 μg methicillin/ml
= methicillin-susceptible strain

Modified from Archer GL. Antimicrobial susceptibility and selection of resistance among *Staphylococcus epidermidis* isolates recovered from patients with infections of indwelling foreign devices. Antimicrob Agents Chemother 1978; 14:353–359.
cfu = colony forming unit

(either intramuscular or intravenous) after an initial series of three 12-hourly doses. A more favorable toxicity profile (less thrombophlebitis, less nephrotoxicity) and the possibility of once-daily intramuscular injections suggest a possible future role in PVE patients infected with gram-positive pathogens. However, intravenous drug abusers display a significantly shorter serum half-life, and some bacteremic patients fail to respond; optimal doses remain to be determined.

The availability of oral ciprofloxacin, a new oral quinolone compound, provides at last an oral agent highly active against methicillin-resistant staphylococci, both MRSA and MRCNS, and *Pseudomonas aeruginosa*. If encouraging results in animal model experimental endocarditis are borne out in clinical practice, this compound (and possibly other new quinolones on the horizon, such as enoxacin and pefloxacin) may prove to be useful (adjuncts) for the oral or parenteral therapy of MRSA or MRCNS PVE and perhaps also in the treatment of resistant gram-negative rod PVE, including infections with *P. aeruginosa*.

SURGERY

Surgery plays an increasingly important role in managing these patients since it is now possible, with aggressive debridement and prolonged postoperative antibiotic therapy, to replace an infected prosthesis during active endocarditis without contaminating the new prosthesis or developing recurrent infection. During the past 10 to 15 years, debridement of infected tissues and restoring valvular function by placing a new prosthesis has become standard therapy for some 50 to 75 percent of patients during their initial period of antibiotic therapy. Some even consider early surgery the primary treatment for PVE, preferring not to wait for complications, since despite prolonged bactericidal antibiotic therapy, cultures of valves at surgery or autopsy are often positive and valve dehiscence is so common a complication, occurring in some 50 percent of patients at surgery or autopsy. Earlier intervention may lower the incidence of dehiscence, according to some investigators. One would ideally like to suppress the infection with appropriate antibiotic therapy for at least 10 to 14 days prior to surgery, but, as is true in NVE, survival is inversely related to the severity of heart failure at the time of surgery, so it is essential to operate before hemodynamic deterioration becomes severe and irreversible.

Surgical intervention must be considered an option in all patients with PVE, since complex surgical techniques, including aortic root reconstructions, are often required due to extensive annular infection and extraannular abscesses. When left ventricular–aortic discontinuity is present, a homograft aortic valve and ascending aorta (as conduit) may rescue an otherwise hopeless situation, illustrating some of the extraordinary surgical techniques possible. The question of if and when has been difficult to resolve. Earlier concerns that reoperation posed formidable technical problems have largely been allayed as cardiac surgical expertise has improved dramatically, and fatality rates for patients treated only medically remain substantial, in the range of 60 to 80 percent. In patients who undergo valve replacement, this figure drops to 15 to 40 percent. Circumstances warranting possible or definite surgical intervention are listed in Table 3.

TABLE 3 Indications for Considering Surgical Intervention in PVE

Hemodynamic complications
  Moderate to severe or rapidly progressive heart failure (N.Y. Heart Association Class III or IV) caused by valvular insufficiency (tissue valves) or valve dehiscence with paravalvular leak (mechanical valves)
  Acute decrease in cardiac output, caused by valve obstruction

Evidence of extending valve infection (annular abscess, myocardial abscess, mycotic aneurysm) suggested by new or progressing conduction system disturbances, or purulent pericarditis; fever persisting > 10 days in the face of appropriate antibiotic therapy

Antibiotic failure
  Persistent fever and/or bacteremia, relapse following apparently "successful" antibiotic therapy, or ineffective or unavailable antimicrobial therapy

Selected organisms associated with increased mortality
  Fungi (definitely)
  S. aureus (debated; consider case by case)
  S. epidermidis (with any feature[s] noted above)

Emboli
  Recurrent or single major (e.g., coronary, cerebral) or new echocardiographic evidence of vegetations
  Emboli associated with any of the features noted above

Adapted from Dismukes WE. Management of infective endocarditis. In: Cardiovascular clinics, 11/3, critical care cardiology. Philadelphia: FA Davis, 1981:189.

Investigators at the Massachusetts General Hospital further analyzed the 116 patients with PVE they treated between 1975 and 1983, employing multivariate analysis to identify risk factors for in-hospital mortality and bad outcome during post-hospital follow-up. Complicated PVE (new or changing murmur, new or worsening heart failure, new or progressive cardiac conduction abnormalities, or prolonged fever during therapy) was present in 64 percent of patients, conditioned primarily by aortic valve infection (odds ratio 4.3, $p = .002$) and onset within 12 months of surgery (odds ratio 5.5, $p = .0001$). In-hospital mortality was 23 percent; complicated PVE patients had a higher mortality than uncomplicated PVE patients (odds ratio 6.4, $p = .0009$). Combined medical-surgical therapy was used in 39 percent of patients, more commonly in patients with complicated PVE (odds ratio 16, $p < .0001$) and in patients infected with coagulase-negative staphylococci (odds ratio 3.9, $p = .0003$). Survival after initially successful therapy was adversely affected by the presence of moderate or severe congestive heart failure at the time of discharge ($p = .03$). Bad outcome during follow-up (death, relapse, or further cardiac surgery) was more common in the medical-therapy-only group ($p = .02$). The presence of complicated PVE is thus a central variable in assessing prognosis and planning therapy, and these patients, for the most part, are best treated with combined medical-surgical therapy. Patients not treated surgically during their initial hospitalization are at high risk for progressive prosthesis dysfunction and require careful follow-up.

The goals of prompt valve replacement are to curtail the extension of infection into vital or inaccessible cardiac structures, prevent or minimize abscess formation, and diminish the possibility of paravalvular leaks, dehiscence, or thrombotic (occlusive) stenosis. In general, I favor an aggressive approach to surgery in almost all patients who develop PVE in the first postoperative year and all patients with fungal endocarditis irrespective of the time interval. However, patients who develop PVE after the initial postoperative year and who are infected with antibiotic-sensitive organisms, such as streptococci and members of the HACEK group (the latter an increasingly important group) quite often respond to antibiotic therapy alone, so strict surgical indications (see Table 3) should be applied in this setting. In general, aortic PVE carries a worse prognosis than mitral PVE, porcine heterografts fare better than mechanical valves, and early PVE consistently demonstrates more risk factors than does late PVE. When the tissues removed at surgery harbor viable organisms or evidence of active inflammation, an additional 6 weeks of antibiotic therapy (dating from the time of surgery) is usually recommended; otherwise 4 additional weeks of therapy is sufficient, at least for more antibiotic-sensitive organisms.

Some investigators urge a careful survey for and repair (if possible) of cerebral mycotic aneurysms before undertaking prosthetic valve insertion, but cardiopulmonary bypass does not appear to exacerbate or provoke neurologic deficits associated with cerebral mycotic aneurysms in most reported medical center experiences. Magnetic resonance imaging (MRI) of the head may prove a useful screening test for those who wish to investigate this possibility.

Anticoagulation

Systemic emboli occur in 15 to 30 percent of patients with infected mechanical or porcine prosthetic valves. Hemorrhagic central nervous system events also complicate PVE, particularly when anticoagulation has been excessive. The role of anticoagulation in patients with PVE is thus highly controversial. In one study, mortality was similar for patients maintained on careful warfarin anticoagulation and those not anticoagulated, but morbidity due to systemic emboli, particularly to the central nervous system, was increased in the non-anticoagulated group. Current guidelines suggest continuing very closely monitored anticoagulation (1.5 times control) during treatment of PVE, but discontinuing warfarin if any cerebrovascular event occurs. If there is no evidence of hemorrhage or a hemorrhagic infarct, cautious anticoagulation can be resumed after 72 hours. Some investigators believe heparin achieves a more stable anticoagulation state than warfarin and prefer it during antibiotic therapy of PVE.

Prophylaxis

Since the infecting organism in most cases of early PVE gains access to the prosthesis during surgery, perioperative antibiotic prophylaxis is employed routinely and is directed against staphylococci, since it is not possible to provide prophylaxis against all potential pathogens. To date there is no well-designed prospective, double-blinded study conclusively proving the benefits of this practice. However, several properly designed studies have demonstrated that short-term (48 hours) use of prophylactic antibiotic during the perioperative period is as effective in preventing PVE as is the use of a prophylactic antibiotic given for a longer period. First-generation cephalosporins (cefazolin, 1 g) or penicillinase-resistant penicillins (oxacillin or nafcillin, 1 to 2 g) should be started just before surgery and continued every 6 hours for no more than 48 hours. However, since most nosocomial *S. epidermidis* strains are methicillin (and cephalosporin)-resistant, the empiric recommendation that substitutes vancomycin (15 mg per kilogram initially preoperatively, followed by 10 mg per kilogram immediately after cardiopulmonary bypass) seems not unreasonable. Some also favor adding gentamicin, 1.7 mg per kilogram intravenously, just before surgery and repeating this dose once 8 hours later.

Persons with prosthetic heart valves are an easily identified population that remains forever at risk for colonization of their prostheses during the transient bacteremias that accompany certain procedures, particularly dental treatments, gastrointestinal and genitourinary manipulations, and gynecologic procedures. The danger of bacteremia from a barium enema is commonly ignored in this setting. Prophylactic regimens derived from in vitro data and the rabbit model of experimental endocarditis suggest that bactericidal antibiotics (penicillin[s], cephalosporin[s], vancomycin) administered prior to the induction of bacteremia can prevent or suppress bacteremia and thus avoid prosthetic infection. A British solution for the problem of prophylaxis for oral procedures, a single 3-g dose of oral amoxicillin 1 hour before the procedure, provides bactericidal blood levels for most oral streptococci for at least 10 hours, almost certainly an adequate margin of safety, since experimental animal models of endocarditis suggest that 9 hours is the critical time following a bacterial challenge in this setting. Although no trials in humans as yet document the efficacy of any prophylactic antibiotic regimen in patients with prosthetic valves who undergo bacteremia-associated procedures, their use is justified on theoretical grounds and carries minimal risk. Prophylaxis should be employed according to the guidelines of the American Heart Association; unfortunately, recent studies indicate very poor physician compliance with these guidelines despite the easy recognizability of this group of high-risk patients. Radiologic departments are notably not aware of these recommendations, particularly in relation to barium enemas, genitourinary instrumentation (e.g., voiding cystogram), or gynecologic procedures (e.g., hysterosalpingogram). The use of an antiseptic mouthwash (such as Betadine; povidone-iodine; 10 to 20 ml for 30 seconds, twice, 2 minutes apart) just before a dental procedure can decrease the frequency of subsequent bacteremia, and should not be neglected, although gingival "degerming" by mouthwash is not a substitute for antimicrobial prophylaxis.

SUGGESTED READING

Calderwood SB, Swinski LA, Karchmer AW, et al. Prosthetic valve endocarditis. Analysis of factors affecting outcome of therapy. J Thorac Cardiovasc Surg 1986; 92:776–783.

Calderwood SB, Swinski LA, Waternaux CM, et al. Risk factors for the development of prosthetic valve endocarditis. Circulation 1985; 72:31–37.

Cowgill LD, Addonizio VP, Hopeman AR, et al. A practical approach to prosthetic valve endocarditis. Ann Thorac Surg 1987; 43:450–457.

Karp RB. Role of surgery in infective endocarditis. Cardiovasc Clin 1987; 17:141–162.

Kotler MN, Goldman A, Parry WR. Noninvasive evaluation of cardiac valve prostheses. Cardiovasc Clin 1986; 17:201–241.

STERNAL WOUND INFECTION AND MEDIASTINITIS

NELSON M. GANTZ, M.D., F.A.C.P.
PATRICK G. FAIRCHILD, M.D.

Postoperative sternal wound infection and mediastinitis are infrequent but potentially devastating complications of a median sternotomy and are associated with considerable morbidity and mortality. The attack rate varies from 0.4 percent to 8.4 percent, with a mortality ranging between 7 percent and 80 percent.

Predisposing factors for infection include obesity, diabetes mellitus, chronic obstructive pulmonary disease, cigarette smoking, length of preoperative hospital stay before cardiac surgery, decreased serum albumin level, and use of corticosteroids. Inadequate antibiotic prophylaxis and improper skin preparation also increase the risk of infection. Other predisposing factors include excessive intrathoracic bleeding, prolonged bypass pump time, early reoperation to manage a complication such as bleeding, closed chest massage, and sustained low cardiac output for more than 24 hours after surgery. Use of an internal mammary artery is associated with an increased incidence of sternal wound infection and mediastinitis.

DIAGNOSIS

The diagnosis is not difficult when the patient has an erythematous incision site with drainage of purulent material from the sternum. Often there are few clinical symptoms and signs and the only clue may be unexplained postoperative fever. The patient may complain of an unexpected degree and persistence of pain at the incision site. Physical findings include instability of the sternum, bubbling of air from the wound, or an audible or palpable mediastinal click or crunching sensation. The first clue of a deep sternal infection may be a slight amount of drainage that mimics a pustule or stitch abscess. Often, the incision site is normal, and the only indication of infection is the report of a positive blood culture.

Conventional radiography is usually of limited value in the establishment of a diagnosis unless there is air or an air-fluid level in the mediastinum. Computed tomography may be helpful in demonstrating an infection. Similarly, a sinogram of a draining sinus tract may provide evidence of a deep collection of pus.

TREATMENT

As soon as infection of the sternum and/or mediastinum is suspected, the entire incision should be reopened and the mediastinum explored. The key to successful therapy depends on adequate debridement and precise identification of the causative organism so that specific therapy can be selected based on the results of cultures and susceptibility testing. The mediastinum must be widely debrided to remove bone wax, fibrin, hematoma, and bone fragments, which can serve as foci for persistent infection. Adequately obtained specimens should be sent for pathologic examination and gram stain as well as culture. A deep tissue specimen should be sent for aerobic and anaerobic culture. Substernal chest tubes are inserted to drain the mediastinum and are kept in place until drainage ceases. Patients requiring extensive debridement may need a vascularized muscle flap to fill the large defect. Local irrigation of the mediastinum with inflow and outflow catheters using various antibiotics has been advocated, but controlled studies with this mode of therapy are not available. Dilute iodophor solutions have also been used for irrigation but again in uncontrolled studies. Irrigation with topical antibiotic solutions may be beneficial, but a risk exists of introducing a resistant organism into the mediastinum via the irrigation tubes.

Parenteral antibiotics based on the results of the Gram stain, culture, and susceptibility data should be administered for 6 weeks in patients with sternal osteomyelitis and/or mediastinitis. If gram-positive cocci are seen on the Gram stain, therapy should be adequate for methicillin-susceptible *Staphylococcus aureus*, methicillin-susceptible *Staphylococcus epidermidis*, methicillin-resistant *S. aureus*, or methicillin-resistant *S. epidermidis*. Vancomycin, 30 mg per kilogram per day intravenously in doses every 6 hours, plus rifampin, 300 mg orally every 8 hours, should be initiated and continued for 6 weeks if the organism is methicillin resistant. Gentamicin in a dose of 1 mg per kilogram intravenously every 8 hours should be added for the initial 2 weeks to the vancomycin, and rifampin, if the organism is susceptible to gentamicin.

Appropriate adjustment of dosages is required in patients with renal insufficiency. Determination of peak and trough levels of vancomycin and gentamicin are essential, and dosages should be adjusted to prevent nephrotoxicity. If the staphylococci are methicillin susceptible, then nafcillin or oxacillin is given in a dose of 2 g intravenously every 4 hours. Gentamicin should be given in a dose of 1 mg per kilogram every 8 hours in a patient with normal renal function for the first 5 days of the nafcillin. In a patient with an immediate type of allergic reaction to a penicillin, vancomycin should be administered for methicillin-susceptible staphylococci. If the patient has a delayed reaction to penicillin, cephalothin is given in a dose of 2 g intravenously every 4 hours or cefazolin in a dose of 1 g intravenously every 6 hours. Cephalosporins should be avoided in patients with methicillin-resistant *S. aureus* or methicillin-resistant *S. epidermidis* infections.

For enterococci, administer aqueous penicillin G in a dose of 3 million units intravenously every 4 hours plus gentamicin, 1 mg per kilogram intravenously every 8 hours. Vancomycin, 30 mg per kilogram per day given in 6-hourly doses, should be substituted for penicillin if there is a history of a penicillin allergy. Against diphtheroids, which are susceptible to gentamicin (MIC $\leq$ 4 μg per milliliter), therapy should include penicillin plus gentamicin or vancomycin along with gentamicin in doses as listed for therapy of enterococci. If the diphtheroids are gentamicin resistant, vancomycin is the drug of choice in a dose of 30 mg per kilogram per day intravenously in 6-hourly doses, when renal function is normal.

For gram-negative enteric infections, combination therapy is administered on the basis of susceptibility data, although controlled studies are unavailable comparing the results of a single-drug with those of a two- or three-drug program. Combination regimens that can be given include a third-generation cephalosporin such as ceftriaxone (2 g intravenously every 12 hours) plus an aminoglycoside such as gentamicin (1.5 mg per kilogram per day intravenously every 8 hours), or imipenem-cilastatin (1 g intravenously every 6 hours) plus an aminoglycoside, or an aminoglycoside plus an extended-spectrum penicillin such as piperacillin (3 g intravenously every 4 hours), or aztreonam (2 g intravenously every 8 hours) plus an aminoglycoside. Ceftazidime (2 g intravenously every 8 hours) can be substituted for ceftriaxone based on the results of susceptibility testing.

Synergistic testing of various combinations of drugs can be performed, but clinical correlations are unavailable. *Pseudomonas aeruginosa* infections should be treated with two drugs based on the results of susceptibility testing. Possible regimens include piperacillin or azlocillin plus tobramycin, ceftazidime plus tobramycin, imipenem-cilastatin plus tobramycin, or aztreonam plus tobramycin. Amikacin in a dose of 7.5 mg per kilogram every 12 hours should be substituted for tobramycin if the organism is resistant to tobramycin. If no organism is identified on culture or by pathologic examination and infection is suspected, empiric therapy with vancomycin, rifampin plus an aminoglycoside, or a third-generation cephalosporin such as ceftazidime may be instituted. Imipenem-cilastatin could be substituted for the ceftazidime. Clinical trials are needed to reveal the comparative success rates of the various regimens.

The importance of adequate surgical debridement in the cure of this infection cannot be overemphasized. The use of irrigation with antibacterial solutions and microvascular surgery using a muscle flap requires further study. Determination of therapeutic but nontoxic drug concentrations as well as close monitoring of the patient for adverse drug reactions is required to achieve an optimal outcome in this difficult infection.

SUGGESTED READING

Acinapura AJ, Godfrey N, Rominta M, et al. Surgical management of infected median sternotomy: closed irrigation versus muscle flap. J Cardiovasc Surg 1985; 26:443–446.

Cheung EH, Craver JM, Jones EL, et al. Mediastinitis after cardiac valve operations: impact upon survival. J Thorac Cardiovasc Surg 1985; 90:517–522.

Nagachinta T, Stephens M, Reitz B, Polk BF. Risk factors for surgical-wound infection following cardiac surgery. J Infect Dis 1987; 156:967–973.

Ottino G, DePaulis R, Pansini S, et al. Major sternal wound infection after open-heart surgery: a multivariate analysis of risk factors in 2,579 consecutive operative procedures. Ann Thorac Surg 1987; 44:173–179.

PERICARDITIS

STEVEN L. BERK, M.D.
ABRAHAM VERGHESE, M.D., F.R.C.P.

Inflammation of the pericardium can be caused by a wide variety of infectious and noninfectious disease processes. These inflammatory processes can result in acute pericarditis (with or without effusion) or chronic pericarditis (which can be effusive-constrictive). Both acute and chronic pericarditis can result in the development of cardiac tamponade, which is a medical emergency. Acute pericarditis is recognized by the classic triad: substernal chest pain, often relieved by sitting up or leaning forward; the presence of a pericardial friction rub; and typical electrocardiogram changes of S-T segment elevation without reciprocal depression and a change in the P-R axis. Chronic

pericarditis with effusion is typically manifested by muffled heart sounds, increased cardiac dullness, or adynamic apical impulse and distention of neck veins in the absence of congestive heart failure. Chest roentgenogram will reveal an enlarging cardiac silhouette, and echocardiogram will confirm the presence of pericardial fluid. Patients who develop cardiac tamponade almost always complain of dyspnea and frequently have substernal chest pain. The hallmarks of cardiac tamponade are rising venous pressure, declining arterial pressure, muffled and quiet heart sounds, tachycardia, and pulsus paradoxus. Although cardiac tamponade can occur with any form of pericarditis, it appears to be uncommon in viral, postmyocardial infarction, and idiopathic pericarditis.

ACUTE BACTERIAL PERICARDITIS

This type of pericarditis has become much less common since the advent of penicillin and other antimicrobial agents in the 1940s. Clinical findings can usually differentiate pyogenic pericarditis from viral myopericarditis. Pyogenic pericarditis usually presents as an acute illness with high fever. The presenting features depend to a large degree on the portal of entry. Pleuropulmonary disease (including postoperative cases) is the commonest source of infection, and in these cases there are symptoms of cough or pleuritic chest pain suggesting the focus of infection. Hematogenous bacterial dissemination is the next-most-frequent source of infection, followed by myocardial abscesses or infective endocarditis. In a febrile patient with pericarditis who appears acutely ill and dyspneic, purulent pericarditis should be assumed to be present, particularly if there is evidence of cardiac tamponade. When the clinical diagnosis of purulent pericarditis has been considered and pericardial fluid has been demonstrated by echocardiogram, pericardiocentesis will be necessary to make an etiologic diagnosis. Fluid obtained by pericardiocentesis usually shows more than 50,000 leukocytes per mm^3, and the pericardial glucose is low (< 35 mg) with an elevated protein level. Fluid tends to accumulate much more rapidly than in viral pericarditis and may reach 1 liter in a few days.

In most cases initial antibiotic therapy will be guided by Gram-stained smear of pericardial fluid. For example, in a patient with pneumonia in whom gram-positive diplococci are seen on smear, high-dose penicillin therapy would be initiated. A quellung reaction could be used to confirm that the organisms seen are *Streptococcus pneumoniae*. Gram-positive cocci in clusters would suggest *Staphylococcus aureus* infection. Since many hospital-acquired infections are caused by methicillin-resistant *S. aureus*, vancomycin is the drug of choice until sensitivity results become available. Treatment of gram-negative bacillary purulent pericarditis has usually necessitated initial therapy with an aminoglycoside. Newer cephalosporins, imipenem-cilastatin, and aztreonam may all have a role in life-threatening infections in some hospitals. High doses of parenteral antibiotics are necessary, and 4 weeks of therapy is prudent. Instillation of antibiotics into the pericardial sac is not recommended.

If pericardiocentesis is delayed or if no organisms are visualized on Gram stain and while awaiting cultures, it is appropriate to begin empiric therapy. Broad-spectrum therapy, which includes coverage of *S. aureus* and gram-negative bacilli, should be initiated. Such therapy must be tailored to the individual patient. In an individual with empyema who develops pericarditis, antibiotic selection based on cultures

of previously obtained pleural fluid is mandatory. A patient with well-documented pneumonia would be treated with a regimen that covers the pathogen causing pneumonia. In a patient with postoperative gram-negative rod infection and pericarditis, information about susceptibility patterns of that hospital's gram-negative bacilli is useful. Prompt drainage of the strategic pericardial space is almost always required. Pericardiocentesis may at times be a sufficient drainage procedure, particularly in pneumococcal disease. However, a pericardial window or pericardiectomy is usually necessary to prevent the development of chronic constrictive pericarditis. Table 1 provides recommended antibiotic regimens for culture-proven bacterial pericarditis.

VIRAL MYOPERICARDITIS

Viruses implicated in pericarditis include group B Coxsackievirus, echovirus type 8, mumps virus, Epstein-Barr virus, influenza virus, poliovirus, and varicella virus. Because serology is infrequently obtained in patients with these diseases, many cases of viral pericarditis are labeled as idiopathic, and conversely many cases of "idiopathic pericarditis" are probably viral. More than half of patients with viral pericarditis give a history of a preceding upper respiratory tract infection. Symptoms include fever, pleurisy, a friction rub, and cough. In most patients with presumed viral myopericarditis, the symptoms are mild, and pericardial effusion is small if it occurs at all. Pericardiocentesis is not worth its inherent risks, and a definitive diagnosis is difficult to make. In patients who do not have an easily identifiable viral symptom complex, noninfectious causes of pericarditis must be included in the differential diagnosis. These include connective tissue disease, uremia, Dressler's syndrome, and the ill-defined entity of idiopathic pericarditis.

Patients with acute pericarditis thought to be viral in etiology should be hospitalized for observation. Paradoxical pulse and distended neck veins should be sought and an echocardiogram obtained. Patients with Coxsackie- or echovirus infection are more likely to have myocarditis with resultant heart failure and marked cardiomegaly. Viral diagnosis may be made by culture of stool and throat washings and in some cases by demonstrating rise in specific antibody titers between acute and convalescent sera. Cardiac enzymes should be monitored to assess myocardial necrosis. Cardiac tamponade is an uncommon event, but it

TABLE 1 Antibiotic Therapy for Purulent Pericarditis

Etiologic Agent	Antibiotic Regimen
Streptococcus pneumoniae	Penicillin G 4 × 10^6 U IV q4h × 4–6 wk
Staphylococcus aureus	Nafcillin 2 g IV q4h × 4–6 wk
Methicillin-resistant *S. aureus*	Vancomycin 500 mg q6h × 4–6 wk
Pseudomonas aeruginosa	Aminoglycoside (gentamicin 3–5 mg/kg/day in 3 divided doses or amikacin 15 mg/kg/day in 2–3 divided doses) *plus* ureidopenicillin (piperacillin 3 g IV q4h)
Other gram-negative enteric pathogens	Aminoglycoside and/or newer semisynthetic penicillin, aztreonam (2 g q8h), imipenem (1 g q6h), ceftazidime (2 g q8h)
Haemophilus influenzae	Ceftazidime or cefuroxime (1.5 g q8h)

can occur. Pericardiocentesis is not indicated in viral pericarditis unless signs of tamponade develop. If pericardiocentesis is performed, the fluid should be cultured for virus and tissue examined by immunofluorescent techniques. Depending on the clinical setting, additional work-up might include testing for antinuclear antibodies; rheumatoid factor; bacterial, tuberculous, and fungal culture; and cytology. Atrial and ventricular arrhythmias and congestive heart failure may require therapy.

In most patients simple supportive treatment is all that is required. The illness tends to last for 1 to 2 weeks, and one or more relapses are not uncommon. Repeated observation throughout the course of the illness should establish the absence of cardiac tamponade or heart failure. Antiviral therapy of any sort has not been proven to be efficacious. Bed rest is strongly advised, and strenuous exercise should be avoided for 1 or 2 months after the illness. Aspirin or indomethacin may be used for symptomatic relief of chest pain. Anticoagulation is contraindicated. In a patient with intense, unrelenting pain, corticosteroid therapy may provide dramatic relief. Prednisone, 80 mg per day in divided doses, is given for 5 days and gradually tapered to be replaced with indomethacin, 50 mg orally every 8 hours, or aspirin, 650 mg every 4 hours. In a patient who might have bacterial pericarditis, corticosteroid use can be hazardous, and it is important to rule out this possibility by every available means.

TUBERCULOUS PERICARDITIS

Tuberculous pericarditis carries a mortality of about 40 percent, and is a difficult disease to diagnose. It is estimated to occur with a frequency of three to four cases per 1,000 cases of tuberculosis. In autopsied cases of pericarditis in which a specific cause is evident, 11 percent of cases are tuberculous. In the last 50 years, the disease has become less common in the young and more common in the middle-aged and elderly. Pathologically, the inflammation produced by the tubercle bacillus tends to cause an initial dry or fibrinous reaction, followed in most instances by progression to an effusive stage, which is characterized by effusions that are frequently bloody and turbid. It is not surprising that constriction occurs when fibrous tissue obliterates the pericardial space as it heals.

The initial clinical symptoms of tuberculous pericarditis can be nonspecific and easily overlooked. Patients are usually recognized in the effusive stage but may go undetected until constriction develops. Cough, low-grade fever, weakness, and fatigability are early symptoms. The four cardinal signs of tuberculous pericarditis in North America are fever, tachycardia, cardiomegaly, and signs of a pleural effusion. The tuberculin skin test is most often positive. This, together with recovery of the organism in pleural fluid or pleural biopsy (which occurs in about one-third of patients with pleural effusion) or in pericardial fluid (in up to 50 percent of patients), is most helpful in making the diagnosis.

Any individual with the signs of pericarditis, a positive tuberculin skin test, and an abnormal chest roentgenogram should be regarded as having tuberculous pericarditis. Empiric therapy with three drugs including isoniazid (INH) (300 mg daily), rifampin (600 mg daily), and ethambutol (15 mg per kilogram daily) should be started pending definitive diagnosis by smear or culture. When primary INH resistance is high (e.g., among Indo-Chinese refugees), triple-drug therapy is especially prudent. Short-course chemotherapy is in vogue for the treatment of pulmonary tuberculosis, and there are a few studies of these regimens in extrapulmonary tuberculosis. Preliminary evidence with limited numbers of patients (including 12 patients with tuberculous pericarditis) suggests that therapy with INH and rifampin for 9 months is as effective as standard regimens in extrapulmonary tuberculosis. Since these series do not include significant numbers of patients with pericarditis, it appears prudent to treat the patient for a minimum of 1½ years.

Retrospective experience with tuberculous pericarditis suggests that therapy with corticosteroids is beneficial in limiting pericardial inflammation, which can lead to rapid accumulation of fluid, induction of arrhythmias, and compromise of an otherwise healthy myocardium. Although controlled trials of corticosteroid use in this situation are lacking, we favor the use of prednisone in a dose of 80 mg daily in divided doses, gradually reducing and discontinuing in 6 to 8 weeks. This appears to curtail continued fluid exudation and cause a decrease in heart size in 72 hours to 2 weeks. Pericardiocentesis may be needed as both a diagnostic and a therapeutic measure. Despite the use of appropriate antituberculous therapy, as well as corticosteroids, many patients will develop a fibrous, unyielding pericardium and pericardiectomy may eventually be needed. The size of the patient's heart should be followed by radiography every 2 weeks, if not more often, and frequent clinical determinations of central venous pressure should be made. If there is a persistently enlarged heart and/or progressive heart failure, pericardiectomy is usually performed. Even if the heart size is regressing but venous pressure begins to elevate, pericardiectomy may be indicated. In patients whose heart size decreases but who have a stable elevated venous pressure, observation is recommended until the venous pressure returns to normal. If heart failure supervenes, or if the venous pressure fails to normalize after 6 months, then pericardiectomy may be beneficial. This procedure appears to be of most benefit when performed early.

SUGGESTED READING

Fowler NO, Manitsas GT. Infectious pericarditis. Prog Cardiovasc Dis 1973; 16:323.

Klacsmann PG, Bulkley BH, Hutchins GM. The changed spectrum of purulent pericarditis. An 86-year autopsy experience in 200 patients. Am J Med 1977; 63:666.

Rooney JJ, Crocco JA, Lyons HA. Tuberculous pericarditis. Ann Intern Med 1970; 72:73.

Spodick DH, ed. Pericardial diseases. Cardiovasc Clin 1976; 7(3):1–297.

BONE AND JOINT INFECTIONS

BACTERIAL OSTEOMYELITIS

JACK L. LeFROCK, M.D.
BRUCE R. SMITH, Pharm. D.
ABDOLGHADER MOLAVI, M.D.

Osteomyelitis continues to pose both diagnostic and therapeutic dilemmas for the clinician, despite recent advances in radionuclide imaging, surgical techniques, and antimicrobial therapy. Intravenous drug abuse, radiation therapy for cancer, and newer orthopaedic procedures, such as total joint replacements, bone grafting, and reconstructive surgery, have broadened the scope of this disease.

Osteomyelitis is an inflammatory process in bone and bone marrow. It is caused most often by pyogenic bacteria but may be caused by other microorganisms including mycobacteria and fungi. Osteomyelitis may be classified on the basis of its pathogenesis as of either hematogenous origin or contiguous focus (with or without peripheral vascular disease) (Table 1). These in turn may be classified as either acute or chronic forms of the disease.

In the past, osteomyelitis usually resulted from hematogenous spread of bacteria to bone and was mostly seen in children with *Staphylococcus aureus* as the causative agent in 80 to 90 percent of the cases. However, in recent years the disease has changed. Hematogenous osteomyelitis is decreasing in frequency while contiguous osteomyelitis and osteomyelitis in association with peripheral vascular disease is increasing. In addition to these changes, there also has been a shift in the age distribution to older patients as well as increasing frequency of unusual bacterial causes, including gram-negative bacilli, anaerobes, and mixed organisms.

HEMATOGENOUS OSTEOMYELITIS

Hematogenous osteomyelitis is generally caused by a single organism, *S. aureus* being responsible for the majority of cases. However, the type of organism may vary with the age of the patient (Table 2). This disease generally occurs in children younger than 12 years, teenagers, and young adults who participate in strenuous physical activities. Bone infection follows bacteremia. The metaphyseal ends of long bones are the most frequent sites of involvement in children and the diaphysis of the long bones in adults.

S. aureus may also cause spinal osteomyelitis with paravertebral abscess formation. This syndrome generally occurs in older men who have had urinary tract manipulation and infection and in drug addicts.

Gram-negative enteric bacteria, *Staphylococcus epidermidis*, may also cause vertebral osteomyelitis secondary to urinary tract infection. Gram-negative bacilli are now isolated more frequently from cases of acute hematogenous osteomyelitis. *Pseudomonas aeruginosa* may cause vertebral, pubic, and clavicular infections in drug addicts, and *Salmonella* species are important in sickle cell disease. Polymicrobial osteomyelitis occurs in 5 percent of patients and is mostly due to *S. aureus* and a streptococcus.

TABLE 1 Classification of Osteomyelitis and Associated Features

	Hematogenous	Secondary to Contiguous Focus of Infection	Due to Vascular Insufficiency
Age distribution	1–20 and >50 years	25–50 years	≥50 years
Usual bones involved	Long bones, vertebrae	Long bones	Small bones of feet
Microbiology	Usually monomicrobial: *Staphylococcus aureus, Streptococcus* (group B)	Usually mixed infections: *Staphylococcus aureus* and *epidermidis*, gram-negative bacilli	Usually polymicrobial: *Staphylococcus aureus* and *epidermidis*, gram-negative bacilli
	Gram-negative bacilli (*Haemophilus influenzae*)		Anaerobes
Associated factors	Trauma, bacteremia, IV drug abuse	Trauma and surgery, soft tissue infections, radiation therapy	Diabetes mellitus, peripheral vascular disease
Clinical features	Fever, local tension and swelling	Fever, swelling and erythema	Fever, swelling, ulceration and drainage

TABLE 2 Osteomyelitis: Commonly Isolated Organisms

Hematogenous osteomyelitis
  Infants <1 year
    Group B *Streptococcus*
    Staphylococcus aureus
    Escherichia coli

  Children 1–16 years
    Staphylococcus aureus
    Group A *Streptococcus*
    Haemophilus influenzae

  Adults >16 years
    Staphylococcus aureus
    Staphylococcus epidermidis
    Gram-negative bacilli
      Pseudomonas aeruginosa
      Serratia marcescens
      Escherichia coli

Contiguous focus osteomyelitis (polymicrobic infection),
  all ages
    Staphylococcus aureus
    Staphylococcus epidermidis
    Group A *Streptococcus*
    Enterococcus
    Gram-negative bacilli
    Anaerobes

CONTIGUOUS OSTEOMYELITIS

Contiguous osteomyelitis is secondary to an adjacent area of infection, as in postoperative infections, direct inoculation from trauma, or extension from an area of soft tissue infection. In contrast to hematogenous osteomyelitis, more than one pathogen is often isolated from the infected bone. *S. aureus* is the most commonly isolated pathogen, but aerobic gram-negative rods and anaerobes also are often isolated. In this form of osteomyelitis, one often finds bone necrosis, compromised soft tissue, and loss of bone stability, which make this type more difficult to treat than acute hematogenous osteomyelitis.

OSTEOMYELITIS ASSOCIATED WITH VASCULAR INSUFFICIENCY

This infection usually develops in diabetic persons as an extension of a local infection either from cellulitis or a trophic skin ulcer. The small bones of the feet, generally the metatarsals and phalanges, are involved. These patients have impaired local inflammatory response that predisposes the involved tissues to infection and necrosis. Multiple aerobic and/or anaerobic pathogens often can be isolated from the infected bone.

CHRONIC OSTEOMYELITIS

Both of the above types of osteomyelitis can become chronic. There are no exact criteria as to when acute osteomyelitis becomes chronic.

DIAGNOSIS

In addition to the historical data and physical findings, cultures of infected material and hematologic and radio-graphic studies are helpful in making a clinical and etiologic diagnosis.

Blood cultures should be performed for all patients with suspected osteomyelitis. Approximately 50 percent of patients with acute hematogenous osteomyelitis have positive blood cultures. Leukocytosis may occur with white blood cell (WBC) counts exceeding 20,000 per cubic millimeter. However, normal or only slightly elevated WBC counts are not uncommon. The erythrocyte sedimentation rate may be normal early in the disease, but usually increases with the duration of illness.

Radiographic changes are often difficult to interpret. Bone density must change at least 50 percent to be detected radiologically. Thus, there may be no definable radiologic changes in osteomyelitis for the first 10 to 14 days in spite of bone destruction or periosteal new bone formation. The initial radiologic findings may be simply soft tissue swelling and/or subperiosteal elevation. Roentgenograms may give misleading information in up to 16 percent of patients and are of no diagnostic value in an additional 23 percent of patients with osteomyelitis. Lytic changes are not seen until 2 to 6 weeks after the onset of disease. Sclerotic changes of periosteal new bone formation (involucrum) denote a more chronic process.

On the other hand, changes are seen on bone scintigraphy as early as 24 hours after the onset of symptoms because of increased bone blood flow and early bone reaction. However, not all patients with acute osteomyelitis have abnormal bone scans. There are reports of normal bone scans, or "subtle" or "cold" defects. In some situations gallium scan shows increased uptake in areas of polymorphonuclear leukocyte infiltration. However, gallium scan does not show bone detail well so it is often difficult to distinguish between bone and soft tissue inflammation. Scanning the infected area with gallium 48 hours after injection and comparing with a ^{99m}Tc bone scan helps resolve this problem. Computed tomography (CT) is useful in identifying areas of dead bone (sequestrum). However, CT cannot be utilized when metal is present in or near the area of bone infection because of the scatter effect, with resultant loss of image resolution. Radiographic follow-up is important in assessing the effectiveness of drug therapy and the need for surgical intervention.

The bacteriologic diagnosis of osteomyelitis rests on isolation of the pathogenic bacteria from the bone or the blood. In chronic osteomyelitis, sinus tract cultures are not reliable in predicting which organism(s) will be isolated from the infected bone because there is a poor correlation between these cultures and those done on bone biopsy material. Bone biopsy specimens should be carefully cultured and stained for aerobes, anaerobes, mycobacteria, and fungi. The biopsied material should also be submitted for histopathologic evaluation.

THERAPY FOR HEMATOGENOUS OSTEOMYELITIS

In acute hematogenous osteomyelitis, a prolonged course of antimicrobial therapy (4 to 6 weeks), with a bactericidal agent, should be directed toward specific causative bacteria isolated by bone biopsy and culture. Therapy based on wound swab cultures of skin and skin structures above the infected bone is often inappropriate. These cultures usually reflect bacterial colonization without accurately identifying the organism in the underlying bone itself. Only the isolation of *S. aureus* from deep wound culture has correlated with its presence in bone.

Oral therapy has been used successfully after 2 weeks of parenteral therapy in the treatment of pediatric osteomyelitis. This method of therapy should be entertained where there is good laboratory backup and close patient monitoring to ensure compliance. Patients casually treated with oral antibiotics often receive inadequate dosage and inadequate monitoring, resulting in a failure rate of 19 percent. For successful therapy, the orally administered antibiotic should be monitored by the measurement of serum bactericidal activity against the causative pathogen. A peak bactericidal dilution of at least 1:8 or greater should be maintained. In children, this form of therapy offers advantages in convenience, comfort, and cost. We treat adults with 6 weeks of intravenous therapy and children with 3 weeks of intravenous therapy followed by 3 weeks of oral therapy.

THERAPY FOR CHRONIC OSTEOMYELITIS

Chronic osteomyelitis secondary to surgery, trauma, or contiguous focal infection must be approached with combined medical and surgical therapy. Debridement should be done as soon as possible to remove all necrotic bone and sequestra. Abscesses or fistulous tracts must be eliminated. Material obtained at the time of surgery should be cultured for aerobes and anaerobes. Internal fixation devices, plates, pins, and screws should be removed. If bone stabilization is required, an external fixation device can be utilized. The wound may have to be debrided every 48 to 72 hours until all nonviable tissue has been removed.

Antimicrobial therapy should be initiated as early as possible, should be directed specifically against the offending pathogen(s), and should be administered intravenously in high doses for 6 weeks after the last debridement. Antimicrobial therapy prior to the time when debridement cultures are obtained should consist of broad-spectrum antibiotics to cover both aerobes and anaerobes. It is advisable to give antibiotics prior to debridement in order to reduce cellulitis or soft tissue swelling and reduce the risk of bacteremia.

There is no good evidence that regional antibiotic perfusion of an extremity or wound irrigation with antibiotics confers an advantage, and irrigation may introduce superinfections with resistant organisms.

THERAPY IN GENERAL

The consequences of inadequate therapy can be grave and lifelong. Knowing the types of organisms producing the osteomyelitis should lead to the use of a specific bactericidal agent except when multiple organisms are involved. Blind therapy is dangerous. Empiric choice of a narrow-spectrum agent not effective against the organism(s) within the bone may lead to treatment failure and chronic relapses. On the other hand, empiric broad-spectrum therapy may unnecessarily expose the patient to excessive or potentially toxic antimicrobial therapy and also inflate the cost of treatment.

The agents chosen for use should be demonstrated to be effective against the organism isolated from bone by in vitro sensitivity tests, such as the minimum inhibitory concentration (MIC) and minimum bactericidal concentration (MBC). Disk sensitivities have been used as the basis of therapy, but disks contain concentrations of drugs in excess of those achievable in bone, and results may not be directly applicable to the clinical situation. The antimicrobial agent chosen should penetrate the involved bone in concentrations greater than those required to be active against the organisms.

We think that serum bactericidal testing should be done to predict the outcome of infection. In patients with acute osteomyelitis, peak serum bactericidal titers have no predictive value; however, trough titers of 1:2 or greater accurately predict cure, whereas trough titers of less than 1:2 predict therapeutic failure. In patients with chronic osteomyelitis, peak serum bactericidal titers of 1:16 or greater and trough titers of 1:4 or greater accurately predict cure, whereas peak titers of less than 1:16 and trough titers of less than 1:2 accurately predict failure.

Hyperbaric oxygen has been used as adjunctive therapy in chronic osteomyelitis, but the value of adding hyperbaric oxygen to conventional surgical and medical management remains debatable.

Soft tissue swelling, periosteal thickening, and periosteal elevation are the earliest changes but are subtle and may be missed. Lytic changes are not seen until 2 to 6 weeks after the onset of disease. Sclerotic changes of periosteal new bone formation (involvarum) denotes a longer process. Radionucleotide scanning (technetium plus gallium or indium) is most helpful in the course of acute disease prior to the development of radiologic changes. Positive scans may be seen as early as 24 hours after the onset of symptoms. CT is useful to identify areas of dead bone (sequestrum).

The bacteriologic diagnosis of osteomyelitis rests on the isolation of the pathogenic bacteria from the bone or the blood. In chronic osteomyelitis, sinus tract cultures are not reliable for predicting which organism(s) will be isolated from the infected bone. There is a poor correlation between sinus tract cultures and bone biopsy cultures. Bone biopsy material should be carefully cultured and stained for aerobes, anaerobes, mycobacterium, and fungus. The bone should also be submitted for histopathologic evaluation.

Antimicrobial therapy should be initiated as early as possible, should be directed specifically against the offending pathogen(s), and should be administered intravenously in high doses for 4 to 6 weeks. Surgical intervention, in the form of bone debridement, is usually required in addition to antibiotics in the therapy of osteomyelitis arising from a contiguous focus of infection, diabetic ulcers, and peripheral vascular disease. In addition, combination intravenous and oral antimicrobial therapy may need to be given for 3 to 6 months in forms of osteomyelitis where extensive bony changes and tissue damage have occurred.

The antimicrobial agent(s) chosen for use should be demonstrated effective against the organism isolated from bone by in vitro sensitivity tests—MIC and MBC. It is best to choose an antibiotic or antibiotic combination that has a low ratio of MIC to MBC relative to its expected serum concentration. We prefer the antibiotic chosen to be able to

TABLE 3 Antibiotic Therapy for Osteomyelitis in Adults

Organism	Antibiotics of First Choice*	Alternative Antibiotics*
Staphylococcus aureus	Nafcillin or oxacillin 2 g q6h	Clindamycin 900 mg q8h, vancomycin 500 mg q6h, cefazolin 1 g q8h
Staphylococcus epidermidis	Nafcillin or oxacillin 2 g q6h	Vancomycin 500 mg q6h, cefazolin 1 g q8h
Nonenterococcal *Streptococcus*	Penicillin G 3 million units q6h	Clindamycin 900 mg q8h, cefazolin 1 g q8h
Enterococcal *Streptococcus*	Ampicillin 2 g q6h *plus* gentamicin 5 mg/kg per day q8h	Vancomycin 500 mg q6h *plus* gentamicin 5 mg/kg per day q12h
Enterobacter species	Cefotaxime 2 g q8h *plus* gentamicin 5 mg/kg per day q8h	Ceftazidime *or* ceftizoxime 2 g q8h *plus* gentamicin 5 mg/kg per day q12h
Escherichia coli	Ampicillin 2 g q6h	Cefazolin 1 g q8h, cefuroxime 1.5 g q8h
Proteus mirabilis	Ampicillin 2 g q6h	Cefazolin 1 g q8h, cefuroxime 1 g q8h
Proteus vulgaris	Cefotaxime 2 g q8h	Cefuroxime 1.5 g q8h, ceftizoxime 2 g q8h
Providencia rettgeri	Ceftazidime 2 g q8h	
Morganella morganii	Ceftazidime 2 g q8h	
Serratia marcescens	Cefotaxime 2 g q8h	Ceftazidime *or* ceftizoxime 2 g q8h, mezlocillin *or* piperacillin 4 g q6h, *plus* gentamicin 5 mg/kg per day q12h
Pseudomonas aeruginosa	Azlocillin 4 g q6h *or* piperacillin 3 g q4h *plus* tobramycin 5 mg/kg per day q8h (in order of choice)	Ceftazidime 2 g q8h *plus* tobramycin 5 mg/kg per day q12h
Bacteroides species	Clindamycin 900 mg q8h IV	Metronidazole 500 mg q8h, cefoxitin 2 g q6h Timentum 3.1 g q8h

* Administered intravenously.

obtain serum levels at least eight times the MIC. Table 3 outlines the choice of antibiotics for the therapy of bacterial osteomyelitis in adults.

On the basis of presently limited available data, ciprofloxacin appears to be useful for bone infections due to susceptible strains of the family Enterobacteriaceae and may be an important alternative for pseudomonal infections. Ciprofloxacin may prove useful as an oral extension of initial parenteral therapy or in patients who are not candidates for intravenous therapy. Careful monitoring for emergence of resistance is advised when treating infections due to *P. aeruginosa*.

SUGGESTED READING

Cierny G, Mader JT, Penninck JJ. A clinical staging system of adult osteomyelitis. Contemp Orthop 1985; 10:17.
Gentry LO. Approach to the patient with chronic osteomyelitis. In: Remington JS, Swartz MN, eds. Current clinical topics in infectious diseases. Number 8. 1987:62.
Raff MJ, Melo JC. Anaerobic osteomyelitis. Medicine (Balt) 1978; 57:279.
Wheat J. Diagnostic strategies in osteomyelitis. Am J Med 1978; 78 (Suppl 6B):218.
Wood MB, et al. Vascularized bone segment transfers for management of chronic osteomyelitis. Orthop Clin North Am 1982; 15:461.

BACTERIAL ARTHRITIS

RALPH TOMPSETT, M.D.

Bacterial arthritis is an infection of the joint space and involves all of the joint structures, including the synovium and the articular cartilage. The joint generally becomes involved by hematogenous infection, through trauma, following joint surgery, or after intra-articular injection of medications. In unusual circumstances the joint may become infected as a result of adjacent disease, such as in fungal or mycobacterial infection. The joint itself may basically be normal, as is usually the case in younger individuals, or it may have underlying structural disease, often rheumatoid arthritis, in older patients.

The possible causative microorganisms are numerous, but the majority of cases are due to just a few species. *Staphylococcus aureus*, *Neisseria gonorrhoeae*, *Haemophilus*, and streptococci of groups A and B are the most commonly encountered organisms. Staphylococcal infections occur at all ages but usually in individuals older than 45 years. Gonococci are found in younger, sexually active patients. *Haemophilus* is almost always encountered in children less than 2 years of age but is also seen occasionally in adults, especially in patients with underlying disease.

The knees are the most commonly involved joints, with fewer cases involving hips, elbows, shoulders, and ankles. The sternoclavicular joints are sometimes involved, particularly in drug addicts. Usually just one joint is affected. In gonococcal infections multiple joints and tendons may become involved, but even in this case the major involvement is frequently restricted to one joint.

DIAGNOSIS

The diagnosis is suspected on the basis of the clinical findings of pain on motion, tenderness about the joint, and signs of acute inflammatory reaction involving the joint. Radiologic examination may be helpful, especially in infants. Fever is usually present. Temporally related infections, such as staphylococcal skin and soft tissue infections or gonococcal urethritis, may give important clues as to the etiology of the arthritis. The diagnosis of septic arthritis may generally be made by examination of the joint fluid. Specific etiology is established by examination of stained smears of joint fluid and by culturing blood and joint fluids. Infected joint fluids usually contain more than 50,000 white blood cells, of which 90 percent or more are neutrophils. The total white blood cell count is a valuable diagnostic laboratory test. Occasionally, in acutely inflamed joints of rheumatoid arthritis or in crystal-induced arthropathy, the cell count reaches this level, but this is not the rule. Glucose concentrations are less than 50 percent of the blood glucose. Gram stains are positive in 40 to 50 percent of the patients and cultures are positive in most. Early diagnosis and initiation of therapy are extremely important in order to prevent joint damage due to the increased pressure in the joint from excessive exudate and to remove fluids containing leukocyte enzymes, which may cause destruction of cartilage.

TREATMENT

The treatment of bacterial arthritis consists of administration of antibiotics and appropriate drainage. If a reasonably certain etiology is established on the basis of the initial examination, including Gram stain of the joint fluid, the most appropriate antibiotic may be chosen from Table 1. If there are no clues as to the probable infecting organism, therapy may be initiated on the first day with intravenous nafcillin and gentamicin. If cultures prove negative and if the clinical response is good, this treatment may be continued. Once the active inflammatory process is under control, therapy may be simplified by changing to ceftriaxone or ciprofloxacin, in that order of preference.

TABLE 1 Antibiotics for Treatment of Bacterial Arthritis

Organism	First-Line Drug	Alternative Drugs
Neisseria gonorrhoeae	Penicillin G 4 million units IV q6h × 3 days, then penicillin V orally 500 mg q.i.d. × 4 days	Ceftriaxone 2 g IV q24h
		Cefoxitin 1 g IV q6h
	Amoxicillin 500 mg orally 4 times daily × 1 week	
Haemophilus influenzae		
Beta-lactamase-negative	Ampicillin 1.5 g IV q6h	Cefuroxime 1.5 g IV q8h
		Cefotaxime 2 g IV q6h
Beta-lactamase-positive	Cefuroxime 1.5 g IV q6h	Cefotaxime 2 g IV q6h
Staphylococcus aureus (coagulase-positive)	Nafcillin 2 g IV q4h	Cefazolin 1 g IV q8h
		Vancomycin 1 g IV q12h
Streptococci, groups A and B, *Streptococcus pneumoniae*	Penicillin 4 million units IV q6h	Cefazolin 1 g IV q8h
		Vancomycin 1 g IV q12h
Pseudomonas aeruginosa	Ticarcillin 3 g IV q4h *plus* gentamicin 1.5 mg/kg IV q8h	Ceftazidime 2 g IV q8h
		Ciprofloxacin 750 mg PO q12h
Organism unknown	Nafcillin 2 g IV q4h *plus* gentamicin 1.5 mg/kg IV q8h	Ceftriaxone 1.5 g IV q8h
		Ciprofloxacin 750 mg PO q12h
Staphylococcus, coagulase-negative	If methicillin sensitive: nafcillin 2 g IV q4h	Cefazolin 750 mg q8h *or*
	If methicillin resistant: vancomycin 1 g IV q12h	Trimethoprim-sulfamethoxazole, 2 double-strength tablets b.i.d.
		Ciprofloxacin
Other organisms	Choice of drug dependent on species of microorganism and sensitivity tests	

General guidelines for duration of therapy in patients without prostheses and with good clinical response: *Neisseria gonorrhoeae,* 1 week; *Haemophilus,* streptococci, and *Streptococcus pneumoniae,* 2 weeks; remainder of organisms, 4 weeks. In patients with a prosthesis, therapy continues for 3 weeks after removal of the prosthetic device. In patients with prompt clinical response and for whom a good oral antibiotic is available, the latter portion of therapy may be accomplished with oral drug.

Repeated aspiration, daily if necessary, should be done over a period as long as a week if the clinical course requires it. If the course is unsatisfactory due to loculation of fluid, irrigation of the joint is appropriate. Irrigation of the knee through the arthroscope may be an excellent means of removing exudate. Open drainage is always required in infections of the hip. It is also required in other joints when despite aspiration and irrigation there is persistent purulent drainage, a persistent positive culture, or continued swelling and tenderness.

In addition to these measures the joints should be rested but not immobilized. Active weight-bearing may be begun early after subsidence of pain and the severe acute inflammatory reaction. Only rarely is synovectomy required.

INFECTION OF PROSTHETIC JOINTS

The problem of infection in prosthetic joints is quite different from that in native joints. A wide variety of microorganisms are found, the most common being coagulase-negative staphylococci, usually *Staphylococcus epidermidis*. Gram-negative rods, particularly *Serratia* and *Pseudomonas*, are common.

Treatment of infection of prosthetic joints usually requires removal of the prosthesis. With this done, appropriate antimicrobial therapy chosen on the basis of sensitivity tests is required for only a relatively short period, that is, for about 2 to 3 weeks. A waiting period thereafter of 3 to 6 months—if this is otherwise feasible—is generally advised before the joint is replaced.

In some patients with prosthetic joint infections, it is impossible to remove the prosthesis (e.g., because of other disease or refusal by the patient). Here, long-term suppressive therapy may be undertaken, and although drainage almost always continues, acute inflammatory episodes may be reduced to a minimum and overt sepsis avoided.

SUGGESTED READING

Carnesdale PG. Infectious arthritis. In: Crenshaw AW, ed. Campbell's operative orthopaedics. 7th ed. St. Louis: CV Mosby, 1987:677.

Smith JW. Infectious arthritis. In: Mandell GL, Douglas RG Jr, Bennett JE, eds. Principles and practice of infectious diseases. New York: John Wiley & Sons, 1985:700.

NONBACTERIAL INFECTIOUS ARTHRITIDES

RICHARD J. MANGI, M.D.

Nonbacterial infectious arthritides include four broad categories: viral, fungal, mycobacterial, and postinfectious (reactive) arthritis. In many cases the underlying infectious process is obvious, and once the physician recognizes that arthritis can be part of the spectrum of disease, additional diagnostic efforts are unnecessary. In other instances, arthritis may be the initial or the only manifestation of the infection. The clinician must, in these cases, consider many diagnoses, including infectious, rheumatologic, traumatic, degenerative, and other disease processes that cause arthritis.

In this chapter the major nonbacterial causes of infectious arthritis are discussed, with a brief approach to the diagnosis and treatment of these diseases.

VIRAL ARTHRITIS

Viruses most often cause arthritis by direct infection of the synovium, as occurs with rubella. In other instances, most notably hepatitis B virus, arthritis results from deposition of immune complexes in synovial tissues. Joint symptoms occur rarely during several other viral infections in which the pathogenesis is not fully understood. Arthritic symptoms usually occur during the prodrome or early in the course of viral disease, commonly with the onset of the viral rash.

Polyarticular involvement is most frequent, involving the joints in a symmetrical manner. Monoarticular disease is less common and usually a manifestation of direct viral infection of the joint.

Viral arthritis is self-limited, and permanent joint damage is rare. Treatment consists of nonsteroidal anti-inflammatory drugs and rest.

Rubella

Rubella is the most frequent cause of viral arthritis, which occurs in up to 50 percent of adult females and 5 percent of adult males with rubella. Joint symptoms begin during the week before or the week after the typical exanthem. Symmetrical polyarticular disease is typical, with involvement of the small joints of (in decreasing order of frequency) the hands, knees, wrists, ankles, and elbows. Arthralgias and morning stiffness are more frequent than frank arthritis. Recent studies indicate that arthritis can persist for several months, with more than 30 percent of adult females experiencing joint symptoms 18 to 24 months after infection.

Rubella arthritis can be confused with rheumatoid arthritis, particularly when the rubella rash is absent. Since many females develop persistent joint symptoms after rubella infection, all patients with seronegative rheumatoid arthritis should be tested for recent rubella infection.

Rubella Vaccine

Arthralgia and, to a lesser extent, arthritis can occur after rubella vaccination. The incidence of arthritis is less than 5 percent in children but up to 13 percent in women.

Arthralgias occur in up to 40 percent of vaccinated women. Symptoms occur from 2 to 6 weeks after vaccination and usually subside within 2 weeks but often last for several months. Symmetrical polyarticular disease is usual, but knee involvement is more common than with natural rubella, followed by fingers, wrists, ankles, and hips. Unlike natural rubella, rubella vaccine can cause relapsing arthritis in up to 5 percent of women and 0.1 percent of all children vaccinated. These epsiodes decrease in frequency and severity with time and probably do not cause any permanent joint damage.

Hepatitis B

Arthritis of hepatitis B virus (HBV) is most likely caused by deposition of immune complexes of HBV surface antigen and antibody (HBsAg and HBsAb) and complement in synovium. Up to 25 percent of patients with HBV have joint symptoms during the prodrome. Polyarticular symmetrical involvement of small joints is most common (proximal interphalangeal joints [PIP], 82 percent; knees, 30 percent; ankles, 24 percent). Monoarticular presentation also occurs. Joint symptoms occur abruptly 6 to 20 weeks after exposure, with striking morning stiffness preceding jaundice by several days or weeks (mean, 2½ weeks) and may occur with anicteric hepatitis. Nausea and vomiting occur in about 25 percent and fever in up to 50 percent of cases of arthritis. Urticaria and maculopapular or petechial rashes occur in 40 percent of patients.

Joint symptoms usually resolve with the onset of jaundice but may persist for several weeks. There is no permanent joint damage. Patients with chronic active hepatitis may have chronic or recurrent joint symptoms.

Liver function abnormalities are present at the onset of arthritis. Peripheral white blood cell (WBC) counts vary from normal to 20,000, and the erythrocyte sedimentation rate (ESR) is usually normal. HBsAg is detectable in the serum, but HBsAb is usually absent at the onset of joint symptoms. Serum complement levels may be depressed or normal. Cryoglobulinemia is common. Joint fluid is inflammatory, with counts of more than 25,000 cells per cubic millimeter usual, representing either a mononuclear or polymorphonuclear leukocyte predominance. Joint fluid glucose concentration is normal, and complement levels are decreased.

Enteroviruses

Coxsackievirus and echovirus occasionally cause polyarticular arthritis, accompanying the rash, fever, and other clinical manifestations of disease. These cases resolve spontaneously within 2 weeks.

Varicella-Zoster

Monoarticular arthritis, most frequently involving the knee, can occur with chickenpox and represents viral septic arthritis. It is self-limiting, resolving within a week. Synovial leukocytosis occurs, usually mononuclear and with fewer than 25,000 cells per cubic millimeter.

Mumps

Arthralgias, morning stiffness, and polyarticular and monoarticular arthritis have all been described during mumps infection. Joint symptoms typically occur during the first 3 weeks after the onset of parotitis but may occur either before parotitis, or with subclinical mumps. Males are affected more frequently than females, and the incidence of orchitis is trebled in patients with arthritis. Fever and mild leukocytosis usually accompany mumps arthritis. Duration of arthritis varies from 2 weeks to 6 months.

Alphaviruses

Five alphaviruses—chikungunya, O'nyong-nyong, Mayaro, Ross River, and Sindbis—frequently cause arthritis. These arthropod-borne viral infections occur in endemic regions (see the chapter *Viral Hemorrhagic Fever*). While each virus has unique features, typical presentation includes fever, rash, and symmetrical polyarticular arthritis. Tendinitis and soft tissue swelling are common. Subcutaneous nodules occur with chikungunya virus. Joint symptoms generally resolve within 1 week but may persist for months.

Other Viruses

Joint symptoms occur less frequently during the following viral infections.

Adenovirus type 7 has been reported to cause polyarticular arthritis following upper respiratory tract symptoms. It is associated with decreased serum complement levels and thought to represent immune complex disease.

Cytomegalovirus monoarticular infection has been documented in a renal transplant recipient.

Epstein-Barr virus has been reported to cause monoarticular arthritis, probably on a direct infectious basis.

Erythema infectiosum frequently causes arthralgias and arthritis of large joints, particularly in adults infected with this virus.

Hepatitis A causes arthralgias preceding or coincident with hepatitis in 11 percent of cases. An additional two cases of arthritis and cryoglobulinemia with relapsing hepatitis have been described.

Herpes simplex virus type 1 disseminated infection has been reported to cause monoarticular arthritis secondary to viral joint infection.

Human immunodeficiency virus (HIV) causes arthralgias and myalgias during the infectious mononucleosis-like acute febrile illness that occurs in up to 90 percent of cases during seroconversion. Headache, lymphadenopathy, and rash are frequent, and the symptoms last 3 to 14 days with no joint sequelae. In addition, an association between HIV and Reiter's syndrome has been described. It is uncertain whether this association is coincidental or whether it is due to diarrheal pathogens or another unrecognized mechanism. Some of these patients are HLA-B27 positive. HIV-Reiter's syndrome is usually progressive and destructive.

FUNGAL ARTHRITIS

Most fungal arthritis is secondary to contiguous spread of infection from adjacent osteomyelitis. Hematogenous fungal infection of joints does, however, occur. *Candida* and *Aspergillus* species occur in immunocompromised hosts. Other cases occur in normal hosts. *Sporothrix schenckii*, *Coccidioides immitis*, *Histoplasma capsulatum*, and *Blastomyces dermatitidis* are the most frequent examples. *Cryptococcus neoformans* can occur in normal or immunocompromised hosts.

Fungi usually cause monoarticular disease of the knee. The majority of cases cause chronic indolent symptoms with relatively few signs of systemic or local inflammation. It is common for the correct diagnosis to be delayed months or years, resulting in permanent joint damage.

Synovial fluid analysis is variable, with total leukocyte counts, usually polymorphonuclear, ranging from a few hundred to more than 100,000 per cubic millimeter, with normal glucose levels. Synovial culture results are superior to those of synovial fluid. It is important that synovial biopsy material be cultured and stained for fungus in all cases of monoarticular or oligoarticular arthritis. Synovial biopsy is usually nondiagnostic with either granulomata or nonspecific inflammation.

The standard treatment for all cases of fungal arthritis is intravenous amphotericin B. Joint fluid levels achieved with 0.8 mg per kilogram given every other day are adequate to treat most fungal infections. There are many anecdotal reports of the use of concomitant direct instillation of amphotericin B for those cases that fail systemic therapy alone. While some physicians routinely use 5-fluorocytosine in combination with amphotericin B for cryptococcal infection, we prefer to use amphotericin B alone and reserve the addition of 5-fluorocytosine for those cases that fail monotherapy. The imidazole antifugal drugs now available commercially, including ketoconazole, are not very effective for fungal arthritis. In addition to medical therapy, most cases should be treated with repeated needle aspiration of joint fluid. Open surgical drainage and debridement may sometimes be necessary, particularly with contiguous osteomyelitis.

Candida

Arthritis can occur in any of the usual settings that predispose patients to candidemia, including immunosuppression, indwelling intravascular lines, prolonged antibiotic therapy, and malignancy. Considering the frequency of candidemia, the incidence of bone and joint infection is extremely low. Symptoms of joint infection are acute or indolent. The organism can usually be cultured from synovial fluid. Most cases respond to repeated needle drainage and intravenous amphotericin B.

Aspergillus fumigatus

Arthritis is a rare complication of *Aspergillus* fungemia and almost always occurs in immunocompromised hosts. Open surgical drainage and intravenous amphotericin B are recommended.

Sporothrix schenckii

Arthritis is rare and usually secondary to direct extension from cutaneous lesions. The hands and wrists are most frequently involved. Disseminated disease secondary to inhalation of *Sporothrix* is unusual but is associated with frequent bone and joint involvement. Some cases occur without pulmonary or systemic signs of infection, leading to a delay in diagnosis that may average more than 2 years. Intravenous amphotericin B is the treatment of choice.

Coccidioides immitis

There are two forms of arthritis: a hypersensitivity reaction occurring during acute disease and septic arthritis associated with disseminated coccidioidal infection. Arthralgias and occasionally arthritis are common during acute disease, resolving spontaneously within a few weeks. Septic arthritis is most frequently secondary to contiguous osteomyelitis, but primary joint infection also occurs. Multiple bone and joint involvement is usual. The delay in diagnosis of monoarticular disease is frequently several years.

Blastomyces dermatitidis

Bone and joint infections often complicate systemic disease. Arthritis can occur from contiguous osteomyelitis or synovial infection. Acute inflammation of the joint is more common than with other fungi, and patients have more systemic signs of infection. Synovial fluid wet mounts and cultures are usually positive.

Cryptococcus neoformans

Joint infection occurs following disseminated disease, and although infection is more frequent in immunocompromised hosts, normal hosts are occasionally infected. Arthritis is usually secondary to spread from adjacent bone infection. The radiographic appearance of cryptococcal osteomyelitis is unique—an osteolytic lesion sometimes mistaken for malignancy.

MYCOBACTERIAL ARTHRITIS

Mycobacterium tuberculosis

M. tuberculosis bone and joint infections occur in about 1 percent of cases in the United States but at a much higher frequency in underdeveloped areas of the world. While vertebral osteomyelitis is the most common site of bone infection, the weight-bearing joints (hip, knee, ankle, in decreasing order) are more frequently involved than the long bones. Radiologic changes occur late in the course of disease. Subchondral erosions and osteopenia precede joint-space narrowing. Signs of joint inflammation are usually minimal, and tuberculosis should be considered in all cases of indolent monoarticular disease.

Synovial fluid cell counts are between 10,000 and 20,000 cells per cubic millimeter, with mononuclear or polymorphonuclear cell predominance. Glucose levels are less than 50 mg per deciliter in little more than 50 percent of cases. Acid-fast smears are positive in about 20 percent of cases, and cultures of synovial fluid positive in about 80 percent. Synovial biopsy may reveal granulomas or nonspecific inflammation.

Tuberculous arthritis should be treated with two drugs, isoniazid, 300 mg per day, and rifampin, 600 mg per day, for 9 to 12 months. Surgical debridement is usually not necessary unless joint destruction is extensive.

Atypical Mycobacteria

Infections of joints, periarticular tissue, and tendon sheaths by atypical mycobacteria occur by direct, surgical, or traumatic inoculation or during intra-articular corticosteroid injection and by systemic dissemination. The hands, wrists, and occasionally the knees are involved. *Mycobacterium kansasii* and *Mycobacterium avium-Mycobacterium intracellulare* are most frequent. Infection is usually indolent, with stiffness and swelling of tendon sheaths or periarticular tissue most common. A delay of several years between the onset of symptoms and diagnosis is frequent. Surgical biopsy and culture of the involved tissue is the best way of making the diagnosis. Joint destruction is unusual in normal hosts but occurs in patients receiving corticosteroids or cytotoxic drugs. Treatment usually requires surgical excision, with chemotherapy directed to the sensitivities of specific organisms. *Mycobacterium marinum* usually causes cutaneous lesions—the "fish tank granuloma"—and rarely causes deeper infection, including arthritis. Infection with this organism should be treated with ethambutol and rifampin for 12 weeks. Less common causes of atypical mycobacterial joint infection are *Mycobacterium fortuitum* and *Mycobacterium szulgari*.

REACTIVE ARTHRITIS (REITER'S SYNDROME)

A reactive inflammatory arthritis occurring after an infection, especially during an epidemic, is termed Reiter's syndrome and is essentially indistinguishable from Reiter's disease, the triad of urethritis, conjunctivitis, and arthritis. There is a long list of infectious agents known to cause Reiter's syndrome (Table 1). *Yersinia enterocolitica* and *Chlamydia trachomatis* are the most frequently implicated pathogens. There is a strong association with HLA-B27 antigen, as there is with other spondyloarthropathies, with 60 to 80 percent prevalence among affected individuals. Only certain enteric pathogens cause disease, and within a species not all serotypes are arthritogenic. For example, *Shigella flexneri*, but not *Shigella sonnei* or *Shigella dysenteriae*, causes disease.

The incidence of postdiarrheal disease is evenly distributed between males and females, while the postvenereal disease favors males in a 9:1 ratio. Disease starts 1 to 4 weeks after diarrhea or sexual exposure. The onset of disease is acute. Urethritis is usually the first symptom, followed by conjunctivitis and arthritis. The knees, ankles, metatarsalphalangeal joint, and wrists are involved in an asymmetri-

TABLE 1 Infectious Agents of Reiter's Syndrome (Reactive Arthritis)

Shigella flexneri, serotype 2a
Yersinia enterocolitica, serotype 3
Yersinia pseudotuberculosis
Salmonella typhimurium
Salmonella enteritidis
Salmonella heidelberg
Salmonella muenchen
Salmonella hador
Campylobacter fetus
Campylobacter jejuni
Chlamydia trachomatis
Chlamydia psittaci
Clostridium difficile
Brucella melitensis
Leptospira icterohaemorrhagiae
Neisseria gonorrhoeae
Neisseria meningitidis
Streptococci
Chronic cutaneous infection (acne fulminans, acne conglobata, hidradenitis suppurativa) ?
Adenovirus
Hepatitis B
Rubella vaccination
HIV ?
Entamoeba histolytica
Giardia lamblia
Strongyloides stercoralis
Ureaplasma urealyticum ?

cal fashion. Heel pain is present in 50 percent and low back pain in 20 percent of cases. Extra-articular manifestations, including keratoderma blenorrhagicum and circinate balanitis, are rare compared with Reiter's disease. Tendinitis and fasciitis are common.

Synovial fluid leukocytosis varies up to 50,000 cells per cubic millimeter, with polymorphonuclear predominance. Glucose levels are normal. About 50 percent of patients experience only one episode of disease, lasting 4 to 12 months. About 30 percent have relapses, with symptom-free intervals lasting months or years, and 20 percent develop chronic, progressive arthritis and spondylitis, usually asymmetrical.

Treatment consists of nonsteroidal anti-inflammatory drugs, rest, and physical therapy. Intra-articular corticosteroids are sometimes effective. Systemic corticosteroids and oral methotrexate are reserved for severe or chronic cases.

PARASITIC ARTHRITIS

Although rare in this country, parasitic rheumatism is well known in endemic areas. *Strongyloides stercoralis*, *Taenia saginata*, *Endolimax nana*, *Schistosoma mansoni*, and filariodes can all cause arthritis. Oligoarticular or monoarticular disease is usual. While parasites can directly invade synovial tissue, immune complex disease is thought to cause parasitic rheumatism. The diagnosis is best entertained by using Doury's criteria (see Suggested Reading, Doury et al, 1983): (1) mono- or oligoarticular disease; (2) history of stay in endemic area; (3) increased ESR; (4) peripheral eosinophilia; (5) parasite identified directly or indirectly in stool, urine, or blood; (6) inflammatory synovial fluid but

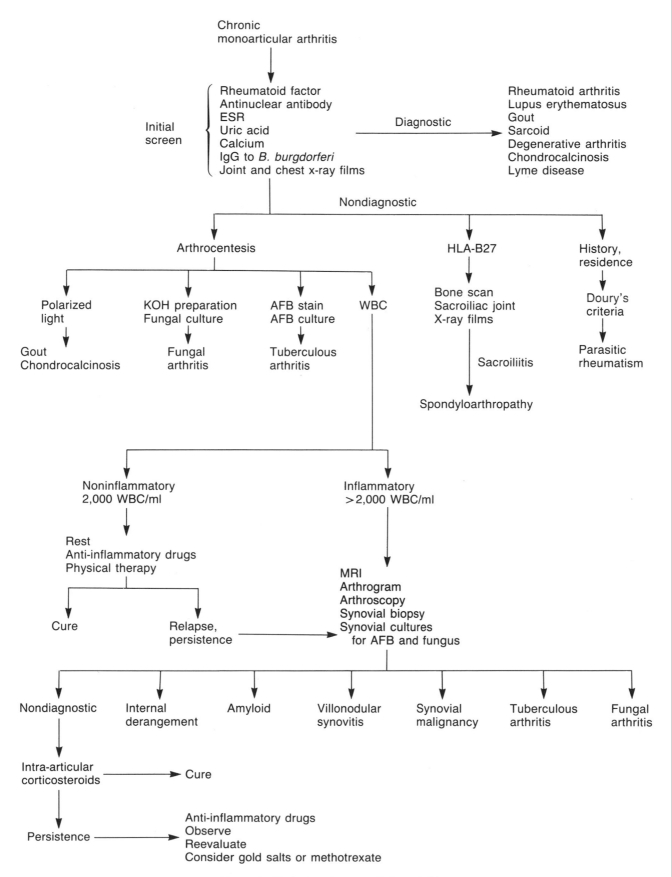

Figure 1 Evaluation of monoarticular arthritis.

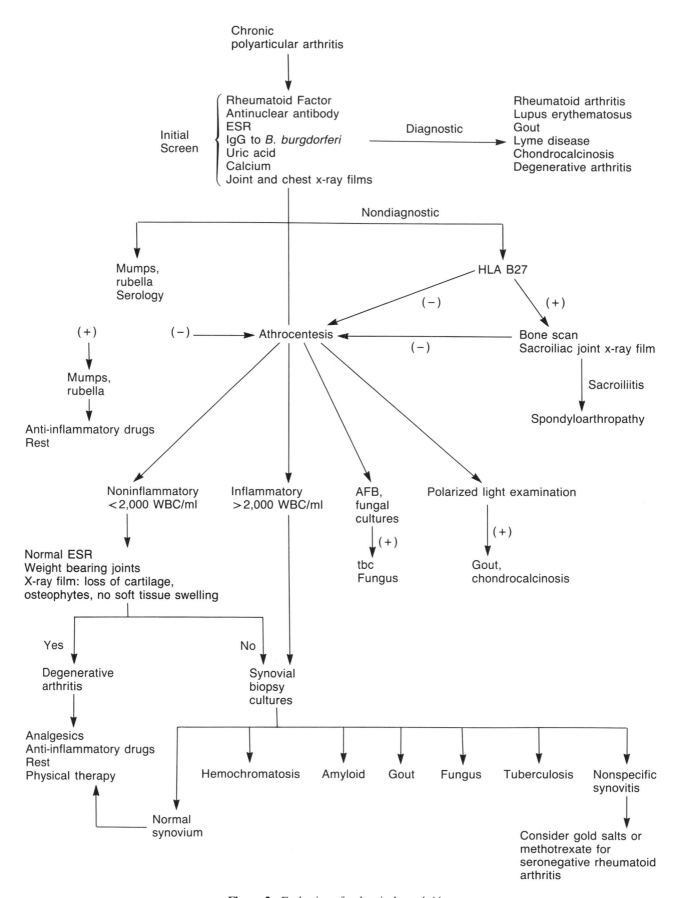

Figure 2 Evaluation of polyarticular arthritis.

no parasite found; (7) no radiologic change; (8) poor response to anti-inflammatory drugs; and (9) dramatic response to antiparasitic drugs.

APPROACH TO MONOARTICULAR ARTHRITIS

Infection is a rare cause of chronic arthritis. Most viral arthropathies are polyarticular. Fungal and mycobaterial disease should, however, be considered in the differential diagnosis of monoarticular or oligoarticular arthritis. The majority of monoarticular arthritides of the knee are noninflammatory, traumatic, posttraumatic, internal knee derangement, or degenerative arthritis. Fungal arthritis and mycobacterial arthritis represent less than 0.1 percent of the cases of swollen knees, and, to compound matters, they often present in an indolent manner, with noninflammatory joint fluid. Small wonder that the infectious diagnosis often escapes detection.

Although this chapter is not intended as a comprehensive rheumatologic approach, the infectious disease clinician should be familiar with a logical approach to the evaluation of arthritis. Figure 1 illustrates the author's approach to chronic (longer than 1 month in duration) monoarticular arthritis. An experienced clinician can make the correct diagnosis on the basis of the history and physical examination in more than 95 percent of cases. Assuming, however, that the diagnosis is not obvious from the history and physical examination, the first step is to obtain the initial screening tests noted (Fig. 1). These tests will uncover most of the common causes of monoarticular arthritis and will be diagnostic in about 50 percent of patients. Although Lyme disease is covered in another chapter, it must be emphasized that antibody screening, preferably ELISA, IgG to *Borrelia burgdorferi*, should be part of every initial screening of mono- and polyarticular arthritis. Lyme disease is probably the most frequently missed infectious cause of chronic arthritis.

The next step is an HLA-B27 screen and an arthrocentesis. A positive HLA-B27 should trigger further tests for spondyloarthropathies, the most frequent inflammatory cause of chronic monoarticular arthritis. Joint fluid analysis should always include an acid-fast (AFB) smear and culture, a potassium hydroxide (KOH) preparation, and a fungal culture. The most important information obtained from the joint fluid is probably the cell count. Patients with noninflammatory cell counts can usually be assigned to a therapeutic trial of conservative management, whereas those with inflammatory fluid require more extensive evaluation.

The magnetic resonance imaging (MRI) technique is the best radiologic method to evaluate monoarticular disease, particularly of the knee. It provides excellent resolution of soft tissue structures, including damaged menisci and cruciate ligaments, and intra-articular tumors. Although this test is expensive, it probably will soon replace arthrograms for radiologic evaluation of chronic knee disease.

Although some rheumatologists prefer to perform closed synovial biopsy, it is my opinion that arthroscopy, in competent hands, provides much more information with a relatively small increase in morbidity. Moreover, in many instances a small meniscal tear or cartilage damage is uncovered during arthroscopy, problems that can be immediately corrected with arthroscopic surgery. For these reasons, I recommend close collaboration with an experienced orthopaedic surgeon to ensure proper diagnostic material during diagnostic arthroscopy.

Even after arthroscopy a significant number of cases remain undiagnosed. Management of these patients is an art. Most clinicians agree with a trial of one or two doses of long-acting intra-articular corticosteroids followed by physical therapy directed at quadricep strengthening.

APPROACH TO POLYARTICULAR ARTHRITIS

The initial screen for diagnosis of polyarticular arthritis is essentially the same as that for monoarticular disease (Fig. 2). The next step is to exclude postviral disease with antibodies to mumps and rubella and an HLA-B27 screen for spondyloarthropathy.

The most important information provided by joint fluid analysis is, once again, differentiation of inflammatory from noninflammatory disease by the cell count. Patients with noninflammatory fluid, a normal ESR, involvement of weight-bearing joints (knees and hips), and radiologic changes compatible with degenerative arthritis should be treated with analgesics and anti-inflammatory drugs, rest, weight reduction, and physical therapy. The rest of the patients should have a synovial biopsy performed upon the largest involved joint—the knee if possible.

Those cases still undiagnosed after synovial biopsy usually fall into two categories: normal synovium, probably degenerative arthritis; and nonspecific synovitis, many of which are seronegative rheumatoid arthritides. The former group should be treated conservatively, but the latter should be more aggressively treated for seronegative rheumatoid arthritis at the discretion of an experienced rheumatologist.

SUGGESTED READING

Arnett FC. Seronegative spondylarthropathies. Bull Rheum Dis 1987; 37(no. 1):1–12.

Bassett LW. Magnetic resonance imaging in musculoskeletal disorders. Bull Rheum Dis 1987; 37(no. 3):1–8.

Blocka KLN, Sibley JT. Undiagnosed chronic monarthritis: clinical and evolutionary profile. Arth Rheum 1987; 30:1357–1361.

Brown JM, Sanders CV. *Mycobacterium marinum* infections: a problem of recognition, not therapy? Arch Intern Med 1987; 147:817–818.

Doury P, Pattin S, Dienot B, et al. Semin Hosp Paris 1983; 53:1359–1363.

Glickstein SL, Nashel DJ. *Mycobacterium kansasii* septic arthritis complicating rheumatic disease: case report and review of the literature. Semin Arth Rheum 1987; 16:231–235.

Imman RD. Rheumatic manifestations of hepatitis B infection. Semin Arth Rheum 1982; 11:406–420.

Tingle AJ, Allen M, Petty RE, et al. Rubella-associated arthritis. I. Comparative study of joint manifestations associated with natural rubella infection and RA 27/3 rubella immunization. Ann Rheum Dis 1986; 45:110–114.

Winchester R, Bernstein DH, Fischer HD, et al. The co-occurrence of Reiter's syndrome and acquired immunodeficiency. Ann Intern Med 1987; 106:19–26.

INFECTIONS AFFECTING MORE THAN ONE SYSTEM CAUSED BY BACTERIA OR VIRUSES

TUBERCULOSIS

ASIM K. DUTT, M.D.
WILLIAM W. STEAD, M.D.

With the dramatic decline of tuberculosis in Western countries, physicians often fail to consider the disease in the differential diagnosis, sometimes with tragic results. The index of suspicion should be especially high when persons in certain groups manifest cough with persistent fever or loss of weight: the elderly, disadvantaged persons, immigrants from developing countries, or immunosuppressed persons (e.g., on corticosteroid therapy or with human immunodeficiency virus [HIV] infection). The clinical presentation may vary over a wide spectrum from virtually no symptoms through symptoms such as mild, persistent fever and loss of weight to severe symptoms including cough, malaise, fever, and even hemoptysis. Isolation of *Mycobacterium tuberculosis* is essential for a firm diagnosis, but a strong clinical suspicion may suffice as an indication for specific chemotherapy.

Once the possibility of tuberculosis is considered, the steps for diagnosis are rather simple. Most important is the collection of secretions and/or biopsy materials for microscopy and culture. Radiologic examination and tuberculin testing are also of importance, but are not diagnostic. A classic roentgenogram of the chest may strongly suggest the disease, but all too often the radiographic presentation is quite atypical, especially when the infection has been acquired recently.

A positive tuberculin reaction by Mantoux test (10 or more millimeters' induration) indicates infection with tubercle bacilli. A compatible clinical presentation and radiographic abnormality increase the possibility of the disease. However, a negative tuberculin test does not necessarily rule out the diagnosis, as 20 to 25 percent of patients who are clinically ill may have an initial negative test. A repeat of the test 2 weeks later may be positive. Some patients are anergic and may not be able to show enough T-cell activity to develop a positive tuberculin reaction. Persons over age 12 years and under 60 years who react to tuberculin should be tested for HIV infection because its presence affects the risk of tuberculosis and the length of therapy.

DIAGNOSIS

Pulmonary Tuberculosis

Spontaneously produced sputum provides necessary material for smear and culture in diagnosis of pulmonary tuberculosis. At least three early-morning sputum specimens should be examined by microscopy (Fig. 1). If one of these is positive, no further collection is necessary. When all are negative on microscopy, at least five specimens should be submitted for culture.

If a patient is unable to produce sputum or is uncooperative, an alternative method is to induce sputum by inhalation of heated aerosol of saline. Other methods are early-morning gastric lavage and laryngeal swab or aspiration; these are not quite as productive.

When microscopy of sputum is negative on at least three specimens, bronchial washing through a fiberoptic bronchoscope may be indicated. In addition, postbronchoscopy sputum specimens should be collected because they often yield positive result. Transtracheal puncture may be necessary as a last resort in unconscious patients with a life-threatening illness. In occasional patients, transthoracic needle aspirate of the lung may be indicated for obtaining necessary material for bacteriology. In rare circumstances the diagnosis is made only by open lung biopsy.

Although fluorescent microscopy is much more sensitive, it is quite nonspecific and must be confirmed by Ziehl-Neelsen or Kenyoun staining. Positive microscopy never confirms the presence of *M. tuberculosis* because other mycobacteria may be present. Therefore, cultural examination is necessary for isolation and identification of *M. tuberculosis*. Furthermore, testing for susceptibility to antituberculosis drugs is useful for identifying the occasional case of primary drug resistance.

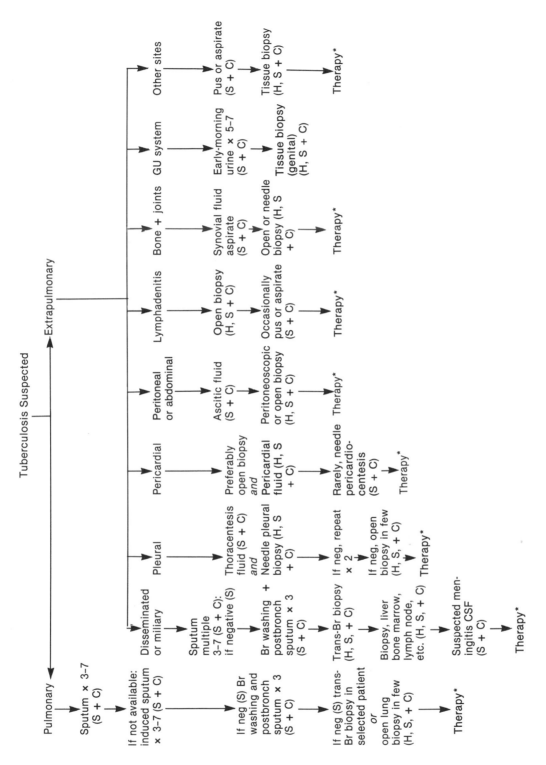

Figure 1 Diagnosis of suspected tuberculosis. Abbreviations: S = smear, C = culture for mycobacteria, H = histology, Br = bronchial, Bronch = bronchoscopy, CSF = cerebrospinal fluid, Bx = biopsy, neg = negative, GU = genitourinary; * therapy started in suspected cases, awaiting cultural results and/or clinical response.

Extrapulmonary Tuberculosis

For the diagnosis of tuberculosis in extrapulmonary sites, secretions and/or biopsy material should be obtained for examination (Fig. 1). In the case of pleural and pericardial effusion, biopsy and/or fluid should be examined and cultured. The yield from culture of pleural fluid is small, presumably because of the relatively small population of organisms present. Cerebrospinal fluid smear and cultural examination are necessary in meningitis, but positive results are found in only 20 to 40 percent of the cases of tuberculous meningitis. Cultural examination of ascitic fluid in tuberculous peritonitis may confirm the diagnosis, but microscopy and culture of a percutaneous biopsy specimen is preferred.

The definitive diagnosis of genitourinary tuberculosis requires the isolation of *M. tuberculosis* by urine culture. An acid-fast stain of an early-morning specimen should be performed on 3 to 5 separate days.

In tuberculosis of joints, bacteriologic examination of synovial fluid is important. Positive synovial fluid culture may be found in approximately 80 percent of cases, and about one-fourth may show the organism in the smear examination. Pus and fluids from discharging sinuses from any site should be submitted for microscopy and culture.

If the microscopic examination of fluid is negative, a definitive diagnosis is delayed for 6 to 8 weeks while cultural results are awaited. Hence, biopsy of the involved tissue, either by needle or exploratory surgery, is often required for early diagnosis.

In cases of the pleural effusion, closed-needle biopsy should be performed to obtain three to four pieces of pleura to submit for both microscopy and culture. The tissue sections should also be stained for acid-fact bacilli. It is common to find a typical granulomatous pleuritis in which no organisms can be found by special staining. Culture of one or two tissue fragments greatly increases the diagnostic yield of the procedure. It is a common error to place all tissue fragments into formalin, which precludes culture. If the first set of biopsies is not diagnostic, at least one more attempt should be made before considering the results negative. Repeated biopsies increase the yield of positive results by 15 to 20 percent. In rare circumstances, surgical biopsy of pleura may be indicated.

Surgical biopsy is preferred for pericardial disease because it is usually a safer procedure and gives enough tissue for examination, while providing drainage of the fluid through a pericardial "window." In disseminated or miliary tuberculosis, needle biopsy of liver and bone marrow is recommended. Hepatic biopsy is positive in more than 80 percent of cases and bone marrow, in more than 50 percent if examined by both microscopy and culture. Miliary pulmonary disease with negative sputum smears is best approached by transbronchial biopsy through a fiberoptic bronchoscope. Rarely, open lung biopsy may be necessary for the diagnosis. Percutaneous biopsy of the peritoneum is generally productive, but open biopsy may be obtained at exploratory laparotomy. Lymph nodes generally require excision biopsy. A Craig-needle biopsy of bone, joint, or vertebra is quite productive if specimens are examined both by microscopy and culture. If results are unsatisfactory, an open surgical biopsy is the next step.

Clinical Diagnosis

A diagnosis of tuberculosis may be justified despite negative bacteriologic results when the clinical picture is strongly suggestive and the clinical situation calls for therapy. Patients with a positive tuberculin test, with compatible abnormal radiographs with or without symptoms, and in whom other possible causes have been reasonably excluded should be given a trial of chemotherapy.

Chemotherapy is initiated only after necessary materials have been submitted for bacteriological studies.

Such patients are observed for the clinical response to therapy. If there is prompt improvement over a few weeks the diagnosis of tuberculosis is likely correct and therapy should be continued to completion. If there is no improvement or worsening over a few weeks, diagnostic efforts to find the correct diagnosis should be undertaken, because tuberculosis is not likely in those circumstances.

CHEMOTHERAPY

Until a few years ago, the standard therapy for tuberculosis consisted of isoniazid (INH) and ethambutol (EMB) with a supplement of 1 to 3 months of streptomycin (SM) in cavitary smear-positive cases. The therapy was effective provided that the drugs were taken for 18 to 24 months. During the past decade, the availability of another oral bactericidal agent, rifampin (RIF), has made it possible to complete therapy much more quickly. By using INH and RIF together, the duration of treatment has been reduced to 9 months. It can even be shortened to 6 months if SM plus pyrazinamide (PZA) or EMB plus PZA are added to the regimen for the first two months.

Bacteriologic Concept of Drug Therapy

Many in vitro and in vivo studies in animals have increased our understanding of the bacterial population in tuberculous lesions and the action of drugs on them. Tubercle bacilli are obligate aerobes and thrive best in an environment with high oxygen tension. There are at least three distinct bacterial populations in a tuberculous lesion: (1) the largest population (ranging from 10^7 to 10^9 organisms) is actively replicating in a neutral or slightly alkaline medium in cavitary lesions; (2) a much smaller population (ranging from 10^2 to 10^5 organisms) exists in a neutral or slightly alkaline milieu of closed caseous and noncaseous lesions where it is metabolically less active or even dormant; (3) a similar small population (ranging from 10^2 to 10^5 organisms) is slowly replicating in the acid medium inside macrophages.

The size and metabolic activity of these bacterial populations is important because tubercle bacilli mutate to drug-resistant forms at a predictable rate irrespective of the presence or absence of antituberculous drug. Mutants resistant to each drug develop independently of other mutations and at a rate of approximately one per 10^{-5} to 10^{-6} replications. Those resistant to two drugs develop rarely, approximately once per 10^{-10} to 10^{-12} replications. Hence, a cavitary lung disease with a bacterial population of 10^7 to

10^9 organisms may contain 100 to 10,000 mutants resistant to any effective drug, and small populations in closed caseous or noncaseous lesions and in macrophages may have few or none. Thus, all cavitary tuberculous lesions harbor a mixture of drug-sensitive and -resistant bacilli, making at least two drugs essential to success.

Tubercle bacilli replicate rather slowly, about every 16 to 20 hours. The antituberculous drugs are effective in killing tubercle bacilli only when the organisms are replicating. Hence, antituberculous drugs are best given in a single daily dose, but must be given for a prolonged period to allow time to kill the entire population, including those that are semidormant and divide only intermittently.

Rapid elimination of the actively multiplying large population of bacilli is essential to prevent emergence of drug-resistant mutants, a process that results in treatment failure. Elimination of smaller populations of intermittently multiplying organisms by extended therapy is necessary to prevent late relapse due to replication of the "persisters."

Drug Action on the Bacilli

The antituberculous drugs are generally classified as bactericidal and bacteriostatic. SM, capreomycin (CAP), RIF, INH, and PZA are considered bactericidal. The bacteriostatic drugs are EMB, ethionamide (ETA), cycloserine (CS), and *para*-aminosalicylic acid (PAS). EMB in a dosage of 25 mg per kilogram is considered by some to be bactericidal and certainly is more effective in eliminating bacilli than in the usually prescribed dose of 15 mg per kilogram.

Among the bactericidal drugs, SM, INH, and RIF are highly active against actively multiplying extracellular bacilli (Fig. 2). With intensive daily therapy, these organisms can be eliminated rapidly. Selection of drug-resistant mutants is avoided and conversion of sputum smears to negative is prompt. Inadequate dosage or irregular ingestion may lead to treatment failure, with emergence of drug resistance.

RIF, INH, and PZA are active against slowly replicating organisms located inside the macrophages or extracellularly (Fig. 2). PZA is particularly effective in the acid environment inside macrophages. RIF is capable of killing bacilli that show even the slightest metabolic activity and, hence, is a useful drug during the continuation phase. With adequate duration of therapy, even the persisters are eliminated, resulting in a permanent cure. Inadequate length of treatment may permit a late relapse due to late replication of the persisters. Such a relapse is usually due to drug-sensitive organisms. It has been shown that most antituberculous drugs are effective when given twice weekly after the initial period of intensive daily administration. The addition of SM or PZA is not generally necessary, but the bactericidal activity of RIF and INH can be intensified by a supplement of SM and PZA to the regimen for the first 2 months. Such a regimen can further reduce the total duration of therapy to 6 months, with an added advantage of being effective even in the presence of INH resistance.

Treatment of Newly Diagnosed Tuberculosis

Before initiation of therapy, four possible clues to the probability of INH resistance should be sought (Fig. 3): (1) Has the patient received antituberculous drugs anytime in the past? (2) Is the patient from a country with a high prevalence of disease and drug resistance, e.g., Southeast Asia, Africa, or Latin America? (3) Is it likely the patient acquired the infection from an individual with a drug-resistant case? (4) Does the patient live in an area where INH resistance is common (more than 5 percent)?

If the answers to all of these inquiries are "no," therapy may safely be initiated with INH, 300 mg, and RIF, 600 mg, daily. In the United States, the incidence of initial drug resistance is low except for a few areas—the Mexican border, large cities, parts of California—where the addition of SM/CAP and PZA should almost be routine. Drug suscep-

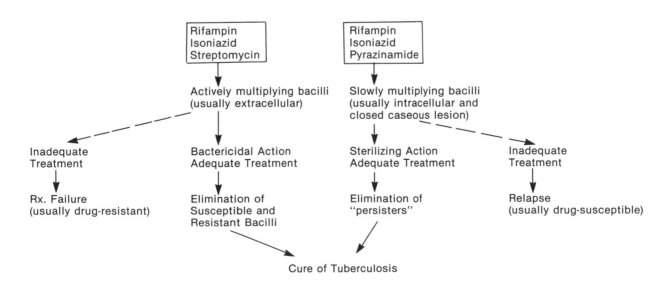

Figure 2 Current principles of tuberculosis chemotherapy.

Pretreatment inquiries:
1. Has the patient ever been treated with drug(s) before?
2. Has the patient acquired infection in countries with high prevalence of drug resistance?
3. Has the patient acquired infection from drug-resistant case?
4. Is the drug resistance high in the area?

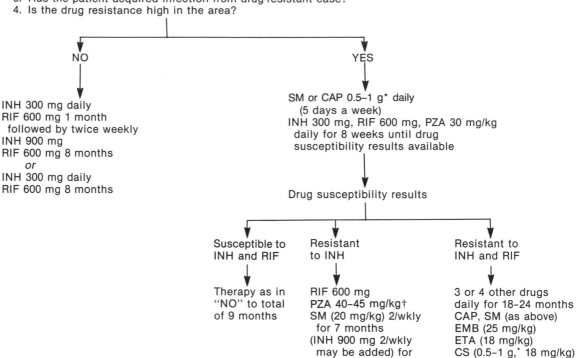

NO

INH 300 mg daily
RIF 600 mg 1 month
 followed by twice weekly
INH 900 mg
RIF 600 mg 8 months
or
INH 300 mg daily
RIF 600 mg 8 months

YES

SM or CAP 0.5–1 g* daily
 (5 days a week)
INH 300 mg, RIF 600 mg, PZA 30 mg/kg
daily for 8 weeks until drug
susceptibility results available

Drug susceptibility results

Susceptible to
INH and RIF

Resistant
to INH

Resistant to
INH and RIF

Therapy as in
"NO" to total
of 9 months

RIF 600 mg
PZA 40–45 mg/kg†
SM (20 mg/kg) 2/wkly
 for 7 months
(INH 900 mg 2/wkly
 may be added) for
 "persisters"

3 or 4 other drugs
daily for 18–24 months
CAP, SM (as above)
EMB (25 mg/kg)
ETA (18 mg/kg)
CS (0.5–1 g,* 18 mg/kg)
PZA (30 mg/kg)

Figure 3 Chemotherapy of tuberculosis. * One gram is preferred; however, in patients who are elderly or weigh less than 100 pounds or have impaired renal function, the dose is revised downward. † Round off dose to tablet size.

tibility should be determined on the initial sputum specimen in each case. We recommend that the drugs be given as combination capsules, e.g., Rifamate (Merrell-Dow) or Rimactizide (Ciba). Each capsule contains INH, 150 mg, and RIF, 300 mg, and thus, two capsules a day in the early morning furnishes the total daily dose. In addition to the convenience of the combination capsule, the patient is precluded from taking only one of the drugs. Both drugs are given daily for 9 months or daily for 1 month followed by INH, 900 mg, and RIF, 600 mg twice weekly, for another 8 months, i.e., two combination capsules and two INH 300-mg tablets twice a week.

Our experience in more than 3,500 patients with the latter regimen has proved successful in more than 95 percent of cases now followed up to 12 years. We have also treated more than 500 patients with various forms of extrapulmonary tuberculosis with similar results and less than 1 percent relapse. Our experience also indicates that the regimen is effective in patients whose tuberculosis is associated with various medical disorders, e.g., diabetes, alcoholism, corticosteroid therapy, malignancy, and cytotoxic chemotherapy.

The addition of a third drug, e.g., EMB or SM, does not add significantly to the bactericidal action of INH and RIF. Such a supplement is recommended by some to ensure against failure in the event of initial INH resistance. We do not routinely add a third drug to our regimen, but add

both SM and PZA if we have a clue that there may be INH resistance (see above). Several recent studies have shown that initial intensive treatment with SM (0.5 to 0.75 g, or about 20 mg per kilogram); INH, 300 mg; RIF, 600 mg; and PZA, 25 to 30 mg per kilogram daily for 2 months, followed by INH, 300 mg, and RIF, 600 mg daily or twice weekly for another 4 months (i.e., total, 6 months), produces similar results. The regimen considerably reduces the duration of therapy.

Drug Therapy in Suspected or Proven INH Resistance

If drug resistance (to INH) is suspected, therapy should be initiated with SM, INH, RIF, and PZA in the dosages mentioned above until the drug susceptibility results are known (usually 2 months) (Fig. 3). Therapy is then changed according to the results. If the organisms prove to be sensitive to INH and RIF, the treatment may be completed with INH, 300 mg, and RIF, 600 mg daily, or INH, 900 mg, and RIF, 600 mg, twice weekly for the remainder of the 9 months. When INH or RIF resistance is found, the therapy is changed to SM (1.0 to 1.5 g; approximately 20 mg per kilogram); PZA, 40 to 45 mg per kilogram; and INH, 900 mg, or RIF, 600 mg (depending on susceptibility) twice weekly for the remainder of the 9 months. INH, 900 mg, is given even in the presence of acquired INH resistance because of its action on the persisters, which generally remain drug susceptible. This regimen ensures effectiveness of at least two bactericidal drugs against the resistant bacilli, i.e., SM and RIF on extracellular rapidly multiplying bacilli and RIF and PZA on the slowly replicating organisms.

In the presence of resistance to both INH and RIF, all drugs are discontinued, and therapy is instituted with three or four other antituberculous drugs. SM or CAP (if SM resistant) is given 5 days a week initially for 3 months along with two other drugs daily from the following: EMB, 25 mg per kilogram; PZA, 25 to 30 mg per kilogram; ETA, 500 to 750 mg (depending on tolerance; 750 mg is preferred, but this drug causes nausea); CS, about 18 mg per kilogram per day, accompanied by pyridoxine, 100 mg twice a day. The latter two are given in divided doses. As these drugs are not bactericidal, the total duration of therapy must be 18 to 24 months.

Preventive Therapy

Persons infected with tubercle bacilli (tuberculin reaction ≥ 10 mm) carry some risk of developing disease that may be prevented with INH preventive therapy. Since infected persons are not all at equal risk and since INH therapy may occasionally cause side effects, the risk and benefit of therapy must be assessed before prescribing preventive therapy. The American Thoracic Society and the Centers for Disease Control recommend the following groups for preventive therapy:

1. Household members and other close contacts of patients with infectious tuberculosis with positive tuberculin test and no previous history of reaction in the past. Contacts under age 4 years with negative tuberculin test should be given preventive therapy for 3 months and assessed again after 3 months with tuberculin test. If negative, the therapy is discontinued; otherwise, the full course is completed.
2. Newly infected persons (tuberculin converters).
3. Persons with a history of inadequately treated tuberculosis
4. Persons with a significant reaction and a stable abnormal chest roentgenogram
5. Positive tuberculin reaction and associated "risk" factors—silicosis, diabetes mellitus, prolonged therapy with costcosteroids, immunosuppressive therapy, hematologic and reticuloendothelial malignancy, acquired immunodeficiency syndrome, end-stage renal disease, and clinical conditions leading to rapid weight loss and chronic undernutrition.
6. Tuberculin skin test reactors under 35 years of age.

Although INH is generally safe, the adverse effect of hepatitis remains a major concern for clinicians. Before initiation of INH therapy, individuals must be screened for the risk factors. Preventive INH therapy of 300 mg daily for adults and 10 to 14 mg per kilogram, not exceeding 300 mg, in children is recommended for 6 to 12 months. Monitoring of preventive therapy for toxicity is no different than for treatment of clinical tuberculosis. Clinical monitoring for symptoms is adequate, obtaining liver function tests only when symptoms indicate. The supply of medication to the patient should not exceed one month's at a time. The patient must be informed of the symptoms of side effects and advised to discontinue therapy on development of symptoms and report immediately to the physician for evaluation.

At present, there is no preventive therapy that has been studied by clinical trial for persons infected with INH-resistant organisms. RIF, 600 mg daily, may be used for 12 months under the almost certain assumption that it would be effective. Similarly, in persons unable to tolerate INH therapy, RIF may be substituted if preventive therapy is strongly indicated.

Preventive therapy with INH has been shown to be 98.6 percent effective among tuberculin converters, both among children and elderly nursing home residents. However, in the treatment of incidentally discovered tuberculin reactors, the efficiency was only about 85 percent and the advantage of therapy more difficult to demonstrate.

Monitoring Adverse Effects of Drugs

The major adverse effect of both INH and RIF is hepatotoxicity, with an incidence of 2 to 4 percent. There is no detectable increase when PZA, another potentially hepatotoxic drug, is included in the regimen. We have encountered hepatotoxicity in 2.5 percent of more than 3,500 patients treated with INH and RIF, even though the majority were elderly and there were many alcoholics. However, prudence dictates that two hepatotoxic drugs should not be used together in patients with active hepatitis. For such persons, we recommend starting treatment with INH and EMB with a supplement of SM if the sputum smear is positive. When the hepatitis subsides, RIF may safely be exchanged for EMB to obtain the advantage of short-course therapy.

Beyond routine baseline biochemical tests for hepatic function, regular biochemical monitoring leads to more confusion than enlightenment, since transient benign elevation of hepatic enzymes is common during therapy. We advise each patient to stop therapy immediately upon development of suspicious symptoms—e.g., anorexia, nausea, vomiting, or scleral icterus—and to report to the clinic for hepatic enzyme estimation. If symptoms are accompanied by elevation of hepatic enzymes of more than five times the base level, drug toxicity is likely. After symptoms have abated and the hepatic enzymes have returned to base line, drugs are reintroduced one at a time, starting with half dosage and monitoring of hepatic enzymes. In this manner, the offending drug can be identified and therapy changed appropriately. It is not uncommon that both drugs can be reintroduced without further adverse effect.

Twice weekly therapy with RIF may give rise to immunologic and hematologic side effects of petechiae and thrombocytopenia. This rarely occurs with a dosage of 600 mg RIF, but was a problem when the dosage 900 to 1,200 mg was used, particularly when the interval between doses was prolonged beyond twice weekly. Petechiae with or without thrombocytopenia has occurred in only 0.5 percent of our patients. The patients should be advised to watch for bruised spots on the legs. RIF should be discontinued if this reaction develops. Twice weekly administration of RIF may also give rise to flu-like syndrome, associated with chills and fever and with considerable aches and pains over the body on the day the medication is taken. This has occurred in 2.5 percent of our patients. The incidence of these adverse effects also increases with the use of higher dosage of RIF (900 to 1,200 mg). The side effect may be eliminated by changing to daily therapy. Other major adverse effects reported in the literature are hemolytic anemia, acute renal failure, and "shock syndrome," but we have not encountered any in our 13 years' experience.

The other side effects are minor, e.g., drug fever, allergies, skin rashes, and gastrointestinal intolerance—these occur in approximately 5 percent of patients. These reactions subside on temporary withdrawal of the drug, which can often be reintroduced slowly without recurrence of symptoms.

SM may cause vestibular damage, but only rarely hearing loss. This adverse effect is dose related and may be reduced by injecting the drug only 5 days a week. Also, the dose of the drug should be cut to 0.5 g for persons older than 60 years of age and for patients with renal failure. Inquiry about dizziness and staggering may detect early toxicity. The drug may also cause allergic rashes and fever, which subside on withdrawal.

EMB is a well-tolerated drug and free from major adverse effects, but is of little value in short-course chemotherapy. The major side effect is optic neuritis (visual disturbances), which rarely occurs with the dose of 15 mg per kilogram, but may occur in 1 to 3 percent of patients receiving the more effective dose of 25 mg per kilogram. Monitoring of the side effect requires regular testing with reading and color charts and referral to an ophthalmologist for opinion in persons in whom toxicity is suspected.

PZA commonly causes flushing and, rarely, a skin rash. Hyperuricemia regularly occurs with PZA therapy, but rarely precipitates clinical gout. This is commoner during daily than during intermittent therapy. Arthralgia is frequent and occurs more often with daily treatment (7 percent) than with twice weekly administration (1 to 3 percent). Arthralgia is usually self-limiting and responds well to analgesics.

During therapy the health care team must remain in close contact with the patients because they may report suspicious symptoms. The patients should be informed about the symptoms of adverse effects and instructed to discontinue therapy if a problem is suspected and to report to the clinic promptly for clinical and laboratory assessment.

Surveillance of Patients During Therapy

Bacteriologic monitoring of patients during therapy is an important aspect in the management of tuberculosis. We suggest that three to five specimens of sputum be submitted for bacteriologic examination initially and that a drug susceptibility test be included. Then a sputum specimen should be submitted every 2 weeks until three specimens are reported to be negative. Thereafter, one specimen a month is adequate for the duration of therapy and for 6 months after completion. During follow-up one specimen every 3 months for another 6 months should be cultured after which the patient is discharged from supervision with the advice to return if symptoms recur.

A satisfactory response to treatment is observed by the gradual decline in the bacterial population of the sputum. Prolonged persistence of organisms in the sputum (more than 5 months) or reversion to positive bacteriology after conversion to negative should raise suspicion of treatment failure. Reevaluation of the patient's compliance and a repeat drug susceptibility test are then indicated in order to make the best choice of a retreatment four-drug regimen.

Frequent roentgenograms of chest are not indicated if bacteriologic studies are done as suggested. The health care team must evaluate whether the patient is taking the medications regularly as prescribed. This is carried out by frequent interviews with the patient, by checking attendance at clinic appointments and picking up of drugs, by surprise pill counts, and by random examination of urine for the color of RIF and for excretion of INH. In patients thought to be noncompliant, direct ingestion of drugs under supervision must be carried out. Twice weekly administration of drugs facilitates direct supervision.

Support by the Health Department

Most health departments provide facilities for collection of sputum specimens and bacteriologic examination. Monitoring of adverse effects of drugs and compliance of patients is provided through the able assistance of public health nurses. Expert advice is also provided by the personnel for difficult problems that may arise during management.

The public health nurses perform contact evaluation, with tuberculin testing and radiography when indicated, after receiving notification of an active case. Delay in notification of the health department may be catastrophic, particularly for children in whom the disease may progress rapidly with fatal results. Busy physicians who undertake to treat tuberculosis are well advised to take advantage of the facilities provided by local health departments in keeping up with patients for the 9 months of therapy.

NONTUBERCULOUS (ENVIRONMENTAL) MYCOBACTERIAL DISEASE IN THE NON–HIV-INFECTED PATIENT

DAVID E. GRIFFITH, M.D., F.C.C.P.
RICHARD J. WALLACE Jr., M.D.

Although most human mycobacterial disease is still caused by *Mycobacterium tuberculosis* or *Mycobacterium leprae*, a number of other mycobacterial species are capable of producing disease in humans. These species are especially important pathogens in certain geographic areas and in some immune compromised conditions, particularly the acquired immunodeficiency syndrome (AIDS). There are currently more than 50 recognized species of mycobacteria other than *Mycobacterium tuberculosis* or *Mycobacterium leprae*. Approximately 16 mycobacterial species are often encountered in large working laboratories. Unfortunately, considerable confusion about these organisms still exists among physicians who do not routinely care for patients infected with them. Part of the confusion rests with both the nonuniformity of labeling of these organisms as a group and a lack of uniformity in nomenclature of individual species. For the former problem, we prefer the term *nontuberculous* or *environmental* mycobacteria, the latter reflecting the fact that the reservoir for these organisms is soil and water. The term *atypical* is still widely used and understood, however. Improved microbiologic techniques with standardized and reliable species identification has fortunately alleviated the latter problem to a large extent.

To add further to this confusion, no simple all-inclusive classification system for environmental mycobacteria exists. The Runyon classification, based on colony pigmentation and rate of growth, is still widely used in laboratories but has significant limitations for the clinician. Rather than focus on a particular classification scheme, we encourage the reader to become familiar with patterns of disease produced by the more common pathogens among the environmental mycobacteria.

Environmental mycobacteria differ from *M. tuberculosis* in a number of ways: (1) Environmental mycobacteria are widely distributed in the environment (e.g., soil, dust, water), whereas *M. tuberculosis* is an obligate human pathogen. (2) Environmental mycobacteria differ from *M. tuberculosis* in their rate of growth, colony morphology, colony pigment formation, biochemical reactivity, and, perhaps, pathophysiology of disease. (3) Infection with environmental mycobacteria rarely, if ever, results from person-to-person transmission.

Isolation of an environmental mycobacterial species does not necessarily indicate that it is responsible for a patient's disease. This is especially true for *Mycobacterium gordoni*, *Mycobacterium scrofulaceum*, *Mycobacterium terrae*, and *Mycobacterium phlei*, species which rarely cause human disease. Conversely, some organisms (*Mycobacterium marinum*, *Mycobacterium kansasii*) are so rarely recovered from the environment and are so commonly associated with disease that their recovery is almost always indicative of human disease. In general, recovery of environmental mycobacterial organisms obtained under sterile conditions, such as percutaneous aspiration or surgical biopsy, is almost always pathognomonic for infection. Isolated colonies of nonpathogenic environmental mycobacteria recovered from nonsterile sites can usually be ignored. Clinical judgement is still required, however, because under the proper circumstances, such as in an immunocompromised host, even relatively nonpathogenic organisms may rarely cause disease.

The question of colonization versus disease can be especially difficult in patients with sputum cultures that are positive for one of the environmental mycobacterial species. This question is of obvious importance in deciding who should receive potentially toxic and perhaps unnecessary drug therapy. Criteria to make the distinction between a contaminant or colonizer and a true pathogen are not uniform. In general, the following are necessary to make the diagnosis of mycobacterial pulmonary disease: (1) clinical evidence of a disease process that can be explained by an environmental mycobacterial species, i.e., apical cavity infiltrates on chest x-ray film; (2) repeated isolation from the sputum of a particular mycobacterial species over time; (3) exclusion of other potential causes or pathogens capable of producing this clinical syndrome; and (4) (optional) a biopsy specimen demonstrating the pathogen and/or a compatible histopathologic picture. Unfortunately, skin testing is not helpful because of unavailability of skin test antigens, extensive cross-reactivity of skin test antigens, and lack of standardization of reactions.

While specific recommendations for therapy will be presented, the reader must remember that environmental mycobacterial disease may be frustrating and difficult to treat even with "ideal" regimens. Patients with the same organisms infecting the same site may require somewhat different approaches to therapy, depending on the severity of disease, the presence of other underlying diseases, and individual responses to therapy. In some instances, in vitro susceptibility of the individual organism is of no consequence in choosing therapy. In other instances, the in vitro sensitivity of the organisms to various antibiotics is critical in terms of the anticipated response of patients. Because it is sometimes difficult to follow simple algorithms for therapy, the reader is encouraged to choose candidates for therapy carefully, monitor therapy closely, and alter therapy as clinical circumstances warrant. For pulmonary disease in particular, prolonged (generally outpatient) and frequently supervised therapy is required.

PULMONARY DISEASE

Mycobacterium kansasii

All patients with established lung disease due to *M. kansasii* should be treated. Because *M. kansasii* is rarely a contaminant or commensal, one positive culture from a wound or two positive cultures from sputum are usually sufficient to establish a diagnosis. Pulmonary disease caused by *M. kansasii* is clinically and radiographically indistinguishable from that due to *M. tuberculosis* (except for the general absence of fever with *M. kansasii*). The typical patient with *M. kansasii* disease is a middle-aged man from the urban Southwest or Midwest with obstructive lung disease.

Successful therapy can be accomplished with either one or two drug regimens (Table 1). The current treatment of choice is daily isoniazid 300 mg, rifampin 600 mg, and ethambutol 15 mg per kilogram for 18 to 24 months. Alternatively, daily isoniazid 300 mg, rifampin 600 mg, and ethambutol 15 mg per kilogram may be given for 12 months if intramuscular streptomycin, 15 mg per kilogram three times weekly is given for the first 3 months of therapy. Surgery plays no role in therapy except in the occasional patient with acquired drug resistance. Therapy with isoniazid and rifampin alone carries a significant risk of development of resistance to rifampin and should be avoided. Pyrazinamide (PZA) has no activity against *M. kansasii*, and hence the current regimen of isoniazid and rifampin for 6 months, with PZA for the first 2 months of therapy, used for *M. tuberculosis* infection is not recommended. The 9-month regimen of isoniazid and rifampin for *M. tuberculosis* is also not recommended for *M. kansasii*. The key to successful therapy for *M. kansasii* disease is in vitro sensitivity to rifam-pin, as susceptibility to isoniazid (1 μg per milliliter) or streptomycin (2 μg per milliliter) does not influence clinical outcome. If rifampin resistance develops (usually as a consequence of noncompliance during therapy), a multiple-drug regimen that includes daily high-dose (900 mg) isoniazid, ethambutol 25 mg per kilogram, sulfamethoxazole 1 g three times daily, and daily streptomycin 10 mg per kilogram can be effective. After 3 months, the streptomycin should be changed to three times weekly to complete a 6-month course. Therapy with the oral drugs should be continued for at least 1 year after sputum conversion.

Mycobacterium avium Complex

The typical patient with pulmonary disease due to *Mycobacterium avium* complex (MAC) is a middle-aged or older man with preexisting lung disease in the rural southeastern United States. The high morbidity and mortality of coexistent lung disease make determination of the natural history and progression of even untreated disease difficult. Repeated isolation of MAC from the sputum over weeks to months, a compatible clinical picture, and exclusion of other reasonable pathogens are particularly important in patients with suspected MAC disease. In equivocal cases, if either 1 to 2 months of chest percussion, postural drainage, bronchodilators, and antibiotics (e.g., trimethoprim-sulfamethoxazole, amoxicillin) or 2 weeks of antituberculous

TABLE 1   Treatment of Environmental (Nontuberculous) Mycobacterial Pulmonary Disease

Species	Drugs*	Dosage	Duration	Toxicity	Monitor
M. kansasii	RIF	600 mg qd	18–24 mo	Liver, hematologic	Liver enzymes
	INH	300 mg qd	18–24 mo	Liver	Liver enzymes
	EMB	15 mg/kg qd	18–24 mo	Optic nerve	Visual acuity, red-green color vision (monthly)
			or		
	RIF, INH, EMB	(As above)	12 mo	(As above)	(As above)
	Streptomycin (IM)	10–15 mg/kg 3 x/wk	First 3 mo of therapy	Ear, renal	BUN, creatinine, check for tinnitus, hearing loss
M. avium complex	RIF	600 mg qd	18–24 mo	(See above)	(See above)
	INH	300 mg qd	18–24 mo	(See above)	(See above)
	EMB	15 mg/kg qd	18–24 mo	(See above)	(See above)
	Streptomycin (IM)	10–15 mg/kg 3 x/wk	First 3 mo of therapy	(See above)	(See above)
	If no sputum conversion in 6 months, consider:				
	INH	(As above)	(As above)	(As above)	(As above)
	EMB	25 mg/kg	(As above)	(As above)	(As above)
	Rifabutin	300–450 mg qd	(As above)	(As above)	(As above)
	Cycloserine	250 mg t.i.d.		Seizures, depression	Clinical assessment
	Ethionamide	250 mg q.i.d.		GI, liver	Liver enzymes
M. chelonae	If isolate resistant to all oral drugs or disease mild, symptomatic care only. For severe or life-threatening disease:				
	Amikacin (IV)	10 mg/kg/qd	3–6 wk	Ear, renal	BUN, creatinine, check for tinnitus and hearing loss
	Cefoxitin (IV)	200 mg/kg/day	3–6 wk	Hypersensitivity, leukopenia	WBC count
	Followed by enteric coated erythromycin	2.0–3.0 g/day	12 mo	GI, liver	Liver enzymes

* RIF =rifampin, INH = isoniazid, EMB = ethambutol.

therapy (see below) *clears* the sputum of the organism, the MAC organism isolated was likely saprophytic.

Antituberculous therapy for MAC disease is frequently frustrating. The species are invariably resistant in vitro to all first-line antituberculous drugs. There are no controlled trials of either medical or surgical therapy. Effects of therapy on morbidity and mortality are difficult to assess because of the frequent association of MAC infection with severe underlying lung disease. We institute drug therapy in patients with extensive lung disease due to MAC, especially those with cavitary disease; patients with progressive radiographic disease; and patients with significant symptoms whose life style is significantly impaired by the MAC disease. In contrast, elderly patients with minimal symptoms and minimal or modest radiographic disease are followed clinically and radiographically with therapy instituted at a later date if the disease is progressive.

The best criteria for therapeutic success of MAC disease is conversion of sputum cultures to negative. The best sputum conversion rates (approximately 60 to 80 percent) and the current treatment of choice for MAC disease is the four-drug regimen: daily isoniazid 300 mg, rifampin 600 mg, and ethambutol 15 mg per kilogram for 18 to 24 months and streptomycin three times a week at a dose of 10 to 15 mg per kilogram intramuscularly (15 mg per kilogram for age less than 50 years, 10 mg per kilogram for age greater than 50 years) for the first 3 months of therapy.

If patients fail to achieve sputum conversion in 6 months on this regimen, some change in drugs is recommended. Rifabutin (formerly called ansamycin and LM-427) is a new rifampin derivative with greater in vitro activity against MAC than rifampin and can be given at a dose of 300 mg or 450 mg instead of rifampin. This drug is available only through the Tuberculosis Control Division of the Centers for Disease Control (CDC). Cycloserine (250 mg three times a day) or ethionamide (250 mg three or four times a day) should be considered as additional agents, although patient intolerance is high. Combined medical therapy with surgical excision offers good results for selected patients with localized disease and adequate pulmonary reserve and may be considered as initial therapy.

Mycobacterium chelonae

The majority of *M. chelonae* lung disease occurs in nonsmokers over the age of 60 years with no underlying lung disease. In most cases, no treatment is necessary or nonspecific treatment is given for clinical flares of disease. Antituberculous drugs are uniformly ineffective. In vitro sensitivities can be used as guides for therapy of aggressive disease. Although no controlled studies of efficacy are available, the following drug regimen for susceptible organisms may be tried: amikacin 10 mg per kilogram in two divided doses plus cefoxitin 200 mg per kilogram intravenously in four divided doses for 2 months, followed by enteric-coated erythromycin orally at a dose of 2.0 to 3.0 g per day in divided doses for an additional 12 months. Surgical resection of limited disease may also be of benefit in selected cases. Unfortunately, the majority of lung disease caused by *M.*

chelonae is due to *M. chelonae* subspecies *abscessus*, which is susceptible in vitro to oral drugs (erythromycin) only 30 percent of the time. The result is that long-term drug therapy is frequently impossible. In patients with minimal disease or symptoms, observation with supportive care may be the best approach.

LYMPHADENITIS

Nontuberculous lymphadenitis generally involves only the cervical or preauricular lymph nodes, although up to 5 percent of other lymph node groups may be involved. The disease is unilateral and presents with a mass of enlarged nodes that are associated with minimal pain or tenderness. Children 1 to 5 years of age are most commonly affected (80 percent of cases) and generally display no constitutional symptoms. Clinical suspicion of the disease is based on a typical presentation and the presence of a partial (less than 10 millimeter) or positive (10 or more millimeter) reaction to intermediate strength PPD. The diagnosis is usually established by histopathologic examination, which shows caseating granulomata. Only about 50 percent of the biopsies will show organisms on acid-fast stain, and only about 50 percent will be culture-positive. MAC is recovered from approximately 70 percent of the culture-positive cases, the remainder usually being due to *M. scrofulaceum*. Because of the frequent subsequent development of a chronically draining sinus and antituberculous drug resistance of this causative organism, simple incision and drainage of the involved nodes with or without antituberculous drug therapy has a failure rate of 80 percent. In contrast, total surgical excision of the obviously enlarged nodes without drug therapy has a greater than 90 percent success rate. Thus for this disease, the treatment of choice is total surgical excision of the involved nodes (Table 2).

SKIN AND SOFT TISSUE INFECTIONS

Mycobacterium marinum

M. marinum is responsible for swimming pool, or fish tank, granuloma. *M. marinum* skin lesions present as small papular or nodular lesions, often with small central ulcerations, at the site of inoculations. The disease is usually self-limited, but without drug therapy the skin lesions may persist for up to 3 years. The diagnosis of disease due to *M. marinum* requires a good clinical history of water or fish exposure during or after an injury with a subsequent high index of suspicion. Diagnosis requires a culture of biopsy material and incubation of the culture material at 28°C to 30°C.

At present, no drug therapy is considered the treatment of choice. Effective drug regimens include: trimethoprim-sulfamethoxazole 800/160 mg twice daily, doxycycline or minocycline 100 mg twice daily, and rifampin 600 mg with or without ethambutol at 15 mg per kilogram daily for a minimum of 3 months.

TABLE 2   Treatment of Environmental (Nontuberculous) Mycobacterial Disease (Nonpulmonary)

Species	Drugs	Dosage	Duration	Toxicity	Monitor
Lymphadenitis					
M. avium complex	Complete surgical excision				
M. scrofulaceum	Complete surgical excision				
Skin and tissue infections					
M. marinum	TMP-SMZ	160/800 mg b.i.d.	3 mo (minimum)	Hypersensitivity, GI, hematologic	CBC
	or				
	Doxycycline*	100 mg b.i.d.	3 mo (minimum)	GI, skin	
	or				
	Rifampin	600 mg/day	3 mo (minimum)	(See above)	(See above)
	Ethambutol	15 mg/kg/day	3 mo (minimum)	(See above)	(See above)
M. fortuitum	Serious or invasive diseases:				
	Amikacin	10–15 mg/kg/day	3–6 wk	(See above)	(See above)
	Cefoxitin	200 mg/kg/day	3–6 wk	(See above)	(See above)
	or	(max 12 g/day)			
	Imipenem	2.0 g/day	3–6 wk	Phlebitis, hypersensitivity, GI	
	Followed by (depending on susceptibilities):				
	Ciprofloxacin	500–750 mg b.i.d.	3–6 mo	GI, CNS, skin	
	or				
	Sulfamethoxazole	1.0 g t.i.d.	3–6 mo	Hypersensitivity, GI, CBC hematologic	
	Doxycycline*	100 mg b.i.d.	3–6 mo	(See above)	
M. chelonae	As for *M. fortuitum;* if isolate not susceptible to any oral agent continue amikacin and cefoxitin for 12 wk; if organism susceptible, enteric-coated erythromycin 2.0–3.0 g/day 3–6 mo; local surgical resection and debridement important				

* Minocycline can be substituted for doxycycline at the same dose.

Rapidly Growing Mycobacteria

Cutaneous disease due to the pathogenic rapidly growing mycobacteria, usually *M. fortuitum* or *M. chelonae*, is relatively common among southern or western coastal states, especially Georgia, Florida, Texas, and California. Skin and soft tissue infections caused by these two species are both community acquired and nosocomial. Community acquired disease (cellulitis, osteomyelitis) follows a skin laceration or puncture wound with environmental contamination. Nosocomial disease follows a surgical procedure. Infected long-term intravenous or peritoneal catheters and wound infections following augmentation mammoplasty or cardiac-bypass surgery are responsible for the majority of these cases. As previously noted, the rapidly growing mycobacteria are resistant to all antituberculous drugs. In vitro drug sensitivities to antibacterial agents are critical in choosing an effective regimen. The treatment of choice for serious or invasive disease is amikacin at 10 to 15 mg per kilogram in divided doses plus cefoxitin at 200 mg per kilogram (up to 12 g per day) in divided doses for 4 to 8 weeks followed by the best available oral agents for a total of 3 to 6 months. For *M. fortuitum*, this oral agent could be ciprofloxacin at 500 to 750 mg twice daily, sulfamethoxazole at 1.0 g three times daily, or

doxycycline at 100 mg twice daily (susceptibility testing must be performed as only 40 percent of *M. fortuitum* are susceptible to doxycycline). For *M. chelonae*, erythromycin in a dose of 2.0 to 3.0 g per day is effective in susceptible organisms; unfortunately, only 30 percent of *M. chelonae* subspecies *abscessus* and 80 percent of subspecies *chelonae* are susceptible or intermediately susceptible to erythromycin. Local surgical resection or debridement of infected tissues is an important adjunct to drug therapy.

SUGGESTED READING

Ahn CH, Lowell JR, Ahn SS, Ahn S, Hurst GA. Chemotherapy for pulmonary disease due to *Mycobacterium kansasii*: efficacies of some individual drugs. Rev Infect Dis 1981; 3:1028–1034.

Iseman MD, Corpe RF, O'Brien RJ, et al. Disease due to *Mycobacterium avium-intracellulare*. Chest 1985; 87(Suppl 2):1395–1495.

Schaad UB, Votteler TP, McCracken GH, Nelson JD. Management of atypical mycobacterial lymphadenitis in childhood: a review based on 380 cases. J Pediatr 1979; 95:356–360.

Wallace RJ Jr, Swenson JM, Silcox VA, et al. Spectrum of disease due to rapidly growing mycobacteria. Rev Infect Dis 1983; 5:657–679.

Wolinsky E. State of the art: nontuberculous mycobacterial and associated diseases. Am Rev Respir Dis 1979; 119:107–159.

LISTERIOSIS

WALTER F. SCHLECH III, M.D., F.A.C.P., FRCPC

Listeriosis is an uncommon bacterial infection caused by *Listeria monocytogenes*, a gram-positive, motile aerobic coccobacillus. The organism is widespread in the environment, and recent epidemiologic evidence suggests that most adult infections are acquired by direct or indirect food-borne transmission. Listeriosis has several presentations, the commonest of which are subacute meningitis in the adult and septicemia or meningitis in the neonate.

Listeriosis can also present in more unusual ways. These include rhombencephalitis, cutaneous infection in veterinarians, cryptogenic liver abscess, aspiration pneumonia, and endocarditis. Neonatal septicemia usually occurs by transplacental infection from the mother. Following a short, febrile bacteremic illness in the mother, the baby may be born prematurely with evidence of disseminated infection. Late-onset neonatal meningitis occurs 7 to 10 days after delivery. In this instance, rectovaginal colonization by *Listeria* in the mother is the source of infection. The susceptibility of neonates to invasive infection reflects the immaturity of their immune system. Similarly in adults, older individuals and immunocompromised patients with cancer or leukemia who are receiving immunosuppressive drugs are most susceptible. Listeriosis has also been a complication of the acquired immunodeficiency syndrome (AIDS), although it is seen less often than expected in this rapidly growing population of compromised patients.

DIAGNOSIS

The diagnosis of listeriosis depends on isolation of the microorganism from appropriate specimens. Cultures of blood and cerebrospinal fluid (CSF) are most likely to yield the organism, and *L. monocytogenes* grows well on routine laboratory media, including those used in automated culture techniques. Once the organism is identified, appropriate specific antimicrobial therapy can be given. Serologic diagnosis and other nonculture techniques for identifying acute infection are not currently available, although recent interest in food-borne listeriosis may lead to new techniques for rapid diagnosis.

THERAPY

Effective therapy for listeriosis depends on the particular clinical syndrome and the relative immunologic impairment of the host. In the commonest form of listeriosis—neonatal sepsis—two patients are usually involved. The mother often develops an influenza-like illness associated with fever, chills, and rigors in the second or third trimester of pregnancy. This is followed by early labor and the delivery of a very ill infant with disseminated infection. In this case, the mother often requires no therapy other than delivery of the fetus. However, early treatment of suspected listerial sepsis in a mother may improve the outcome in the infant. Therefore, prior to delivery, the mother should be given ampicillin, 2 g every 4 hours intravenously, if renal function is normal. After delivery and when the fever has resolved, oral amoxicillin, 500 mg three times daily, is substituted, for a total course of antibiotic therapy of 1 week. A number of other agents are active against *L. monocytogenes* in vitro and in vivo. An alternative regimen for a penicillin-allergic mother would be erythromycin, 500 mg every 6 hours intravenously, until defervescence, followed by oral erythromycin, for a total of 1 week.

An infant with neonatal sepsis should be treated with ampicillin, 100 mg per kilogram per day intravenously in divided doses every 12 hours, depending on age. Gentamicin, 5 mg per kilogram daily every 12 hours, should be added. It should be noted that ampicillin is not a bactericidal agent against *Listeria*, and in vitro and in vivo studies suggest that ampicillin and aminoglycoside combinations may be synergistic against *L. monocytogenes* and lead to a more rapid resolution of bacteremia. This has not been studied in controlled clinical trials, and ampicillin alone may be equally effective when there is a relative contraindication to the use of aminoglycosides.

Infants with late-onset listeriosis usually develop acute bacterial meningitis with or without sepsis. Treatment of this syndrome should also be with ampicillin, 100 mg per kilogram per day in divided doses every 6 hours. CSF levels of ampicillin above 1 μg per milliliter are achieved with this regimen and are approximately twice the inhibitory concentration for most strains of *L. monocytogenes*. Systemic aminoglycoside therapy should also be employed, recognizing that CSF concentrations are likely to be low but might aid in clearing foci of infection outside the central nervous system. Intrathecal therapy by the ventricular or lumbar route is usually not warranted but might be considered for infants with persistently positive CSF cultures after 72 hours of therapy.

In the normal healthy adult, except in the epidemic setting, listerial meningitis is vanishingly rare. It is most commonly seen in patients with profound degrees of cell-mediated immunosuppression. Treatment of listerial meningitis is difficult in these patients because the patient cannot contribute to the inhibitory activity of antibiotics against this facultative intracellular parasite.

Ampicillin remains the drug of choice for immunosuppressed adults in a dose of 2 g every 4 hours. Aminoglycosides do not appear to add any therapeutic benefit despite the in vitro synergy studies noted above. If the patient fails to respond, as manifested by clinical deterioration and/or continued positive CSF cultures in spite of therapy, a change to trimethoprim-sulfamethoxazole (TMP/SMZ) (80 mg of the trimethoprim base every 6 hours intravenously) should be considered. The pharmacokinetic profile of TMP/SMZ and its improved CSF penetration, compared with ampicillin or ampicillin-aminoglycoside combinations, make this drug attractive first-line therapy for listerial meningitis. However, experience with this regimen is limited, and ampicillin remains the drug of choice for listerial meningitis in immunocompromised patients.

The duration of therapy of listerial meningitis in the immunocompromised host is uncertain. Relapses have been described after 2 weeks of antibiotic therapy, and the combination of intravenous therapy for 2 weeks followed by 2 weeks of oral therapy with the appropriate equivalent oral agent (amoxicillin, 500 mg three times daily, or TMP/SMZ [160 mg of TMP base] twice a day) should be employed in most instances.

Patients with AIDS and listeriosis should probably remain on therapy indefinitely, and because of the increase in adverse effects associated with sulfonamide therapy in these patients, amoxicillin is the drug of choice to prevent relapse. No cases of penicillin allergy complicating the treatment of listerial infection in AIDS patients have been reported, and alternative regimens have not been studied. An attractive alternate agent in this setting might be rifampin, 600 mg twice a day. This drug has the advantage of excellent tissue penetration and low inhibitory concentrations against *L. monocytogenes*. The drug is not bactericidal in vitro, but resistance has not developed in animal models of listeriosis treated with rifampin alone. Rifampin therapy might also be added to ampicillin or TMP/SMZ as an alternative to aminoglycosides when failure to respond to either drug alone is noted. In vitro the combination of ampicillin and rifampin may be synergistic or antagonistic, but antagonism has not been demonstrated in animal experiments.

Because *L. monocytogenes* is sensitive to a wide variety of antimicrobial agents, other drugs that have been considered or used in treatment of listeriosis include erythromycin, tetracyclines, and vancomycin. Combinations of these agents may be effective in treating listeriosis but have not been studied in humans. In vitro data and animal experiments have generally demonstrated that these agents are no more effective than ampicillin or TMP/SMZ, and their use should be reserved for the rare cases when neither of these agents can be used as first-line therapy. These drugs, if considered for use, should be scrutinized carefully for their toxicity profile, pharmacokinetic properties including penetration into tissues, and previous anecdotal clinical experience.

Of particular importance for physicians having limited experience with listeriosis is the inactivity of cephalosporins against *L. monocytogenes*. This includes new third-generation cephalosporins such as ceftriaxone and imipenem. Quinolones also have unpredictable activity against *Listeria*. These increasingly popular antibiotics, of which the most recently released are norfloxacin and ciprofloxacin, also have no place in the management of listerial sepsis or meningitis.

The rarer forms of listeriosis can be treated with the same agents used for sepsis and meningitis. Cutaneous infection, which occurs among farm workers or veterinarians handling infected calves or lambs at birth, can be treated with oral antibiotics alone for 7 days. Listerial hepatitis and rhombencephalitis should be treated with regimens designated for sepsis and meningitis, respectively. Endocarditis requires prolonged intravenous therapy for at least 4 weeks. Although no data exist to document its utility, monitoring of therapy with serum bactericidal and inhibitory levels against the patient's organism may be helpful in making adjustments to dosing or examining potential combinations of antibiotics for in vivo synergy. These studies should not be ordered routinely if a rapid clinical response is evident. They might be useful in patients who have had relapsing central nervous system infections as well.

There are no controlled studies of adjunctive therapy for patients with listeriosis. Central nervous system infection complicated by encephalitis, particularly involving the rhombencephalon, might benefit from corticosteroid therapy or mannitol if CSF pressures are high. High-dose (4 mg per day), short-term (4 days) dexamethasone therapy should be strongly considered if life-threatening focal abnormalities are present on initial evaluation. However, there is no evidence that use of corticosteroids or mannitol alters the outcome when appropriate antibiotics are used. Hydrocephalus is an uncommon complication, and CSF shunting is usually unnecessary.

Careful follow-up of the therapeutic response in all forms of listeriosis is important so that alterations in therapy can be made if necessary. Clinical parameters to follow closely are the disappearance or persistence of fever, the progression or loss of focal neurologic abnormalities for patients with significant encephalitic features, a deterioration or improvement in the level of consciousness, and an improvement in CSF findings, including cell count, glucose, and positive or negative cultures. The CSF should be examined 48 to 72 hours after initiation of treatment if clinical improvement does not occur. For patients with listerial sepsis, repeat blood cultures should be obtained at the same interval to document clearance of the organism from the blood. Persistently positive cultures should prompt an alteration in initial therapy, with a change in or the addition of antibiotics among the many to which *L. monocytogenes* is usually susceptible.

SUGGESTED READING

Larsson S, Walder MH, Cronberg SN, et al. Antimicrobial susceptibility of *L. monocytogenes* strains isolated from 1958 to 1982 in Sweden. Antimicrob Agents Chemother 1985; 28:12–14.

Moellering RC, Medoff G, Leech I, et al. Antibiotic synergism against *Listeria monocytogenes*. Antimicrob Agents Chemother 1972; 1:30–34.

Neiman RE, Lorber B. Listeriosis in adults: a changing pattern. Report of eight cases and review of the literature, 1968–1978. Rev Infect Dis 1980; 2:207–227.

Richards J, Swann RA, Ponton AWG. Recurrence of *Listeria monocytogenes* meningitis. J Infect 1988; 16:65–71.

Spitzer PG, Hammer SM, Karchmer AW. Treatment of *Listeria monocytogenes* infection with trimethoprim-sulfamethoxazole: case report and review of the literature. Rev Infect Dis 1986; 8:427–430.

TETANUS

DONALD L. BORNSTEIN, M.D.

Tetanus, a potentially lethal neurotoxic illness characterized by intense muscular spasm and rigidity, is caused by the action of tetanospasmin, a potent neurotoxin released by *Clostridium tetani*. Spores of this organism are ubiquitous in soils and dust and can be introduced into the body by major trauma or by trivial or even inapparent penetrations of the skin. The disease is totally preventable by active immunization, and in the United States fewer than 100 cases have been reported annually for the last decade. However, tetanus is still rampant in developing countries, and it is estimated to cause from 160,000 to 900,000 deaths per year, primarily in newborns (tetanus neonatorum) whose mothers have not been immunized.

PATHOGENESIS

C. tetani is an obligate anaerobe and will not germinate after introduction in the human body unless there is accompanying tissue necrosis, anoxia, foreign material, or microorganisms. Spores have lain dormant months to years after the initial seeding only to be reactivated by trauma or surgery (latent tetanus). When conditions permit germination of the spores, tetanospasmin, a 150,000-dalton neurotoxin is released into the local tissues, where it is picked up by lymphatics and carried into the circulation. The toxin binds to motor nerve endings in local and distant muscle fibers and ascends within the axon or perineural sheath to the neuronal cell body in the spinal cord or the brain stem. There it blocks synaptic transmission of motor inhibitory stimuli from interneurons, which are required for coordination of agonistic and antagonistic signals into purposeful motor activity. The toxin appears able to ascend along sympathetic nerve fibers as well. It is no longer believed that the toxin reaches the CNS directly from the bloodstream or that the toxin exerts a significant direct effect on acetylcholine release at the neuromuscular junction. Like strychnine, tetanospasmin blocks inhibitory regulation of motor neurons; it does not stimulate excitation directly.

The wounds that introduce tetanal spores are usually minor and occur around the home or in the garden. They include splinters, thornpricks, minor burns, abrasions, scratched dermatitis, and, especially in older persons, contaminated varicose ulcers, as well as sealed puncture wounds, crush injuries, major lacerations, gun-shot wounds, open fractures, and other major trauma accompanied by soil contamination—the so-called tetanus-prone wounds. Drug addiction has caused serious cases of tetanus, especially among "skin-poppers" who use subcutaneous rather than intravenous injection. In the United States, more than two-thirds of cases occur in persons over 50 years of age. In other parts of the world the umbilical stump, the postpartum uterus, and the middle ear (chronic otitis media with perforation of the tympanic membrane) represent major portals of entry. In more than 25 percent of cases in the United States, no wound or site of entry can be identified by examination or by history, which indicates how little inflammation or necrosis is required for the production of lethal amounts of this deadly toxin.

CLINICAL PRESENTATION

The first manifestations of tetanus appear from 3 days to 3 weeks after a known injury, usually between the fifth and tenth day. The commonest presenting symptom is tightness in jaw and facial muscles and in the neck, with or without malaise, headache, or other systemic complaints. Over the next 36 to 72 hours, these symptoms progress to trismus (spasm of the masseters, which prevents opening the mouth), spasm of the facial muscles, which produces a characteristic grimacing facies (risus sardonicus), pain and dysfunction on swallowing, and pain and spasm in the neck and back. In another day or two, the back and trunk muscles and the extremities are tense, rigid, and extended, and the abdomen is board-like. Waves of uncoordinated tonic spasms follow, accompanied by great pain and anxiety, causing opisthotonos, an arching of the spine due to extensor spasm severe enough to fracture vertebral bodies and to tear abdominal muscle fibers. Bowel and bladder function is impaired; swallowing is impossible; laryngeal spasm can occur. The unsedated patient is in terror of the recurrent spasms, exhausted, perspiring excessively, calling out in pain, unable to take fluids or nutrition, and, most important, in danger of asphyxia and anoxia because of aspiration, immobility, rigidity of the chest wall, constriction of the airway, and the more frequent spasms that cause long apneic periods. In the more severe cases, marked sympathetic overactivity is seen, with tachyarrhythmias, hyperthermia, hypertensive episodes, and sometimes refractory hypotension.

In most cases, symptoms and signs reach a plateau after the first 5 days or so and persist at that level until the effects of the fixed neurotoxin wear off, which usually takes from 4 to 6 weeks. Tetanus leaves no permanent neural injury, and if the serious complications accompanying 3 to 6 weeks of intensive hospital care are avoided, full recovery can be expected.

Trismus is an early and almost invariable finding (more than 90% of cases) because toxin carried to myoneural junctions in the masseters has a much shorter intra-axonal path to the CNS than is true for muscles of the arms or legs. Short incubation periods (fewer than 7 days) and rapid development from first symptoms to the first major spasms (less than 3 days) correlate with more severe illness and more complications.

More than 90 percent of cases seen in the United States are generalized. There are a few patients who have partial immunity or have a minor intoxication whose symptoms are limited to rigidity and spasm of the muscles around the site of injury. These patients with local tetanus generally do well, but the disease can become generalized later in its course if not recognized and treated effectively. Another group of patients acquire tetanus after an injury to the head, face, or neck or from a chronic eardrum perforation. In these cases the incubation period is short because the path to the CNS is shorter than from an extremity. Cephalic tetanus has a poorer prognosis, in part from a delay in recognition. Cranial nerve involvement is commonly seen along with trismus.

DIAGNOSIS

There is no laboratory test or pathologic finding that can establish the diagnosis of tetanus; diagnosis rests purely on clinical grounds. It is possible to recover spores of *C. tetani* from wounds in patients without the disease, and organisms are recovered from debrided wounds in only about 30 percent of cases. The clinical diagnosis is distinctive and, except in the earliest stages or in unusual mild cases in persons with partial immunity, is readily distinguishable from other causes of muscular rigidity and spasms. The differential diagnosis of trismus as an isolated finding includes local pathology such as dental abscess, subluxation of the temporomandibular joint, retropharyngeal abscess, and mumps. Painful spasms similar to those in tetanus are seen in strychnine poisoning, but here the muscles are relaxed and not rigid between spasms. There has been some confusion with patients receiving phenothiazine drugs, who may be somewhat rigid, but these patients tend to be dystonic to some degree and have a history of drug ingestion, and their muscular symptoms are rapidly reversible with diphenhydramine, 50 mg intravenously. Hysterical reactions can easily be distinguished by the lack of generalized rigidity, trismus, or true spasms.

TREATMENT

The goals of therapy are twofold: to neutralize unbound toxin while removing any residual nidus of *C. tetani* and to provide optimal physiologic support until the effects of the bound toxin dissipate. The first goal is easily accomplished; the second poses major problems for even the most skilled hospitals and intensive care facilities.

When the diagnosis of tetanus is first made, the patient should be transferred to an intensive care unit with full facilities for cardiovascular and pulmonary monitoring and ventilatory support because the disease progresses rapidly from the initial presentation and emergency intervention may be required.

Human tetanus immune globulin (TIG) should be administered, 3,000 units intramuscularly, in several sites; infiltration of a portion of the TIG around the wound of entry is recommended for a particularly contaminated wound. It is customary to begin penicillin G (1 million units intravenously every 4 hours). If a site of entry is found, it should be thoroughly debrided 30 minutes or more after antitoxin has been injected, cultured, and left open. Manipulation may release more toxin into the blood, so it is important to wait until TIG is absorbed into the circulation. Penicillin should be continued for 7 days, if no site can be identified for debridement, to prevent further germination of *C. tetani*. Cefazolin, 1.0 g every 8 hours intravenously, or tetracycline, 0.5 g orally every 6 hours, can be used for those with hypersensitivity to penicillin. Antibiotics alone provide little protection from tetanus, however.

Since a lethal dose of tetanus toxin is much smaller than an immunizing dose, clinical tetanus does not confer protective immunity. It is therefore important to administer a first dose of alum-adsorbed tetanus toxoid, at a different site from the TIG. When the patient is ready to leave the hospital, the first booster dose is administered, and arrangements should be made for a second booster dose 6 months later.

The major cause of death in tetanus is respiratory compromise and failure. The chest wall is fixed and rigid, with low compliance and poor respiratory excursions. Recurrent spasms of chest wall, pharyngeal muscles, or the larynx can produce long apneic periods and hypoxia. Impaired swallowing and deep sedation lead to aspiration of mouth contents and risk of aspiration pneumonia. Immobility and prolonged bed rest favor atelectasis. The result is alveolar hypoventilation, hypoxemia, and respiratory acidosis.

At the first clinical or laboratory signs of respiratory compromise, a cuffed endotracheal tube or, preferably, a tracheostomy tube should be placed, with the patient under appropriate sedation and general anesthesia. This will protect against the dangers of laryngeal spasm and of aspiration and allow for effective suctioning. For most patients who require intubation the duration of need is such that an endotracheal tube would have to be replaced by a tracheostomy tube in any case. Because of the spasticity of the chest wall, protecting the patency of the airway may not be enough, and ventilating the lungs mechanically will be necessary. The stiffness of the chest usually requires total paralysis of skeletal muscle for adequate ventilator function. Paralysis is effected with the nondepolarizing neuromuscular blocker D-tubocurarine by intravenous drip or intramuscularly, about 15 mg per hour. This regimen—paralysis and mechanical ventilation—is the most effective and successful for serious cases, but carries with it grave monitoring responsibilities to ensure that the paralyzed patient is never accidentally disconnected from the respirator, an accident that would cause fatal or crippling anoxic brain damage. In addition, the quality of the nursing care, and especially of tracheostomy care, will determine the course of the recovery in most cases.

The patient will require medication to relieve anxiety, rigidity, and painful spasms, since these patients are mentally alert. Diazepam in the form of a continuous intravenous drip or intermittent intravenous bolus (5 to 20 mg every 3 to 4 hours, as required) has proved to be effective for these problems and for preventing the nightmares that paralyzed but inadequately sedated patients can suffer after recovery. Diazepam is very irritative if it infiltrates; only a secure intravenous line should be used. Painful spasms may require more powerful analgesia, and narcotics may be required. Chlorpromazine is sometimes helpful for its calmative effects, and it is sometimes alternated with diazepam, at doses of 25 to 50 mg (as required) every 6 hours intravenously or intramuscularly. Short-acting barbiturates such as pentobarbital, 50 mg to 100 mg intramuscularly every 6 hours, are generally used for sedation in addition to diazepam. The choice of sedatives and muscle relaxants will depend upon the overall strategy for dealing with respiratory support. If paralysis and ventilator support are required, as in most cases today, these choices may be less critical than when total control of spasm depends on these drugs. It is also important to limit unnecessary stimuli to the patient since minor stimulation can trigger a painful spasm in a lightly sedated patient.

With good control of ventilation and spasms by paralysis and sedation, successful management of the patient rests on avoiding the complications that attend immobility and paralysis in an intensive care setting for the 3- to 6-week period that will pass before the effects of tetanus toxin wear off adequately to allow a simpler regimen. Dedicated nursing care is required to prevent serious decubitus ulcers, atelectasis, contractures, and infections around infusion sites, and to keep the tracheostomy stoma clean and the airway clear. Many complications known to occur in such patients can be prevented or recognized and treated promptly. Low-dose heparin is often used to prevent pulmonary embolism; it is appropriate especially in obese or elderly patients (5,000 units every 12 hours by deep subcutaneous injection with a 25-gauge needle using concentrated [10,000 units per milliliter] heparin). Antacids may prevent stress ulcers; daily weighings can help assess fluid losses (which are always much greater than is appreciated) thus avoiding a dangerous degree of hypovolemia; and enteral feeding via a nasogastric tube—or, if necessary, a gastrostomy or jejunostomy tube—can prevent the severe catabolic state and wasting that can otherwise occur. Frequent chest roentgenograms and urine examinations can help detect urinary tract and pulmonary infections at an early stage.

Autonomic dysregulation, a hallmark of the most serious cases, represents the major complication of tetanus after ventilation has been secured. Beginning about 7 to 10 days after admission, or sometimes even earlier, there are episodes of sympathetic hyperactivity with marked and rapid swings of blood pressure, signs of myocardial irritability, hyperthermia, and profuse sweating. Refractory hypotension, bradycardia, and cardiac arrest are late and ominous signs. Propanolol (10 mg orally every 3 to 6 hours) or other beta-blockers can control the tachycardia and some other catechol effects. The hypertension may on occasion require phentolamine; the hypotension may respond to stimulating the patient and correcting for hypovolemia. Some patients have had several episodes of cardiac arrest and resuscitation. Aggressive cardiovascular monitoring is required to guide management.

Untreated, more than 80 percent of patients would die; overall, our mortality rates are about 40 percent. In intensive care units, however, this can be reduced to about 10 percent. The role for intrathecal human TIG in severe cases has been claimed, but not substantiated as yet. Hyperbaric oxygen, once advocated by some, is clearly useless and dangerous in this disease.

PREVENTION

Immunization prevents this lethal disease. Cases occur only in unimmunized or partially immunized persons. Yet despite the safety and the wide availability of tetanus toxoid, recent surveys in the United States reveal that 11 percent of young adults and 49 percent to 60 percent of persons over the age of 60 years lack protective levels of antibody. After an immunizing series of three DPT injections in infancy and a booster dose of DPT at age one and on entering school, a booster dose of tetanus toxoid should be administered every 10 years, at age 15, 25, 35, and so on. Since immunity to diphtheria is lost over time, the recommended form of tetanus toxoid for adults (Td) contains a small amount of diphtheria toxoid (2 flocculation units) as well. Whenever a patient is seen with a puncture wound or other penetrating wound or laceration and the possibility of introduction of tetanus spores is considered, the history of the patient's tetanus immunization must be carefully reviewed. If an immunizing course of three injections of toxoid has been received, as in persons with U.S. military service or with childhood immunizations, and if the last booster dose has been administered within 10 years, no further immunization is necessary for minor wounds. If the last booster dose was received within 5 years, no further toxoid is required for major wounds. Since a booster dose of toxoid is innocuous except in the very rare patient with marked hypersensitivity to previous toxoid doses, in most emergency rooms the practice is to boost for minor wounds and for major wounds if the interval since the previous booster dose has been 5 years or 1 year, respectively, although this is probably not necessary.

Persons with a wound who have not been immunized, or whose immunization history is partial or uncertain, require three doses of toxoid, the second following in a month and the third in 6 to 12 months. Since the first injection of Td will not offer protection for the current wound, passive immunization with TIG is additionally required for anything other than innocent, clean, minor wounds. The usual dose is 250 units intramuscularly, but for more serious tetanus-prone wounds, 500 units or as much as 1,000 units are sometimes used, depending on the severity of the wound. Arrangements to complete the immunization series should be made at this time. Infants born of unimmunized mothers should also receive a dose of TIG to prevent the rare and avoidable cases of tetanus neonatorum.

SUGGESTED READING

Adams EB, et al. Tetanus. Oxford: Blackwood Publications, 1969.
Ashley MJ, Bell JS. Tetanus in Ontario: a review of the epidemiological and clinical features of 102 cases (1958–1967). Can Med Assoc J 1969; 100:798.
Simpson LL. Molecular pharmacology of botulinum toxin and tetanus toxin. Ann Rev Pharmacol Toxicol 1986; 26:427.
Stanfield JP, Galazka A. Neonatal tetanus in the world today. Bull WHO 1984; 62:647.
Veronesi R. Tetanus—important new concepts. Amsterdam: Excerpta Medica, 1981.

GRAM-NEGATIVE ROD BACTEREMIA

DONALD E. CRAVEN, M.D.
WILLIAM R. McCABE, M.D.

Gram-negative rod bacteremia connotes the isolation of gram-negative bacilli from blood cultures. This term is usually reserved for bacteremia caused by members of the families Enterobacteriaceae and Pseudomonadaceae; *Salmonella* and *Haemophilus* species are not included. By comparison, *gram-negative rod sepsis* is a term often used to described a clinical condition characterized by fever, chills, and impaired tissue perfusion, irrespective of whether bacteremia has been documented.

Gram-negative rod bacteremia was uncommon in the preantibiotic era, but since 1950 it has become one of the commonest infectious disease problems in medical centers throughout the United States. Rates of bacteremia as high as one episode per 100 hospital admissions have been reported in university teaching hospitals, but lower rates have been reported from smaller community hospitals. Common etiologic agents include *Escherichia coli*, species of *Klebsiella, Enterobacter, Serratia, Proteus,* and *Bacteroides*, as well as *Pseudomonas aeruginosa*. Fifteen to 20 percent of gram-negative bacteremias are mixed or polymicrobial. Fatality rates for gram-negative rod bacteremia vary depending on the patient's underlying disease, but overall fatality rates are in the range of 25 percent.

EPIDEMIOLOGY

Gram-negative bacillemia may be categorized as hospital-acquired (nosocomial) or community-acquired. Community-acquired bacteremia usually originates from the genitourinary or gastrointestinal tracts and is frequently caused by *E. coli* sensitive to many antibiotics. Some "community-acquired" bacteremias, acquired during earlier hospitalization or during residence in nursing homes, may be caused by bacteria that are more antibiotic resistant. Hospital-acquired infections that account for approximately 75 percent of cases, may originate from the urinary tract, gastrointestinal tract, respiratory tract, skin, or mucous membranes. Nosocomial bacteremia may be associated with prior surgery or the use of invasive devices and are generally caused by more antibiotic-resistant species of bacteria.

The increasing frequency of gram-negative rod bacteremia over the last three decades can be attributed to several factors. Enteric gram-negative rod bacilli are relatively avirulent and have limited invasive capacity in the normal host, but they comprise the major aerobic flora of the gastrointestinal and female urogenital tract and readily colonize the hospital environment. Nosocomial gram-negative bacilli are known for antibiotic resistance. *P. aeruginosa* is inherently resistant to many antibiotics, whereas other species of gram-negative bacilli acquire antimicrobial resistance from plasmids or R-factors. Plasmids are extrachromosomal fragments of DNA that may rapidly transmit resistance to several antibiotics. Gram-negative bacilli resistant to multiple antimicrobial agents are a continuous problem in hospitals.

The increasing incidence of gram-negative bacteremia over the last 30 years also reflects changes in medical management and the hospital population (Table 1). Patients are older and often have chronic disease. Radical surgery, immunosuppressive therapy, and extensive use of devices that violate natural host barriers have become an integral part of modern medical management.

CLINICAL MANIFESTATIONS

The clinical manifestations of gram-negative rod bacteremia are protean and may vary from fulminant and lethal disease to infections that may go unrecognized for days. Clinical findings suggestive of gram-negative rod bacteremia are shown in Table 2. Many of these symptoms and clinical signs are nonspecific. Therefore, it is imperative to maintain a high index of suspicion and draw blood for cultures whenever bacteremia is suspected.

The classic triad of shaking chills, high fever, and hypotension occurs only in approximately one-third of patients. Fever, although a nonspecific sign, is usually present unless the patient is elderly, uremic, or receiving treatment with corticosteroids. In patients with leukemia or gastrointestinal disease, or those who have had genitourinary tract manipulation, fever may be the only indication of bacteremia.

Approximately 40 to 50 percent of patients with bacteremia develop shock—defined as a decrease in blood pressure to 90/60 mm Hg or less. Shock usually occurs 4 to 10 hours after the initial signs of bacteremia caused

---

TABLE 1 Factors That Predispose to Development of Gram-Negative Rod Bacteremia

Underlying host diseases
  Diabetes mellitus
  Cancer
  Congestive heart failure
  Hepatic disease
  Renal failure
  Granulocytopenia
  Thermal injury
  Multiple organ failure
Devices
  Intravascular catheters
    (peripheral, central, tunneled, and arterial)
  Indwelling bladder catheter
  Tracheostomy
  Endotracheal tube
  Nebulization equipment
  Prosthetic devices
Treatment factors
  Surgery
  Steroids
  Cytotoxic drugs
  Irradiation

TABLE 2   Clinical Manifestations of Gram-Negative Rod Bacteremia

Fever, chills, hypotension
Fever alone (in a patient with a malignancy, hematologic disorder, urinary tract disease, an intravenous or urinary tract catheters)
Hypotension*
Tachypnea, hyperpnea, and respiratory alkalosis*
Change in mental status (confusion, stupor, agitation)*
Oliguria or anuria*
Acidosis*
Hypothermia*
Thrombocytopenia*
Disseminated intravascular coagulation*
Adult respiratory distress syndrome*
Evidence of a urinary tract or pulmonary infection

*Without an alternative cause.

by gram-negative bacilli. Because of the high frequency of shock associated with gram-negative rod bacteremia, it is essential that the etiology of any episode of shock be clearly elucidated and the possibility of bacteremia considered.

Two types of hemodynamic alterations have been noted in patients with gram-negative rod bacteremia. "Warm shock" is characterized by evidence of a hyperdynamic circulation. Increased cardiac output with decreased peripheral resistance is characteristically associated with a high or normal central venous pressure, hyperventilation, and lactate accumulation in the initial phase of sepsis. Patients in "cold shock" are usually pale, are cyanotic, and have cold and clammy extremities. Cold shock tends to occur late in the course of septic shock. Physiologic alterations in cold shock include decreased cardiac output, increased peripheral vascular resistance associated with decreased central venous pressure, hyperventilation, and lactate accumulation. Respiratory alkalosis usually occurs early and may evolve to a metabolic acidosis, which carries a poorer prognosis.

The combination of hyperpnea, tachypnea, and respiratory alkalosis in the absence of pulmonary abnormalities is an important early clinical sign of bacteremia. In elderly patients, unexplained oliguria, increased confusion, or stupor also may be the only signs of sepsis.

Leukocytosis is common, although some patients may manifest normal or low leukocyte counts. Gram-negative rod bacteremia is a frequent complication of antineoplastic chemotherapy producing granulocytopenia (less than 1,000 neutrophils per cubic millimeter). Neutropenia secondary to bacteremia is an infrequent consequence in patients with normal hematopoietic function.

Mild to moderate thrombocytopenia occurs in about 70 percent of patients. Disseminated intravascular coagulation (DIC), characterized by decreased levels of clotting factors II, V, and VIII, together with hypofibrinogenemia, thrombocytopenia, and circulating fibrin split products is found in approximately 12 percent of patients but only about one-fourth of these patients exhibit clinical manifestations attributable to DIC.

PATHOPHYSIOLOGY

Endotoxin, or lipopolysaccharide (LPS), a major constituent of the gram-negative cell envelope, is generally thought to initiate the changes observed during bacteremia. However, several careful experimental and clinical studies have indicated that factors other than free endotoxin liberated from the bacterial cell wall contribute to the manifestations of such infections. Irrespective of the role of endotoxin, a variety of vasoactive materials have been implicated as potential mediators of the circulatory changes observed in bacteremic shock. These include endogenous pyrogen (interleukin-1), Hageman factor, plasmin, complement components, kinins, serotonin, histamine, prostaglandins, endorphins, catecholamines (epinephrine and norepinephrine), and tumor necrosis factor (cachectin). However, precise delineation of the role and interaction of these mediators in human disease is limited.

Available evidence suggests that the activation of the coagulation, fibrinolysis, kinin, and complement systems may contribute to the hemodynamic and other pathophysiologic alterations seen in gram-negative rod bacteremia. Activation of Hageman factor (Factor XII) by either intact bacilli or endotoxin results in sequential activation of the intrinsic coagulation system and the conversion of plasminogen to plasmin. Circulating gram-negative bacilli, endotoxin, and plasmin are all capable of activating the complement system through the classical or alternate pathways. Anaphylatoxins (C3a and C5a) cause peripheral vasodilation and increased vascular permeability. Plasmin and activated Hageman factor also activate the kinin pathway, resulting in vascular permeability and early peripheral vasodilatation in shock. Bradykinin, in turn, increases the release of prostaglandins PGE_2 and PGF_2.

Endotoxin may also release prostaglandins, prostacycline, or thromboxane. Studies have suggested that prostaglandins and endorphins may contribute to the pathogenesis of septic shock. Inhibitors of prostaglandin synthesis such as ibuprofen and indomethacin have ameliorated endotoxin-induced hypotension in experimental animals and humans.

Endorphins may also contribute to the pathogenesis of shock. The endorphin antagonist noxalone appears to reduce hypotension in animals. One uncontrolled clinical study of patients in shock reported improvement in blood pressure following the intravenous administration of 1.2 mg of the endorphin inhibitor naloxone, but a recent, randomized, placebo-controlled clinical study of patients in septic shock at our institution was unable to confirm any beneficial effect of this dose of naloxone in septic shock.

Cytokines are soluble proteins from stimulated cells that are important mediators of inflammatory response during gram-negative rod bacteremia. Recent interest has

TABLE 3 Initial Choice of Antibiotics for Suspected Gram-Negative Rod Bacteremia by Site of Infection

Site of Infection	Likely Etiologic Agent	Initial Antibiotic of Choice
Urinary tract: Community-acquired	E. coli K pneumoniae P. mirabilis	Aminoglycoside* or Cephalosporin†‡
Urinary tract: Hospital-acquired	K. pneumoniae Proteus species P. aeruginosa	Aminoglycoside* or Aztreonam or Third-generation cephalosporin‡
Gastrointestinal tract: Colon	E. coli Bacteroides species K. pneumoniae Proteus species P. aeruginosa	Aminoglycoside* or Aztreonam plus Clindamycin or Metronidazole or Cefoxitin
Biliary tract	E. coli K. pneumoniae Proteus species	Aminoglycoside* plus Ampicillin
Female reproductive tract:	E. coli K. pneumoniae Bacteroides species	Aminoglycoside* plus Clindamycin or Cefoxitin alone
Lower respiratory tract: (patient with tracheostomy or endotracheal tube)	P. aeruginosa Acinetobacter species Serratia species E. coli K. pneumoniae	Aminoglycoside* or Aztreonam plus Third-generation cephalosporin‡
Aspiration (in hospital)	E. coli Bacteroides species Fusobacterium species K. pneumoniae Acinetobacter species Serratia species	Aminoglycoside* or Aztreonam plus Penicillin or Clindamycin
Decubitus ulcers	E. coli Bacteroides species K. pneumoniae Proteus species P. aeruginosa Enterobacter species	Aminoglycoside* or Aztreonam plus Clindamycin or Cefoxitin or Third-generation cephalosporin‡
Burns	P. aeruginosa Enterobacter species	Aminoglycoside* or Aztreonam or Aminoglycoside* plus Carbenicillin§ or Third-generation cephalosporin‡
Intravascular device	P. aeruginosa Acinetobacter species Serratia species	Aminoglycoside* or Aztreonam or Third-generation cephalosporin‡

Table continues on the following page

TABLE 3 *Continued*

Site of Infection	Likely Etiologic Agent	Initial Antibiotic of Choice
Neutropenic patient (< 100 PMN/mm³)	*E. coli* *Klebsiella* species *P. aeruginosa*	Aminoglycoside* *plus* Carbenicillin§

* Because of their toxicity, aminoglycosides may be replaced by aztreonam or third-generation cephalosporins such as cefotaxime, ceftriaxone, or ceftazidime. An initial loading dose for amikacin = 8 mg/kg, gentamicin = 2 mg/kg, or tobramycin = 2 mg/kg. Modify dosage in patients with renal insufficiency. Reevaluate antibiotic regimen after culture and sensitivity data are available and treat with least toxic drug to which the organism is sensitive.
† Patients having a recent hospitalization or indwelling bladder catheters, or residents of nursing homes should initially receive an aminoglycoside.
‡ If the organism is sensitive. Resistant nosocomial gram-negative bacilli or *P. aeruginosa* bacteremia may be treated with an aminoglycoside or aztreonam. Possible third-generation cephalosporins include cefotaxime, cefoperazone, ceftazidime and ceftriaxone.
§ Ticarcillin, mezlocillin, azlocillin, or piperacillin may be used interchangeably with carbenicillin.

been directed at tumor necrosis factor, a 17,000-dalton cytokine released from macrophages that appears to reproduce many of the clinical and metabolic changes observed in gram-negative rod bacteremia and sepsis. Furthermore, antibody to tumor necrosis factor appears to protect animals against shock and death following the administration of endotoxin. Recent data in humans indicate that endotoxin also elicits detectable tumor necrosis factor, which is accompanied by fever, tachycardia, and systemic symptoms, but further studies are needed to define more clearly its role in the pathogenesis of septic shock.

ANTIBIOTIC TREATMENT

Because of the nature of the disease, therapy for gram-negative rod bacteremia is usually initiated before the etiologic agent and antibiotic sensitivities are known. Initial treatment should be based on the type of infection (community-acquired or nosocomial), the probable site of infection, and the bacterial flora residing at that site. Basic principles of management include prompt recognition of the clinical signs and symptoms of bacteremia and identification of the source of infection. Blood cultures, Gram stains, and cultures of infected sites should be performed to identify the etiologic agent and determine antibiotic sensitivity. Fluids, oxygen, and adequate doses of an appropriate antibiotic should be administered promptly. In addition, management of complications such as shock, hypoxia, and hemorrhage is of paramount importance. Any abscess should be drained and infected foreign bodies removed as soon as possible.

Once the source of infection is identified, appropriate antimicrobial therapy designed to cover all the pathogenic flora at that site should be instituted (Table 3). Aminoglycosides such as gentamicin, tobramycin, or amikacin have a broad spectrum of activity against aerobic gram-negative bacilli, including *P. aeruginosa*. The type of aminoglycoside selected (Table 4) will depend on the condition of the patient, the type and location of infection, and the specific antibiotic resistance pattern of

the hospital flora. At Boston City Hospital we presently recommend gentamicin for initial coverage of gram-negative rods because it is less expensive and the number of gentamicin-resistant gram-negative bacilli is low. Initial therapy with tobramycin or amikacin may be more appropriate in other hospitals, depending on the general patterns of bacterial resistance. Doses of aminoglycosides should be altered for patients with renal failure, and blood levels should be monitored in a person who has impaired renal function or no response to therapy, or in whom long-term therapy is required. Because of their well-known ototoxicity and nephrotoxicity, aminoglycosides may be replaced by less toxic antibiotics if the organism is sensitive.

Infections originating from the gastrointestinal tract or the female reproductive tract may involve aerobic gram-negative bacilli and anaerobic organisms such as *Bacteroides fragilis*. For this reason, combinations of antibiotics such as an aminoglycoside (chosen as indicated above) and clindamycin or metronidazole would be indicated for initial therapy.

A cephalosporin may be used for initial therapy only if the organism is likely to be susceptible. First-generation cephalosporins—such as cephalothin or cefazolin—have activity against community strains of *E. coli*, *Klebsiella pneumoniae*, and *Proteus mirabilis*, but some strains are resistant and activity is lacking against many of the nosocomial gram-negative bacilli, making this group of agents inappropriate for initial therapy of suspected gram-negative bacteremia. Second-generation cephalosporins, such as cefoxitin, have a greater spectrum of activity against aerobic gram-negative bacilli. Cefoxitin also has activity against *B. fragilis*, but second-generation cephalosporins have no activity against *P. aeruginosa*. Third-generation cephalosporins—such as cefotaxime, ceftriaxone, ceftazidime, and cefoperazone—have activity against a variety of enteric gram-negative bacilli. Cefoperazone and ceftazidime have activity against *P. aeruginosa*. These antibiotics have a high therapeutic-toxicity ratio and serum blood levels do not need to be monitored. Consequently, they are easier to use and are less toxic than aminoglycosides.

TABLE 4 Parenteral Antibiotics That May Be Prescribed for the Treatment of Gram-Negative Rod Bacteremia

Antibiotic	Dose*	Comments
Aminoglycosides		
Gentamicin	1.7 mg/kg IM or IV q8h	Aminoglycosides have a good spectrum against aerobic gram-negative bacilli, including *P. aeruginosa*
Tobramycin	1.7 mg/kg IM or IV q8h	
Amikacin	7.5 mg/kg IM or IV q12h	
Cephalosporins		
First-generation		
Cephalothin	2 g IV q4h	Activity limited to *E. coli, K. pneumoniae,* and *P. mirabilus*; should not be used unless sensitivity of organism is known
Cefazolin	2 g IV q8h	
Cephradine	2 g IV q6h	
Cephapirin	2 g IV q4h	
Second-generation		
Cefoxitin	2 g IV q4h	Cefoxitin provides good coverage against *B. fragilis* and most aerobic gram-negative bacilli except *P. aeruginosa*
Cefamandole	2 g IV q4h	
Third-generation		
Cefotaxime	2 g IV q4h	Third-generation cephalosporins have broad-spectrum activity against *P. aeruginosa*; Cefoperazone and ceftazidime have good activity.
Cefoperazone	3 g IV q6h	
Ceftriaxone	1 g IV q12h	
Ceftazidime	2 g IV q8h	
Extended-spectrum penicillins		
Carbenicillin	5 g IV q4h	Useful in combination with an aminoglycoside for treating *P. aeruginosa* bacteremia or for treating patients with neutropenia
Ticarcillin	3 g IV q4h	
Piperacillin	3 g IV q4h	
Mezlocillin	3 g IV q4h	
Azlocillin	3 g IV q4h	
Monobactams		
Aztreonam	2 g IV q8h	Good coverage for gram-negative bacilli, including *P. aeruginosa*
Other beta-lactams		
Imipenem-cilastatin	500 mg of each drug IV q6h	Good coverage for aerobic gram-negative bacilli and *B. fragilis*
Trimethoprim-sulfamethoxazole	2 ampules IV q8h	Effective against many resistant nosocomial gram-negative bacilli

* Doses are the maximum for patients with bacteremia and normal renal flow. Doses should be adjusted after organism and antibiotic activity are known or if patient has impaired renal function.

Extended-spectrum penicillins—such as ticarcillin, carbenicillin, azlocillin, mezlocillin, and piperacillin—are generally used in combination with an aminoglycoside for treating patients with neutropenia or serious infections caused by *P. aeruginosa*. It should be emphasized that once the sensitivities of the offending organism are known, the least toxic and least expensive antibiotic to which the organism is sensitive should be prescribed. The duration of therapy depends on the source of infection. In general, antibiotics should be continued for a minimum of 5 afebrile days or longer if a local source of infection persists.

Aztreonam is a monobactam that has broad-spectrum activity against all aerobic gram-negative bacilli except *Acinetobacter* species. Aztreonam has activity similar to the aminoglycosides but is less toxic and more expensive.

Imipenem-cilastatin has a wide spectrum of activity against anaerobic and aerobic gram-negative bacilli as well as many gram-positive bacteria. It may be particularly useful for treating some of the more resistant nosocomial pathogens but has a limited spectrum against strains of *P. aeruginosa*.

More recently, the oral quinolone antibiotics have been released, which have excellent activity against most aerobic gram-negative bacilli, and intravenous preparations are being evaluated in clinical trials. Development of resistance may occur and some strains of *P. aeruginosa* may be resistant.

MANAGEMENT OF SHOCK

Shock is the most frequent complication of gram-negative rod bacteremia. Shock in patients with gram-negative rod bacteremia is associated with a sevenfold increase in fatality. Therefore, goals for treating patients with gram-negative rod bacteremia include early diagnosis and therapy to prevent shock and rapid correction of any hemodynamic alterations that occur. Optimal care requires the prompt institution of appropriate antibiotics as well as maintenance of an adequate intravascular volume. A

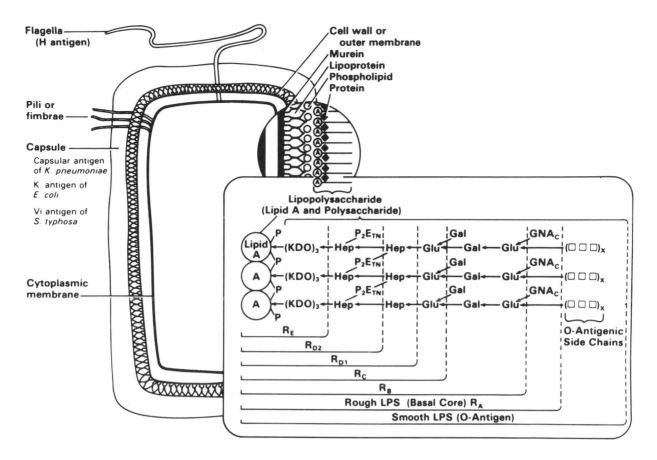

Figure 1 Schematic depiction of structure and antigens of gram-negative bacilli and the chemical structure of the lipopolysaccharide (LPS) of smooth (S) and rough (R) Salmonella. R mutants, Ra, Rb, Rc, Rd$_1$ Rd$_2$, and Re are shown in order of increasing roughness produced by progressive deletion of sugars of the core portion of LPS. GNAc = N-acetylglucosamine; Glu = Glucose; Gal = Galactose; Hep = Heptose; KDO = 2-keto 3-deoxyoctulosonate; P = Phosphate. (From McCabe WR. Endotoxin: microbial, chemical, pathophysiological, and clinical correlation. In: Weinstein L, Fields BN, eds. Seminars in infectious disease. New York: Thieme and Stratton, 1980.)

central venous pressure (CVP) catheter or a Swan-Ganz catheter inserted to measure pulmonary artery wedge pressure (PAWP) are valuable aids for monitoring intravascular fluid expansion. Furthermore, an indwelling bladder catheter (using sterile precautions and a closed drainage system) is usually inserted to measure urinary output and renal perfusion.

Initially fluid (5 percent dextrose in normal saline) should be infused at a rate of 10 to 20 ml per minute for 10 to 15 minutes. If the CVP or PAWP does not increase by a level of 5 cm H$_2$O or 2 mm Hg, respectively, further fluid should be administered. If the need for further fluid volume is established, either colloid or crystalloid may be used at a rate of 10 to 20 ml per minute. Signs of fluid overload and cardiac decompensation include a sudden progressive increase in the CVP of more than 5 cm H$_2$O, a CVP of more than 12 to 14 cm H$_2$O, or an increase of PAWP of more than 8 mm Hg or an absolute level of 8 to 12 mm Hg.

If volume expansion does not produce prompt improvement, vasoactive agents should be added to increase cardiac output further. Dopamine is usually given by constant infusion in a dose of 2 to 20 μg per kilogram per minute. If there is no response to dopamine, isoproterenol in a dose of 2 to 8 μg per minute or dobutamine in a dose of 2 to 15 μg per kilogram per minute should be instituted to enhance cardiac output and increase urine output.

In the past, many clinicians have administered corticosteroids to patients in septic shock, but two recent double-blind placebo-controlled studies demonstrated that steroids were no more effective than placebo. Neither study found any beneficial effect in reversing hypotension or increasing survival. Furthermore, there was a suggestion that the patients treated with steroids had more complications with bacterial infections than the patients receiving placebo. Therefore, steroids should only be administered to patients with gram-negative rod bacteremia if there is a suspicion of adrenal insufficiency.

Clinical evidence of disseminated intravascular coagulation (DIC) occurs in less than 5 percent of patients with gram-negative bacteremia, and these patients are invariably in shock. Heparin has been suggested for treatment, but enthusiasm for heparin therapy must be tempered by evidence that such treatment failed to reduce fatalities in either experimental models or humans despite improvement in coagulation factors. For treatment of

DIC, we suggest that maximal efforts be directed at replacing blood products and reversing the cause of shock.

Hypoxia occurs frequently in septic shock, and monitoring of arterial blood gases is essential to maintain proper tissue oxygenation. Patients who develop adult respiratory distress syndrome (ARDS) often require mechanical ventilation with a volume-cycled ventilator. Patients who have a progressive decrease in their PaO_2 despite the use of increasing oxygen concentrations, may benefit from positive end-expiratory pressure (PEEP).

Oliguric renal failure is another complication of septic shock. If the urine flow is less than 30 ml per hour, the patient should be treated with an intravenous infusion of 12.5 g of mannitol over 5 minutes. If there is no response, this dose should be repeated in 2 hours. Individuals failing to respond to mannitol can be given furosemide intravenously.

IMMUNIZATION AND PREVENTION

The search for an effective vaccine against gram-negative rod bacteremia has been limited by the large number of distinct organisms causing disease. However, different species of gram-negative bacilli share common antigens present in the core region (Ra-Re) of the lipopolysaccharide in the outer membrane (Fig. 1). There is no program for actively vaccinating humans at risk for gram-negative rod bacteremia. However, hyperimmune serum obtained from persons following immunization with an Rc mutant of *E. coli* has demonstrated increased survival rates of patients in septic shock compared with a controlled group of patients given preimmune serum. Further, multicenter trials of hyperimmune monoclonal antibodies directed against the lipid A portion of the lipopolysaccharide are in progress. Although more research is needed, there may be a role for immunotherapy in addition to antibiotic therapy for the treatment of gram-negative rod sepsis.

Specific efforts should be directed at preventing gram-negative rod bacteremia. Since the majority of gram-negative rod bacteremias are nosocomial in origin, the use of proper handwashing, consideration of barrier precautions in the critical care unit, along with careful evaluation of the need for and care of invasive devices such as the indwelling bladder catheter, endotracheal tube, and central venous and intravenous catheters should reduce the frequency of nosocomial infection and bacteremia. Additional measures should include rational use of antibiotics as well as the appropriate collection and feedback of surveillance data used to monitor nosocomial infection.

SUGGESTED READING

Bone RC, Fisher CJ Jr, Clemmer TP, et al. A controlled clinical trial of high dose methylprednisolone in the treatment of severe sepsis and septic shock. N Engl J Med 1987; 317:653–659.

DeMaria A, Craven DE, Heffernan JJ, et al. Naloxone versus placebo in treatment of septic shock. Lancet 1985; 1:1363–1365.

DuPont HI, Spink WW. Infections due to gram-negative organisms: an analysis of 860 patients with bacteremia at the University of Minnesota Medical Center, 1958–1966. Medicine 1969; 45:307–332.

Klein BS, Perloff WH, Maki DG. Reduction of nosocomial infection during pediatric intensive care by protective isolation. N Engl J Med 1989; 320:1714–1721.

Kreger BE, Craven DE, McCabe WR. Gram-negative bacteremia. III. Re-assessment of etiology, epidemiology, and ecology in 612 patients. Am J Med 1980; 68:332.

Kreger BE, Craven DE, McCabe WR. Gram-negative bacteremia. IV. Re-evaluation of clinical features and treatment in 612 patients. Am J Med 1980; 68:344.

McCabe WR. Endotoxin: microbial, chemical, pathophysiological and clinical correlation. In: Weinstein L, Fields BN, eds. Seminars in infectious disease. Vol III. New York: Thieme and Stratton, 1980:38.

McCabe WR, Jackson CG. Gram-negative bacteremia. II. Clinical, laboratory, and therapeutic observations. Arch Intern Med 1962; 110:856–864.

McCabe WR, Olans RN. Shock in gram-negative bacteremia. In: Remington JS, Swartz MN, eds. Current clinical topics in infectious disease. Vol 2. New York: McGraw-Hill, 1981; 121.

Michie HR, Manogue KR, Spriggs DR, et al. Detection of circulating tumor necrosis factor after endotoxin administration. N Engl J Med 1988; 318:1481–1486.

The Veterans Systemic Sepsis Collaborative Study Group. Effect of high-dose glucocorticoid therapy on mortality in patients with clinical signs of systemic sepsis. N Engl J Med 1987; 317:660–665.

Young LS. Gram-negative sepsis. In: Mandell GL, Douglas RE Jr, Bennett JE, eds. Principles and practices of infectious diseases. New York: John Wiley 1985; 452.

Ziegler EJ. Tumor necrosis factor in humans. N Engl J Med 1988; 318:1533–1535.

Ziegler EJ, McCutchan JA, Fierer J, et al. Treatment of gram-negative bacteremia and shock with human antiserum to a mutant of *Escherichia coli*. N Engl J Med 1982; 307:1225–1230.

RICKETTSIAL INFECTION

THEODORE E. WOODWARD, M.D., M.A.C.P.

Rickettsiae cause three major groups of illness: the spotted fevers (including Rocky Mountain spotted fever), the typhus group (including classic typhus and murine typhus), and Q fever. Rash is a characteristic feature of all except Q fever. The following discussion focuses on the rickettsial diseases causing rash that are commonest in the United States.

DIAGNOSIS

Differential Diagnosis

The suspicion of Rocky Mountain spotted fever (RMSF) should be raised for a patient with fever, prostration, headache, and a history of tick bite or tick exposure while engaged in work or recreation in a rural or wooded area of known endemicity (Fig. 1). Early in the febrile illness before the rash has appeared, differentiation from other acute infections is confusing. The rickettsial rash is initially pink macular, fades on pressure, and becomes petechial or ecchymotic more slowly over several days. This exanthem is not sensitive to palpation. Meningococcemia and measles are common mistaken diagnoses.

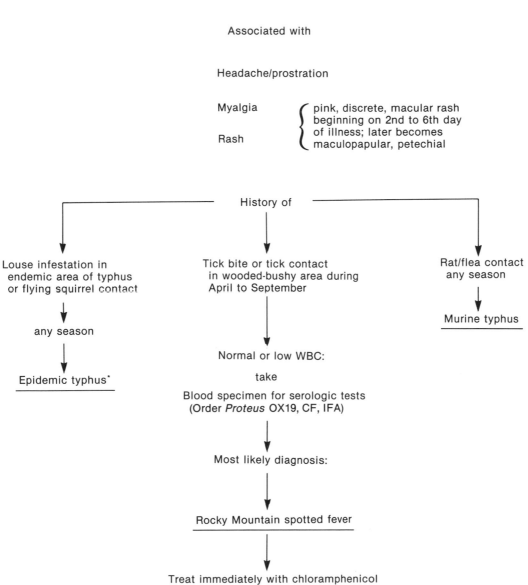

Fever (usually high and continuous)

Associated with

Headache/prostration

Myalgia

Rash

{ pink, discrete, macular rash beginning on 2nd to 6th day of illness; later becomes maculopapular, petechial

History of

Louse infestation in endemic area of typhus or flying squirrel contact

any season

Epidemic typhus*

Tick bite or tick contact in wooded-bushy area during April to September

Normal or low WBC:

take

Blood specimen for serologic tests (Order *Proteus* OX19, CF, IFA)

Most likely diagnosis:

Rocky Mountain spotted fever

Treat immediately with chloramphenicol or tetracycline

Rat/flea contact any season

Murine typhus

Figure 1 Salient epidemiologic, clinical, diagnostic, and therapeutic features of the major rickettsial diseases. * Serology as for Rocky Mountain spotted fever.

The rash of meningococcemia simulates RMSF and epidemic typhus in certain features since it may be macular, maculopapular, or petechial in acute or subacute forms and either petechial, confluent, or ecchymotic in more acute types. Usually the hemorrhagic, purplish, necrotic exanthem develops rapidly in fulminant meningococcemia and is tender to palpation. Significant leukocytosis favors meningococcal infection. The features of gonococcemia resemble those of meningococcemia.

Measles, more often an autumn- and winter-occurring illness, is associated with coryza, cough, conjunctival injection and photophobia, and a characteristic cephalocaudal progression of the rash. It appears about 3 days after onset—first in the face and neck as pink macules—soon becomes maculopapular and extends within a day or two to the trunk and extremities. Petechiae or ecchymoses may occur; Koplik's spots are distinctive. In rubella (German measles), the rash is frequently a flush, not unlike scarlet fever, which soon spreads from the face and neck to the trunk and extremities. It is less extensive and of shorter duration than measles with mild constitutional manifestations. Postauricular adenopathy and absence of Koplik's spots suggest rubella.

The initial lesions of varicella or variola are first exanthematous and later become vesicular. Rose spots in the typhoid fevers are usually on the upper abdomen and lower chest and remain delicate, without hemorrhagic characteristics. The macular lesions in RMSF, in contrast to typhoid, begin on the periphery of the body and later become petechial. The rash of infectious mononucleosis (uncommon except when associated with sensitivity to drugs) is usually morbilliform on the trunk and rarely becomes petechial. In pharyngitis, the presence of a whitish membrane, lymphadenopathy, and atypical lymphocytes in the blood are differentiating features.

Drug rashes, including that of erythema multiforme, often cause fever. Yet such patients are less toxic in their appearance than are those with RMSF, and the rash is frequently diffusely erythematous; the individual lesions are larger, raised, and vesicular.

Epidemic typhus frequently causes all of the pronounced clinical, physiologic, and anatomic alterations noted in cases of RMSF: hypotension, peripheral vascular failure, cyanosis, skin necrosis and gangrene of digits, renal failure with azotemia, and neurologic manifestations. However, the rash of classic typhus occurs initially in the axilla and on the trunk and later extends peripherally, rarely involving the palms, soles, and face. Classic or epidemic typhus occurs in the United States as Brill-Zinsser disease (recurrent epidemic typhus fever) and an endemic type associated with contact with flying squirrels. Each is usually milder than cases of classic typhus.

Murine typhus is a milder disease than RMSF and epidemic typhus, the rash is less extensive, nonpurpuric, and nonconfluent, and renal and vascular abnormalities are uncommon. Differentiation among these three major rickettsial diseases must often await the results of specific serologic tests.

An illness that simulates RMSF is caused by *Rickettsia canada,* a member of the typhus group. Rickettsialpox, caused by a member of the spotted fever group of organisms, is easily differentiated from RMSF by the initial lesion, the relative mildness of the illness, and early vesiculation of the maculopapular rash.

Q fever is the one rickettsial infection unassociated with a rash. Usually the illness is mild to moderate. It is manifested by fever for about a week to 10 days, severe headache, and pneumonitis in about 50 percent of cases. The roentgenographic findings are nonspecific and may resemble those of influenza or the atypical pneumonias. Occasionally, a dense infiltrate may suggest a neoplasm. An acute form of hepatitis, with or without jaundice, may progress to chronic granulomatous hepatitis. A chronic form of Q fever endocarditis is becoming clinically significant. In chronic hepatitis or endocarditis, antibodies to phase I antigens are present, which confirm the clinical diagnosis. The Weil-Felix reaction is negative.

Confirmatory Laboratory Diagnosis

In ordinary practice, the available serologic tests are adequate for laboratory confirmation of the rickettsioses provided that two and preferably three serum samples are examined during the first, second, and fourth to sixth weeks of illness. This allows demonstration of a rise in titer of specific antibody during convalescence.

Weil-Felix Test

The Weil-Felix test, using *Proteus* strains of OX19, gives positive results in many patients with RMSF and epidemic and murine typhus and negative or nonspecific results in those with rickettsialpox, Q fever, and scrub typhus. In Brill-Zinsser disease (recurrent typhus), *Proteus* OX19 titers are usually negative or low. Proteus OXK agglutinins appear in more than 50 percent of patients with scrub typhus. Although the *Proteus* reaction is a dependable screening test for the presence of certain rickettsioses, it does not distinguish between the spotted fever and typhus groups. A single convalescent serum titer of 160 to 320 is usually diagnostic, but demonstration of a rise in titer is of greater value. Approximately 10 percent of patients with either RMSF or typhus may fail to show *Proteus* OX19 agglutinins, and when specifically acting antibiotics are given early in the first week of illness, the titers may be delayed, but usually reach diagnostic levels. False-positive reactions may occur in urinary tract infections or bacteremia caused by *Proteus* organisms and in enteric, relapsing, and rat-bite fevers, leptospirosis, brucellosis, and tularemia.

Complement-Fixation Reaction

Group-specific rickettsial antigens clearly differentiate the rickettsial disease group (the typhus fevers, spotted fevers, and Q fever). Using nonspecific, washed rickettsial antigens, it is possible to distinguish among the various member diseases of the spotted fever group (RMSF, rickettsialpox, fièvre boutonneuse, North Asian tick-borne rickettsioses, and Queensland tick typhus).

Complement-fixing antibodies appear during the second or third week in patients who receive no specific therapy and may be delayed when illness is shortened by vigorous antibiotic treatment initiated within several days after onset of fever.

Antibodies present after response to a primary infection of RMSF and typhus are usually 19S globulins (IgM). In Brill-Zinsser disease, antibodies appear rapidly, several days after onset, and are of the 7S (IgG) type. Q fever antigens are usually diagnostic. In acute Q fever infections, such as with pneumonitis, antibodies to phase II antigen appear.

Coxiella burnetii undergoes antigenic phase changes similar to the rough-smooth variation of bacteria. In nature, *C. burnetii* is found only in the smooth phase I. It possesses a cell wall–associated surface antigen. Phase I antigen is antiphagocytic and appears to be related to virulence. Phase II antigen develops after adaptation to growth in chick embryos; the organism lacks a surface phase I antigen and is of lesser virulence than the parent strain. The phase phenomenon is reversible; phase II organisms revert to phase I by passage in animals. High phase I complement-fixing titers are considered pathognomonic of chronic Q fever, such as hepatitis or endocarditis.

Other Specific Serologic Tests

The following serologic tests are becoming standard procedures and are more reliable than the Weil-Felix or complement-fixation tests. Specific diagnoses of RMSF, other tick-borne rickettsioses, and the typhus fevers may be achieved by the rickettsial microagglutination and the indirect fluorescent antibody (or hemoagglutination) reactions.

Early Diagnosis by Identification of Rickettsiae in Tissues

Rickettsia rickettsii are identified by the indirect fluorescent antibody reaction in pink macular skin lesions obtained by biopsy as early as the third day or in ecchymotic lesions as late as the tenth day. The organisms show an identifiable morphology and staining properties. This technique may be used with formalized tissue. Organisms can be demonstrated on heart valves of patients with Q fever endocarditis caused by *Coxiella burnetii*. Undoubtedly, such techniques would apply for epidemic and murine typhus as well as others.

THERAPY

There are important physicochemical changes that merit understanding in planning a therapeutic regimen for patients seriously ill with the spotted fever-typhus group of rickettsioses. Often there is circulatory collapse, oliguria, anuria, azotemia, anemia, hyponatremia, hypochloremia, hypoalbuminemia, edema, and coma. Management is much less complicated in mildly and moderately ill patients when these alterations are absent. The principles of treatment of all rickettsioses are specific chemotherapy and supportive care.

Specific Treatment

Chloramphenicol and the tetracyclines are specifically effective; they are rickettsiostatic and not rickettsicidal. When therapy is initiated during the early stages coincident with appearance of the rash, there is prompt alleviation of clinical signs. Response is less dramatic when therapy is delayed until the rash becomes hemorrhagic and diffuse.

Optimal antibiotic regimens are: chloramphenicol, in an initial oral dose of 50 mg per kilogram body weight, or tetracycline, 25 mg per kilogram body weight. Either is acceptable. Subsequent daily doses are calculated as the initial oral dose divided equally and given at 6- to 8-hour intervals. Antibiotic treatment is given until the patient improves and has been afebrile for about 24 hours. In patients too ill to take oral medication, intravenous preparations are employed for the loading and subsequent doses. All patients with rickettsioses respond promptly to antibiotic treatment when it is initiated early in illness, before serious tissue changes have occurred. Clinical improvement is obvious in 36 to 48 hours, with defervescence in 2 to 3 days. In scrub typhus, the response is even more dramatic.

Clinical improvement is slower and fever extends over longer periods in those patients first treated during the latter stages of illness. Large, single oral doses of chloramphenicol (50 mg per kilogram) have been effective in patients with RMSF and scrub typhus, although this regimen is not recommended. A single oral dose of 200 mg of doxycycline (a lipotropic tetracycline derivative that produces sustained high blood and tissue levels) has been shown in field trials to be practically effective for treatment of louse-borne typhus fever.

Tetracycline and chloramphenicol are quite effective for treatment of patients with the acute manifestations of Q fever. Recovery is usually prompt. Endocarditis is difficult to treat since the vegetations are rather large and the broad spectrum antibiotics are rickettsiostatic and not rickettsicidal. Long-term treatment is necessary; this favors tetracycline as the antibiotic of choice. As a general rule, surgical intervention with valve replacement is necessary for cure. A few patients have recovered following extended antibiotic treatment.

Steroid Treatment

Large doses of adrenal cortical steroids (e.g., prednisone, 1.0 mg per kilogram, or Solu-Cortef, 5.0 mg per kilogram) given for about 3 days in combination with specific antibiotics are recommended in patients critically ill with spotted fever or with typhus that is first observed late in the course of severe illness. Temperature abates more rapidly than usual, as do the toxic manifestations. Steroids are not recommended for mild or moderately ill patients.

Supportive Treatment

Mouth care—swabbing of the oral cavity and use of mouth washes—may help prevent gingivitis and parotitis. Frequent turning of the patient will help prevent aspiration pneumonia and avert pressure sores over bony prominences.

A generous intake of protein supplements with frequent feedings is useful. Protein intake of up to 2.0 g per kilogram normal body weight, with adequate carbohydrate and fat sufficient to make the diet palatable, is usually well tolerated. In uncooperative patients, when there is no abdominal distention, hourly liquid protein feedings by gastric tube are helpful, but such measures are usually obviated by proper intravenous alimentation. Attention is given to parenteral alimentation with glucose and amino acid supplements in critically ill patients with enhanced capillary permeability, edema, and vascular decompensation. Dialysis is indicated if there is clear-cut evidence of acute tubular necrosis.

SUGGESTED READING

Harrison. Principles of internal medicine. New York: McGraw Hill Company, 1989.
Weatherall DJ, ed. Oxford textbook of medicine, 2nd ed. Oxford: Oxford Medical Publications, 1987.

NONSUPPURATIVE SEQUELAE OF GROUP A STREPTOCOCCAL INFECTION

ALAN L. BISNO, M.D.

Group A streptococci (*Streptococcus pyogenes*) are the cause of a wide variety of acute infections in humans, including tonsillopharyngitis, otitis media, sinusitis, scarlet fever, erysipelas, pyoderma, cellulitis, lymphangitis, endometritis, pneumonia, septicemia, and localized abscesses. This organism is distinguished from other pyogenic bacteria, however, by the occurrence of delayed nonsuppurative sequelae during convalescence from the acute infectious process. The two major nonsuppurative sequelae of group A streptococcal infection are acute rheumatic fever (ARF), which follows streptococcal upper respiratory tract infection, and poststreptococcal acute glomerulonephritis (AGN), which may be a consequence of either upper respiratory or cutaneous infection. Other nonsuppurative disorders, such as Schönlein-Henoch purpura and erythema nodosum, have been attributed to group A streptococci, but an exclusive and specific relationship between Schönlein-Henoch disease and such streptococci has not been established; erythema nodosum is associated with a wide variety of infectious and noninfectious disorders.

ACUTE RHEUMATIC FEVER

The incidence of ARF has declined dramatically in North America, western Europe, and many other highly developed countries during the last few decades. Within the past 4 to 5 years, however, there has been a resurgence of the disease in a number of communities in the United States, and ARF epidemics have been reported in military camps in California and Missouri.

Diagnosis

The diagnosis of ARF can at times be difficult because the clinical presentation is quite variable and there is no diagnostic laboratory test. Certain manifestations, however, are so highly characteristic of the disease that they have been designated as major manifestations in the set of diagnostic criteria developed many years ago by T. Duckett Jones. The five major manifestations are migratory polyarthritis, carditis, erythema marginatum, subcutaneous nodules, and Sydenham's chorea. Certain other clinical and laboratory findings occur frequently in ARF but are too nonspecific to be utilized except as supporting evidence for the diagnosis. These minor manifestations include fever, arthralgia, previous rheumatic fever or rheumatic heart disease, prolonged P-R interval on the electrocardiogram, leukocytosis, and the presence of acute-phase reactants in the blood (elevated C-reactive protein level, accelerated erythrocyte sedimentation rate).

The presence of two major criteria—or of one major and two minor criteria—makes the diagnosis of ARF highly probable, provided that there is supporting evidence of recent group A streptococcal infection. Such evidence may consist of a throat culture positive for group A streptococci or a documented recent bout of scarlet fever. In most instances, however, the evidence is provided by an elevated serum titer of one or more antibodies to group A streptococcal extracellular products, e.g., antistreptolysin O, antideoxyribonulcease B, or antihyaluronidase. Failure to demonstrate an elevated titer of antistreptococcal antibodies or a significant titer rise by a battery of the above tests makes the diagnosis of ARF most unlikely.

Streptozyme (Carter-Wallace Laboratories) is a rapid and sensitive slide agglutination test that is widely used to screen for streptococcal antibodies. The antigens responsible for the Streptozyme hemagglutination reaction, however, are poorly characterized, and some investigators have reported considerable lot-to-lot variation in the titers obtained. The test cannot, therefore, be recommended at this time.

The Jones criteria, even when accompanied by evidence of recent streptococcal infection, are not infallible. The criteria are particularly subject to error when satisfied by polyarthritis as a single major manifestation accompanied by minor criteria indicative of acute inflammation. In those geographic locales wherein the incidence of ARF remains quite low, other infectious and vasculitic disorders may be more frequent causes of acute polyarthritis than is ARF. Thus, diseases such as gonococcal arthritis and Still's disease, to name only two, must be ruled out by therapeutic maneuvers or by careful follow-up before the diagnosis of ARF can be established with confidence.

Therapy: General Measures

The management of patients with ARF depends to a significant extent upon the predominant clinical manifestations. Some patients experience polyarthritis, some carditis, some chorea, and some various combinations of the three. Chorea tends to appear after a latent period that is variable but, in general, longer than that of the other major manifestations. It may occur as an isolated disorder ("pure" chorea) but, mercifully, rarely occurs simultaneously with arthritis. Polyarthritis is usually accompanied by considerable fever and toxicity; patients with pure chorea may present no evidence of acute inflammation; carditis may be fulminant or indolent.

Patients should be placed at bed rest during the acute febrile portion of the illness or while experiencing active carditis. The pulse rate should be carefully monitored; a tachycardia that persists during sleep after fever has abated strongly suggests carditis. Routine base-line laboratory studies should include a complete blood count, erythrocyte sedimentation rate, C-reactive protein determination, throat culture, urinalysis, streptococcal antibody assays, chest roentgenogram, and electrocardiogram. An echocardiogram is useful in detecting subtle pericardial effusions or valvular abnormalities and in establishing a base line for further evaluation. Synovial fluid analysis is frequently indicated, particularly in problem cases in which other rheumatologic or infectious causes of arthritis are strongly suggested.

In cases in which gonococcal or other forms of septic arthritis are major considerations, the response to a brief (3-day) trial of appropriate antibiotic therapy should, in most instances, precede institution of anti-inflammatory agents. Indeed, in early cases wherein the diagnosis is not clear-cut, it is best to withhold anti-inflammatory agents (treating pain only with codeine) until the disease process has had an opportunity to declare itself. Such management does not influence the long-term prognosis of the rheumatic process. It is important that the diagnosis of ARF be as secure as possible because it has major implications for the patient's long-term management.

Antistreptococcal and Anti-inflammatory Therapy

Once the diagnosis of ARF has been established, the patient should be given an adequate course of antistreptococcal therapy. In the absence of penicillin allergy, the treatment of choice is a single intramuscular injection of benzathine penicillin G—600,000 units for children weighing less than 27 kg (60 lb) and 1.2 million units for heavier individuals. The penicillin-allergic patient should receive erythromycin. Prescribing information for various formulations should be consulted for the precise dosage. For most preparations, the dosage is 40 mg per kilogram per day, not to exceed a total of 1 g. The antibiotic is administered orally in two to four equally divided doses. Throats of family contacts should be cultured; contacts harboring group A streptococci in the pharynx should receive a course of antistreptococcal therapy.

The two time-honored anti-inflammatory agents for use in ARF are salicylates and corticosteroids. Both drugs quiet the acute inflammation when given in adequate doses, but corticosteroids are more potent. The choice of agents depends upon the nature of the rheumatic process and the patient's tolerance of high doses of salicylates. Data on the use of nonsteroidal anti-inflammatory agents are inadequate to allow formulation of firm recommendations regarding their use.

Patients whose only manifestation is mild arthritis may be managed with analgesics such as codeine. Avoiding the use of anti-inflammatory agents allows a better assessment of when the attack has actually terminated and avoids posttherapeutic rebounds. For patients with moderate to severe arthritis without carditis, aspirin is the drug of choice. The initial dose of 100 mg per kilogram (not to exceed 6 to 7 g per day) is designed to produce serum levels in the range of approximately 25 mg per deciliter. Aspirin should be given every 4 hours around the clock for the first 1 to 2 days and then in four doses equally spaced through the waking hours. Small amounts of milk given with the aspirin will reduce gastric irritation. Large doses of sodium bicarbonate should be avoided, as they result in decreased blood levels of acetylsalicylic acid. Data are lacking as to the efficacy of enteric-coated aspirin preparations in ARF, but these formulations have been of value in management of patients with inflammatory arthritides of other types. Absorption of the enteric-coated products may be less predictable than that of regular aspirin, but this problem can be circumvented by careful monitoring of serum salicylate levels.

Once the acute signs and symptoms of arthritis have abated and the temperature has returned to normal, the aspirin dose may be reduced to two-thirds of the original dose and maintained at this level until laboratory manifestations of acute inflammation are normal. (The C-reactive protein is a particularly useful measure in this regard.) Thereafter, the dose may be reduced to one-half of that used initially. The total duration of therapy should be at least 6 weeks. Patients with rheumatic carditis who do not exhibit significant cardiomegaly and who do not have congestive heart failure may also be treated with salicylates, but the duration of therapy should be at least 8 weeks.

The above treatment schedules represent general guidelines that must be individualized from patient to patient. The aspirin dose must be titrated against clinical response and patient tolerance. If the patient exhibits severe gastrointestinal intolerance or signs of salicylism (e.g., hyperpnea, tinnitus) at required dosage levels or if the clinical response is inadequate, it is advisable to switch to corticosteroids.

Patients with carditis associated with high fever, prominent systemic toxicity, or congestive heart failure should receive corticosteroids. In very ill patients with carditis, the profound anti-inflammatory effects of corticosteroids may be critical in controlling congestive failure. Authorities differ as to the advisability of using corticosteroids in patients with carditis manifested by cardiomegaly but without overt congestive heart failure; I favor the use of steroids in this situation. An initial starting dose of 40 to 60 mg of prednisone may be varied according to the patient's response. In particularly severe cases intravenous methylprednisolone may be instituted. Steroids are continued in full dosage for 2 to 3 weeks, at which time salicylates are added while steroids are gradually tapered over an additional 1 to 3 weeks. Aspirin, in a dosage sufficient to suppress clinical and laboratory manifestations of inflammation, is continued for at least 1 month after termination of the steroids to minimize the chances of a rebound.

Treatment of Heart Failure

The usual measures of bed rest, sodium restriction, oxygen as necessary, sedation, and diuretics are indicated in management of congestive heart failure associated with acute rheumatic carditis. As indicated above, corticosteroids, by quieting inflammation and damping fever, decrease the demand on the heart. Although there has been some debate in the past as to the risk-to-benefit ratio of digitalis in acute rheumatic carditis, this drug should be used if the modalities listed above fail to bring congestive heart failure under control.

Rebound of Rheumatic Activity

As anti-inflammatory therapy is reduced or terminated, a flare of rheumatic activity may occur. These exacerbations usually appear within the first 2 weeks, and virtually always within 5 weeks, after cessation of therapy. At times rebounds may be detectable only by monitoring of acute-phase reactants in the blood. Clinically overt rebounds may be mild, consisting of fever, arthralgia, or mild arthritis, or they may be even more severe than the initial attack. A rebound of rheumatic carditis may be manifested by cardiomegaly, appearance of new murmurs, pericarditis, and congestive heart failure. The severity of the rebound seems related to the profundity of suppression of the rheumatic process. Thus, rebounds are thought to occur more frequently and to be more severe in steroid-treated than in salicylate-treated patients. Mild rebounds usually require no specific treatment. In more severe rebounds, reinstitution of anti-inflammatory therapy is indicated, and this should be with aspirin if possible to avoid further rebounds. In patients treated initially with steroids, the occurrence of severe rebounds may be minimized by instituting aspirin therapy while corticosteroids are being tapered.

Sydenham's Chorea

Patients with this disorder should be placed in a quiet, supportive environment and protected from inadvertent physical injury caused by their involuntary movements. Often sedation with phenobarbital or tranquilization with drugs such as diazepam, chlorpromazine, or haloperidol is required. The choice must be individualized, depending on the severity of the chorea and the patient's clinical response to the various agents.

Prevention of Rheumatic Fever

Prevention of the first attack of ARF is accomplished by accurate diagnosis and appropriate therapy of group A streptococcal upper respiratory infections (so-called primary prevention). Because the signs and symptoms of group A streptococcal and viral pharyngitis overlap, it is advisable to obtain throat cultures in patients with acute tonsillopharyngitis. Although the throat culture does not distinguish reliably between true streptococcal pharyngitis and asymptomatic streptococcal carriage, it does prevent unnecessary treatment of the majority of patients with sore throat who will have negative throat cultures.

A number of commercial kits are now available which utilize immunologic methods for detection of group A streptococcal carbohydrate directly from throat swabs. The direct antigen tests are simple, rapid, and highly specific. A positive test for group A antigen can typically be obtained in a matter of minutes, thus obviating the need for a throat culture. Unfortunately, the antigen tests are somewhat less sensitive than are throat cultures, and for this reason it is advisable to confirm a negative result with a culture. This caveat is of particular importance in areas wherein the incidence of ARF appears to be again on the increase.

Patients with acute pharyngitis and positive throat cultures or direct antigen tests for group A streptococci should be treated with penicillin if they are not allergic. A single intramuscular injection of benzathine penicillin G, 600,000 units for children weighing less than 60 lb (27 kg) and 1.2 million units for heavier individuals is highly effective. In epidemiologic settings wherein the risk of ARF is low, a full 10-day course of penicillin V by mouth is sufficient. The standard dosage regimen is 250 mg three times a day. Penicillin-allergic individuals should receive oral erythromycin in the dosage indicated above in the section Antistreptococcal and Anti-inflammatory Therapy. Oral cephalosporins are also acceptable alternatives in the penicillin-allergic patient, provided that the patient is known to be able to tolerate these drugs. Oral cephalosporins should not be used in the patient with immediate hypersensitivity to penicillin. The efficacy of these oral regimens, of course, depends on patient fidelity, which is a serious consideration because the signs and symptoms of acute pharyngitis ordinarily abate long before the 10 days are over.

Individuals who have experienced an attack of ARF are inordinately susceptible to repeated attacks following group A streptococcal infections, and such recurrences may lead to progressive cardiac damage. Thus, they should be protected from intercurrent streptococcal infections by continuous antimicrobial prophylaxis (secondary prevention). The most effective form of prophylaxis is benzathine penicillin G, 1.2 million units intramuscularly every 4 weeks. Oral prophylaxis is less reliable, and fidelity is difficult to assure. Oral regimens include sulfadiazine, 0.5 g once a day for children weighing less than 60 lb and 1 g once a day for heavier patients, or penicillin V, 250 mg twice a day. For the rare patient who is allergic to both penicillin and sulfadiazine, erythromycin, 250 mg twice a day, may be prescribed.

In general, benzathine penicillin G should be used for prophylaxis of patients at greatest risk of recurrence of ARF and of development of progressive cardiac damage. Risk factors include presence of rheumatic heart disease, previous recurrences, and less than 5 years since the most recent attack. Individuals with intensive exposure to school-aged children at home or at work are obviously at increased risk of acquiring streptococcal infection. The rate of ARF recurrence declines with age. Thus, as age and changing epidemiologic circumstances lower the risk, it is permissible to switch from parenteral to oral prophylaxis. Although few patients maintain rheumatic fever prophylaxis for life (especially in the absence of significant rheumatic heart disease), there are no firm guidelines as to when prophylaxis may be discontinued. This decision should be taken only after careful appraisal of the risks and in consultation with the patient. From a personal viewpoint, I consider discontinuing prophylaxis in patients who have reached their mid-20s, have had only a single ARF attack that occurred at least 5 years previously, have no evidence of residual rheumatic heart disease, are not intimately exposed to primary schoolchildren at home or by the nature of their occupation, and can be counted upon to seek medical attention should they develop acute pharyngitis. As stated above, the decision to discontinue prophylaxis in less optimal circumstances must be individualized.

ACUTE GLOMERULONEPHRITIS

Poststreptococcal AGN is an inflammatory disease of the renal glomerulus that follows upper respiratory tract or cutaneous infection with certain nephritogenic group A streptococcal strains belonging to a limited number of M-protein serotypes. (Rare common-source outbreaks of group C streptococcal infection have also been reported to be associated with AGN.) The pathology of AGN is characterized by diffuse proliferative glomerular lesions and clinically by edema, hypertension, hematuria, and proteinuria.

The clinical spectrum of AGN ranges from asymptomatic hematuria and hypocomplementemia to severe clinical disease with volume overload and hypertensive encephalopathy. In cases severe enough to require hospitalization, the most immediate problem is usually that of circulatory overload. The patient is placed at bed rest; salt and fluids are restricted, and if required, a diuretic is administered. Digitalis is usually not indicated for management of the circulatory problems associated with AGN because myocardial function is normal. In most instances specific antihypertensive therapy other than diuretics is unnecessary. Antihypertensives should be used, however, if the clinical situation dictates. If severe hypertension and hypertensive encephalopathy ensue, potent parenteral agents may be required. Acute pulmonary edema or severe and prolonged oliguria occur in a small percentage of patients with AGN and are managed by the measures conventionally employed in these conditions.

The occurrence of a case of AGN signals the presence of a nephritogenic streptococcus in the patient and, often, in his family contacts. Thus, the patient should receive antistreptococcal therapy, preferably with a single intramuscular injection of benzathine penicillin G, or if the patient is penicillin-allergic, with erythromycin. Dosages to be employed are the same as those indicated above for primary prevention of ARF. Family contacts should be screened for asymptomatic nephritis with urinalysis and serum C3 complement determinations. In addition, the contacts should have cultures of the pharynx and any pyodermal lesions. Individuals harboring group A streptococci should receive appropriate therapy in order to eradicate the nephritogenic strain. Although this is an important measure from the epidemiologic standpoint, such treatment will not modify the course of preexistent AGN, nor is it likely to abort the disease in a patient who is within the latent period.

Most patients with AGN are children, and for them the prognosis appears quite good. Death during the acute attack is fortunately rare, but a small percentage of AGN patients never resolve the acute attack. In them, the disease enters a subacute phase, resulting in virtually complete loss of renal function within a few months to 2 years. For the vast majority of pediatric patients, however, the disease appears to resolve completely and does not lead to either chronic glomerulonephritis or hypertension in later life. The data on adult patients are more limited. It does appear, however, that the prognosis for adults may be poorer.

Unlike ARF patients, those with AGN are not at increased risk of repeated attacks, and continuous antistreptococcal prophylaxis is not indicated.

SUGGESTED READING

Bisno AL, Shulman ST, Dajani AS. The rise and fall (and rise?) of rheumatic fever. JAMA 1988; 259:728–729.
Committee on Rheumatic Fever, Endocarditis, and Kawasaki Disease, American Heart Association. Prevention of rheumatic fever. Circulation 1988; 70:1118A–1121A.
Stollerman GH, ed. Rheumatic fever and streptococcal infection. New York: Grune & Stratton, 1975:336.
Veasey LG, Weidmeier SE, Orsmond GS, et al. Resurgence of acute rheumatic fever in the intermountain area of the United States. N Engl J Med 1987; 316:421–427.

DIPHTHERIA

CARLOS H. RAMIREZ-RONDA, M.D., F.A.C.P.

Diphtheria is an acute, infectious, preventable, and potentially fatal disease caused by *Corynebacterium diphtheriae*. The infection is usually localized to the upper part of the respiratory tract and the skin; the infection gives rise to local and systemic signs. These signs are the result of a toxin elaborated by the microorganisms multiplying at the site of infection. The systemic complications particularly affect the heart and the peripheral nerves.

Diphtheria is distributed worldwide, with a higher incidence in temperate climates. The disease occurs predominantly under poor socioeconomic conditions where crowding is common and where many persons are either not immunized or inadequately immunized.

The only significant reservoir of *Corynebacterium diphtheriae* is the human host. The organism is transmitted directly from one person to another, and intimate contact is required. The usual habitat for the microorganism is the respiratory tract. There are extrarespiratory locations of diphtherial infection, which include skin, wounds, buccal mucosa, the vagina, and the conjunctiva. Disease spreads from asymptomatic or convalescent carriers, who constitute a reservoir. The organism can multiply in the mucous membranes of the respiratory tract of the immunized host without causing clinical disease. Transmission is usually by way of infected droplets of nasopharyngeal secretions. Infective skin exudate is also involved in human-to-human transmission. Transmission may also be by animals, fomites, or milk.

Morbidity and mortality are highest in children younger than 14 years. In the United States, attack rates are highest in blacks and Mexican-Americans between 5 and 14 years old and are higher for unimmunized household members and contacts of an index case.

Immunity against the disease depends upon the presence of antitoxin in the host's blood. Antitoxin is formed by immunization or by clinical or subclinical infection, including skin infections. The Schick test consists of an intradermal injection of 0.1 ml of purified diphtheria toxin dissolved in buffered human serum albumin. This is injected into the volar surface of one arm, and 0.1 ml of purified diphtheria toxoid is used as a control in the other arm. The test can be used to assess the immune status of the subject. A positive reaction (reaction to toxin but not to toxoid) is interpreted to mean that the patient is susceptible to diphtheria; a negative reaction (no reaction at site of toxin or toxoid injection) indicates that the patient is immune and that levels of antitoxin exceed 0.03 unit per milliliter. The test provides only an estimate of immunity. The lack of ability to perform it should not delay the treatment of asymptomatic contacts of diphtheria. The Schick test is not used prior to adult immunization.

CLINICAL FEATURES

Diphtheria may be a symptomless state or a rapidly fatal disease. The incubation period varies from 1 to 7 days, but is most commonly from 2 to 4 days.

Anterior Nares Diphtheria

The infection is localized to the anterior nasal area and is manifested by unilateral or bilateral serous or serosanguinous discharge that erodes the adjacent skin, resulting in small crusted lesions. The membrane may be seen in the nose.

Tonsillar (Faucial) Diphtheria

This is the commonest presentation and includes the most toxic forms. The onset is usually sudden, with minimal fever (rarely exceeding 38°C), malaise, and mild sore throat. The pharynx is moderately injected, and a thick whitish gray tonsillar exudate is frequently seen. There is enlargement of the tonsillar and cervical lymph nodes. The exudate may extend to other areas and result in nasopharyngeal diphtheria and massive cervical lymphadenopathy ("bullneck" appear-

ance). The commonest complaints reported are sore throat (in 85 percent), pain on swallowing (23 percent), nausea and vomiting (25 percent), and headache (18 percent).

Pharyngeal Diphtheria

This form is diagnosed when the membrane extends from the tonsillar area to the pharynx.

Laryngeal and Bronchial Diphtheria

This type involves the larynx. The voice becomes hoarse, and inspiratory and expiratory stridor may appear. Dyspnea and cyanosis occur, and the accessory muscles of respiration are used. Tracheotomy or intubation is needed.

Cutaneous Diphtheria

Classically described as diphtheria in tropical areas, this form now is seen in nontropical areas. It takes the form of a chronic, nonhealing ulcer, sometimes covered with a grayish membranous exudate. Another form is secondary infection of a preexisting wound. Finally, superinfection with *C. diphtheriae* may occur in a variety of preexisting skin lesions such as impetigo, insect bites, ectyma, or eczema.

COMPLICATIONS OF DIPHTHERIA

Myocarditis

Although electrocardiographic changes have been described in up to 25 percent of cases, overt clinical myocarditis is less common. The onset is insidious, occurring in the second or third week of the infection. The patient exhibits a weak rising pulse, distant heart sounds, and a profound weakness and lethargy. More overt signs of heart failure can occur. The most common electrocardiographic changes are T-wave flattening or inversion, bundle branch block or intraventricular block, and several disorders of rhythm. Serial determination of SGOT levels identifies most patients with myocarditis. The prognosis is poor, especially when heart block supervenes. Management should be aggressive in intensive care areas.

Peripheral Neuritis

The commonest form of cranial nerve palsy is paralysis of the soft palate. There may be nasal regurgitation and/or nasal speech. The condition is usually mild and recovery occurs within 2 weeks. Ciliary paralysis and oculomotor paralysis are the next commonest forms. Peripheral neuritis affecting the limbs may appear during the fourth to the eighth week. It is usually manifest by weakness of the dorsiflexors and decreased or absent deep-tendon reflexes. Diphtheritic polyneuritis has been described after cutaneous diphtheria.

DIAGNOSTIC APPROACH

Diagnosis is made on clinical grounds and can be confirmed by laboratory tests (Fig. 1). The clinical features of a fully developed diphtheritic membrane, especially in the

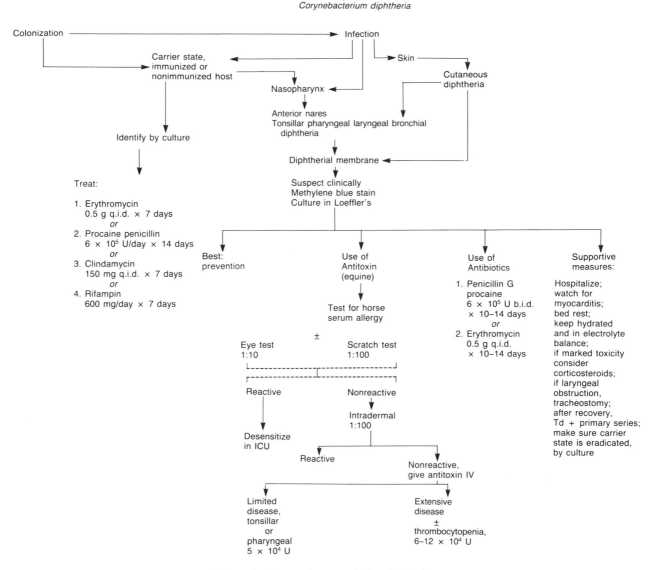

Figure 1 Diagnostic approach for diphtheria.

pharynx, are sufficiently characteristic to suggest the possibility of the disease and for treatment to start immediately.

A definite diagnosis of diphtheria requires culture of the microorganism and the demonstration of toxin production.

Specific diagnosis of diphtheria depends completely on demonstration of the organism in stained smears and their recovery by culture. Methylene blue–stained preparations are positive in experienced hands in 75 to 85 percent of cases. The presence of deeply stained granules with methylene blue (metachromatic granules) is suggestive of *C. diphtheriae*. The bacilli can be recovered by culture in Loeffler's medium within 8 to 12 hours if patients have not been receiving antimicrobial agents. The lesion or a piece of membrane should be cultured on Loeffler's medium plus a tellurite plate and a blood agar plate before antibiotics are given. The presence of β-hemolytic streptococci does not rule out the diagnosis of diphtheria, since such streptococci are recovered in 20 to 30 percent of patients with diphtheria.

Since a patient may have a nontoxigenic bacilli, efforts should be made in the laboratory to determine toxigenicity of cultured diphtheria-like organisms. Tests that can be used are the Elek-plate method, guinea pig inoculation, and others.

The differential diagnosis of tonsillar-pharyngeal diphtheria should include streptococcal pharyngitis, adenoviral exudative pharyngitis, infectious mononucleosis, and Vincent's angina, among others (Table 1).

THERAPEUTIC APPROACH

The best and most effective approach to diphtheria is prevention by immunization with diphtheria toxoid, since this is a preventable disease. The most important aspect of treatment is to administer antitoxin as soon as diphtheria is suspected clinically, without awaiting laboratory confirmation. The patient should be hospitalized and isolated at bed rest for 10 to 14 days (see Fig. 1).

TABLE 1   Differential Diagnosis of Diphtheria

Localization	Other Condition
Nasal	Sinusitis, foreign body, "snuffles" of congenital syphilis, rhinitis
Faucial and pharyngeal	Streptococcal or adenoviral exudative pharyngitis, ulcerative pharyngitis (herpetic, coxsackieviral), infectious mononucleosis, oral thrush, peritonsillar abscess, retropharyngeal abscess, Vincent's angina, lesions associated with agranulocytosis or leukemia
Laryngeal	Laryngotracheobronchitis, epiglottitis
Skin	Impetigo, pyogenic ulcers, herpes simplex infection

Use of Antitoxin

The diphtheria antitoxin is of equine origin, and the minimal effective dose remains undefined; therefore, dosage is based on empiric judgments. It is usually accepted that for patients with mild or moderate cases, including those with tonsillar and pharyngeal membrane, 50,000 units, injected intramuscularly, is enough (for a child, 30,000 units). In severe cases, such as with a more extensive membrane and/or thrombocytopenia, 60,000 to 120,000 units is the recommended dose, depending on severity, at least half of it being given by slow intravenous infusion in critically ill patients.

Before administration of antitoxin, any history of allergy or reactions to horse serum or horse dander must be determined. All patients must be tested for antitoxin sensitivity. The test is carried out by diluting horse antitoxin in saline and performing an eye test with a 1:10 dilution. This is followed by a scratch test with a 1:100 dilution; if negative in ½ hour, the scratch test is followed by an intradermal test, 1:100 dilution. If all tests are negative, antitoxin can be given. The intravenous route is recommended, first a slow intravenous infusion of 0.5 ml of antitoxin in 10 ml of saline, followed in ½ hour by the balance of the antitoxin dose in a dilution of 1:20 with saline, infused at a rate not to exceed 1 ml per minute. Others give the antitoxin dose intramuscularly—in mild to moderate cases only.

If the patient is sensitive to horse serum, desensitization should be carried out with care, preferably in an intensive care unit. Epinephrine should be available as well as intubation equipment and respiratory assistance. The following doses of horse serum antitoxin should be injected at 15-minute intervals, if no reaction occurs: (1) 0.5 ml of 1:20 dilution subcutaneously; (2) 0.10 ml of 1:10 dilution subcutaneously; (3) 0.3 ml of 1:10 dilution subcutaneously; (4) 0.1 ml of undiluted antitoxin subcutaneously; (5) 0.2 ml of undiluted antitoxin subcutaneously; (6) 0.5 ml of undiluted antitoxin subcutaneously; (7) remaining estimated therapeutic dose intramuscularly.

During all tests and injections of antitoxin, a syringe containing epinephrine, 1:1,100 dilution in saline, should be at hand to be used immediately in a dose of 0.01 ml per kilogram subcutaneously or intramuscularly at any sign of anaphylaxis. A good precaution is to have a venous access with normal saline prior to the test. If needed, a similar amount of epinephrine diluted to a final concentration of 1:10,000 in saline may be given slowly, intravenously, and repeated in 5 to 15 minutes. Other information and instructions in the package insert accompanying the antitoxin should be observed.

Antibiotic Use

C. diphtheriae is susceptible to several antimicrobial agents. After cultures have been performed, antibiotics should be administered to prevent multiplication of the microorganisms at the site of infection and to eliminate the carrier state. Penicillin G is the drug of choice and is usually given as procaine penicillin, 600,000 units intramuscularly every 12 hours for 10 days. Erythromycin is also active against the diphtheria bacillus and is given in a dose of 2.0 g per day divided in four doses for the same period. Resistance to erythromycin has been reported. Other antimicrobial agents with activity against *C. diphtheriae* include tetracycline, rifampin, clindamycin, and ampicillin; data on their clinical use are scarce. Antimicrobial therapy may be discontinued after the antibiotic course and when three successive daily cultures from both nose and throat are negative.

Supportive Measures

Bed rest is essential during the acute phase of the disease. Return to physical activity must be carefully guided by the physician and will depend on the degree of toxicity and the presence of cardiac involvement.

Complications such as dehydration, malnutrition, and congestive heart failure should be promptly diagnosed and treated. The pulse and blood pressure should be measured frequently. The use of digitalis in heart failure associated with diphtherial myocarditis has been questioned and should be individualized on a case-by-case basis (e.g., for an elderly patient with rapidly progressing myocarditis).

In cases of severe laryngeal involvement, marked toxicity, and/or shock, corticosteroids (prednisone, 5 mg per kilogram per day) have been advocated, but there are no hard data on their effectiveness; I use corticosteroids in this situation, but only until the inciting cause has been relieved.

In cases of laryngeal obstruction with respiratory stridor, a tracheotomy is necessary and should be performed promptly.

Before the patient is discharged, specimens from throat and nose or local lesion should be cultured; at least two, and preferably three, consecutive negative cultures should be obtained.

After recovery, toxoid against tetanus and diphtheria (Td) should be administered to complete a primary series if the patient has not been immunized.

APPROACH TO CARRIERS

The chronic carrier state may occur despite immunity, derived from either clinical disease or immunization. The carrier state occasionally occurs and persists in the absence of antecedent disease. Erythromycin (in adults, 0.5 g orally four times a day for 7 days) is the drug of choice for treatment of the carrier state and probably also the acute disease. Alternative antibiotics are procaine penicillin G, 600,000 units intramuscularly daily for 14 days; clindamycin, 150 mg orally four times a day for 7 days; or rifampin, 600 mg by mouth daily for 7 days.

APPROACH TO EPIDEMICS

The approach to epidemics is as follows:

1. Identify all primary cases, hospitalize, and treat.
2. Use toxoid in all the population at risk.
3. Culture all contacts for diphtheria, and treat all persons with *C. diphtheriae* in throat, nose, or skin lesions with erythromycin for 7 days to eliminate carrier state (see Prevention, below).
4. Watch primary contacts closely during the first week of exposure and treat at first signs or symptoms. Alternatively, all susceptible primary contacts can be given 1,500 to 3,000 units of diphtheria antitoxin intramuscularly, using the same precautions for antitoxin administration as previously stated, in addition to toxoid. This low-level dose will boost individuals while they are forming their own antibody.

PREVENTION

Prevention of diphtheria has been achieved mainly by active immunization of all children in the population. Primary immunization of children 6 years of age and younger should be carried out with a mixture of diphtheria and tetanus toxoids and pertussis vaccine (DTP), according to the following schedule: 2 months, DTP; 4 months, DTP; 6 months, DTP; 18 months, DTP; 4 to 6 years, DTP; 14 to 16 years,

Td (adult type). For primary immunization of children older than 6 years of age, adult type tetanus and diphtheria toxoids (Td) should be used. This combination contains no more than 2 flocculation units (Lf) of diphtheria toxoid per dose, in contrast to 7 to 25 Lf in DTP and is less likely to produce reactions in older recipients. Complete immunization is accomplished with two doses at least 8 weeks apart followed by a third dose a year later.

Children who have had a complete course of primary immunization with DTP may be given a booster injection on exposure to diphtheria. This is done in cases of outbreaks but not routinely. Antibiotic prophylaxis is highly effective.

Household and other close contacts of a patient with diphtheria should be observed attentively for 7 days. They should receive either an intramuscular injection of 1.2 million units of benzathine penicillin or a 7-day course of erythromycin by the oral route. Cultures should be performed before and after treatment. An injection of toxoid appropriate for age and immunization status can also be given. Susceptible close contacts who have had no (or only one) prior injections of toxoid should promptly be given 3,000 to 10,000 (depending on body size) units of antitoxin, with the usual precautions being followed. When indicated, active immunization with toxoid should be continued to completion.

SUGGESTED READING

Koopman JS, Campbell J. The role of cutaneous diphtheria infections in a diphtheria epidemic. J Infect Dis 1975; 131:239–245.
McCloskey RV. *Corynebacterium diphtheriae* (diphtheria). In: Mandell GL, Douglas RG Jr, Bennett JE, eds. Principles and practice of infectious diseases. New York: John Wiley, 1985:1171.
McCloskey RV, Eller JJ, Green M, et al. The 1970 epidemic of diphtheria in San Antonio. Ann Intern Med 1971; 75:495–500.
Zalma VM, Older JJ, Brooks GF. The Austin, Texas, diphtheria outbreak. Clinical and epidemiological aspects. JAMA 1970; 211:2125–2128.

PERTUSSIS

SARAH S. LONG, M.D.

DISEASE CHARACTERISTICS

Appropriate treatment strategy for a case of pertussis requires the dual appreciations that the patient is the sentinel of a larger problem and that the disease is not an infection but a toxicoinfection. Pertussis is one of the most contagious of infectious diseases, with clinically apparent disease occurring in 90 percent of unimmunized exposed individuals.

Complete immunization (three doses in a primary series in the first year of life or two doses in the second year of life, plus a reinforcing dose 6 months after completion of a primary series) confers 80 to 90 percent protection against clinical pertussis after exposure. Neither the disease nor immunization confers lifelong immunity, clinical pertussis occurring not infrequently in exposed adults whose antibody level has waned. Furthermore, recent data show that subclinical or atypical infection occurs in as many as 90 percent of immunized household members when a case is identified (usually an unimmunized child with classic symptoms). Subclinical infections may in fact contribute propitiously to persistent clinical immunity. They probably also constitute the reservoir of *Bordetella pertussis*, an obligate and exclusive parasite of ciliary epithelium of the human respiratory tract.

Pertussis is at least a 6-week illness for most individuals with 2-week periods of incubation, catarrhal infective phase (mild upper respiratory tract symptoms and maximal contagion), paroxysmal toxic phase (incapacitating coughing spells and diminishing contagion), and convalescent phase (diminishing episodes of coughing when the organism can no longer be recovered). Mortality from apnea, hypoxemia, toxic encephalopathy, central nervous system hemorrhage, or secondary pneumonia occurs in the paroxysmal phase in 0.7 percent of infants less than 1 year old with pertussis in the United States.

B. pertussis is by far the most common cause of the pertussis syndrome, other agents such as adenovirus, *Bordetella parapertussis*, *Bordetella bronchiseptica*, and *Chlamydia* being causative infrequently. The incidence of pertussis has increased in the Untied States since 1981, probably reflecting an actual increase in the number of cases (especially in young adults with only vaccine-induced immunity from childhood) and an increase in accuracy of diagnoses.

DIAGNOSTIC TESTS

Confirmation of cases of pertussis is dependent on the quality of specimens and the laboratory's enthusiasm for doing so. Culture of *B. pertussis* requires expeditious inoculation of nasopharyngeal mucus, collected by a swab, on special agar. Regan-Lowe medium—with sheep red blood cells, charcoal to absorb toxic fatty acids, and cephalexin to inhibit growth of nasopharyngeal flora—is probably superior to Bordet-Gengou agar. Early identification of tiny glistening colonies 2 to 5 days after inoculation is aided by use of specific fluorescence antibody testing of suspect colonies. The direct immunofluorescence test of patients' nasopharyngeal secretions is a useful rapid test but requires performance by experienced personnel and strict quality control to avoid false-positive results.

Both tests are most likely positive in patients in the late incubation through the catarrhal phase into the early paroxysmal phase of illness. Both tests are affected by patients' prior treatment with antibiotics. In situations in which specimens are collected on site and in which laboratories have expertise in performing both tests, culture is the more sensitive. Fluorescence testing of nasopharyngeal mucus has the advantages of forgiving a time delay in processing slides prepared at the bedside and allowing transport to a reference laboratory. Transport medium containing casamino acids is used when culture inoculation is delayed for a few hours. There is no single serum or secretory antibody test that is both sensitive and specific for the diagnosis of pertussis.

Lymphocytosis of up to 80 percent of a total peripheral white blood cell count of 20,000 to 100,000 is a manifestation of pertussis toxin's "anti-homing" effect on lymphocytes. Notably, cells are small, normal lymphocytes, not the sticky vacuolated large atypical lymphocytes characteristic of viral infection. Very young infants, adults, and immunized individuals with pertussis have only modest lymphocytosis; eosinophilia is a common response in young infants. Chest radiograph is remarkable only for peribronchial streaking with patchy atelectasis and overaeration unless secondary pneumonia has occurred.

TREATMENT

B. pertussis neither invades tissue nor disseminates to extrarespiratory sites. Symptoms in the paroxysmal phase are primarily the effect of pertussis toxin. Toxin is irreversibly bound, is internalized, and alters function of certain cells.

It is not surprising then that antibacterial and antitoxic therapies have little clinical effect. The thrust of treatment is to prevent complications during the paroxysmal phase in infants, to abort disease in infected contacts, and to halt contagion of cases and contacts.

Care of the Patient

Infants less than 1 year of age usually should be hospitalized during the early paroxysmal phase to assess severity and frequency of coughing spasms; to monitor for hypoxemia and hypercapnia; to provide intermittent oxygen therapy as required; to assure adequate nutrition and fluid; to remove asphyxiating concretions of organisms, denuded cilia, and mucus when necessary; and to correct metabolic derangements. Secondary bacterial otitis media and pneumonia, hypoglycemia, and excessive secretion of antidiuretic hormone are recognized complications.

Providing necessary medical care without violating the preemptive rule of therapy for pertussis, which is, "Don't bother the baby" and risk inducing a paroxysm, requires extraordinary educational efforts in the modern high-technology hospitals. A startling light, noise, jarring, or awakening, as well as the obvious agitation caused by physical examination, blood letting, suctioning, administering of medicines, and even oral feedings can induce a life-threatening coughing spell and post-tussive vomiting. Small-volume frequent feedings in a quiet, darkened room are usually successfully taken. Occasionally, parenteral alimentation is required for fluid and nutrition, and paralysis and mechanical ventilation are necessary if paroxysms cause anoxia or apnea. A mist tent (if it does not cause anxiety), or a humidifier is useful to loosen secretions and to prevent a dry airway from inducing cough. Hospitalized children should be strictly isolated under respiratory precautions.

The principles of therapy for older individuals in the home setting are similar. Smoke must be completely excluded from the environment. Ambulatory patients can be allowed to return to day care, school, or work after 5 days of antimicrobial therapy (see below). Occasional paroxysmal cough, as well as dramatic exacerbations during viral respiratory illnesses, occurs during the year following pertussis.

Erythromycin is the most effective bactericidal agent against *B. pertussis* in vitro. No resistance to erythromycin has developed. Erythromycin given during the incubation period aborts the clinical disease. If given during the catarrhal phase it shortens symptoms. It is difficult to show clinical efficacy when it is given during the paroxysmal phase. Erythromycin is the most effective agent yet studied in eliminating organisms from the nasopharynx, rendering the patient noncontagious. Erythromycin estolate (50 mg per kilogram per day administered in four divided doses orally; maximum daily dose, 1 g) for 14 days is universally successful.

Therapies using other doses, other erythromycin preparations (ethylsuccinate, stearate, or base), for shorter durations (5, 7, or 10 days) do not have the record of efficacy attained by erythromycin estolate for this purpose. It is expected that higher dosages of the other erythromycin preparations that accrue concentrations in respiratory secretions similar to that of the estolate would be effective. Unlike other preparations of erythromycin, in which food interferes with drug absorption, absorption of the estolate appears to be enhanced when taken with food. This may reduce gastric irritation and drug intolerance. Cholestatic hepatitis (very rare in children receiving a 14-day course) is probably not more commonly associated with the estolate preparation, as was formerly believed.

In a recent small study, twice daily administration of erythromycin ethylsuccinate orally (50 mg per kilogram per day for 14 days) was effective in eliminating colonization, suggesting that a high level of bactericidal activity, even though less frequently present, is effective. It is not clear whether the relative success of 14 days of therapy is due to the final elimination of all organisms or to suppression of growth until the time when specific secretory antibody is produced. Alternative drugs such as ampicillin, tetracycline, and trimethoprim/sulfamethoxazole have in vitro efficacy against *B. pertussis*, but there is less clinical experience with their therapeutic or prophylactic efficacy.

The use of glucocorticoids has been studied in two controlled trials, showing efficacy in reducing the number, severity, and duration of paroxysms. Relative paucity of experimental and experiential data suggests limiting the use of glucocorticoids to a brief period and for only the most severe cases. A dosage could be 2 mg per kilogram per day of prednisone in two doses for 3 days.

Small studies and anecdotal reports of the use of orally administered β_2-agonists, such as albuterol or salbutamol, in treatment of pertussis have appeared in the literature in recent years. It is reasoned that prevention of bronchial obstruction might lessen coughing spells. Although no study to date fulfills the criteria of large numbers of patients with disease of similar clinical severity who are studied in a blinded, placebo-controlled, and cross-over fashion, the more stringent the test, the less an effect is shown. Their use should not be routine and must be undertaken with the knowledge of adverse effects, lack of proven efficacy, and lack of approval for use in infants or for the indication of pertussis. Dosages used in reports to date are 0.3 to 0.6 mg per kilogram per day divided into four doses orally for 2 days' duration.

Pertussis immune globulin (human) is of no value in the amelioration of symptoms of pertussis and is no longer commercially available.

Antitussive medicines should not be used as they have no proven beneficial effect, may be drying, may have behavioral effects in infants, and can impair the ability of the patient to cough up obstructive plugs of thick mucus from the respiratory tract.

A patient with a confirmed case of pertussis need not receive pertussis immunization(s) in the future.

Sequelae from pertussis are related to complications of the paroxysmal phase, such as necrotizing secondary bacterial pneumonia or damage to the central nervous system from hypoxia or hemorrhage.

Care of Exposed Contacts

Household, day care, classroom, and other close contacts less than 7 years of age who have had at least four doses of pertussis vaccine should receive a booster dose of vaccine, usually as DTP, unless a dose has been given within the past 3 years. Additionally, erythromycin estolate (50 mg per kilogram per day divided into four doses) should be given for 14 days because immunity against infection and protection against disease manifestations are not absolute. Those children with no or less than full immunization should receive DTP and erythromycin estolate and then continue on a recommended primary or "catch-up" immunization schedule. For household and other close contacts 7 years of age or older, erythromycin estolate (50 mg per kilogram per day divided into four doses, or comparable doses of other preparations; see "Care of Case") should be given for 14 days to abort an incubating case or render the asymptomatically infected person noncontagious. Immunization is not usually recommended for individuals 7 years of age or older. Symptomatic contacts should not return to school or work for 5 days after beginning antibiotic therapy.

PREVENTION

Many assessments of cost effectiveness of immunization against pertussis, data on the prevention of morbidity and mortality, as well as knowledge gleaned from "experiments" of countries where routine immunization was suspended all affirm the wisdom of universal immunization in infancy. It is not surprising for a disease such as pertussis, in which clinical infection does not confer long-lasting immunity, the mechanisms of pathophysiology have not been completely delineated, the basis for immunity cannot be established, and the bacterium's toxin is associated with both the efficacy and reactogenicity of vaccine products, that prevention by vaccine is imperfect. Recent evaluation of a candidate acellular pertussis vaccine containing pertussis toxoid and fibrial hemagglutinin revealed diminished, minor adverse effects but clinical efficacy of only about 70 percent.

SUGGESTED READING

Bass JW. Erythromycin for treatment and prevention of pertussis. Pediatr Infect Dis J 1986; 5:154–157.
Eichenwald HF. Adverse reactions of erythromycin. Pediatr Infect Dis J 1986; 5:147–150.
Krantz I, Norrby SR, Trollfors B. Salbutamol vs. placebo for treatment of pertussis. Pediatr Infect Dis J 1985; 4:638–640.
Pittman M. The concept of pertussis as a toxin-mediated disease. Pediatr Infect Dis J 1984; 3:467–486.
Steketee RW, Wassilak SGF, Adkins WN Jr, et al. Evidence for a high attack rate and efficacy of erythromycin prophylaxis in a pertussis outbreak in a facility for the developmentally disabled. J Infect Dis 1988; 157:434–440.

ANTHRAX

BORIS VELIMIROVIC, M.D., D.T.P.H.

Anthrax is an acute disease caused by the aerobic, spore-forming, gram-positive, toxin-producing rod *Bacillus anthracis*. It is the oldest known zoonosis with worldwide distribution: very infrequent in the industrialized countries, only very sporadic in the United States, moderately frequent in southern Europe, very rare in central and northern Europe, and common in the USSR, tropical and subtropical Africa, Asia, the Caribbean, and South America. The incidence has decreased considerably in all countries. The usually quoted numbers, which come from a well-known reference paper more than 30 years old, are not valid any longer.

EPIDEMIOLOGY

The ability to form spores permits the organism to survive environmental and disinfective measures that destroy most other bacteria. Public health problems largely arise from its long persistence in the soil (90 years proved). Infection of the skin comes about by contact with contaminated goat hair, wool, hides, bones, and other similar products during processing, spinning, and wearing, or by direct contact with infected tissues, i.e., meat.

Inhalation anthrax results from aspiration of *B. anthracis* or spores via small aerosolized bacillus-bearing particles. Less than 5 μm in size, the spores germinate in the alveoli and multiply. They are ingested by alveolar macrophages and carried to the regional lymph nodes.

Gastrointestinal anthrax results from ingestion of contaminated meat and occurs in explosive outbreaks. Spores are ingested and absorbed through intestinal mucosa, and vegetative forms multiply in the regional lymph nodes. If transported through oral mucosa, they can produce a cervical form. There is no evidence that milk from infected animals transmits the disease. Biting flies and other insects may serve as mechanical vectors. Incubation is usually 48 hours but may be longer.

For epidemiologic purposes, the disease is divided into agricultural and industrial anthrax (occupational history is important). Particularly exposed or at potential risk are veterinarians, veterinary assistants, herders, agricultural and ranch workers, slaughterhouse employees, tannery and textile industry workers, home craftsmen using imported yarn from endemic areas, and people handling bonemeal fertilizer.

PATHOGENESIS

The anthrax bacilli proliferate at the site of entry and are numerous beneath the central necrotic area of the skin lesion. They are transported to the regional lymph nodes, producing a hemorrhagic lymphadenitis. If they penetrate the bloodstream, septicemia can occur and can cause metastatic lesions.

The virulence of the organism is variable and is determined by at least two factors: an extracellular toxin and the capsular polypeptide. The number of organisms in the initial inoculum also plays a role. The toxin causes vascular permeability, edema and fluid loss, and oligemic shock, which is the mechanism of death. The toxin consists of at least three components—edema factor, protective antigen, and lethal factor—each of which is nontoxic but acts synergistically. Differing concentrations of individual toxins in any given strain of *B. anthracis* lead to varying pathogenicity and virulence. In the pulmonary form, primary lesions are in the bronchopulmonary lymph nodes (hemorrhagic lymphadenopathy), not in alveoli or bronchi, but there may be secondary involvement of alveoli.

CLINICAL PICTURE

Infection occurs in three distinct main forms: cutaneous, pulmonary, and intestinal.

Cutaneous

The commonest form accounts for up to 98 percent of all cases. There are two forms: dry and edematous. A small red papule develops, after an incubation period of 1 to 7 days, at the entry points on the exposed parts of the skin—a minor injury, a cut or an abrasion—or after active rubbing in the skin by the fingers, usually of the hand or other parts of the upper extremities, in the face (about half of all cases), lips, eyebrows, or neck (but also the feet, upper chest or back, breast, penis, and scrotum). This papule progresses within 12 to 48 hours to a fluid-filled blister. The fluid in the vesicle is initially clear, but soon it becomes dark and bluish black. The blister is surrounded by inflammation, extensive hard induration and edema in the adjacent deeper tissues, lymphadenitis, and lymphadenopathy. There is no carbuncle. Fever is mild. The lesion is not painful. Double lesions do occur. Satellite vesicles can develop near the initial lesion. The vesicle ruptures and develops into a pustule (pustula maligna), the tissue necrotizes and progresses to a lesion that is relatively painless, and then it becomes a dark-colored or black eschar (anthrax is Greek for "black") of about 1 to 3 cm in diameter or larger. This heals and the scab falls off, leaving a scar.

In untreated (or unrecognized) cases, there may be hematogenous spread via regional lymph nodes, bacteremia (fever), and toxemia, which may lead to death in 5 to 20 percent of cases (localization on the head or neck has a more serious prognosis). Eighty percent of cases of cutaneous anthrax can heal spontaneously without treatment.

Pulmonary

The pulmonary form is initially manifested by a mild upper respiratory tract infection with a nonproductive cough suggestive of atypical pneumonia, influenza, or mild bronchopneumonia. Roentgenograms may show mediastinal widening. After several days and often after a temporary improvement from the primary phase (at which there is a surprising discrepancy between subjective and objective findings: the patient is well oriented, alert, not agitated), there is a sudden onset of acute dyspnea, cyanosis, stridor, signs of pleural effusion, and an elevated temperature due to septicemia. The patient usually dies of toxemia and suffocation within 24 hours of onset of this second stage. Postmortem findings are of massive pulmonary edema, hemorrhagic mediastinitis, and hydrothorax. The first stage may not be clearly observed and the disease is noted in the second stage, which is also called the septicemic form.

Not all persons exposed to inhalation of spores develop the clinical disease. Subclinical infection, as assumed on the basis of serologic tests, may provide some protection against a new challenge.

Intestinal

The usually not clinically recognized intestinal form appears 2 to 5 days after ingestion of meat contaminated with spores of *B. anthracis* and the penetration of the intestinal mucosa. The local ulcerative lesions in the gut, most frequently in the ileocecal region but also in the jejunum, are similar to those of the cutaneous form and are accompanied by nonspecific symptoms such as nausea, vomiting, dizziness, anorexia, slight fever, abdominal pain, splenomegaly or bloody diarrhea, and hemorrhagic ascites (even several liters) in the absence of liver damage. There is progression to generalized septicemia, toxemia, shock due to massive fluid loss (hypovolemia) and renal failure, and death in about 50 percent of cases. Local lesions, hemorrhagic spots in the serosa, and a typical septic, soft, small necrotic spleen (no splenomegaly) are characteristic postmortem findings. The gastric form is extremely rare.

Other Forms

The meningeal form generally occurs following an initial cutaneous disease in up to 3 to 5 percent of cases; it rarely occurs as a primary infection, or it may result from inhalation. Clinically, typical symptoms of bacterial meningitis are present and lead almost invariably to death in 2 to 4 days.

Milder or subclinical cases in cutaneous and pulmonary forms and chronic cases in the intestinal form can occur, but their incidence is unknown. Any differential diagnosis of anthrax must consider staphylococcal contagious pustular dermatitis; in the tropics, cutaneous diphtheria and plague in cutaneous form; any pneumonia in respiratory form; and various enteric infections and sepsis in intestinal form. Recently a renal form has been described.

LABORATORY DIAGNOSIS

Diagnosis is by microscopic confirmation of *B. anthracis* in films made from pus, exudates from lesions, cerebrospinal fluid, or discharges, or by direct microscopic examination. In the gastrointestinal form the organism can be demonstrated in vomitus or feces, and in the pulmonary form in hemophysis. Bacilli are usually not present in the bloodstream in large numbers (except in septicemia) until just before death, but a blood specimen must be cultured. The bacillus can be identified by fluorescent antibody techniques in tissue sections. Examination of paired sera by indirect

microhemagglutination or ELISA may be helpful. (The *B. subtilis* group may resemble *B. anthracis* and *B. cereus,* and the differentiation may be impossible. All reactions are the same except urease production, which is negative in *B. anthracis.* It has been found to produce a clinical picture milder but similar to cutaneous anthrax). The use of radioactively labeled antibodies for rapid detection (indirect immunoradiometric assay) has been reported.

TREATMENT

Treatment should start on suspicion, without waiting for laboratory culture results. Procaine penicillin remains the drug of choice: 1 to 2 million units daily, divided into two intramuscular injections initially and continued as single daily doses thereafter for 7 days. However, in the cutaneous form a shorter course may be equally effective. If penicillin G is used, doses should be increased. Benzylpenicillin or intravenous crystalline penicillin could also be given. Complete sterilization of the wound is achieved in cutaneous anthrax within 24 hours. The edema resolves within about 5 days; it may increase in the first 24 to 48 hours because of the release of toxin from disintegrating bacilli. In pulmonary and septicemic forms, which have an unfavorable prognosis, up to 10 million (even 30 to 40 million) units of penicillin in infusion have been recommended. Other broad-spectrum antibiotics, such as tetracyclines, 0.5 g every 4 hours, chlortetracycline, erythromycin, 0.2 g every 4 hours, chloramphenicol, aureomycin, achromycin, 3 g per day for 6 to 7 days, and streptomycin, 30 mg per kilogram per day divided in two intramuscular injections, cephalosporins, and also trimethoprim-sulfamethoxazole, are fully effective. In plague-endemic areas, streptomycin or tetracycline is recommended if diagnostic doubts exist. In milder forms oral penicillin can be given. Correction of the electrolyte balance in the intestinal form may be necessary.

There is only limited experience with the newer aminoglycoside antibiotics. With antibiotic treatment, there should be no fatal cases with cutaneous anthrax. However, antibiotics have no effect on the toxin already produced and on the course of existing skin lesions in cutaneous anthrax. Prophylactic antibiotics should be considered if a person is known to have eaten contaminated meat. Antiserum is no longer used, but recently there have been suggestions that it may be useful in the initial phases of the disease. Antitoxin preparations are not available. Antibiotic ointments have no influence on the healing process. Skin transplantation after extensive cutaneous lesions may be necessary.

PREVENTION

Prevention of cutaneous and probably inhalation anthrax is possible by immunization of persons potentially at high risk (e.g., veterinarians in endemic areas, workers in imported-wool processing plants and textile factories) with a cell-free vaccine prepared from a culture filtrate of a nonvirulent, nonencapsulated strain containing the protective antigen absorbed to aluminum hydroxide gel. The vaccine is given parenterally, three doses at 2-week intervals followed

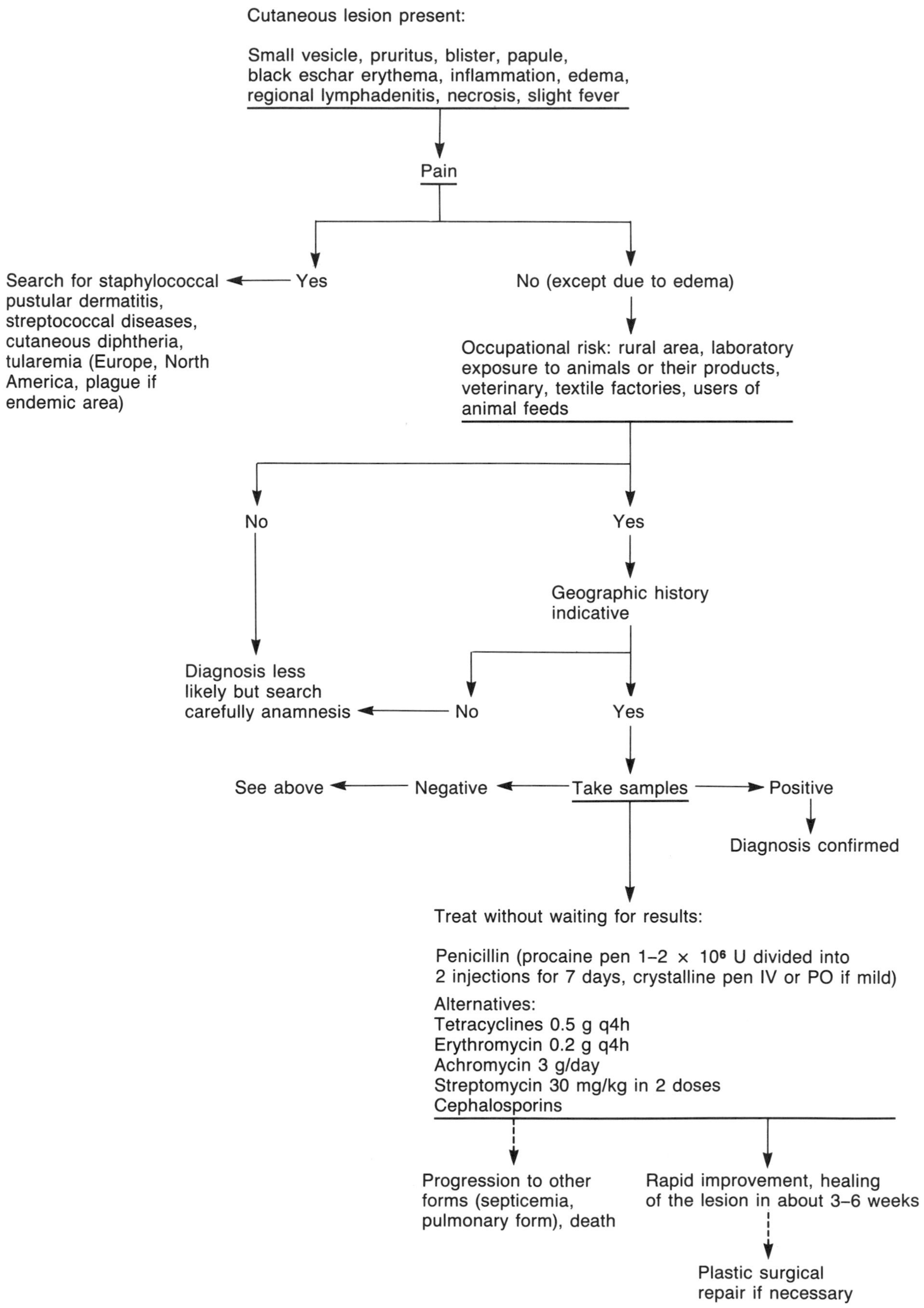

Cutaneous lesion present:

Small vesicle, pruritus, blister, papule, black eschar erythema, inflammation, edema, regional lymphadenitis, necrosis, slight fever

↓

Pain

Yes → Search for staphylococcal pustular dermatitis, streptococcal diseases, cutaneous diphtheria, tularemia (Europe, North America, plague if endemic area)

No (except due to edema)

↓

Occupational risk: rural area, laboratory exposure to animals or their products, veterinary, textile factories, users of animal feeds

No → Diagnosis less likely but search carefully anamnesis

Yes

↓

Geographic history indicative

No → Diagnosis less likely but search carefully anamnesis

Yes

↓

See above ← Negative ← Take samples → Positive

Positive → Diagnosis confirmed

↓

Treat without waiting for results:

Penicillin (procaine pen 1–2 × 10⁶ U divided into 2 injections for 7 days, crystalline pen IV or PO if mild)

Alternatives:
Tetracyclines 0.5 g q4h
Erythromycin 0.2 g q4h
Achromycin 3 g/day
Streptomycin 30 mg/kg in 2 doses
Cephalosporins

Progression to other forms (septicemia, pulmonary form), death

Rapid improvement, healing of the lesion in about 3–6 weeks

↓

Plastic surgical repair if necessary

Figure 1 Management of cutaneous anthrax.

Signs of pneumonia:

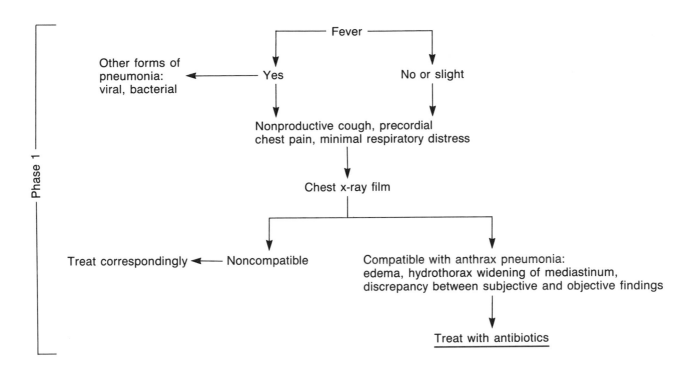

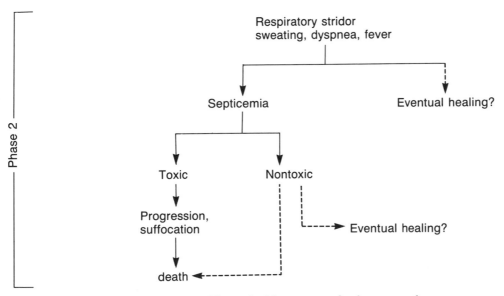

Figure 2 Management of pulmonary anthrax.

by three booster inoculations at 6-month intervals and then annual booster inoculations.

The best control measure is the immunization of animals in endemic areas. For the purchase of large quantities of vaccine contact the Bureau of Disease Control and Laboratory Services, Michigan Department of Public Health, P.O. Box 30035, 3500 North Logan Street, Lansing, Michigan 48909, in the United States, or in Europe, the Pasteur Institute, 28 Rue du Docteur Roux, 75724 Paris, Cedex 15, France (telephone 1–45.68.80.00). Regarding individual patients, contact the Biologic Drugs Division, Bureau of Laboratories, Centers for Disease Control, Atlanta, Georgia 30333.

LEPROSY

BURTON C. WEST, M.D.

Innumerable unanswered questions about leprosy exist because *Mycobacterium leprae* has never been cultivated in vitro. This is particularly ironic because leprosy was among the first diseases to be correctly attributed to a microorganism. Hansen made those landmark observations on tissues from leprosy patients in 1873. Because major efforts to culture *M. leprae* have been unsuccessful, clinicians and investigators have developed practical, but extraordinary techniques and methods for dealing with *M. leprae* and with leprosy patients, making leprosy unique among infectious diseases.

Leprosy is not understood, as are other infectious diseases, with regard to its epidemiology, reservoir, source, transmission, natural history, host-parasite interactions, prevention, and cure. Furthermore, the clinical microbiology, identification of therapeutic agents, assessment of therapy, susceptibility, and drug resistance depend on noncultural methods. In the absence of a method of culture, other methods are important. Since the organism replicates in mouse foot pads, antimicrobial susceptibility or resistance is determined by a labor- and time-intensive bioassay, which costs in excess of $800. The recent discovery of phenolic glycolipid-1 (PGL-1), a substance uniquely specific for *M. leprae*, is extremely important. Although also labor- and time-intensive, measurement of PGL-1 by enzyme-linked immunosorbent assay (ELISA) using monoclonal antibody and measurement of antibody to PGL-1 in human serum are beginning to increase the understanding of many aspects of leprosy. Furthermore, the nine-banded armadillo, which has been shown to harbor a naturally occurring infection with *M. leprae*, is susceptible to experimental infection, and it has become the prime experimental animal for the study of leprosy.

CLINICAL EPIDEMIOLOGY

Nonetheless, much is known about leprosy. Ten to 15 million people are clinically infected in the world today. Although uncommon in the United States, it has been increasing in frequency. In the early 1970s, about 140 new cases per year were identified. In the mid-1980s, nearly 400 per year were being reported. More than 90 percent of persons with leprosy were foreign-born and immigrated from endemic areas, the majority from Asia and Pacific islands. A significant minority are Hispanic, most having entered the United States from Mexico. Indigenous cases continue to account for less than 10 percent of the total cases and are reported from Hawaii, California, Texas, and Louisiana, but not recently from Florida. Because of immigration and travel, nearly all states have reported leprosy in the past 15 years. Most large cities are the home to dozens of active cases.

Supported in part by grants from the Ed E. and Gladys Hurley Foundation and from American Leprosy Missions, Inc.

Fifty to 70 percent of patients with leprosy do not know of any contact with another human case. However, transmission from an infected to a susceptible human being is generally thought to be the way leprosy is spread. Household contact with an untreated human with leprosy is an important risk factor. Some evidence of spread involving insects, soil, water, vegetation, armadillos, and even naturally infected monkeys exists but is not generally accepted.

Classification of leprosy is useful in dealing with the spectrum of its clinical and other manifestations. Ridley and Jopling provided five clinicopathologic categories ranging from polar lepromatous leprosy (LL), characterized by large numbers of *M. Leprae*, and little evidence of immunity, to polar tuberculoid leprosy (TT), characterized by few or no *M. leprae* by ordinary methods of examination and the presence of active cell-mediated resistance, i.e., granulomatous inflammation. Intermediate forms are borderline lepromatous leprosy (BL), borderline leprosy (BB), and borderline tuberculoid leprosy (BT). Untreated patients with large numbers of organisms are considered contagious to susceptible persons.

Practically speaking, the person from any area endemic for leprosy is at higher risk than others to develop it. Birth or prolonged residence in Indochina, Samoa, the Philippines, Mexico, or another endemic country is a risk factor. Of adults with lepromatous leprosy, men outnumber women. Generally, rural persons are more likely to develop leprosy than city dwellers.

Patients with tuberculoid leprosy mount a fairly normal immune response, whereas those with lepromatous leprosy exhibit defective cell-mediated immunity. Conversely, persons with known defects in immunity do not appear to be at increased risk for leprosy. The question of susceptibility to leprosy is complex. Of at-risk, unrelated household members exposed to an active case, not more than 4 or 5 percent actually develop leprosy. Thus, only 4 or 5 percent of persons are apparently susceptible, unless subclinical infection occurs. Recently, an association between leprosy and HLA antigens DR2 and DQw1 has been found to exist across a wide range of populations. Surprisingly, to date only one man with acquired immunodeficiency syndrome has been reported to have developed leprosy. More are expected to be complicated by this infection, despite its generally not being opportunistic in the usual sense.

DIAGNOSIS

Although the clinical epidemiology is useful in assessing specific findings, it is skin and nerve lesions that alert the clinician to the possibility of Hansen's disease or leprosy. Table 1 summarizes the major clinical presentations of leprosy in its various forms. Skin lesions are the most common initial complaint or physical abnormality. Some are only seen with thorough examination of all skin under natural light. Confusing lesions include localized edema, tender papules, and macules thought to be vitiligo. Commonly, presentation occurs with macules that variously are erythematous or hypopigmented and anesthetic. Invariably, there is a differential diagnosis of other skin diseases; it is best resolved by biopsy.

Nearly as commonly, there will be a peripheral nerve presentation (Table 1). Anesthesia of solitary or multiple macules is a strong clue to the diagnosis. Large-nerve involvement, a mononeuritis multiplex, is also relatively common. Deformities and self-induced, inadvertent trauma develop when medical care is not sought or the diagnosis is missed. Sadly, sometimes they develop anyway.

A variety of other lesions can develop through the presence of local infection or immunologic reactivity in a specific organ (Table 1). Of note is the frequency of false-positive VDRL serologic screening tests for syphilis.

The definitive diagnosis requires biopsy of the affected tissue, usually the skin (Table 2). The bacterial index (BI) is used to quantify the bacteria in a biopsy and is useful in following the response to treatment of lepromatous leprosy. The morphologic index (MI) is considered more sensitive than the BI for following response to treatment. Here, experienced pathologists note treatment-induced changes in the morphology of wild-type *M. leprae*. In diagnosed patients, "tissue juice" from various sites stained for acid-fast bacilli is used to assess the extent of disease and the response to therapy. The clinical use of PGL-1 and antibody to PGL-1 is just beginning and shows considerable promise. One report documents a patient's healthy contact whose serum contained detectable PGL-1 fully 2 years before the first clinical skin lesions of leprosy appeared. Although PGL-1 and antibody to PGL-1 might become the standard for diagnosis and follow-up of patients with leprosy, at present, a relatively deep, Fite-stained, properly interpreted skin biopsy specimen is essential for the diagnosis of leprosy and for its classification.

TABLE 1   The Clinical Diagnosis of Leprosy

Clinical Suspicion	Skin Lesion(s)
Born or lived in endemic country or state	Solitary or multiple macules
Family member or friend with leprosy	Multiple papules
Male gender	Anesthetic to touch and pinprick
Rural habitation	Anhidrosis
	Tender papules
	Localized edema
	Localized erythema
	Loss of eyebrows
	Thickened, lumpy, smooth skin
	Hypopigmented macules
	Traumatized or burned digits

Nerve Lesions	Miscellaneous Lesions
Palpable nerves	Bone lesions
Peripheral neuropathy	Glomerulonephritis
Motor	Testicular atrophy
Sensory	Conjunctivitis, keratitis, iridocyclitis, or corneal ulcer
Cranial nerve neuropathy, especially of nerve V or VII	Destructive upper airway lesions
Focal anesthesia in skin macule	Epistaxis
Claw-like flexion deformities	False-positive VDRL test (at least 10%)
Foot drop	Amyloidosis
Pressure ulcers	

TABLE 2   Confirmation of the Clinical Diagnosis of Leprosy

Skin biopsy with Fite stain, which shows characteristic histology, including acid-fast bacilli (AFB), except in otherwise typical tuberculoid cases where granulomas are the hallmark; some AFB are in nerves, often some are in clumps; these tissues should be culture-negative for mycobacteria

Experimental: measurement of detectable PGL-1 or antibody to PGL-1 in serum

Ancillary: superficial skin incision, e.g., from earlobe, yielding AFB in stained smears of "tissue juice"

THERAPY

Therapy should generally not be undertaken without a biopsy-proven diagnosis. Empiric therapy is ill-advised because of the far reaching implications of the diagnosis and the many years of treatment currently recommended for all forms of the disease. Dapsone resistance is an increasing problem, and it has led the World Health Organization (WHO) study group to recommend multidrug regimens for all forms of leprosy.

In many parts of the world, indeterminate leprosy is a clinical diagnosis. Indeterminate leprosy is generally quite limited and lacks clinical or histologic conclusiveness about its classification. It sometimes resolves without treatment. Perhaps here measurement of PGL-1 will prove useful. If indeterminate leprosy is diagnosed histologically and if the patient is closely followed, dapsone should suffice (Fig. 1). However, if indeterminate leprosy is diagnosed clinically or is not carefully followed, then two drugs are recommended, as for other paucibacillary leprosy including tuberculoid (TT) and borderline tuberculoid (BT) leprosy (Fig. 1). The WHO study group recommends that dapsone be given daily (1 to 2 mg per kilogram) and that rifampin be administered under supervision at an oral dose of 600 mg once per month for 6 months. This will suffice in many cases, but in the United States, daily therapy with two drugs for a 3-year period is recommended (Fig. 1).

Recommended therapy for LL, BL, and BB leprosy is initially quite similar: two drugs, initially including dapsone and rifampin, are given daily (Fig. 1). Therapy for such multibacillary cases is generally continued for more than 3 years. In lepromatous leprosy, rifampin is recommended for 5 to 7 years, and dapsone is generally recommended for life. The WHO study group, however, responding to the needs of emerging countries (which include the cost of drugs and dapsone resistance), has recommended a three-drug regimen, including dapsone, 100 mg daily; rifampin, 600 mg monthly; and clofazimine, 50 mg daily and 300 mg monthly. The monthly doses of rifampin and clofazimine are to be administered under supervision.

Because of adverse effects from dapsone or rifampin, it is sometimes necessary to substitute another active drug for one or even both of them. The best alternative drug currently is clofazimine, 100 mg per day. A good drug, but with significant hepatotoxicity, is ethionamide. It can be used in place of a first-line drug to provide a two- or three-drug regimen.

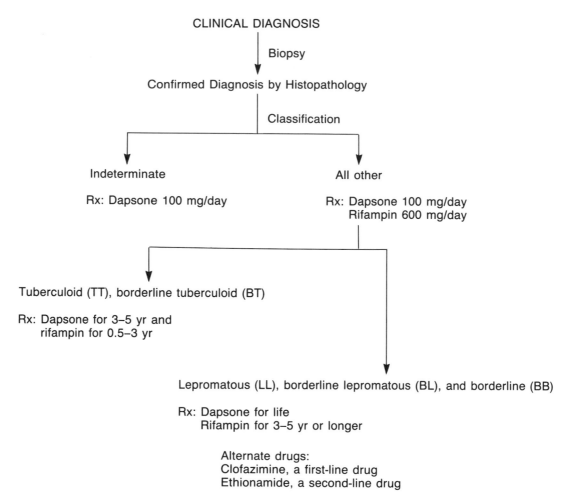

Figure 1   Therapy for leprosy classified according to the Ridley-Jopling method. Children should receive the following doses: dapsone, 1 mg per kilogram per day; rifampin 10 mg per kilogram per day; and/or clofazimine 1 mg per kilogram per day.

At present, no other drugs are as good or as well demonstrated to be safe and effective in the treatment of leprosy. However, several agents demonstrate activity against *M. leprae* in animal studies and to a limited extent in humans with leprosy. A problem with controlled clinical trials in leprosy is that to determine effectiveness and relapse rate, a trial must be continued for 10 to 15 years. Acedapsone, a long-acting, injectable dapsone-like drug, has been undergoing trials. Ansamycin, a congener of rifampin, has shown promise. Certain aminoglycosides, e.g., amikacin, are known to have activity but are not used because the prolonged treatment results in toxicity. With the possible exception of thiacetazone (not available in the United States), other antituberculosis drugs are not effective. A few β-lactam antibiotics, e.g., cefoxitin, cefuroxime, and mezlocillin, have shown limited activity in mouse foot-pad testing as have some macrolides; most show none. Some quinolones, e.g., ofloxacin (not licensed), have shown activity when tested in mice. None of these drugs is recommended for the treatment of leprosy at present.

Many specialized forms of treatment exist for leprosy. Because of the frequency of foot ulcers and injuries due to sensory neuropathy, careful attention must be paid to the feet.

After ulcers are healed, custom-made shoes can be made to protect the feet from further injury. A variety of surgical procedures have been devised for the treatment of flexion deformities, e.g., claw-hand, for nerve entrapment syndromes, and for ophthalmic leprosy. Nutrition, physical therapy, occupational and vocational rehabilitation, and psychological counseling and reassurance should be provided whenever possible. Screening of household and other close contacts for both an index case and possible secondary cases must be considered. Each case should be reported to the public health authorities.

DRUGS AND ADVERSE EFFECTS

Reactions during therapy take three forms: first, there are drug reactions; second, there is erythema nodosum leprosum (ENL); and third, there are reversal reactions.

Dapsone or diaminodiphenyl sulfone (DDS) has the potential of having sulfonamide-like side effects. Rashes, nausea, hypersensitivity reactions, and agranulocytosis are among the many described. Dapsone reactions may be confused with reactional states. Persons with glucose-6-

phosphate dehydrogenase deficiency will hemolyze at doses of 50 mg per day and will become anemic at higher doses. Testing for the enzyme deficiency is recommended. While normal persons may hemolyze mildly from dapsone, recently described is Heinz body hemolytic anemia in the presence of hemoglobin E trait. Certain Indochinese have a 36 percent prevalence of hemoglobin E, putting them at risk for hemolytic anemia while they are receiving dapsone.

Rifampin is a broad-spectrum antibiotic with effects on the immune system. It is one of few drugs that enters phagocytes, which may account for its effectiveness against the intracellular parasite *M. leprae*. Although rifampin is capable of causing hepatitis, reactional states can yield a similar complication, making assessment of the contribution of rifampin difficult to judge. Serious adverse effects such as renal failure must be considered during the prolonged therapy that is recommended. Rifampin causes orange discoloration of the urine, tears, and other body fluids, which should be explained to patients to avoid undue concern. More important, hepatic metabolism is speeded up, which sometimes interferes with the action of oral contraceptives and warfarin, for example. Because of multiple possible drug interactions, the physician is advised to review any nonleprosy treatment with regard to such potential complications.

Clofazimine is also a dye, which accounts for its most troublesome side effect, brown skin discoloration. This can become a major cosmetic problem for white and nonwhite patients alike, especially those who must take the high dose, i.e., 300 mg per day, for the treatment of reactions. Gastrointestinal intolerance may also limit its use.

REACTIONS DURING THERAPY

Classically, erythema nodosum leprosum (ENL) is a common one of many so-called lepra reactions that occur during the course of untreated multibacillary leprosy. Rarely today, leprosy presents with ENL. Now this distressful complication commonly occurs in the first year of treatment of multibacillary leprosy. Clinically and histopathologically it is similar to erythema nodosum. In addition to painful and tender red nodular skin lesions that are not limited to the lower extremities, fever and toxicity are frequent and are occasionally associated with jaundice and prostration. Rarely, ENL is life-threatening. Local inflammation involving joints, nerves, eyes, testes, or other organs may occur. Each nodular lesion contains features of allergic and vasculitic inflammation, which, taken as a crop, could be described as a multifocal Arthus reaction. However, the molecular stimulus for ENL is unknown. As outlined in Figure 2, treatment includes adrenal corticosteroids, either parenterally with methylprednisolone or orally with prednisone in doses initially of 60 to 80 mg per day. When this is insufficient or when the steroids cannot be successfully tapered after a few weeks, thalidomide is recommended. Since it causes phocomelia and other major birth defects, thalidomide is contraindicated in women of child-bearing age and absolutely contraindicated in pregnancy. It is a sedative. It can be obtained from the Gillis W. Long Hansen's Disease Center (Carville, Louisiana 70721; telephone 504–642–8325) as an investigational drug, following local hospital committee approval. If thalidomide is not available, does not work, or cannot be used because of pregnancy, then clofazimine, 300 mg per day, may be helpful (Fig. 2).

Reversal reactions constitute a complex and varied complication of leprosy treatment. Patients with borderline leprosy, after several months of treatment, may develop indurated inflamed skin lesions, but with fewer organisms than seen originally. The lesions may ulcerate. Reversal refers to the associated, seeming improvement in immune status. Steroids may be helpful, but because of the chronicity of the reactions, clofazimine 300 mg per day may be required to help control the reaction (Fig. 2).

In conclusion, treatment of leprosy was revolutionized in 1941 by dapsone. No longer is isolation needed to treat the patient or stigmatization required to protect the rest of society. Skillful early diagnosis of leprosy and chemotherapy

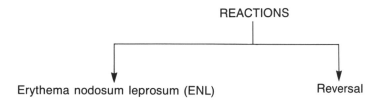

Figure 2 Therapy for reactions occurring during treatment of leprosy.

can prevent physical deformity and emotional stigma. The routine and initial use of two- or three-drug regimens hastens improvement and prevents the further emergence of dapsone resistance. It is no surprise that the slowest mycobacterium to replicate is the slowest to respond to chemotherapy, initially requiring monthly physician visits and sometimes requiring life-long therapy.

SUGGESTED READING

Blake LA, West BC, Lary CH, Todd JR. Environmental non-human sources of leprosy. Rev Infect Dis 1987; 9:562–577.

Lachant NA, Tanaka KR. Case report: dapsone-associated Heinz body hemolytic anemia in a Cambodian woman with hemoglobin E trait. Am J Med Sci 1987; 294:364–368.

Neill MA, Hightower AW, Broome CV. Leprosy in the United States, 1971–1981. J Infect Dis 1985; 152:1064–1069.

Thomas DA, Mines JS, Thomas DC, et al. Armadillo exposure among Mexican-born patients with lepromatous leprosy. J Infect Dis 1987; 156:990–992.

West BC, Todd JR, Lary CH, et al. Leprosy in six isolated residents of northern Louisiana: time-clustered cases in an essentially non-endemic area. Arch Intern Med 1988; 148:1987–1992.

WHO Study Group. Chemotherapy of leprosy for control programmes. WHO Tech Rep Ser 1982; 675:7–33.

NOCARDIAL INFECTION

MICHAEL C. BACH, M.D., FRCPC

Nocardia, an aerobic actinomycete, is an important though relatively uncommon pathogen that primarily causes pneumonia, brain abscess, and rarely, primary skin infections. It affects immunocompetent as well as immunodeficient patients. The antimicrobial susceptibility pattern is significantly different from that of other infectious pathogens, and thus specific recognition and identification of *Nocardia* is necessary.

MICROBIOLOGY

The organism grows aerobically. On Gram stain, it appears as branching gram-positive beaded thin hyphae (Fig. 1). When 1 percent H_2SO_4 is used as the decolorizer with the acid-fast stain, the hyphae are acid-fast. Specific species are identified by further biochemical tests. The organism is a slow grower (48 to 72 hours), and laboratories need to

be alerted to its potential presence so culture plates may be held an additional 2 to 3 days to detect its presence in mixed cultures.

CLINICAL PICTURE

A number of clinical conditions are associated with nocardia infection (Table 1). The commonest presentation is pneumonia. It may also present as a pulmonary nodule, which often cavitates (Fig. 2). Histologically, the cellular response is an acute suppurative process with polymorphonuclear leukocytes and necrosis. Empyema is a well-recognized complication, as is septic pericarditis.

Brain abscess, the result of hematogenous dissemination, is the commonest complication. It may become clinically apparent as the patient is being treated for infection in another organ (Fig. 3). Skin lesions can be seen as part of systemic dissemination or as primary inoculation disease. The organism can also invade other parenchymal organs such as bone, liver, and kidney.

THERAPY

Routine microbiologic sensitivity testing is difficult because of the slower growth of the organism and its tendency to clump when inoculated in liquid media. It is recommended that the organism be sent to reference laboratories for antimicrobial sensitivity testing since the need for alternative therapies may not be apparent when standard therapy is initiated.

A sulfonamide remains the drug of choice for *Nocardia*. Sulfisoxazole, 2 g every 6 hours orally, is an inexpensive and effective agent. Measurement of sulfonamide levels in blood drawn 2 hours after a dose is useful early in therapy

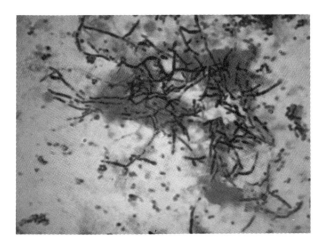

Figure 1 Gram stain of sputum from a renal transplant recipient suffering from nocardial pneumonia, illustrating the thin branching hyphae characteristic of *Nocardia*.

TABLE 1 Conditions Associated With Nocardiosis

Normal host
Pulmonary alveolar proteinosis
Corticosteroid therapy
Organ transplant recipients
Underlying neoplastic disease
Acquired immunodeficiency syndrome

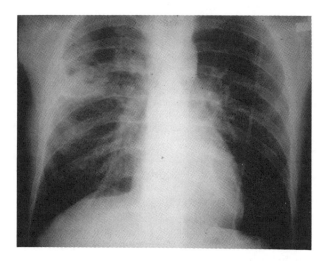

Figure 2 Chest roentgenogram showing a right upper lobe cavitating infiltrate that began as a nodule in a patient with acquired immunodeficiency syndrome.

to be sure that an adequate blood level of between 100 and 150 mg per liter has been achieved. Therapy should be continued for 6 months. In patients with AIDS, it may be necessary to consider longer therapy or, occasionally, long-term smaller-dose maintenance therapy. Although many authors recommend the combination of trimethoprim and sulfamethoxazole, there is no convincing evidence that this combination is more effective than the sulfonamide component alone.

For patients who are allergic to sulfonamides or who do not appear to be responding to therapy, there are some alternatives (Table 2).

Minocycline in a dose of 200 mg twice daily orally may be useful and has been shown to be clinically effective. Vestibular nerve irritation resulting in vertigo may curtail the drug's use in certain individuals. In selected patients unable to tolerate sulfonamides or minocycline and where in vitro susceptibility tests show the organism to be susceptible, the combination of amoxicillin and erythromycin has been shown to be clinically effective. This should not be considered first-line therapy. In seriously ill patients for whom paren-

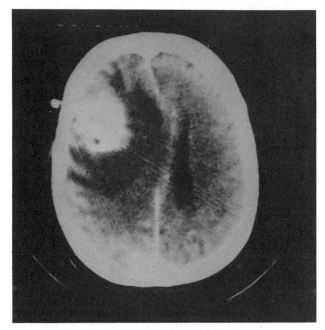

Figure 3 Computed tomogram of the head showing a large frontoparietal lobe abscess becoming clinically apparent while the patient was responding to therapy for nocardial pneumonia.

teral therapy other than intravenous trimethoprim-sulfamethoxazole must be used, amikacin, 7.5 mg per kilogram twice daily, or imipenem-cilastatin, 500 mg every 6 to 8 hours, may be used until the patient can be switched to oral therapy.

Because of the propensity of this organism to form abscesses, failure of response may be due not to drug failure but to purulent collections that require surgical drainage. Monitoring of therapy during the required prolonged treatment period should consist of episodic checks on blood cell count and liver and kidney function to be sure there are no adverse effects from the medications. In the case of amikacin therapy, blood levels 30 minutes after a dose should be in the 15 to 25 μg per milliliter range. Imipenem-cilastatin should be used carefully when renal dysfunction is present,

TABLE 2 Therapy for Nocardial Infection

Drug	Dose	Duration	Adverse Effects
Sulfisoxazole	2 g PO q6h	6 months	Crystalluria, fever, leukopenia, rash
Minocycline	200 mg PO q12h	6 months	Vestibular toxicity, nausea
Amoxicillin* and Erythromycin*	500 mg PO tid 500 mg PO q6h	6 months	Rash, diarrhea, nausea
Amikacin	7.5 mg/kg IV q12h	Until able to take oral medications	Nephrotoxicity, VIII nerve
Imipenem-cilastatin	500 mg IV q6h	Until able to take oral medications	Seizures (dose-related with renal dysfunction)

* If susceptible on in vitro testing.

and the dosage should be modified according to the manufacturer's package insert.

Patients suffering from nocardial infection will generally show a good clinical response to antimicrobial therapy within a few days. Since these patients are often immunocompromised, persistent fever in spite of appropriate therapy should dictate a full reevaluation to include the possibilities of drug fever, undrained septic foci, and most important, the presence of another opportunistic infection.

SUGGESTED READING

Bach MC, Sabath LD, Finland M. Susceptibility of *Nocardia asteroides* to 45 antimicrobial agents in vitro. Antimicrob Agents Chemother 1973; 3:1–8.

Curry WA. Human nocardiosis. A clinical review with selected case reports. Arch Intern Med 1980; 140:818–826.

Dewsnup DH, Wright DN. In vitro susceptibility of *Nocardia asteroides* to 25 antimicrobial agents. Antimicrob Agents Chemother 1984; 25:165–167.

ACTINOMYCOSIS

J. JOHN WEEMS Jr., M.D.

Actinomycosis refers to infection caused by filamentous, anaerobic to microaerophilic gram-positive bacteria belonging to the family Actinomycetaceae. The actinomycetes are classified in the same order as the *Mycobacterium* and *Nocardia* species. *Actinomyces israelii* accounts for most cases of human infection, but actinomycosis has also been reported to be caused by four other species of this genus (*A. naeslunelii, A. viscosus, A. odontolyticus,* and *A. meyerii*) and one species of a closely related genus, *Arachnia proprionica.*

Actinomycosis is characterized by a chronic, suppurative focus of infection that extends directly across tissue planes, causing marked fibrosis and the formation of sinus tracts or fistulae. Classically, the disease is divided into three categories based on the primary anatomic area of involvement: cervicofacial, thoracic, and abdominal and pelvic. Other sites of infection, including the central nervous system and the extremities, are also described but occur much less frequently.

The actinomycetes are a prominent part of the endogenous oral flora. The pathogenesis of actinomycosis, therefore, is thought to be related to invasion of soft tissues through breeches in normal gastrointestinal and respiratory mucosal barriers. Although actinomycosis has been recognized since the late nineteenth century, the diagnosis continues to be elusive. This description, therefore, emphasizes the earlier recognition and diagnosis of actinomycosis.

CLINICAL MANIFESTATIONS

Cervicofacial actinomycosis can present either as a slowly developing, indurated mass below the mandible or as a more rapidly progressive inflammatory process in any of the soft tissue spaces of the head and neck. Draining sinuses are more commonly associated with the chronic form. Fistulae may occasionally drain internally to oropharyngeal mucosal surfaces. Thoracic disease usually is discovered during the evaluation of an abnormality on the chest radiograph, which may take the form of a mediastinal, hilar, or peripheral

mass; a parenchymal infiltrate; or a pleural effusion. Draining chest wall sinuses are rare in the modern era. Abdominal and pelvic actinomycosis is perhaps the most insidious of the three. The ileocecal region is the most common area of infection, although any segment of the gastrointestinal tract may be involved. Direct extension from the bowel wall can involve mesentery, abdominal wall, pelvic organs, the retroperitoneal space, liver, or spleen. Presentations are therefore varied and may include abdominal or pelvic pain, obstruction, mass, perirectal abscess, and fistula-in-ano. Abdominal wall sinus tracts are not uncommon.

DIFFERENTIAL DIAGNOSIS

Perhaps the most important element in the recognition of actinomycosis is remembering to include the condition in the differential diagnosis of more common conditions that may have similar clinical presentations. In cervicofacial infection, the main condition for which actinomycosis may be mistaken is head and neck neoplasm, including primary tumor of bone. Features that suggest actinomycosis in this setting include a history of recent dental manipulation or trauma (including natural eruption of a tooth), poor dental hygiene, or periodontal disease. Careful inspection for external or internal sinus tracts should be performed. As opposed to neoplastic or other inflammatory processes in the head and neck, actinomycosis usually does not produce adenopathy unless nodes are directly involved by the primary lesion. The acute form of cervicofacial actinomycosis may closely resemble other pyogenic processes in this location, but the lack of confinement to anatomic spaces and involvement of bone favor actinomycosis.

Thoracic actinomycosis may simulate almost any chronic inflammatory or neoplastic process in the chest. Again, the presence of poor dental hygiene or periodontal disease is suggestive. Although chronic disease of the airways is associated with pulmonary actinomycosis, this manifestation is unlikely to be helpful in distinguishing actinomycosis from other conditions. The most likely source of a clue to the presence of thoracic actinomycosis is the chest radiograph. A focal pulmonary lesion that extends directly across an interlobar fissure or through the chest wall should definitely alert the clinician to the possibility of actinomycosis. In addition, the involvement of bone (sternum, rib, or vertebrae) adjacent to a pulmonary lesion is highly suggestive of the diagnosis. Because tuberculosis also may involve vertebrae adjacent to a pulmonary lesion, it should be pointed out that, in distinction to tuberculosis, actinomycosis usually spares the intervertebral disk space. Abdominal actinomycosis can present much like Crohn's disease, diverticulitis, chronic appendicitis, gastrointestinal tuberculosis, and carcinoma of the colon (particularly cecal). In this setting, a history of previous surgery, bowel perforation, or penetrating or ingested foreign body should lead one to consider the diagnosis of actinomycosis. Any refractory intra-abdominal abscess should raise the suspicion of actinomycosis. Pelvic actinomycosis should be ruled out when chronic pelvic inflammatory disease is associated with a current or previous history of an intrauterine device.

LABORATORY FEATURES

The diagnosis of actinomycosis also depends on the use of specific microbiologic techniques and the recognition of unique histologic findings in the actinomycotic lesion. Cultures of material, preferably obtained directly from a suppurative focus, must be incubated anaerobically and may require 5 to 10 days for growth. Cultures of lesions may yield a mixture of actinomycetes and other bacterial species, termed associates. The identity of the associates reflects the flora of the site of the primary lesion. In cervicofacial and thoracic disease, they are primarily endogenous oral flora, while in abdominal lesions, they are more likely to be enteric gram-negative aerobes or anaerobes. The pathogenic role of associates remains unclear.

Because prior antibiotic therapy may lead to negative cultures, the diagnosis of actinomycosis can hinge solely on histologic findings. The unusual combination of acute inflammation with marked fibrosis should alert the pathologist to the possibility of actinomycosis. The pathologic hallmark of actinomycosis is the sulfur granule. These can occasionally be seen with the naked eye and appear microscopically as masses of radially arranged club-shaped filaments. With careful searching, granules can be detected in approximately 90 percent of actinomycotic lesions but may be few in number and require multiple sections to be demonstrated.

Although actinomycetes are not uncommonly recovered on culture or observed on smears of various specimens, the diagnosis of actinomycosis should be made only after the pathologic demonstration of an inflammatory reaction in association with the organisms or at least a positive culture obtained from a clinically suggestive lesion.

TREATMENT

The therapeutic approach to actinomycosis has remained essentially unchanged for the last 25 years. The antibiotic of choice is penicillin. For most cases of cervicofacial infection, treatment should begin with intravenous aqueous penicillin G in a dose of 12 million units per day divided in six doses. For thoracic and intra-abdominal disease as well as severe cervicofacial infection, a dose of 18 million units per day in six doses is recommended. The rare case of disseminated or central nervous system infection may require 24 million units per day. If treatment is being provided in an outpatient setting, a 6-hour dosing interval would be acceptable and more convenient. Intravenous therapy should continue for at least 4 weeks and until the primary focus of infection has largely resolved. At that point, the patient should be placed on a regimen of oral phenoxymethyl penicillin (penicillin V) in a dose of 4 g per day to continue for 6 months after all evidence of active infection has resolved. Gastrointestinal symptoms may limit the dose of penicillin V to 2 g per day. A careful and realistic assessment of the likelihood of compliance to oral therapy should be made before discontinuing intravenous penicillin.

As mentioned, the pathogenic role of associates remains unclear. Generally, it is not necessary to direct antimicrobial therapy at these isolates. However, in abdominal disease, coexistent abscesses involving penicillin-resistant gram-negative aerobes or enteric anaerobic organisms may require the addition of a broader-spectrum agent.

The indications for surgery in actinomycosis, in addition to diagnostic tissue biopsy, include providing for adequate drainage of abscesses and occasionally the resection of actively infected tissue that is refractory to an adequate trial of antibiotic therapy. There appears to be little risk of relapse associated with areas of fibrosis that remain present after antibiotic therapy has been completed, and therefore resection of such tissue is usually not necessary. In cervicofacial disease, both the satisfactory results of antibiotic therapy alone and the risk of cosmetic damage indicate a very conservative approach to surgery in this area.

In the penicillin-allergic patient, there are only a few alternative regimens for which adequate experience is available. (1) Intravenous tetracycline, 2 g per day divided in four doses, probably has few advantages over orally administered drug and is associated with venous sclerosis, which may be particularly problematic when used for a long term. Tetracycline is, of course, contraindicated in children less than 8 years old and during pregnancy. (2) Clindamycin, 2,400 mg per day intravenously divided in four doses followed by 1,200 mg per day orally in four doses, may be given. Diarrhea, with or without antibiotic-associated colitis, may limit the usefulness of this approach. Some strains of actinomycetes other than *A. israelii* may be relatively resistant to clindamycin. (3) Erythromycin, 2 g per day divided in four doses, may be used. For all of these alternative regimens, the duration of therapy should be determined according to the guidelines outlined for penicillin. None of the alternative drugs can be recommended for involvement of the central nervous system.

Although there is abundant documentation of the in vitro susceptibility of the actinomycetes to a number of other β-lactam agents, there is inadequate clinical experience to recommend them for the therapy of actinomycosis. There are few data on the activity of quinolones against the actinomycetes, although the poor activity of the currently available agents in this class against anaerobic organisms indicates that they would be unlikely to be useful for therapy in actinomycosis. There is no clinically significant difference in the antibiotic susceptibility of the pathogenic actinomycetes. Acquisition of resistance during therapy has not been documented to occur with the actinomycetes.

SUGGESTED READING

Eastridge CE, Prather JR, Hughes FA Jr., et al. Actinomycosis: a 24-year experience. South Med J 1972; 65:839–843.
Lerner PI. *Actinomyces* and *Arachnia* species. In: Mandell GL, Douglas RG Jr., and Bennett JE, eds. Principles and practice of infectious diseases. New York: John Wiley & Sons, 1985:1427.

Lerner PI. Susceptibility of pathogenic actinomycetes to antimicrobial compounds. Antimicrob Agents Chemother 1974; 5:302–309.
Schiffer MA, Elguezabel A, Sultana M, et al. Actinomycosis infections associated with intrauterine contraceptive devices. Obstet Gynecol 1975; 45:67–72.
Weese WC, Smith IM. A study of 57 cases of actinomycosis over a 36-year period. Arch Intern Med 1975; 135:1562.

TULAREMIA

BURKE A. CUNHA, M.D.

Francisella tularensis is an obligate, intracellular, gram-negative aerobic bacillus that is the etiologic agent of tularemia. Tularemia is an important and underappreciated zoonotic infection, primarily affecting individuals in the northeastern, southeastern, and western United States. Tularemia was initially described as causing a plague-like illness in rodents and today remains an important infection in wild mammals. Tularemia may be transmitted to humans via inhalation, ingestion, insect bite, or direct contact.

The clinical manifestations of tularemia are determined, in part, by the mode of transmission of the organism. Six clinical varieties of tularemia are commonly recognized: glandular, ulceroglandular, oropharyngeal, gastrointestinal, oculoglandular, and typhoidal. Tularemic pneumonia most commonly complicates typhoidal or ulceroglandular tularemia but may be associated with any tularemic presentation. Similarly, tularemic meningitis rarely may be associated with ulceroglandular or typhoidal tularemia. The incubation period is ordinarily 3 to 7 days, and the initial clinical manifestations are in large part determined by the initial site of infection; i.e., ingestion of tularemic organisms may result in oropharyngeal or gastrointestinal tularemia, whereas contact exposure involving an extremity may result in glandular, ulceroglandular, or typhoidal tularemia.

DIAGNOSIS

The diagnosis of tularemia is usually suggested by an appropriate epidemiologic history and clinical presentation; direct isolation of the organism from clinical specimens is inadvisable because of its potential infectivity to laboratory personnel. Gram stains of *Francisella* from clinical specimens are usually nondiagnostic because the organism does not stain well by Gram's method.

Definitive diagnosis is usually by retrospective serology using tube agglutination techniques. A tularemia tube agglutination titer of 1:160 or higher in the appropriate setting with a disease compatible to tularemia is considered diagnostic of tularemia. Tube agglutination titers peak in 4 to 8 weeks, but only 50 percent of patients have rises in antibody levels within the first 2 weeks of illness. It should be remembered that there is some degree of cross-reactivity with patients with brucella or yersinia infections. However, the magnitude of the serologic response of cross-reactions is invariably of lesser magnitude than the antibody response to *Francisella*, thereby making diagnosis relatively straightforward.

Since a definitive diagnosis by serologic methods usually requires some time, tularemia is usually diagnosed on clinical grounds and empiric antimicrobial therapy directed against tularemia is initiated on the basis of clinical findings. Rabbit-associated, glandular or ulceroglandular tularemia usually occurs in fall or winter and predominantly affects the lymph nodes of the upper extremities. Tick-borne tularemia usually affects the inguinal nodes draining the lower extremities and alternatively may affect nodes of the axilla or head and neck. The typhoidal form of tularemia may occur after *Francisella* organisms are acquired from any source and is a particularly difficult infectious disease to diagnose, since there are no localizing signs and a history of animal or tick contact is often lacking.

It is useful to approach patients with tularemia as having either a mild-to-moderate disease or severe, life-threatening infection. This permits a logical therapeutic approach to the disease. Mild-to-moderate tularemia may be treated with streptomycin or gentamicin. Classically, streptomycin has been used, in a dose of 500 mg intramuscularly every 12 hours for 7 to 10 days. Since streptomycin is potentially ototoxic, gentamicin may be substituted for streptomycin and may be given by the intravenous or intramuscular route. Gentamicin may be given intramuscularly or intravenously in a dose of 1.5 to 5 mg per kilogram per day, in three equally divided doses every 8 hours. Care should be taken to avoid high-dose gentamicin in patients with ototoxic potential. Nephrotoxicity is not an issue with 80 mg of gentamicin (intravenous or intramuscular) every 8 hours for 7 days. In theory, other aminoglycosides may be used in place of gentamicin, but there are no data to support their use at present.

A tetracycline regimen or chloramphenicol may be used in conjunction with aminoglycoside therapy in the treatment of tularemia. Doxycycline and minocycline are preferred to chloramphenicol because of their better records of safety and compliance. The relapse rate with tetracycline or chloramphenicol is related to inadequate duration of therapy or to beginning treatment at the onset of disease in conjunction with aminoglycoside therapy. It is important to remember that a tetracycline regimen or chloramphenicol should not be started initially with aminoglycoside therapy but should only be started, preferably, 3 days into the treatment regimen. Patients should not relapse with a tetracycline regimen or chloramphenicol when these antibiotics are started well after aminoglycoside therapy has begun. Any tetracycline

TABLE 1 Therapeutic Approaches to Tularemia

Postexposure prophylaxis

    Not recommended, only prolongs incubation period; does not prevent disease

Mild/moderate tularemia

Streptomycin	0.5 g IM q12h or 30 mg/kg/day in 2 divided doses IM q12h × 7 days
or	
Gentamicin	80 mg or 1.5 mg/kg IV/IM q8h × 7 days
and (optional)	
after 3 days:	
Tetracycline	Loading dose of 30 mg/kg followed by 500 mg IV/PO q6h × 7 days
or	
Doxycycline	Loading dose of 200 mg followed by 100–200 mg IV/PO q12h × 7 days
or	
Chloramphenicol	1 g IV q6h × 7 days

Typhoidal/life-threatening tularemia

Streptomycin	0.5–1 g IM q12h or 40 mg/kg/day in 2 divided doses IM q12h × 72 h followed by a maintenance dose of 0.5 g IM q12h or 20 mg/kg/day in 2 divided doses IM q12h for a total of 14 days
and after 3 days:	
Tetracycline	Loading dose of 30 mg/kg followed by 500 mg IV/PO q6h × 7 days
or	
Doxycycline	Loading dose of 200 mg followed by 100–200 mg IV/PO q12h × 7 days
or	
Chloramphenicol	Loading dose of 30 mg/kg IV/PO followed by 500 mg IV/PO q6h × 7 days

analogue may be used, but doxycycline is preferable on the basis of its pharmacokinetic profile; i.e., its long half-life permits 12-hourly dosing versus 6-hourly dosing with tetracycline. After an initial loading dose of 200 mg of doxycycline, 100 to 200 mg may be given intravenously or by mouth every 12 hours for 7 days. Since there is virtually no mortality associated with mild-to- moderate tularemia, there is no justification at present for including chloramphenicol in the treatment regimen. If chloramphenicol is used, it should be started no sooner than 3 days into the illness and continued for 7 days. Ordinarily, treatment is continued for 7 to 10 days. The preferred approach is to use an aminoglycoside for the initial 7 days combined with a tetracycline regimen beginning 3 days into the illness, providing for 10 total days of therapy. Fortunately, both aminoglycosides and tetracyclines are active against *F. tularensis*. Since obligate intracellular pathogens usually require a longer duration of therapy than extracellular infections, 10 days of therapy is preferred.

Severe typhoidal, life-threatening tularemia should be treated with 500 mg to 1 g of intramuscular streptomycin twice daily for 72 hours, followed by a maintenance dose of 500 mg intramuscularly twice daily for a total of 14 days. The addition of a tetracycline regimen or chloramphenicol 3 days after the aminoglycoside treatment has begun is advised (Table 1). Chloramphenicol is particularly useful in treating tularemic meningitis since the penetration of aminoglycosides into the central nervous system is suboptimal by the parenteral route. For tularemic meningitis in adults, 2 g of chloramphenicol intravenously every 6 hours should be given with parenteral streptomycin in the usual doses. Life-threatening tularemia and tularemic meningitis should be treated for a total of at least 14 days.

SUGGESTED READING

Penn RL, Kinasewitz GT. Factors associated with a poor outcome in Tularemia. Arch Intern Med 147:265–268, 1987.

Sanford JP. Tularemia. JAMA 250:3225–3226, 1983.

Schmid GP, Kornblatt AN, Connors CA, et al. Clinically mild tularemia-associated tick-borne *Francisella tularensis*. J Infect Dis 148:63–67, 1983.

Teutsch SM, Martone WJ, Brink EW, et al. Pneumonic tularemia on Martha's Vineyard. N Engl J Med 301:826–828, 1979.

Young LS, Bicknell DS, Archer BG, et al. Tularemia epidemic: Vermont, 1968. N Engl J Med 280:1253–1260, 1969.

LEPTOSPIROSIS

GEORGE WATT, M.D., DTM&H

Leptospirosis is a worldwide zoonosis with diverse clinical findings ranging from asymptomatic infection to renal failure and death. Severe icteric infection is commonly referred to as Weil's disease. The causative agent, *Leptospira interrogans*, is a single species of spirochete with multiple serotypes that are arranged in antigenically related groups. More than 170 serovars and 18 serogroups have been identified. Making the diagnosis depends on having strong suspicion in the presence of key epidemiologic and clinical findings. Laboratory confirmation is available, but the results of established tests are rarely obtained in time to aid in patient management. Since newer rapid methods of serodiagnosis are not in widespread use, the prompt verification of leptospirosis remains a problem. Recent work has established the value of antibiotic therapy in patients with leptospirosis. Figure 1 outlines the diagnosis and management of suspected *L. interrogans* infection.

EPIDEMIOLOGY

Leptospirosis has greatest impact in the tropics, though its distribution is worldwide. The disease is of considerable veterinary importance in the United States, but only 50 to 150 human cases are reported annually. Most infections go unrecognized and unreported because leptospirosis is often confused with other entities, and, even when suspected, confirmation of the diagnosis can be difficult. In the past, different names were given to various clinical or epidemiologic syndromes in the belief that they were linked to specific serotypes or serogroups. We now know that leptospires belonging to unrelated serogroups can cause similar clinical syndromes, and conversely, infections caused by members of the same group can be very different. Old terms such as peapicker's disease, swineherd's disease, and canicola fever are therefore inaccurate and confusing and should no longer be used.

The transmission of infection from animals to humans usually occurs through contact with contaminated water or moist soil. Less frequently, leptospirosis is acquired by direct contact with the blood, urine, or tissues of infected animals. Organisms enter through abrasions of the skin or through mucosal surfaces. People working in a milieu that associ-

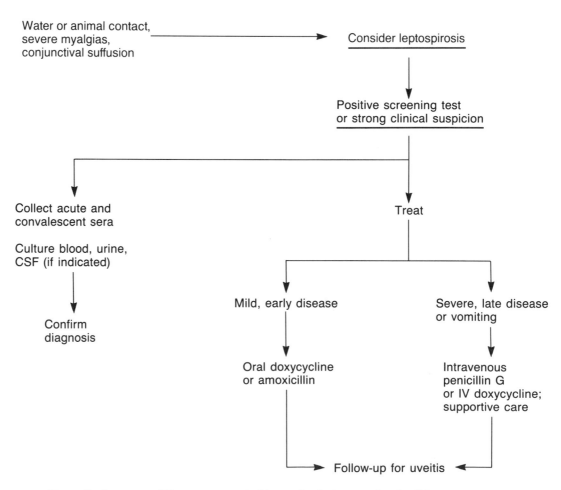

Figure 1 Summary of the management of leptospirosis (see text for details).

ates rats or infected livestock with water are especially susceptible to infection. Certain agricultural laborers are at high risk, as are abattoir workers, fish and poultry processors, butchers, sewer workers, and soldiers undergoing jungle training. However, epidemiologic patterns in the United States and United Kingdom have changed—recreational exposure and animal contact at home have replaced occupational exposure as the chief source of disease.

GENERAL CLINICAL FEATURES

Table 1 summarizes the clinical features of the disease; Table 2 illustrates the salient differences between severe (Weil's disease) and anicteric leptospirosis. Subclinical infection is common, and less than 10 percent of symptomatic infections result in severe, icteric illness. Even relatively virulent serovars such as icterohemorrhagiae lead more often to anicteric than to icteric disease. The incubation period has shown extremes of 2 and 26 days, but the standard interval is 1 to 2 weeks, and the average, 10 days. The duration of the incubation period has no prognostic significance.

Once symptoms develop, they are said to follow a biphasic course: after an initial febrile illness, there is defervescence of fever and symptomatic improvement, followed by a second period of disease. However, a clear demarcation between the first and second stages is atypical of severe leptospirosis, and in mild cases the distinction can be unclear or the second stage may never occur. Thus a history of a biphasic illness supports the diagnosis of leptospirosis, but its absence does not rule it out.

TABLE 1   The Most Common Clinical Manifestations of 208 Patients With Leptospirosis

	Percentage of Cases		
	Anicteric (n = 106)	Icteric (n = 102)	Whole Group (n = 208)
Symptoms			
Fever	100	99	99
Myalgia	97	97	97
Headache	82	95	91
Chills	84	90	85
Sore throat	72	87	79
Nausea	71	81	75
Vomiting	65	75	69
Eye pain	54	38	46
Diarrhea	23	30	27
Decreased urine	20	30	25
Cough	15	32	24
Hemoptysis	5	14	9
Signs			
Conjunctival injection	100	98	99
Muscle tenderness	70	79	75
Hepatomegaly	60	60	80
Pulmonary findings	11	36	24
Lymphadenopathy	35	12	24
Petechiae and ecchymoses	4	29	16

Adapted from Diaz-Rivera RS, et al. Leptospirosis in Puerto Rico. Zoonoses Res 1963; 2:152–227.

TABLE 2   Salient Differences Between Anicteric and Severe Leptospirosis (Weil's Disease)

	Severe (Weil's Disease)	Anicteric
Jaundice	+++	−
Leukocytosis	+++	−
Hemorrhage	+	−
Renal failure	+	−
Death	+	−
Aseptic meningitis	−	+
Disturbances of consciousness*	+	+

(−) = rare or absent; (+) = can occur; (+++) = characteristic.
* Due primarily to uremia in severe disease and to encephalitis in anicteric cases.

DIFFERENTIAL DIAGNOSIS

As illustrated in Table 1, the varied manifestations of *L. interrogans* infection can lead to a bewildering number of possible diagnoses. The key is to suspect leptospirosis when typical features are present: a history of contact with animals or contaminated water, severe myalgias, and conjunctival suffusion. Particular attention will be devoted to the differential diagnosis of suspected Weil's disease in patients returning from the tropics. Not only is leptospirosis a common tropical infection, but American physicians may be unfamiliar with some infections acquired overseas with which it can be confused.

Conjunctival suffusion is the most characteristic and diagnostically helpful physical sign (see Table 1). It usually appears 2 or 3 days after the onset of fever and involves the bulbar conjunctiva, and redness decreases in intensity towards the cornea. It is not a conjunctivitis. Pus and serous secretions are absent, and there is no matting of the eyelashes and eyelids. Suffusion gradually fades over 3 days to 3 weeks. The marked variation in the reported incidence of this finding is due more to the diligence with which suffusion is sought than to true differences in the frequency with which it occurs. Mild suffusion can easily be overlooked.

Muscle pain can be excruciating and occurs most commonly in the thighs, calves, lumbosacral region, and abdomen. Some leptospirosis patients have intense abdominal wall pain associated with tenderness and fever that mimic an acute surgical abdomen. There are numerous reports of inappropriate surgical interventions, particularly appendectomies.

Understandably, atypical or mild cases are often confused with other entities, but because of a low index of suspicion and the disease's protean manifestations, the diagnosis is often missed even in typical cases. *L. interrogans* infection was included in the admitting differential diagnosis in less than 25 percent of more than 1,000 confirmed cases reported by the Centers for Disease Control since 1949, and in another series of 483 proven cases, only 17 percent of patients were initially thought to have leptospirosis. Aseptic meningitis is the most common clinical impression in leptospirosis patients, while fever of unknown origin, influenza, appendicitis, and gastroenteritis are other frequent diagnoses.

The differential diagnosis is more critical in patients with Weil's disease—a dramatic, life-threatening illness. Conjunctival suffusion, severe myalgias, and a history of water or animal contact are very helpful diagnostic clues in jaundiced patients as they are in anicteric individuals. Viral hepatitis is a particularly common misdiagnosis in patients with icteric disease. Leukocytosis, elevated serum bilirubin levels without marked transaminase elevations, and renal dysfunction are typical of leptospirosis but unusual in hepatitis.

Malaria, typhoid fever, scrub typhus, and Hantaan virus infection (hemorrhagic fever with renal syndrome) are important differential diagnoses in patients returning from the tropics. Marked leukocytosis and a negative malaria smear argue against *Plasmodiun falciparum* infection; jaundice, severe renal dysfunction, and leukocytosis against typhoid fever. Differentiating leptospirosis from scrub typhus and Korean hemorrhagic fever in areas where thses diseases coexist is more difficult. Both are associated with animals and both can cause conjunctival suffusion. Splenomegaly and generalized lymphadenopathy are characteristic of scrub typhus but not leptospirosis, while jaundice and leukocytosis are unusual in *Rickettsia tsutsugamushi* infections. Korean hemorrhagic fever is transmitted by infected rodent urine, and mixed infections with *L. interrogans* and Hantaan virus have been reported. Liver disease is not usually a prominent manifestation of Korean hemorrhagic fever.

Pediatric leptospirosis shares many features with adult disease but has several distinct clinical features. Hypertension, acalculous cholecystitis, pancreatitis, abdominal causalgia, and skin lesions that may desquamate or become gangrenous have been reported. Cardiopulmonary arrest sometimes occurs. Some of these features suggest Kawasaki disease (mucocutaneous lymph node syndrome).

POSITIVE DIAGNOSIS

Confirmation of leptospirosis is usually serologic. Classic methods rely on rises in antibody titers between acute and convalescent sera and are only performed at reference centers such as the Centers for Disease Control. Though effective in establishing a diagnosis, results are not available in time to influence patient management. Similarly, isolation procedures are not difficult, but leptospires grow so slowly that results may be delayed for up to 8 weeks. Direct examination of blood or urine by dark-field microscopy is not only insensitive but often erroneous; it should not be performed except by highly skilled specialists.

Recent studies have established the utility of rapid serodiagnostic procedures, but these methods are not yet in general use. In practice, when confronted with a case of suspected leptospirosis, clinicians must inquire whether a rapid test is available. If not, acute and convalescent sera should be obtained and isolation of the organism attempted as described below.

Isolation of leptospires from blood or cerebrospinal fluid (CSF) is possible during the first 10 days of clinical illness. Organisms usually appear in the urine during the second week of illness and may persist for several months, thus permitting diagnosis by urine culture in untreated patients even after clinical illness is over. Leptospires are not difficult to isolate, providing that specialized medium is used; organisms will not grow in the standard media used for isolation of pathogens from blood or urine. If specialized media are not immediately available, leptospires will remain viable for up to 11 days in blood anticoagulated with sodium oxalate. Repeated attempts at isolation will increase the diagnostic yield.

Isolations are usually made from urine, but too much urine inhibits growth. Best results are obtained by diluting 0.1 ml of urine obtained as sterilely as possible with 0.9 ml of buffered saline and then making four additional dilutions. These different concentrations are then inoculated into 5 ml of Fletcher's or EMJH semisolid medium and incubated at 28°C to 30°C in the dark for at least 5 to 6 weeks. For either blood or CSF the same procedures are followed, beginning with from one to four drops of sample liquid. Isolates can be sent to reference centers for identification of the responsible serovar. Animal inoculation offers no greater chance than culture for recovery of leptospires.

The microscopic agglutination test is considered the serodiagnostic method of choice for leptospirosis, but its complexity limits its use to reference laboratories. Dilutions of patient sera are applied to live, pathogenic leptospires. The results are viewed under dark-field microscopy and expressed as the percentage of organisms cleared from the field by agglutination. To ensure detection of antibodies that may be provoked by any of the large number of different serovars, it is necessary to use a battery of antigens, usually 24. This test does not reliably identify the infecting serovar because of frequent cross-reactivity. Agglutinating antibodies generally do not reach detectable levels until the sixth to 12th day of illness and rise to maximal levels by the third or fourth week. It is usually necessary therefore to obtain acute and convalescent sera, and a fourfold or greater rise in antibody titer after the onset of a disease compatible with leptospirosis is considered a confirmed case.

Rapid serodiagnostic tests rely on the detection of genus-specific antibody by a nonpathogenic antigen. These tests have the advantage of being simple—only one antigen is needed—and safe— nonpathogenic organisms are employed. Both the IgM-specific dot-ELISA (enzyme-linked immunosorbent assay) and the genus-specific microagglutination test were shown recently to be effective in diagnosing leptospirosis in an endemic area, and test results were available the same day. Single high titers (e.g. >1:400) or positive dot-ELISAs are diagnostic.

The macroscopic slide agglutination test is the only serologic method that is commercially available. Killed or formalinized organisms are combined into several antigenic pools. This test is less sensitive and specific than the microagglutination test but can serve as a screening test if nothing else is available.

SUPPORTIVE THERAPY

Prompt recognition and appropriate management of renal dysfunction in severe leptospirosis is the key to patient survival. Life-threatening renal failure is a complication of icteric disease, though all forms of leptospirosis may be associated with mild kidney involvement. With adequate supportive care, the case fatality rate is less than 10 percent. Meticulous attention must be paid to fluid and electrolyte balance, and patients aggressively rehydrated when necessary. Ensuring adequate renal perfusion prevents renal failure in the majority of oliguric individuals, in whom there is usually increased urine output in response to fluid challenge. There is rapid progression to acute tubular necrosis and anuria if hypovolemia is not corrected. Rarely, patients present late in the course of disease with symptomatic uremia and anuria. Such individuals rarely respond to conservative measures and have a high risk of death. Peritoneal dialysis is preferred to hemodialysis in patients who require it. Renal failure in leptospirosis is hypercatabolic, so frequent dialysis may be necessary.

Massive hemorrhage is uncommon in leptospirosis, but lesser amounts of bleeding occur frequently and decrease renal perfusion by worsening hypovolemia. A careful search should be made for sources of occult blood loss, blood should be transfused as necessary, and parenteral vitamin K should be administered in the event of a prolonged prothrombin time.

ANTIBIOTIC TREATMENT

A wide range of antibiotics are active against *L. interrogans* both in vitro and in experimental infections in animals. The list includes penicillin, ampicillin, the tetracyclines, some third-generation cephalosporins, and some quinolones. Whether antibiotics are effective in the treatment of human disease has been debated for more than 40 years because of conflicting data from uncontrolled trials. However, in recent double-blind, placebo-controlled studies, doxycycline shortened the course of early leptospirosis, and intravenous penicillin decreased the duration of both fever and renal dysfunction in severe, late disease. Antibiotics should therefore be given to all patients with leptospirosis, regardless of when in their disease course they are seen.

Doxycycline, 100 mg orally twice a day for 1 week, is the only regimen proven effective for mild, early disease. Patients who are vomiting or seriously ill require parenteral therapy. Intravenous penicillin G is administered as 1.5 million units every 6 hours for 7 days (150,000 units per kilogram per day for children). Reports that a Jarisch-Herxheimer reaction occurs within 4 to 6 hours after initiation of penicillin treatment have not been confirmed.

Alternate regimens have not been clinically tested. Pregnant women, children under 9 years of age, or tetracycline-allergic patients with mild disease could be given oral amoxicillin in doses of 500 mg every 8 hours for 1 week (40 mg per kilogram per day in divided doses every 8 hours for children less than 20 kg). Penicillin-allergic adults and children older than 12 years who require parenteral treatment should be given 200 mg per day of intravenous doxycycline for 1 week. Children weighing less than 100 pounds in whom tetracyclines are not contraindicated receive 2 mg per pound per day. Parenteral nephrotoxic tetracyclines are to be avoided in the treatment of Weil's disease.

Defervescence, return to normal of serum creatinine levels, and resolution of hepatic percussion tenderness are useful parameters of successful therapy. Jaundice and abnormalities in urinalysis are not—they may persist for several months. Individuals who survive severe leptospirosis eventually have complete recovery of hepatic and renal function. Patient follow-up should concentrate on the detection of uveitis, a late complication with a generally favorable prognosis. Although it is seen as early as the third week of illness, the average time is after 4 to 8 months.

PREVENTION

Doxycycline (200 mg) taken once a week prevents infection by *L. interrogans*. Widespread use of doxycycline prophylaxis is not indicated but can benefit those at high risk for a short time, such as military personnel or certain agricultural workers.

The efficacy and safety of human leptospiral vaccines have yet to be conclusively demonstrated. Surface decontamination, the wearing of protective clothing, and rodent control are preventive methods applicable to some work environments.

SUGGESTED READING

Berman SJ, Tsai CC, Holmes KK, et al. Sporadic anicteric leptospirosis in South Vietnam. Ann Intern Med 1973; 79:167–173.
Feigin RD, Anderson DC. Human leptospirosis. CRC Crit Rev Clin Lab Sci 1975; 5:413–465.
Johnson RC. The biology of parasitic spirochetes. New York: Academic Press, 1976.
Takafuji ET, Kirkpatrick JW, Miller RN, et al. An efficacy trial of doxycycline chemoprophylaxis against leptospirosis. N Engl J Med 1984; 310:497–500.
Watt G, Padre LP, Tuazon L, et al. Placebo-controlled trial of intravenous penicillin for severe and late leptospirosis. Lancet 1988; 1:433–435.

PLAGUE

ROYCE H. JOHNSON, M.D., F.A.C.P.

Plague is a bacterial infection caused by *Yersinia pestis*, which is currently common only as an enzootic infection with incidental transmission to humans. The commonest clinical form of *Y. pestis* human infection is bubonic plague. This form is characterized by striking regional lymphadenopathy. Less frequent is pneumonic or septicemic plague.

For centuries *plague* has been a term applied to any of a number of illnesses resulting in significant morbidity. In the restricted sense, plague is the illness we now recognize as being caused by *Y. pestis*. Numerous epidemics and pandemics punctuate the history of the last two millennia. No disease has brought such terror as has bubonic plague.

Plague currently has an extensive geographic distribution, including major portions of Southeast Asia, Africa, and South America. Plague is a widely distributed zoonosis in the western United States, the largest number of cases occurring in New Mexico, Arizona, California, Colorado, and Oregon. The animals usually involved are squirrels, chipmunks, deer mice, wood rats, prairie dogs, and marmots. Human infections occur as the result of direct contact with the fleas of these animals or with the infected animal tissues. Human infections may also occur when domestic animals such as dogs or cats bring fleas from infected rodents. Domestic animals may become infected, and the tissues of the animal serve to infect the human host.

PRESENTATION

The clinical presentation of *Y. pestis* infection in more than 90 percent of cases is as bubonic disease. The incubation period for this form of the disease ranges from 2 to 6 days. The majority of patients present with fever and painful lymphadenopathy. Lymphadenopathy may be subtle or dramatic. Erythema and edema may be present in the tissues overlying the bubo. The inguinal and femoral nodes are involved in more than 50 percent of cases. Axillary and cervical nodes are less frequently involved. Other sites are rarely involved.

Septicemic plague is a form of *Y. pestis* infection characterized by bacteremia and toxemia without notable lymphadenitis. The clinical picture is one of bacterial sepsis without apparent cause.

Pneumonic plague is caused by *Y. pestis* transmitted from respiratory secretions of pulmonary infections. It has a shorter incubation period than the bubonic form, usually 1 to 3 days. Sputum is frequently scanty at the onset, with later development of mucoid and finally bloody secretions. The untreated individual usually deteriorates rapidly, and death occurs in 36 to 48 hours.

Other less-frequent manifestations of *Y. pestis* infection include meningitis and endophthalmitis. Skin lesions can be noted in *Y. pestis* infections. The initial site of inoculation from the flea bite may be discerned. Other patients may have a macular-papular rash or even lesions that suggest ecthyma gangrenosa.

DIAGNOSIS

Laboratory abnormalities include leukocytosis, with white blood cell counts as high as 50×10^9 per liter. Mean white blood cell counts of 18×10^9 per liter are more usual. Thrombocytopenia has been noted along with other abnormalities suggestive of disseminated intravascular coagulation. Abnormalities of liver function may also be noted.

The microbiologic examination of patients with suspected *Y. pestis* infection should be done with caution. There should be direct examination of lymph node aspirate. Instillation of nonbacteriostatic saline should be done if no material is readily aspirated from nodes. Sputum and buffy coat are also suitable for direct examination by Gram stain, methylene blue, or the preferred Wayson's stain (carbol fuchsin–methylene blue). These materials may yield a rapid diagnosis if they show the classic bipolar "safety pin" morphology of the organisms. *Y. pestis* grows well in ordinary laboratory media both aerobically and anaerobically.

Suspected cases should have appropriate clinical specimens or isolates referred to local or state health departments for definitive identification.

Plague most often presents as an acute lymphadenitis. Other diagnoses that might be considered are streptococcal or staphylococcal lymphadenitis, cat-scratch disease, tularemia, lymphogranuloma venereum, syphilis, mycobacterioses, actinomycosis, and appendicitis. Additionally, noninfectious diseases such as lymphoma are in the differential diagnosis.

Septicemic plague presents a more confusing and difficult problem. Most early diagnostic thoughts would be aimed at gram-positive and gram-negative bacterial sepsis. The suspicion of plague would depend on a recent history of possible exposure. Differential diagnosis of pneumonic plague would be that of acute fulminant pneumonia.

THERAPY

The therapy of plague in the early bubonic form is relatively simple and effective. Treatment of more advanced cases with pneumonia, meningitis, sepsis, and shock frequently meet with little success. The mortality rate of untreated cases is more than 50 percent. Early treatment can reduce mortality to 5 percent. Various treatment regimens are recommended, but none has been subjected to a controlled trial. Streptomycin has been used since 1948 with great success. Thirty + mg per kilogram per day in divided doses is recommended.

High doses of tetracycline HCl or chloramphenicol, with reduction of doses as improvement occurs, are also appropriate. Oral tetracycline, 15 mg per kilogram to a maximum of 1 g is given as initial therapy. This is followed by 30 mg per kilogram per day in four divided doses for 10 days. If intravenous tetracycline is required, 15 mg per kilogram per day in divided doses should be given until oral therapy can be substituted. Chloramphenicol, 75 mg per kilogram per day in four doses given orally or intravenously for 10 days, may be substituted. The use of streptomycin in addition to tetracycline or chloramphenicol as primary therapy is recommended. Chloramphenicol is preferred over tetracycline in meningitis, pediatric cases, and pregnancy.

Sulfonamides, trimethoprim-sulfamethoxazole, and aminoglycosides are probably effective, but experience is limited. Some in vitro data suggest that later-generation cephalosporins are effective, but no clinical data are available.

PREVENTION

Prevention of plague requires public awareness of the epidemiology. Avoidance of sick or dead animals in the endemic area and the use of insect repellents is recommended. Domestic animals should be kept out of plague-infested areas. If domestic animals are necessarily brought to such areas, use of flea powders or collars is mandatory. Persons or animals in contact with cases of primary or secondary plague pneumonia should be given prophylactic oral tetracycline, 500 mg four times daily for 7 to 10 days. Although there has been no controlled trial of prophylaxis, it may be

one of the reasons that no pneumonic cases have occurred through contact with active cases in more than 50 years. Patients with active pneumonia or draining lesions should be isolated. Proven or suspected cases should be reported promptly to public health authorities.

A vaccine is available and is probably effective; however, it is not recommended for general use to protect against an infection as rare as that with *Y. pestis* unless individuals are specifically at high risk.

SUGGESTED READING

Butler T, Mahmoud AAF, Warren KS. Algorithms in the diagnosis and management of exotic diseases. XXV. Plague. J Inf Dis 1977; 136:317–320.

Connor JD, Williams RA, Thompson MA. Plague in San Diego—interdepartmental conference—University of California Medical Center and Childrens Hospital and Health Center, San Diego; and Department of Public Health, County of San Diego (speciality conference). West J Med 1978; 129:394–406.

Hull HF, Montes JM, Mann JM. Septicemic plague in New Mexico. J Inf Dis 1987; 155:113–118.

Florman AL, Spencer RR, Sheward S. Multiple lung cavities in a 12-year-old girl with bubonic plague, sepsis, and secondary pneumonia. Am J Med 1986; 80:1191–1193.

BABESIOSIS

MARK R. ECKMAN, M.D.

EPIDEMIOLOGY

Babesiosis, a protozoan disease, has been common for centuries in wild and domestic animals (including cattle, horses, dogs, and rodents). In 1957 the organism was found to be responsible for human disease. Since 1969, a constellation consisting of the vector deer tick (*Ixodes dammini*), the white-footed mouse, and the white-tailed deer on Nantucket Island, Massachusetts, has supplied an endemic focus of murine *Babesia microti* leading to disease among summer visitors to this resort area.

The majority of detected infections have been discovered in the Northeast coastal area of the United States. However, babesiosis is not limited to this part of the United States. Clinical cases and serologic surveys have suggested at least the potential for infection with various *Babesia* species in several parts of the world, including the eastern coast of the United States from Massachusetts to Georgia, Minnesota, Wisconsin, and California; Canada; the USSR; Mexico; Taiwan; Nigeria; and Europe, especially Ireland, Scotland, France, and Yugoslavia.

Cases reported from Europe have been due to bovine species of *Babesia* and carry high morbidity and mortality, whereas nearly all American cases have been due to the murine *B. microti* species, which has yet to cause mortality unless it is associated with comorbid conditions. Most human

infections have minimal or no symptoms, but severe cases manifesting as fever, chills, and hemolysis occur especially in those with prior splenectomy, corticosteroid therapy, or defective T cell immunity. Human immunodeficiency virus (HIV) antibody–positive individuals will likely provide an attractive human host, and an increasing frequency of babesial infections is sure to follow the epidemic of HIV.

An additional confounding infection associated with the *Ixodes* ticks is provided by the Lyme disease spirochete (*Borrelia burgdorferi*). Fatal pancarditis has been reported in a 66-year-old man from Nantucket Island. His peripheral blood smear showed *B. microti* in 3 percent of his erythrocytes, and at autopsy after sudden death. *Borrelia* spirochetes were demonstrable in the myocardium. These instances provide a clear warning to consider both diseases in patients suspect of either babesiosis or Lyme disease. Endemic foci overlap along eastern Long Island, Shelter and Fire Islands in New York, and Nantucket, Massachusetts. Serologic evidence for both diseases was found in 66 percent of randomly selected patients with Lyme disease from those areas endemic for both diseases. The midwestern (Minnesota, Wisconsin) focus of Lyme disease has a much lower prevalence of babesial infections, but two people reported there with babesial infection also had positive serologic tests for *B. burgdorferi* infection.

CLINICAL MANIFESTATIONS AND DIAGNOSIS

The clinical manifestations mirror those of malaria and include chills, intermittent fever, anorexia, headache, lassitude, and myalgia (Fig. 1). Physical findings may be normal or may include jaundice, pallor, and hepatomegaly. Laboratory findings include anemia, thrombocytopenia, relatively

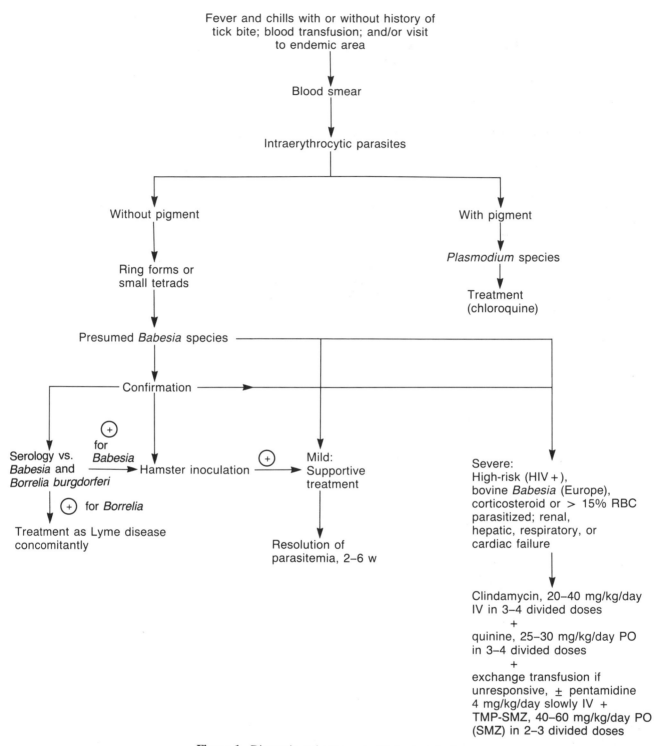

Figure 1 Diagnosis and treatment of babesia infection.

low or normal leukocyte count with a left shift, increased serum bilirubin and creatinine levels, reduced haptoglobin level, hemoglobinuria, signs of disseminated intravascular coagulation, and most importantly, a positive blood smear. Differentiation from the more common *Plasmodium falciparum* is critical. The hemozoin pigment usually found within red cells parasitized by *P. falciparum* is not seen with babesial infection. Cruciate, Maltese cross, or tetrad forms are diagnostic. The *Babesia* do not produce circulating schizonts or gametocytes. The percentage of red blood cells parasitized has prognostic significance and should be determined. Intraperitoneal hamster inoculation of the patient's blood is more sensitive and specific. Contact with the state health department or Centers for Disease Control (CDC, Atlanta) will provide information on research laboratories capable of performing these studies. Serology by indirect immunofluorescence testing is useful. Titers are generally well above the diagnostic threshold of 1:64 and gradually decline over months after the infection is cleared.

TREATMENT

The murine variety (B. microti) most common in the United States is self-limited in the majority of cases. Toxic, expensive therapy may be avoided with good supportive care. Monitoring the parasitemia percentage will provide a clinical guidepost for the introduction of antimicrobial agents or exchange transfusion. Experience in human infection suggests that levels below 1 percent may be associated with significant morbidity. Despite this, the day-to-day variation in percent parasitemia will often provide reassurance that the disease is clearing. Parasitemia levels in the range of 85 percent have been seen in surviving patients with B. microti. The European experience with babesial infections has suggested a more virulent parasite of bovine origin (Babesia divergens) with high mortality in splenectomized patients. The B. microti infections prevalent in the United States have been reported fatal rarely (the above-mentioned case and an elderly patient with aplastic anemia who died of a myocardial infarction). The reporting of serologic surveys of B. microti asymptomatic infections has probably made them seem to occur more commonly in patients with an intact spleen compared with the occurrence of infection due to other Babesia species.

Chemotherapy for human babesiosis has had limited success. Earlier reports on chloroquine, often chosen because of diagnostic confusion with P. falciparum, seem optimistic when viewed from the perspective of later studies on human and animal parasitemia showing no response. Experimental disease with B. microti in hamsters developed levels of parasitemia equal to those of control animals after 3 weeks of chloroquine. Perhaps early clinical responses were secondary to its anti-inflammatory effect or to spontaneous regression of the infection assisted by host response.

Clindamycin combined with quinine was serendipitously discovered in a case of transfusion-transmitted babesial infection originally thought to be falciparum malaria in an 8-week-old infant reported in 1982. Clindamycin alone was effective against B. microti in hamsters but had no effect on parasitemia in Mongolian jirds. Quinine alone has been reported ineffective in humans and animals, but combined with clindamycin in hamsters it has proved more effective than clindamycin alone. In 1983 this combination was reported to have been used in two more B. microti cases, with a decrease in parasitemia documented more rapidly than with other chemotherapy. Subsequent failure to infect hamsters with blood from these patients is strong evidence for eradication of the organism, rather than suppression below the level detectable by blood smear.

Further experience in humans was reported in 1985, with a slower clinical course in a 54-year-old asplenic Wisconsin resident infected with B. microti. He was unable to tolerate more than 2 days of quinine and received 12 days of clindamycin, 300 mg intravenously every 6 hours. Parasitemia declined from 2.5 percent to 1.6 percent by day 6, and he became afebrile in 9 days of treatment. Subsequent blood smears were negative, although he required later treatment with tetracycline for Lyme disease. The first failure of the clindamycin-quinine regimen was reported in 1986 in a New Hampshire man with transfusion-associated B. microti who was also receiving corticosteroids, which were started on day 5 for treatment of red blood cell aplasia. His quinine was stopped on day 10 while Babesia were still present, because of the development of thromboyctopenia. Two weeks after concluding 12 days of clindamycin, a one percent parasitemia was noted, and he died of cardiac disease 2 weeks later. The optimism of 1983 was quelled somewhat with another 1987 report of recurrent symptomatic parasitemia 8 months after the apparently successful treatment with the combination—clindamycin, 1.2 g intravenously every 12 hours, and quinine, 650 mg orally every 8 hours—of a patient with antibody to HIV. Control of symptoms with prolonged continuous therapy, as seen in HIV antibody–positive patients with other infections such as toxoplasmosis, cryptococcosis, salmonellosis, and cytomegalovirus, seemed to be possible.

Two aromatic diamidines have been somewhat successful, but their use is limited by their toxicity, accessibility to investigational drugs, and a lack of favorable reports of use in humans. Diminazene aceturate (Berenil, Hoechst-Roussel) appears effective in reducing parasitemia in hamsters infected with B. microti, but relapses were noted. It has been used successfully against other species of Babesia, but use in humans has lagged consequent to one report of Guillain-Barré syndrome after its use. Ironically, this may have been a consequence of co-infection with B. burgdorferi rather than a drug reaction. Pentamidine (Pentam-Lymphomed) does not appear to be effective alone. Success was reported with pentamidine, 240 mg intravenously daily, combined with cotrimoxazole (trimethoprim-sulfamethoxazole), 3 g per day. Lack of fever and clear blood smears after 72 hours of treatment were noted in an asplenic patient with the more virulent B. divergens infection. American experience with pentamidine has been marred by poor tolerance—renal toxicity in 25 percent of the recipients—and prolonged morbidity with intramuscular injection–associated abscesses and pain.

Exchange transfusions in B. microti infection have been reported three times with some measure of success. Each effort has produced a remarkably prompt improvement in symptoms. The risks of exchange transfusion, especially in patients with cardiovascular disease, and the risk of infectious agents in the transfused blood must be carefully balanced versus the potential benefits.

Currently, supportive therapy without antimicrobial agents should probably be utilized for many patients with B. microti infection. In patients with special risk factors, including splenectomy, HIV infection, or corticosteroid therapy, early intervention with clindamycin combined with quinine seems reasonable. The use of exchange transfusions should probably be reserved for patients with parasitemia of at least 15 percent.

The approach to the European variety of babesial infections is less clear and should be more aggressive. A trial of clindamycin-quinine therapy is warranted, but if unsuccessful, pentamidine with trimethoprim-sulfamethoxazole, with or without exchange transfusion, should probably be attempted.

PREVENTION

Individuals at known special risk, including splenectomized or HIV antibody-positive patients and patients receiving corticosteroids, should probably avoid areas infected by *I. dammini* ticks during the May to September season. Long-sleeved garments and diethyltoluamide tick repellant may provide some measure of protection. Removal of any embedded ticks as promptly as they are found with a fine forceps placed close to the point of attachment may also be protective, as studies have shown transmission can occur within 24 hours of engorgement.

Prevalence studies in high-risk people have shown antibody to *B. microti* in as many as 6.9 percent, so individuals from known endemic areas should be screened for infection before they are accepted as blood donors.

SUGGESTED READING

Centers for Disease Control. Epidemiologic notes and reports: clindamycin and quinine treatment for *Babesia microti* infections. MMWR 1983; 32:5, 65–72.
Miller LH, Neva FA, Gill F. Failure of chloroquine in human babesiosis (*Babesia microti*): case report and chemotherapeutic trials in hamsters. Ann Intern Med 1978; 88:200–202.
Rosner F, Zarrabi MH, Benach JL, Habicht GS. Babesiosis in splenectomized adults: review of 22 reported cases. Am J Med 1984; 76:696–701.
Rowin KS, Tanowitz HB, Wittner M. Therapy of experimental babesiosis. Ann Intern Med 1982; 97:556–558.
Teusch SM, Juranek DD. Babesiosis [letter]. Ann Intern Med 1981; 95:241.

HUMAN BRUCELLOSIS

M. J. WINSHIP, M.D.

Brucellosis (undulant fever) is a disease of the genitourinary tract of domestic and wild animals. It is a zoonotic illness in which humans are incidentally infected. Human brucellosis is not common in developed countries, but remains a problem worldwide where brucellosis in domestic animals has not been controlled. Human infections caused by brucellosis are related to occupation, avocation, food habits, and standards of hygiene. The infection occurs from direct contact with infected animals and/or their products, and an increased risk is seen in farmers, veterinarians, abattoir workers, laboratory personnel, and hunters. No human-to-human transmission of the disease occurs except with the exchange of blood products, such as transfusions. A history of animal contacts or of drinking or eating of unpasteurized milk or milk products should be sought in suspected cases of brucellosis. In many patients, the symptoms are mild, and the diagnosis may not be considered even in severe infections.

PATHOGENESIS

Four of the six known *Brucella* species cause human disease (*B. abortus*, *B. melitensis*, *B. suis*, and *B. canis*). Additionally, strain 19 vaccine for cattle causes human disease when accidentally injected. Brucellae are intracellular organisms that have the ability to survive and divide within phagocytic cells. This intracellular survival in phagocytic cells aids in its spread throughout the body and also protects the bacteria against antimicrobial agents that do not penetrate

into phagocytic cells. Activated macrophages appear to be the principal defense against *Brucella* and other intracellular pathogens.

CLINICAL MANIFESTATIONS

Brucellosis is a spectrum of diseases, ranging from asymptomatic brucellosis to relapsing brucellosis, to strain 19 disease, and lastly to the somewhat controversial chronic brucellosis. The incubation period is usually 4 weeks for the acute illness, with a range of 1 week to 4 months. The symptoms are influenza-like, with shaking chills, fever, tiredness, headache, night sweats, fatigue, and anorexia, which may be acute in onset but at times can also be insidious. Acute influenza-like symptoms are seen in approximately one-half of the cases, and the fever in these cases usually occurs in the afternoon and subsides in the morning. Additionally, pain is noted across the back, arms, and legs, and the feeling of extreme tiredness persists. These symptoms persist for several weeks, and they are usually of longer duration than in true influenza. Gastrointestinal symptoms may be present in one-third of cases. Physical signs are scarce, and occasionally there is enlargement of the cervical and intraaxillary lymph nodes in the acute phase. Occasionally, enlargement of the spleen and liver is seen.

Antimicrobial agents ameliorate the symptoms, which recur if the drugs are not given for a long enough time or if an inappropriate agent has been chosen. The duration of antimicrobial therapy should be 3 to 4 weeks. If brucellosis is unrecognized and antimicrobial agents are not given, the fever may recur, with waves of duration from 2 to 3 weeks, accompanied by constitutional symptoms. Recovery occurs in a number of patients without antimicrobial agents in 2 to 3 months, but relapses are common.

"Chronic" brucellosis persists or occurs for more than 1 year, by definition. "Recurring flu" is a common label in patients with this form of the disease. The symptoms are nonspecific, with fatigue and headache. However, a peculiar type of muscle ache across the top of the shoulders with radiation down the arms and also in the low back region is present in a large number of these cases. It mimics polymyalgia rheumatica, but the sedimentation rate is normal. Some patients with chronic brucellosis do have recurring fever. Depression is often a common diagnosis in these cases as well as in those cases without fever, and these are often labeled as psychosomatic. A few signs and symptoms occur quite commonly: night sweats and a unique tiredness, occurring in the afternoon.

Systemic complications include localized brucellosis such as spondylitis, osteomyelitis, testicular and epididymal involvement, and central nervous system involvement with headache, convulsions, and meningitis. Other areas of the body rarely infected are the cardiovascular and pulmonary systems. Veterinarians may experience a localized allergic reaction when they come into contact with *Brucella* while vaccinating or attending a *Brucella*-infected animal.

In infected animals, brucellae cause abortions, but human abortions are not common because the human placenta lacks a growth factor (erythritol) for *Brucella*. In up to 25 percent of men with brucellosis, epididymitis and orchitis may occur. Microscopically, *Brucella* cause nonspecific, noncaseating granulomas in the liver, lymph nodes, and other tissues rich in reticuloendothelium.

DIAGNOSIS

Any patient who has had a fever for more than 1 week, generalized myalgia, and arthralgia with a history of exposure should be considered for diagnosis of brucellosis (Fig. 1). Blood cultures are the definitive test, but it takes 3 to 4 weeks for the organism to grow. In acute illness, up to 70 percent of the blood cultures will be positive, although the range

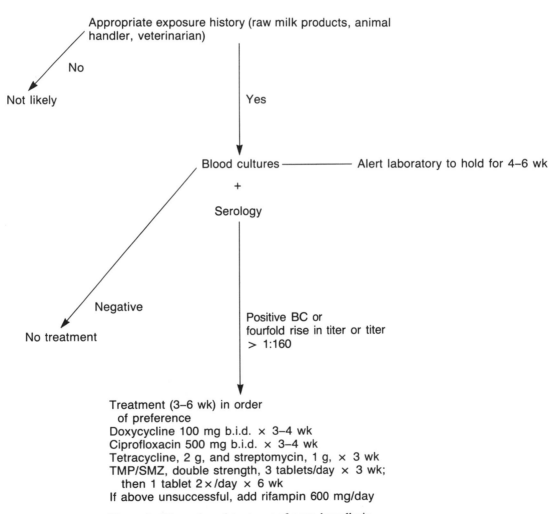

Figure 1 Diagnosis and treatment of acute brucellosis.

is usually 20 to 30 percent. In areas where brucellosis is common, laboratory workers have been exposed to the organism and are relatively immune. In developed countries where brucellosis is uncommon, it is an easily acquired laboratory infection. The laboratory personnel should be alerted to the possibility of brucellosis so the blood cultures can be held for a longer time. Precautions must be taken to prevent the acquisition of brucellosis in the laboratory. Other sources for culture include bone marrow and other tissues rich in reticuloendothelium.

In the absence of culture, serologic methods are used seeking the rise of specific antibodies. The antibody tests should be run in a reference laboratory that uses standardized procedures. The febrile agglutination panel commonly used in hospitals will miss 50 percent of cases, probably because of the prozone phenomenon. A variety of tests have been used including the tube agglutination (IgM and IgG), 2-mercaptoethanol (IgG only), and complement fixation. A titer of 1:160 or higher or a fourfold rise in antibodies indicates acute brucellosis.

The diagnosis of chronic brucellosis does not rest on the laboratory alone. It requires a clinical pattern of illness, and the laboratory only supports the diagnosis much as in the rheumatologic disorders. Commonly, marked fatigue, malaise, peculiar shoulder girdle aches, and depression, often with little response to antidepressants, occur in chronic brucellosis. The erythrocyte sedimentation rate is normal, separating it from polymyalgia rheumatica. The antibody titer is usually 1:160 or greater and of the IgG class.

TREATMENT

A number of therapeutic trials have been reported in the literature, but there are no controlled double-blinded studies. Relapse rates have been as high as 70 percent with sulfonamides alone, and as low as 1 to 10 percent, with a combination of streptomycin and tetracycline. Tetracycline inhibits the majority of the *Brucella* strains, but the drug is not bactericidal. High-dose tetracycline, 40+ g total dose, has an acceptable relapse rate of 6 to 10 percent. Doxycycline is probably preferable in that it can be given fewer times a day, and there is likely to be greater compliance. I recommend doxycycline, 200 mg once a day for 3 to 6 weeks. The greatest mistake in the treatment of brucellosis is stopping therapy too early. It may be helpful to add intramuscular streptomycin, 1 g per day for 1 to 3 weeks. Gentamicin is more active in vitro than streptomycin, but there are no controlled comparative studies. I rarely use aminoglycosides unless the patient is quite ill. The usual doses are 5 mg per kilogram per day of gentamicin and 15 mg per kilogram per day of streptomycin. Trimethoprim-sulfamethoxazole (TMP/SMZ) double strength (160 mg of TMP, and SMZ, 800 mg) three tablets a day for 3 weeks followed by one tablet twice a day for a total of 6 weeks has a low relapse rate of 5 percent.

Rifampin has shown promise in the treatment of brucellosis and has been used in combination with other antimicrobial agents to eradicate the organism in laboratory mice. It should be used with tetracycline or TMP/SMZ but never alone.

The penicillins and first- and second-generation cephalosporins have little activity against the organism. They may mask the fever, only to have it return when the antimicrobial agent is stopped. In vitro, some of the newer β-lactam drugs do show some activity.

The new fluoroquinolones such as norfloxacin and ciprofloxacin have excellent activity against *Brucella*. Ciprofloxacin, given twice a day for 3 to 4 weeks, or norfloxacin, given three times a day, which is higher than standard doses, is curative in the chronic stage as well as being very therapeutic in the acute stage. There have been several anecdotal reports of cure of brucella endocarditis without surgery. Complications such as meningitis and endocarditis remain difficult therapeutic problems. Treatment of these conditions is still in evolution.

Chronic brucellosis is a controversial area at present in some areas of the world. The main controversy revolves around the definition of the illness. It should be defined clinically with the laboratory supporting but not making the diagnosis. It is usually present for longer than 6 months to 1 year. There are a number of individuals with laboratory titers that are in the chronic brucellosis range who are asymptomatic, yet others whose titers are slightly lower who have marked clinical symptoms. Treatment has improved recently with the use of the new fluoroquinolones. Symptoms have improved, and the serologic titers have decreased with the use of these drugs.

PREVENTION OF HUMAN BRUCELLOSIS

Prevention and control will occur only through improvement in food hygiene, environmental protection, personal hygiene, and education. Occupation is clearly a primary risk factor. Brucellosis is prevalent where large herds of cattle, sheep, or goats are maintained and the population consumes available raw milk and milk products. Farm sanitation with disinfectants such as chloramine is recommended as well as disinfection of farm implements. Animal husbandry practices such as animal vaccination and depopulation are essential. In developed countries laboratory workers must be aware of the infectious nature of brucellosis in the laboratory environment.

SUGGESTED READING

Elberg SS, ed. A guide to the diagnosis, treatment, and prevention of human brucellosis. World Health Organization.
Young EJ. Human brucellosis. Rev Infect Dis 1983; 5:821–842.
Young EJ, Corbel MJ. Brucellosis: clinical and laboratory aspects. Boca Raton, Fla: CRC Press, 1988.

PSITTACOSIS

DAVID W. GREGORY, M.D.
WILLIAM SCHAFFNER, M.D.

Firmly rooted in more than a century of use, the term *psittacosis* and its even more colorful pseudonym, *parrot fever,* refer to human infection caused by *Chlamydia psittaci.* This zoonosis is widely distributed among avian species, including parrots, parakeets, cockatiels, canaries, and even ducks and turkeys. Because of this extensive involvement of the bird kingdom, some authorities prefer the more general name, *ornithosis. C. psittaci* has been overshadowed in recent years by the other chlamydial strain pathogenic for humans, *Chlamydia trachomatis,* a major cause of sexually transmitted diseases. A newly recognized strain of chlamydia currently known as TWAR has been associated with respiratory infections, including pneumonia, in both college students and older adults.

Chlamydia were once believed to be viruses, but they are now considered unusual bacteria that have cell walls resembling those of gram-negative bacilli. Chlamydia contain both RNA and DNA, but are incapable of generating energy. They are dependent on ATP produced by the infected host cell and are, therefore, obligate intracellular parasites. Thus, chlamydia cannot be recovered on the routine media available in hospital microbiology laboratories. In reference laboratories, *C. psittaci* can be grown in embryonated yolk sacs and in cell culture systems.

PATHOGENESIS

The incubation period for psittacosis is usually 7 to 15 days. Two pathogenetic routes are illustrated in Figure 1. The longer-incubation, two-stage process is thought to occur more commonly. Although a systemic infection occurs, the lungs are affected most prominently. The resultant pneumonitis can involve both the alveolar and the interstitial spaces, producing a mononuclear cell exudate, edema, and hemorrhagic necrosis. Inflamed airways may become occluded with mucus and debris. In severe cases, these lesions can result in anoxia and cyanosis.

EPIDEMIOLOGY

Between 100 and 200 cases of psittacosis are reported annually in the United States, but the disease probably is considerably more common than the reports would indicate. Most sporadic cases occur among bird fanciers and pet store employees who come in contact with canaries or cockatiels. Outbreaks among workers in poultry processing plants have implicated infected turkey flocks.

Adult birds that appear well can carry and excrete the organism for prolonged periods. Exotic birds that are imported from abroad are required to remain for 30 days in quarantine while they are fed medicated feed. Many imported birds that have passed through quarantine have, nonetheless, subsequently transmitted infection to their new owners. Under the stressful conditions of importation, quarantine, and distribution, asymptomatic birds may become ill with lethargy, poor feeding, ruffled feathers, nasal discharge, and diarrhea. Humans acquire the chlamydia via inhalation of small aerosols of dried, but still infective, avian excreta or by handling sick birds. Although person-to-person transmission has been described, this mode of spread seems to be unusual. Food-borne transmission from eating poultry or wild birds has not been documented.

CLINICAL FEATURES

Common clinical features of psittacosis are listed in Table 1. The disease usually begins suddenly with chills and spiking fever; the pulse may be slow relative to the height of the fever. Headache is often prominent. The cough is hacking and persistent, but sputum production is scant. Although signs of lobar consolidation occur in some patients, the majority have only fine rales on auscultation. Approximately one-third of patients have splenomegaly, which, when present, is a distinctive clue that should suggest the diagnosis. Chest radiographic findings may surprise the physician because they usually are more extensive than anticipated by the results of the physical examination. Mild forms of psittacosis resemble influenza. Less common and more severe clinical features are listed in Table 2.

The diagnosis of psittacosis often is considered only after patients with a "nonspecific pneumonia" have failed to respond to therapy with penicillin or other β-lactam antibiotic. The differential diagnosis includes the various causes

Figure 1 Two pathogenetic mechanisms of psittacosis are recognized. In both, the organism is inhaled and establishes an infection in the epithelial cells of the lower respiratory tract. On occasion rapid direct local invasion of the pulmonary parenchyma occurs, resulting in disease with a short incubation period (1 to 3 days). More commonly, the epithelial infection produces a primary bacteremia that infects the reticuloendothelial cells of the liver and spleen. A secondary bacteremia then occurs that infects the lung. This two-stage process has the effect of producing longer incubation periods (1 week or longer).

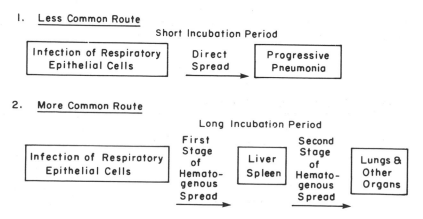

TABLE 1 Common Clinical Features of Psittacosis

Fever, chills, slow pulse
Headache, myalgia, arthralgia
Cough, scant sputum, occasional hemoptysis
Fine lower lobe rales, splenomegaly
Disproportionately abnormal roentgenography

TABLE 3 Treatment of Psittacosis

Treatment	Agent	Dose	Duration	Adverse Effects
Preferred	Tetracycline	0.5 g PO q6h	3 wk	Vaginal candidiasis, sun sensitivity
Alternate	Erythromycin	0.5 g PO q6h	3 wk	Nausea, vomiting, abdominal pain

of a "penicillin-resistant pneumonia," most prominently, legionnaires' disease, pneumonia due to *Mycoplasma pneumoniae,* and pulmonic tularemia.

DIAGNOSIS

The diagnosis of psittacosis is not usually made incidentally or casually. The physician must consider psittacosis as a possible cause of community-acquired pneumonia and should ask all patients about possible exposure to birds. Routine laboratory tests provide little assistance to the clinician. Roentgenograms of the chest are likewise not sufficiently specific to be diagnostic.

Conventional clinical laboratories do not undertake the somewhat hazardous procedure of attempting to isolate *C. psittaci* from human or avian specimens. Reference laboratories, such as those at the Centers for Disease Control, may accept specimens if they are contacted in advance.

In routine clinical practice the diagnosis of psittacosis is established by demonstrating a fourfold rise in complement-fixing serum antibodies measured in specimens taken during the acute illness and during convalescence. A single convalescent-phase titer of 1:32 or greater provides presumptive evidence of psittacosis. Serum antibodies usually appear in the second week of illness but may be delayed by antimicrobial therapy. Therefore, in order to establish the diagnosis definitively, it may be necessary to obtain a late convalescent serum specimen when the patient returns to the physician's office a month or two after being discharged from the hospital.

TREATMENT

Table 3 lists the preferred antimicrobial regimen for the treatment of psittacosis as well as an alternate drug regimen. Tetracycline is the drug that has been most successful, and many patients show improvement within 72 hours after initiation of treatment. However, some patients respond more slowly, and tetracycline cannot be used for a "therapeutic

TABLE 2 Unusual Clinical Features of Psittacosis

Dyspnea, cyanosis, pleurisy, consolidation
Seizures, stupor, focal neurologic signs, encephalopathy
Pancreatitis, jaundice
Renal failure
Endocarditis, pericarditis
Disseminated intravascular coagulation

trial." Termination of treatment at less than the recommended 3 weeks risks relapse. The substantial mortality (20 to 40 percent) observed in patients before antimicrobial treatment was available has been reduced to the current level of approximately 1 percent.

PREVENTION

Natural immunity to *C. psittaci* is short-lived, and a vaccine is not available. Therefore, pet owners, pet store employees, and other persons with ongoing contact with birds are at risk of repeated infection.

The benefit of regulated importation of pet birds is circumvented in part by a brisk trade in exotic birds smuggled into the United States from Latin America. Legally acquired birds that have been fed tetracycline-containing seed for 30 days while in quarantine may still harbor chlamydia and be capable of transmitting infection. In addition, imported birds may be mixed with domestically reared birds during both wholesale and retail operations, offering opportunities for horizontal transmission of *C. psittaci.*

Psittacosis is a notifiable disease, and all cases should be reported promptly to local public health authorities. Investigations may uncover illicit bird smuggling.

TWAR

Recent investigations have identified a new chlamydial organism, TWAR, as an important cause of respiratory infections in several populations. Its unusual name was derived from the laboratory codes used for the first two isolates. At first, TWAR was thought to be a variant of *C. psittaci,* but more recent studies of DNA homology have demonstrated that *C. psittaci* and TWAR are distinct organisms.

TWAR causes several respiratory syndromes of varying severity, of which pneumonia and bronchitis are most common. It can also produce a biphasic illness: an episode of pharyngitis and laryngitis which, after resolving spontaneously, is followed by pneumonia and/or bronchitis 2 or 3 weeks later. The illnesses usually are mild, but a few cases of severe pneumonia have been described.

Seroepidemiologic studies in Seattle and in Denmark indicate that TWAR is a rather common infection; by middle age, 40 to 60 percent of individuals have TWAR antibodies. Humans are thought to be the reservoir and the mode of transmission is likely person to person, but the data on these points are scanty.

Diagnostic reagents still are restricted to research laboratories, but interest in TWAR is high, and we are likely to learn much more about these infections in the near future.

SUGGESTED READING

Bowman P, Wilt JC, Sayed H. Chronicity and recurrence of psittacosis. Can J Publ Health 1973; 641:167–173.

Byrom MP, Walls J, Mair HJ. Fulminant psittacosis. Lancet 1979; 1:353–356.

Grayston JT, Kuo C, Warg S, et al. A new *Chlamydia psittaci* strain, TWAR, isolated in acute respiratory tract infections. N Engl J Med 1986; 315:161–168.

Schaffner W, Drutz DJ, Duncan GW, et al. The clinical spectrum of endemic psittacosis. Arch Intern Med 1967; 119:433–443.

LYME DISEASE

GARY P. WORMSER, M.D.

Lyme disease, also known as Lyme borreliosis, is a newly recognized infectious disease caused by the spirochetal organism, *Borrelia burgdorferi*. It is spread by the bite of *Ixodes* ticks, and rodents are the principal reservoir of infection in nature. Lyme disease is the most common tickborne disease in North America as well as the most common borrelial infection. Although infection is widespread, having been reported from at least 43 states of the United States and from much of Europe, most cases are clustered geographically and temporally, mirroring both the regional and seasonal prevalence and the activity of the vector tick species. For example, over 90 percent of reported cases in the United States occur in just nine states—New York, Connecticut, New Jersey, Pennsylvania, Massachusetts, Wisconsin, Minnesota, Rhode Island, and California—and the overwhelming majority of acute cases occur during the months of June and July, when the nymphal stage of *Ixodes dammini* is most abundant.

NATURAL HISTORY OF LYME DISEASE

Lyme disease, like the spirochetal diseases syphilis and relapsing fever, has protean clinical manifestations typically expressed in a pattern of acute exacerbations and spontaneous remissions, with variable periods of latency. Like syphilis, certain manifestations may first appear many months to years after infection.

The most specific clinical feature of Lyme disease is the characteristic skin rash, erythema migrans, which occurs approximately 7 days after the tick bite (3 days to a month or more). Beginning as an erythematous macule or papule, it may rapidly expand over the course of several days to an annular lesion, with diameters varying from as little as 2 cm to well in excess of 20 cm. The lesion is surprisingly asymptomatic, but a diagnostic hallmark is the presence of central clearing. However, erythema migrans may be completely homogeneous or may have a wide variety of other appearances including a pattern of concentric rings or target-like lesions (Fig. 1). On occasion, the center of the lesion may be vesicular, necrotic, or more intensely erythematous, or it may have a bluish cast. In some patients, erythema migrans is indistinguishable from ordinary bacterial cellulitis, although some of the favored anatomic locations such as the upper arm, axillary area, neck, groin, chest, or abdomen would be unusual for staphylococcal or streptococcal infections.

The pathogenesis of erythema migrans is local cutaneous infection with *B. burgdorferi* at the site of inoculation by the tick. In 15 to 25 percent of patients in the United States and in a lesser number in Europe, one or more secondary erythema migrans lesions will develop at sites remote from the tick bite, thought to be due to hematogenous dissemination of *B. burgdorferi* to other areas of the skin.

Flu-like symptoms including headaches and fever occur concomitantly with erythema migrans in 60 to 80 percent of cases. Other nonspecific symptoms are also common (Table 1). An unknown percentage of patients do not have a rash and only manifest a flu-like illness. Available data indeed suggest that subclinical infection associated with seroconversion is at least as common as recognized erythema migrans.

If the patient is untreated, erythema migrans will spontaneously resolve in about 3 weeks (longer in the European experience) but may recur later. Only approximately 20 percent of untreated patients, however, will remain completely well over a mean follow-up period of 6 years. Instead, 80 percent develop neurologic, cardiac, rheumatologic, or other manifestations of Lyme disease (see Table 1).

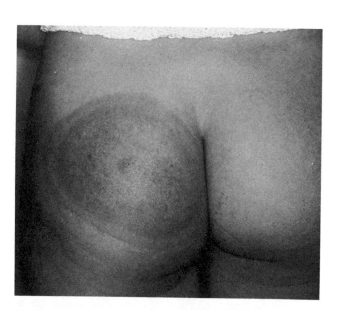

Figure 1 Erythema migrans on left buttock with a target-like appearance.

TABLE 1 Clinical Manifestations of Lyme Disease

Cutaneous	Cardiologic	Neurologic	Rheumatologic	Miscellaneous
Erythema migrans	Heart block	Cranial nerve	Arthralgias	Fever
	Myocarditis	palsy (esp.		
Lymphocytoma	Pericarditis	facial nerve)	Arthritis	Fatigue
	Arrhythmia	Radiculopathy		
Acrodermatitis		Meningitis	Myalgias	Sore throat
chronica		Encephalitis		
atrophicans	Cardiomegaly	Peripheral	Myositis	Conjunctivitis
	Syncope	neuropathy		Hepatitis
Malar rash		Plexopathy	Enthesopathy	Lymphadenopathy
	Dizziness	Chorea		Splenomegaly
Urticaria	Shortness of	Multineuritis	Baker's cyst	Hepatomegaly
	breath	multiplex		Testicular
Septal panniculitis		Transverse myelitis	Tendinitis	swelling
	Chest pain	Cerebellar ataxia		Nausea, vomiting
		Pseudotumor cerebri		Iritis
	Palpitations	Guillain-Barré		Panophthalmitis
		like syndrome		Cough
	Gallops	Optic neuritis		Hoarseness
	Friction rubs	Multiple sclerosis–		
		like illness		
		Seizures		
		Dementia		
		Cranial arteritis		
		Arygyll Robertson		
		pupil		
		Psychosis		
		Anorexia nervosa–		
		like illness		
		Headaches		
		Photophobia		
		Stiff neck		
		Dysesthesias		
		Paresthesias		
		Diplopia		
		Irritability		
		Poor concentration		
		Hearing loss		
		Sleep disturbances		
		Hemiparesis		
		Paraparesis		
		Emotional lability		

Typically, within a few weeks to several months after infection, approximately 15 percent of untreated patients manifest neurologic complications, most commonly facial nerve palsy (which may be bilateral), aseptic meningitis, or radiculopathy. Without therapy, spontaneous resolution will usually take place over the course of several months, but some complications may become chronic and, on occasion, irreversible despite antimicrobial treatment. It has also been recently recognized that certain neurologic manifestations may first appear several years after infection.

Approximately 8 percent of untreated patients (with or without neurologic complaints) are recognized to have cardiac involvement. Cardiac complications occur early after infection, within weeks to several months, and are self-limited. Myocarditis is the principal cardiac manifestation of Lyme disease, potentially resulting in varying degrees of heart block, arrhythmias, syncope, or in rare instances, death. In contrast to rheumatic fever, endocardial involvement and valvular lesions are not a recognized feature of Lyme disease.

The most common sequelae of Lyme disease are rheumatologic, with up to 80 percent of untreated erythema migrans patients developing either frank arthritis (60 percent) or arthralgias without arthritis (20 percent). Arthritis is typically a late manifestation appearing for the first time an average of 6 months after infection, although the range of time intervals when these symptoms may arise is broad (4 days to 2 or more years). Episodic monoarticular or asymmetric oligoarticular arthritis is the most common pattern of joint involvement. The joint most frequently involved is the knee. Temporomandibular joint arthritis is also relatively common, while involvement of the sacroiliac joints is distinctly unusual. Except for cases in children, most Lyme patients with arthritis do not have fever or the classic "hot joint" more typically associated with other bacterial causes of arthritis. A small percent of patients will develop a chronic synovitis lasting continuously for a year or more, possibly resulting in loss of articular cartilage and erosions of the articular cortex. Like most other complications of Lyme disease, spontaneous resolution of joint symptoms can occur without antibiotic treatment.

DIAGNOSIS

The three keys to diagnosis of Lyme disease are clinical suspicion, recognition of the characteristic signs and symptoms, and appropriate utilization of tests for antibody to *B. burgdorferi*. The vast majority of cases of early Lyme disease occur in the summer months among residents of, or travelers to, endemic areas. Recollection of a recent tick bite is a useful historical clue, but the absence of that history should never exclude the diagnosis, since only 20 to 30 percent of patients with confirmed cases recall such bites. The presence of erythema migrans (or its occurrence within the immediate past) is diagnostic of early Lyme disease. Serologic testing is neither necessary nor helpful at this stage since there is up to a 50 percent false negativity rate. Thus, early Lyme disease in the absence of erythema migrans, for example with a flu-like syndrome only, can be extremely difficult to diagnose. In addition, prompt antibiotic therapy may prevent a rise in antibody titer between tests done on acute and convalescent sera.

In endemic areas patients who develop facial nerve palsy, aseptic meningitis, radiculopathy in the absence of intervertebral disk disease, unexplained heart block, or an arthritis of any type should be carefully evaluated for Lyme disease (see Table 1). Fortunately, the majority of patients with these later manifestations of Lyme disease have a positive antibody test for *B. burgdorferi*. Culturing of clinical material for this organism has too low a yield and is too labor intensive and slow to serve as a practical diagnostic tool for Lyme disease. Other laboratory studies are only useful for the purpose of excluding alternative diagnoses.

A few caveats should be remembered in regard to optimal use of Lyme disease serology. First, early in the course of disease, specific tests for IgM antibody to *B. burgdorferi* are more sensitive than IgG tests. Second, because of lack of standardization of testing and interlaboratory variability of test results, a single negative antibody test result should never be interpreted as excluding Lyme disease in clinically suspicious cases. In these instances, repeat serologic testing should be performed, ideally by a second laboratory using a different testing methodology. In some patients with neurologic manifestations, specific antibodies are present in cerebrospinal fluid selectively and are absent in serum.

Immunoblotting or an antibody-capture enzyme immunoassays are more sensitive antibody assays than standard enzyme-linked immunosorbent assays (ELISA) or indirect immunofluorescent assays (IFA) but at present are available only in research facilities. Therefore, in selected patients who are seronegative, a strongly compatible clinical picture may nevertheless justify an empiric trial of antimicrobial therapy.

False-positive tests for antibody to *B. burgdorferi* may occur in other spirochetal diseases, particularly syphilis. Usually the clinical picture is sufficiently distinctive to avoid diagnostic confusion. If not, the diagnosis of syphilis is supported by a positive VDRL test (or other anticardiolipin antibody test), since this test is usually negative in Lyme disease.

TREATMENT

Optimal treatment for Lyme disease is unknown. A comparison of antimicrobial efficacy based on studies done in vitro, in infected laboratory animals, and in humans is shown in Table 2. Results of in vitro testing of antimicrobial agents against *B. burgdorferi* should be viewed cautiously as there is no standardized method of testing and no proven correlation with clinical effectiveness. For example, erythromycin is consistently among the most active drugs in vitro, but studies in laboratory animals and clinical trials in humans have suggested a relatively lower degree of activity. Studies comparing antibiotic efficacy in infected laboratory animals are limited by the failure to demonstrate comparability of dosing regimens on the basis of pharmacokinetic parameters and antibiotic blood levels.

Accumulating data based on recovery of *B. burgdorferi* from culture of clinical specimens suggest that most objective manifestations of Lyme disease are associated with viable organisms, underscoring the importance of defining exactly what constitutes curative antimicrobial therapy. The author's approach to treatment according to disease manifestation is found in Table 3.

Studies in adult patients with erythema migrans suggest that oral dosing regimens, consisting of 10-day treatment courses of 1 g daily doses of either penicillin preparations or tetracycline, are effective in shortening the course of the skin infection and in reducing the frequency of later manifestations of disease. Approximately 15 percent of patients treated in this manner develop a Jarisch-Herxheimer-like response with an intensification of symptoms during the first 24 hours of therapy. Because erythromycin (given as a 1-g daily dose) was significantly less effective in clearing erythema migrans than either penicillin or tetracycline at the same dosage, and because the latter two therapies were themselves associated with a failure rate of about 15 percent based on the need for retreatment or development of later sequelae, the author empirically recommends that standard oral therapy with all three drugs be increased to 2 g per day. Whether other oral antibiotics, such as ampicillin, amoxicillin, amoxicillin–clavulanic acid, cephalosporins, doxycycline, minocycline, or the addition of probenecid to a β-lactam regimen, are equally satisfactory or possibly superior therapies is not known. The optimal duration of therapy has not been established, although in one study of adult patients with erythema migrans, a 20-day course of tetracycline was no better than a 10-day treatment regimen.

The role of oral therapy for other manifestations of Lyme disease is less clear and less well studied. Patients with facial nerve palsy without overt signs of meningitis or other neurologic involvement may be treated orally and in almost all patients the palsy will completely resolve, with an average time to resolution of 24 days. However, this rate of resolution is no faster than has been seen in similar patients with Lyme disease who did not receive any antibiotic treatment. Thus, prevention of later sequelae of Lyme disease is the main reason to give antimicrobial therapy for patients with facial nerve palsy.

Higher-dose intravenous therapy with penicillin or the third-generation cephalosporin ceftriaxone, given for 10 to

TABLE 2 Antimicrobial Activity in Vitro, in Laboratory Animal Models, and in Clinical Lyme Disease from Published Studies

	Activity		
Antimicrobial Agent	In Vitro	Animal Models	Human Disease
Amikacin	0	NA	NA
Ampicillin	++	NA	NA*
Amoxicillin	++	++	++
Amoxicillin–clavulanic acid	++	++	++
Cefotaxime	+++	++	NA*
Ceftriaxone	+++	++	++
Ciprofloxacin	+	NA	NA
Chloramphenicol	+	NA	NA*
Doxycycline	++	NA	NA*
Erythromycin	+++	+	+
Gentamicin	0	NA	NA
Imipenem	++	++	NA
Mezlocillin	++	NA	NA
Minocycline	+++	NA	++
Ofloxacin	+	NA	NA
Oxacillin	++	NA	NA
Penicillin	+	+	++
Rifampin	0	NA	NA
Tetracycline	++	++	++
Trimethoprim-sulfamethoxazole	0	NA	NA

NA = not available; 0 = not active; +, ++, +++ = degrees of activity, from least to most.
* Effective in anecdotal cases.

14 days, has been successfully used in patients with other neurologic complications such as meningitis or encephalitis. Headache, stiff neck, and radicular pain improve rapidly with these therapies but motor deficits resolve much more slowly.

High-dose therapy with either penicillin or ceftriaxone is also effective for the majority of patients with Lyme arthritis, although it is possible that some of these patients would respond just as well to an oral antibiotic regimen. Lyme arthritis typically resolves slowly over the course of several weeks, and prolonged follow-up is necessary to evaluate outcome accurately because of the potential for late relapses. The relative efficacy of high-dose penicillin versus ceftriaxone is not established, but it is clear that some patients will respond to ceftriaxone who have previously failed a course of intravenous penicillin.

Few data are available to guide antibiotic therapy specifically for patients with cardiac involvement. Parenteral therapy, as for neurologic or rheumatologic disease, would seem appropriate. Perhaps the most important measure to be taken on behalf of these patients is the placement of a temporary cardiac pacemaker for patients with advanced heart block.

Benzathine-Penicillin Preparations

Benzathine-penicillin G, which gives prolonged but very low blood levels of penicillin after intramuscular administration, has been successfully used to treat both early and late manifestations of Lyme disease. As penicillin blood levels are actually higher with oral therapy, this preparation cannot be recommended.

PREGNANCY

The precise risk to the developing fetus of maternal Lyme disease during pregnancy is unknown, although it is well established that fetal infection can occur and may have serious outcomes, including malformations and death. Since anecdotal experience has suggested that oral antibiotic therapy does not invariably protect the fetus, this author prefers high-dose intravenous penicillin for pregnant women with active Lyme disease.

ASSESSMENT OF RESPONSE TO THERAPY

Assessing the adequacy of treatment for Lyme disease poses special problems because of the organism's latency and the intermittent pattern of exacerbations and remissions in the natural history of untreated infection. Furthermore, approximately 50 percent of patients with erythema migrans who apparently respond to antibiotic therapy based on prompt resolution of the skin manifestations and the absence of serious late complications over a several year follow-up nevertheless remain unwell, complaining of intermittent arthralgias, myalgias, headaches, or fatigue that may last from a few months to several years. Anecdotal observations of retreatment with high-dose intravenous penicillin did not show improvement in these complaints. Furthermore, there is no established laboratory test to follow, such as the VDRL in syphilis, to judge the adequacy of therapy in Lyme disease.

Two additional concerns arise in determining the response to therapy. First, reinfection with B. burgdorferi, leading to recurrence of clinical disease, is well documented. Reinfection in a recently treated patient could easily be misinterpreted as a treatment failure. Secondly, the tick vector

TABLE 3 Author's Approach to the Therapy of Lyme Disease

Manifestation of Lyme Disease	Recommended Treatment Regimen
Skin	
Erythema migrans	Regimen A
Lymphocytoma	Regimen A
Acrodermatitis chronica atrophicans	Regimen A or B
Neurologic	
Cranial nerve palsy, e.g., facial nerve palsy	Regimen A
Meningitis	Regimen B
Encephalitis	Regimen B
Radiculopathy	Regimen A or B
Cardiac	
Pericarditis/myocarditis	Regimen B
Heart block	Regimen B, insertion of temporary pacemaker to be considered
Rheumatologic	
Arthralgias	Regimen A
Arthritis	Regimen B
Miscellaneous	
Flu-like illness	Regimen A
Asymptomatic, seropositive; never previously treated	Regimen A (or observation)
Tick bite in endemic area, asymptomatic	Observation
Tick bite in a pregnant woman, asymptomatic	Regimen A (do not give tetracycline)
Lyme disease during pregnancy, any manifestation	Regimen B (do not give tetracycline)
Interstitial keratitis	Topical corticosteroids

Regimen A

Adults
  Preferred
    Tetracycline 500 mg PO q.i.d. x 10–14 days
        or
    Phenoxymethyl penicillin 500 mg PO q.i.d. x 10–14 days
  Alternative
    Erythromycin 500 mg PO q.i.d. x 10–14 days

Children
  Preferred

>8 yr	*<8 yr*
Tetracycline 12.5 mg/kg PO	Phenoxymethyl penicillin 12.5 mg/kg PO q6h x 10–14 days (up to 2 g/day)
q6h x 10–14 days (up to 2 g/day)	

        or
    Phenoxymethyl penicillin 12.5 mg/kg PO q6h x 10–14 days (up to 2 g/day)
  Alternative
    Erythromycin 12.5 mg/kg PO q6h x 10–14 days (up to 2 g/day)

Regimen B

Adult
  Preferred
    Penicillin G 3–4 x 10^6 U IV q4h x 10–14 days
        or
    Ceftriaxone 2 g IV/day x 10–14 days
  Alternative
    Tetracycline 500 mg PO q6h x 30 days

Children
  Preferred
    Penicillin G 4 x 10^4 U/kg IV q4h x 10–14 days (up to 24 x 10^{6}U/day)
        or
    Ceftriaxone 37.5 mg/kg–50 mg/kg q12h IV/day x 10–14 days (up to 2 g/day)
  Alternative

>8 yr	*<8 yr*
Tetracycline 12.5 mg/kg PO q6h x 30 days (up to 2 g/day)	Erythromycin 12.5 mg/kg PO q6h x 30 days (up to 2 g/day)

of Lyme disease may simultaneously transmit other infectious agents, such as *Babesia* in the United States or tick-borne encephalitis virus in Europe. These agents cause illnesses with symptoms that may overlap with those of Lyme disease but which would not respond to the standard antibiotic therapies used for Lyme disease.

ADJUNCTIVE THERAPY

Nonsteroidal anti-inflammatory medications are useful adjuncts for controlling muscle or joint pains in Lyme disease. Previously, systemic corticosteroids were widely used to treat various neurologic, rheumatologic, or cardiac manifestations of Lyme disease. Evidence now exists, however, that these drugs may have a deleterious effect on the outcome of Lyme disease for some patients, and thus they should be used cautiously, if at all.

Arthroscopic synovectomy may sometimes be useful for arthritic patients in whom antibiotic treatment has not given relief, especially for those with knee involvement.

PREVENTION

Prevention of Lyme disease is a challenging problem in areas where infected ticks are abundant. Various methods of reducing tick numbers in the environment are under intensive investigation. Useful advice for individuals living in these areas is to wear light-colored protective clothing during outdoor activities, to consider spraying the surface of pants' legs and socks with an insect repellent containing either diethyltoluamide (DEET) or permethrin, and to inspect carefully the entire body surface and scalp at the end of each day for ticks. Household pets should be similarly scrutinized. As is the case with Rocky Mountain spotted fever, transmission of *B. burgdorferi* from tick to host is not immediate and can be prevented if ticks are promptly removed.

SUGGESTED READING

Anonymous. Treatment of Lyme disease. Med Lett 1988; 30:65–66.
Dattwyler RJ, Halperin JJ, Volkman DJ, Luft BJ. Treatment of late Lyme borreliosis—randomized comparison of ceftriaxone and penicillin. Lancet 1988; 1:1191–1194.
Duffy J. Lyme disease. Infect Dis Clin North Am 1987; 1:511–527.
Steere AC, Schoen RT, Taylor E. The clinical evolution of Lyme arthritis. Ann Intern Med 1987; 107:725–731.
Wormser GP. Treatment of Lyme disease—state of the art. N York Med Q 1985; 5:110–115.

HERPES SIMPLEX VIRUS INFECTIONS

MARY ALICE HARBISON, M.D.
SCOTT M. HAMMER, M.D.

Infections with herpes viruses are among the most common of human infections. The herpes simplex viruses (HSV) can cause a wide range of illness, from minor but irritating fever blisters and painful, recurrent genital ulcers to severe encephalitis and disseminated infections in neonates and immunocompromised hosts. Fortunately, treatment of HSV infections has been an area of signal medical progress in the last 10 years, and indeed, HSV has been the primary target of the first truly successful systemic antiviral agents, vidarabine and acyclovir.

MECHANISMS AND PHARMACOKINETICS

Vidarabine is an analogue of adenine and, following intravenous administration, is rapidly deaminated by adenosine deaminase to arabinosyl hypoxanthine. The latter possesses antiviral activity, but it is severalfold less active than the parent compound. Vidarabine is converted to its active form, vidarabine triphosphate, by cellular kinases. This compound then acts as a competitive inhibitor of the viral DNA polymerase. Incorporation into the growing viral DNA chain and DNA chain termination may both occur. The hypoxanthine metabolite, which is the measurable drug in serum, has a half-life of 3.5 hours and can accumulate in renal failure. Thus, dosage adjustments are necessary when there is renal insufficiency.

Acyclovir is an analogue of guanine that possesses an acyclic side chain instead of an intact ribose moiety. Antiviral specificity is conferred by the fact that it is selectively taken up by HSV-infected cells, and the first step in its activation (conversion to acyclovir monophosphate) is catalyzed by the virally specified enzyme, thymidine kinase. Subsequent conversion to the active form of the drug, acyclovir triphosphate, is completed by cellular enzymes. The triphosphate, in turn, inhibits the viral DNA polymerase and may also act as a viral DNA chain terminator. The much greater affinity of this agent for the HSV DNA polymerase than for the cellular α-polymerase confers further targeting specificity. The half-life of acyclovir is 2.5 to 3.9 hours following intravenous or oral administration. Oral bioavailability is low, however, being approximately 20 percent. Levels in cerebrospinal fluid (CSF) are approximately 50 percent of those in serum, and the drug is hemodialyzable. Acyclovir is largely excreted by renal mechanisms, and thus dosage adjustments are indicated when the creatinine clearance falls below 50 ml per minute. For creatinine clearances of 25 to 50 and 10 to 25 ml per minute, the normal intravenous dosing interval should be increased from 8 to 12 and 24 hours, respectively. Under 10 ml per minute, half of a single dose can be given every 24 hours. Redosing after hemodialysis is indicated.

MUCOCUTANEOUS HERPES SIMPLEX INFECTIONS IN NORMAL HOSTS

HSV syndromes may be divided into initial and recurrent episodes. Initial disease may be further subdivided into primary and nonprimary infections. Primary infections are those that occur in individuals who are seronegative for both type 1 and type 2. Nonprimary, initial infections are those that represent the first clinical episode of herpes in a patient who is seropositive at the outset. This is most commonly seen clinically in two settings: the individual with a past history of herpes labialis who acquires genital herpes and the individual who has not recognized mild earlier episodes of the disease. The differentiation is important, as true primary disease is typically more severe, often with systemic signs of fever, malaise, and myalgias, and with more local pain, more lesions, greater adenopathy, and a longer time to healing.

Oral herpes infections are usually caused by HSV type 1 and genital infections by type 2 virus strains, although 10 to 15 percent of cases at either anatomic site will be caused by the opposite virus type. Typing of virus isolates can be done simply by monoclonal antibody staining or by more involved techniques such as restriction endonuclease mapping. The latter can be used to compare individual virus strains for epidemiologic purposes. Typing of the isolate is of clinical relevance with regard to providing prognostic advice to patients concerning the pattern of recurrences. HSV type 1 recurs with greater frequency when it infects oropharyngeal sites, and HSV type 2 tends to recur more frequently when it infects the genital region. The reason for this difference in biologic behavior is unexplained.

The diagnosis of mucocutaneous HSV infection can usually be made on clinical grounds from the history and the presence of typical vesicular or ulcerated lesions on an erythematous base. Diagnosis should always be confirmed by culture of the lesions and/or by cytologic smear, using the Tzanck technique or direct immunofluorescent staining with monoclonal antibodies. The cytologic methods have the advantage of making an immediate diagnosis, whereas cell cultures may take from 24 to 72 hours to show typical cytopathic effects. When specimens are properly prepared and testing is done by experienced personnel, the immunofluorescent staining method approaches cell culture in diagnostic sensitivity and specificity for genital lesions. Because antibodies to HSV are prevalent, serologic testing is not generally useful diagnostically except to document primary episodes. However, new antibody tests are under development that may reliably distinguish between type 1 and type 2 infections.

Treatment of genital herpes infections continues to be the subject of active research, and recommendations are consequently still evolving. Initial studies focused on primary episodes and demonstrated that intravenous acyclovir was highly effective in shortening the period of viral shedding, the formation of new lesions, and the healing time, although it had no effect on the establishment of latency or the rate of subsequent recurrences. Oral acyclovir has also been shown to be similarly effective, and is now in general the drug of choice for both primary and recurrent attacks.

Because of their tendency to be more severe and prolonged, virtually all primary episodes of genital herpes should be treated with acyclovir, and the duration of therapy should be longer than for recurrent episodes. The usual dose of oral acyclovir for primary attacks is 200 mg every 4 hours (five times a day) for 10 days. Topical acyclovir ointment (5 percent) has some proven efficacy in the treatment of primary genital infection but has been largely supplanted by the oral preparation. Other more convenient oral dosing regimens are currently being tested. Severe cases with neurologic involvement (i.e., urinary retention or aseptic meningitis) may require hospitalization, and intravenous therapy (5 mg per kilogram every 8 hours) should then be considered until improvement occurs.

Recurrent episodes of genital herpes can be effectively treated with a 5-day course of oral acyclovir. Recently 800 mg twice a day has been found to be as effective as the more standard course of 200 mg five times daily for treatment of recurrent attacks. Many studies have shown that treatment of recurrences is most effective when initiated by the patient at the first prodromal symptoms; education of patients about their disease and its management is therefore a crucial part of therapy. Certainly not every recurrent episode requires drug treatment; in deciding upon a treatment protocol the clinician must take into account the frequency and severity of recurrences, the degree of inconvenience and discomfort to the patient, and psychosocial factors.

For patients with fewer than six recurrences per year, each attack is probably best managed individually. Patients with a higher number of recurrences should be considered potential candidates for chronic suppressive acyclovir treatment. Several studies have now shown that continuous administration of oral acyclovir can markedly decrease the rate of genital herpes recurrences for up to 2 years, with about 50 percent of patients experiencing no recurrences at all in any given year and about 30 percent remaining disease free for 2 years. Breakthrough episodes can occur but tend to be mild attacks. A total daily dose of 600 to 800 mg as a single or divided dose appears most effective for long-term suppression; lower daily doses and intermittent dosing (i.e., "weekend" therapy) have not proved satisfactory.

Minimal drug toxicity has been noted in these studies, and routine laboratory monitoring of patients does not appear necessary. However, patients should be advised about the cost of therapy ($2 to $3 per day), and female patients must be cautioned to use strict birth control measures for the duration of suppressive treatment. No congenital defects due to inadvertent acyclovir administration in pregnancy have been reported, but the long-term genetic effects of this nucleoside analogue remain to be determined. In two small studies, no effects were seen on white cell chromosomes or on sperm count and morphology after several months of continuous acyclovir. The current U.S. Food and Drug Administration recommendations for suppression with acyclovir extend only for 6 months, but in light of the accumulating data on the safety and continued efficacy of longer treatment, these recommendations are likely to change. Most authors still recommend interrupting suppressive therapy after 6 to 9 months to determine whether the natural frequency of recurrences has diminished.

In contrast to genital herpes, attempts to develop effective treatment for oral HSV infections in normal hosts have been mostly disappointing. One trial of oral acyclovir suspension in children with primary herpes stomatitis has been reported, in which an antiviral effect was documented but little clinical benefit obtained. Acyclovir is therefore not generally recommended for treatment of primary gingivostomatitis in otherwise healthy children, although the occasional severe case which might require hospitalization and intravenous hydration may warrant a trial of intravenous acyclovir therapy.

While other controlled trials have shown that continuous use of topical or oral acyclovir was helpful in preventing and minimizing the severity of recurrences of herpes labialis in adults who suffer frequent attacks, neither form of the drug was helpful in decreasing pain or duration of lesions when used for treatment of individual episodes. Again, therefore, for most patients with infrequent, uncomplicated attacks of herpes labialis, acyclovir treatment is not indicated. However, recent studies have shown that short-term oral acyclovir therapy with 400 mg twice daily can prevent recurrences of herpes labialis in patients with predictable recurrences, such as skiers with sun-related attacks, or patients undergoing trigeminal ganglion surgery or dermabrasion.

Acyclovir is also proving useful for treatment of other cutaneous HSV infections, and the list of indications will undoubtedly continue to expand as more experience is gained. For example, the hand is a common site of inoculation with both HSV 1 and 2, and oral acyclovir when taken in the prodrome has been shown to shorten the duration of primary episodes and to prevent recurrences. Individuals with atopic eczema and other skin conditions can develop a widespread cutaneous HSV infection known as eczema herpeticum. In children the condition can be severe, resulting in large areas of erosion, dehydration, secondary infection, and even death. Intravenous acyclovir, 5 mg per kilogram every 8 hours for 5 days, has been anecdotally successful and should be used in children and severely ill adults. Milder cases in adults have also responded to some degree to oral acyclovir 200 mg five times a day; 400 mg five times a day may be a more prudent dose to employ. Erythema multiforme is another rare but potentially serious complication of HSV infection. Oral acyclovir can abort recurrent attacks when started with the first prodromal symptoms, and some individuals with extremely frequent attacks have benefitted from chronic suppressive therapy for up to 6 months.

OCULAR HSV INFECTIONS

Superficial and deep structures of the eye can be involved in both primary and recurrent HSV infections. The cornea is by far the most commonly involved site, and recurrent HSV keratitis is the most common cause of infectious blindness in the United States. Treatment of ocular HSV infections should always be undertaken with qualified ophthalmologic consultation. However, it is important for all practitioners to consider HSV infection in patients with eye pain or corneal lesions, since delay in treatment or incorrect management (e.g., steroid treatment in superficial

HSV keratitis) can have devastating consequences. Currently two topical antiviral agents are licensed for use in ocular HSV infections: vidarabine and trifluorothymidine. Trifluorothymidine is the more potent and more soluble agent with better penetration into the cornea and is therefore usually the drug of choice. Topical acyclovir has been used extensively in Europe with some success but is not yet licensed for ocular use in the United States. Anecdotal reports also indicate that oral and intravenous acyclovir may be useful in treating deep ocular infections.

HERPES SIMPLEX ENCEPHALITIS

Herpes simplex encephalitis (HSE) is certainly one of the most devastating forms of HSV infection and virtually the only life-threatening form to occur regularly in normal hosts beyond the neonatal period. HSV is the most frequent cause of fatal, sporadic encephalitis in the United States today, with an estimated annual incidence of 1,000 to 2,000 cases, or one case per 250,000 to 500,000 population. HSE must be differentiated from the aseptic meningitis seen in association with genital herpes, which is a benign and self-limited condition.

Patients with HSE generally have abrupt onset of fever, headache, altered behavior and mentation, and focal neurologic deficits, reflecting the common involvement of the temporal lobes. CSF profiles usually show elevated protein levels and a lymphocytic pleocytosis, but the formulas are not diagnostic. The availability of effective treatment for HSE, first with vidarabine and now with acyclovir, has dramatically escalated the debate over whether to perform a brain biopsy for diagnosis. Proponents of early biopsy argue that it is crucial to establish a firm diagnosis early, in order to be confident of the need for antiviral therapy and to rule out other treatable causes of encephalitis, which may be present in up to 20 to 30 percent of cases. Opponents argue that there is little harm in overtreating with acyclovir; that brain biopsy cannot possibly be done in every patient in whom HSE is considered; that the procedure itself may add morbidity; and that effective treatment may be delayed, especially in smaller institutions, while waiting for biopsy to be done. Rapid laboratory methods of diagnosis, such as measuring herpes simplex antigen in the CSF, are under development but not generally available. An elevated ratio of CSF to serum antibody or a fourfold rise in CSF HSV antibody titers correlates well with proven HSE, but these cannot be helpful diagnostically until at least the second week of illness. Recently, magnetic resonance imaging (MRI) has proven capable of identifying extremely early focal anatomic lesions in HSE; computed tomograms (CT) generally do not show defects before the fourth to fifth day of illness.

In the double-blind, placebo-controlled trial of vidarabine published in 1977 by the National Institute of Allergy and Infectious Disease (NIAID) Collaborative Antiviral Study Group, mortality in untreated cases of HSE was 70 percent at 6 months, with only 11 percent of survivors returning to a normal neurologic status. Vidarabine was proven to reduce mortality to 40 percent at 6 months and to increase the fraction of normal survivors to 20 percent. However, subsequent trials of acyclovir versus vidarabine have clearly established acyclovir as the drug of choice for HSE, reducing the 6-month mortality rate to 20 percent and further benefitting the survivors, with 30 to 60 percent regaining normal function. Age, Glasgow coma score, and duration of illness were important determinants of outcome; patients who were comatose when treatment started had no better prognosis than placebo-treated controls. Hence prompt diagnosis and treatment remain essential to ensure optimal results.

A prudent course to take with patients presenting with a febrile, focal encephalitis compatible with HSE is as follows: (1) MRI or CT should be done immediately, followed by a lumbar puncture if threatening cerebral edema is not seen. If focality is not demonstrated initially, an electroencephalogram, technetium brain scan, and early follow-up MRI or CT should be considered to see if focality develops. (2) In patients with a strongly suggestive presentation, acyclovir should be immediately administered intravenously at a dose of 10 mg per kilogram every 8 hours (if renal function is normal). (3) If a focal abnormality is demonstrated by one of the above techniques, a brain biopsy to confirm the diagnosis and exclude other treatable etiologies should be strongly considered in centers with appropriate neurosurgical and virologic support. Transfer to regional centers with such expertise is often appropriate. However, it should be reiterated that treatment should not be delayed pending either a diagnostic work-up or transfer of the patient, if an acceptable neurologic outcome is to be expected. Administration of acyclovir for 24 to 48 hours will not affect the diagnostic yield of biopsy if viral antigen testing in addition to viral culture is included. If HSE is confirmed, acyclovir treatment should continue for at least 10 to 14 days and possibly longer, depending on the clinical course. Rare cases of relapsing infection after acyclovir therapy have been reported, which may respond to a second course of treatment. A demyelinating postinfectious encephalomyelitis has also been recognized, which has a characteristic appearance on brain biopsy; partial responses to steroid treatment have been reported.

HSV INFECTIONS IN IMMUNOCOMPROMISED PATIENTS

In contrast to the situation in normal hosts, endogenous reactivation of HSV causes severe morbidity and mortality in patients with many forms of immune suppression. Sixty to eighty percent of seropositive transplant recipients and patients undergoing chemotherapy for hematologic malignancies will reactivate HSV, usually within the first 6 weeks of treatment. Oral HSV mucositis can be difficult to distinguish from (or may coexist with) candidiasis or drug-induced mucositis in such settings, so the clinician must be alert to this possibility. Individuals with the acquired immunodeficiency syndrome (AIDS) also suffer a high rate of HSV recurrences, which can be chronic, indolent, and difficult to manage. All such episodes can be prolonged and painful, with lesions taking twice as long to heal as in normal hosts, and relapses are frequent when therapy is stopped. HSV can also disseminate viscerally in immunosuppressed patients, causing hepatitis and pneumonia, and, by interrupting the normal skin barriers, can pose a risk of secondary infection.

It is now well established that intravenous and oral acyclovir are both effective treatments for HSV reactivations of all types in immunocompromised patients. The choice of drug route should depend on the overall condition of the patient and the ability to tolerate oral medications. The usual intravenous doses used are 250 mg per square meter (5 mg per kilogram) every 8 hours. Effective oral doses are somewhat higher than necessary in normal hosts, usually 400 mg five times a day. Length of treatment may depend somewhat on the response of lesions, but should be for at least 7 to 10 days.

Since HSV reactivation occurs commonly and often predictably in immunocompromised patients, acyclovir can also be used successfully as prophylaxis against recurrences. Several controlled studies have shown reactivation rates of 0 to 10 percent in acyclovir-treated patients compared to 60 to 80 percent in controls, with breakthrough episodes frequently being mild or consisting of asymptomatic viral shedding. Acyclovir prophylaxis is therefore now routine practice in many centers for seropositive patients undergoing bone marrow transplantation, induction therapy for leukemia, and solid organ transplantation. Both 250 mg per square meter (5 mg per kilogram) intravenously every 8 hours and 200 mg orally every 6 hours are generally effective, and treatment should continue from the day of conditioning, induction, or transplantation for 4 to 6 weeks. Indications for prophylaxis in patients with AIDS are not as well defined. Anecdotal experience has shown that higher oral doses may be required to maintain suppression in AIDS patients, i.e., 400 mg three to four times daily.

NEONATAL HSV INFECTIONS

Most neonatal HSV infections are acquired perinatally from infected genital secretions of the mother and are consequently caused by HSV type 2. It is estimated that 10 to 40 percent of exposed infants will become infected, but methods for identifying precisely which mothers and infants will be at risk at the time of delivery have not been perfected. The annual incidence in the United States is approximately one case per 2,500 to 5,000 live births.

HSV infection must be suspected in neonates with rash, with sepsis or meningoencephalitis without a bacterial source, and especially in those with a maternal history of genital herpes or cultures positive for HSV. Seventy to eighty percent of affected infants will have a vesicular rash from which virus can be isolated; the rest may have virus cultured from the oropharynx, eyes, or buffy coat. Three patterns of neonatal infection are seen: mucocutaneous disease limited to the skin, eyes, and oropharynx; disseminated infection with visceral involvement; and encephalomyelitis. Mortality rates in the latter two forms range from 50 to 80 percent without treatment, and even those infants with "only" mucocutaneous disease have a 30-percent incidence of subsequent neurologic deficits. Progression from mucocutaneous disease to disseminated infection and/or encephalitis can occur in up to 80 percent of infants; therefore, a major goal of therapy is prompt recognition and treatment to halt further progression. Hence, all neonates with any form of HSV infection should be treated.

Preliminary data from the most recent comparative trial from the NIAID Collaborative Antiviral Study Group has shown that vidarabine and acyclovir at doses of 30 mg per kilogram per day are probably equally efficacious in neonatal HSV infections. Mortality was decreased from 60 to 80 percent in untreated cases to 20 percent, and the fraction of normal survivors increased from 20 to 55 percent overall. As in the encephalitis trials, the duration of illness before institution of therapy had a major impact on outcome. No differences in short-term side effects or drug toxicities were noted, but the long-term follow-up from this latest comparative trial remains incomplete as yet.

Current recommendations are therefore to treat all neonates with any form of HSV infection with either acyclovir 10 mg per kilogram intravenously every 8 hours, or vidarabine 30 mg per kilogram administered intravenously over 12 hours at a concentration of 0.5 mg per milliliter. Duration of treatment with either drug is 10 days. Many children will develop recurrent skin vesicles within several months of treatment, but these do not require repeat therapy unless signs of systemic involvement are present.

Rapid identification of women at risk of transmitting HSV at delivery is a major area of ongoing research. Classic practice has been to perform caesarean section in all women with genital lesions or positive viral cultures at delivery, as well as in any woman with primary genital infection during the last trimester, provided that surgery was feasible before or within 12 hours of rupture of membranes. No controlled trials of acyclovir prophylaxis in peripartum mothers or in exposed neonates have yet been conducted because of ongoing concern over the possibility of long-term adverse effects. When more experience is gained with acyclovir in children, the potentially considerable benefits of prophylaxis in certain infants may eventually be realized.

ADVERSE EFFECTS

Vidarabine has numerous potential side effects. Its relative insolubility makes fluid management difficult in individuals with HSE and concomitant cerebral edema. Gastrointestinal and hematologic toxicities are not uncommon. Further, it possesses a significant neurotoxic poten-

TABLE 1 Therapy of HSV Infections

Host/Syndrome	Treatment	Alternatives	Comments
Immunocompetent hosts			
Primary herpes genitalis	Acyclovir (ACV) 200 mg PO 5 ×/day ×10 days	ACV 400 mg PO b.i.d. × 10 days *or* ACV 5 mg/kg IV q8h (if severe) *or* ACV 5% ointment (topical)	
Recurrent herpes genitalis	ACV 200 mg PO 5 ×/day × 5 days	ACV 400 mg PO b.i.d. × 5 days	Consider chronic suppression if ≥ 6 recurrences/yr
Primary herpes gingivostomatitis	Supportive in most cases	ACV 200 mg PO 5 ×/day *or* ACV 400 mg PO b.i.d. *or* ACV 5 mg/kg IV q8h (if severe)	
Recurrent herpes labialis	Supportive		Short-term prophylaxis for specific indications can be considered
Cutaneous syndromes:			
Herpetic whitlow	ACV 200 mg PO 5×/day × 5 days	ACV 400 mg PO b.i.d. × 5 days	
Eczema herpeticum	ACV 5 mg/kg IV q8h	ACV 400 mg PO 5 ×/day (if mild)	
HSV-associated erythema multiforme	ACV 400 mg PO 5 ×/day (if mild)		Chronic suppressive therapy may be indicated
Keratitis	1% trifluorothymidine solution (topical)	3% vidarabine (VDB) ointment (topical)	Ophthalmologic consultation advised
Encephalitis	ACV 10 mg/kg IV q8h × 10–14 days	VDB 15 mg/kg IV qd × 10–14 days	
Immunocompromised hosts			
Mucocutaneous disease	ACV 5 mg/kg IV q8h × 7–10 days (if severe)	ACV 200–400 mg PO 5×/day × 7–10 days (as follow up to IV treatment or if less severe)	Higher oral doses indicated for patients with AIDS
Visceral involvement (pneumonia, hepatitis, meningoencephalitis, etc.)	ACV 10 mg/kg IV q8h × 10–14 days	VDB 15 mg/kg IV qd × 10–14 days	
Neonatal disease	ACV 10 mg/kg IV q8h × 10–14 days	VDB 30 mg/kg IV qd × 10–14 days	Superiority of ACV not yet established

Oral doses given are for adults. Doses recommended are for individuals with normal renal function; adjustments for renal insufficiency are necessary (see text). See text for discussion of prophylaxis/chronic suppression.

tial, especially in individuals with preexisting neurologic insults, renal compromise (with subsequent drug accumulation), and concomitant allopurinol therapy.

Acyclovir is a much better tolerated agent. The most common side effects are minor: headache and nausea. More significant toxicities have been reported and include reversible renal dysfunction secondary to crystalluria, if the drug is too rapidly infused, and occasional neurotoxicity. High doses, preexisting neurologic disease, or concomitant therapies all may predispose to acyclovir-associated neurotoxic reactions.

ACYCLOVIR RESISTANCE

As with antibacterial therapy, there is much interest and concern whether resistance to antiviral agents will occur as they become widely used. Resistance of HSV strains to acyclovir is known to occur, but its precise frequency and its ultimate clinical importance are not fully defined. The most common mechanism of resistance demonstrated by HSV isolates is diminished thymidine kinase activity, but these strains are inherently less pathogenic and have a diminished capacity to establish latency in animal models. Other mechanisms of resistance include an intact viral thymidine kinase with an altered substrate specificity, so that the drug is not phosphorylated, and strains with an altered DNA polymerase that is no longer inhibited by acyclovir triphosphate.

In normal patients on chronic suppressive therapy for recurrent genital herpes, no overall increase in resistance of the HSV isolates has been observed. In immunocompromised patients, resistant isolates have been reported with increasing frequency in patients with AIDS, and this has correlated with a lack of clinical response. The situation is complex, however, as some lesions may heal despite the isolation of a resistant strain. Also, lack of response may not always indicate resistance to the antiviral agent, as host immune factors may be more crucial to the outcome. As a practical matter, one should use acyclovir prudently, but widespread resistance has not yet emerged as a major problem since its licensure. However, in a serious clinical situation, if a patient is not responding to adequate doses of acyclovir, resistance should be considered. Isolates can be tested for resistance in a number of research laboratories, and alternative treatment with vidarabine or foscarnet (an experimental agent) should be considered.

CONCLUSIONS

A summary of treatment recommendations for the major forms of HSV infection is shown in Table 1. In the past 5 years the availability of oral acyclovir has revolutionized the treatment of many mucocutaneous HSV infections. While treatment of primary HSV episodes with acyclovir does not prevent the establishment of latent infection and does not affect the rate of subsequent recurrences, alleviation of individual attacks and long-term prevention of many forms of recurrent infection are now feasible both in normal and immunocompromised individuals. Additionally, intravenous acyclovir remains the treatment of choice for all severe forms of HSV infection, including encephalitis and neonatal infections. Rapid diagnosis and prompt initiation of treatment are the cornerstones of successful therapy.

It is likely that acyclovir will remain the drug of choice for HSV for the foreseeable future. Meanwhile, the development of therapies that can prevent the establishment of viral latency, eradicate latent virus from neural tissue, or prevent reactivation of latent genomes are important and formidable goals for future investigation. Active research in HSV vaccine development continues and has been encouraging, but this form of preventive therapy remains a more long-term objective.

SUGGESTED READING

Dorsky DI, Crumpacker CS. Drugs 5 years later: acyclovir. Ann Intern Med 1987;107:859–874.

Gold D, Corey L. Acyclovir prophylaxis for herpes simplex virus infection. Antimicrob Agents Chemother 1987;31:361–367.

Liesegang TJ. Ocular herpes simplex infection: pathogenesis and current therapy. Mayo Clin Proc 1988;63:1092–1105.

Lietman PS, Fiddian P, Chapman SK, eds. The Wellcome International Antiviral Symposium. Am J Med 1988;85(no. 2A).

VIRAL HEMORRHAGIC FEVER

CLARENCE J. PETERS, M.D.
ALEXIS SHELOKOV, M.D.

Several RNA viruses transmitted to humans from animals or arthropods may cause a syndrome referred to as viral hemorrhagic fever or VHF (Table 1). The target organ in the VHF syndrome is the vascular bed; cor-

The views of the authors do not purport to reflect the positions of the US Department of the Army or the US Department of Defense.

respondingly, the dominant clinical features are usually a consequence of microvascular damage and changes in vascular permeability. Common presenting complaints are fever, myalgia, and prostration; clinical examination may reveal only conjunctival injection, mild hypotension, flushing, and petechial hemorrhages. Full-blown VHF typically evolves to shock and generalized mucous membrane hemorrhage and often is accompanied by evidence of neurologic, hematopoietic, or pulmonary involvement. Hepatic involvement is common, but a clinical picture dominated by jaundice and other evidence of hepatic failure is only seen in some cases of Rift Valley fever, Crimean-Congo hemorrhagic fever (HF), Marburg HF, Ebola HF, and yellow fever. Renal failure is proportion-

TABLE 1 Recognized Viral Hemorrhagic Fevers of Humans

Viral Group	Disease (Virus)	Natural Geographic Distribution	Source of Human Infection*	Incubation Period (Days)
Arenavirus	Lassa fever	Africa	Rodent (nosocomial)	5–16
	Argentine HF (Junin)	South America	Rodent (nosocomial)	7–14
	Bolivian HF (Machupo)	South America	Rodent (nosocomial)	7–14
Bunyaviridae				
Phlebovirus	Rift Valley fever	Africa	Mosquito (slaughter of domestic animal)	2–5
Nairovirus	Crimean-Congo HF	Europe, Asia, Africa	Tick (slaughter of domestic animal; nosocomial)	3–12
Hantavirus	HF with renal syndrome (Hantaan and related viruses)	Asia, Europe; possibly worldwide	Rodent	9–35
Filovirus	Marburg and Ebola HF	Africa	Unknown (nosocomial)	3–16
Flavivirus (mosquito-borne)	Yellow fever	Tropical Africa, South America	Mosquito	3–6
	Dengue HF	Asia, Americas, Africa	Mosquito	†
Flavivirus (tick-borne)	Kyasanur Forest disease	India	Tick	3–8
	Omsk HF	Soviet Union	Tick (muskrat-contaminated water)	3–8

*Usual source in nature (other routes in parentheses).
†Unknown for DHF, but 3 to 15 days for uncomplicated dengue.

al to cardiovascular compromise, except in hemorrhagic fever with renal syndrome (HFRS), where it is an integral part of the disease process. Mortality may be substantial, ranging from 5 to 20 percent or higher in recognized cases.

EPIDEMIOLOGY

Because these viruses are all zoonotic agents, exposure to a rural reservoir is necessary for human infection (see Table 1). Several exceptions exist: (1) Dengue typically is an urban disease, although a sylvatic cycle exists. (2) Yellow fever may develop an urban transmission cycle by involving *Aedes aegypti* mosquitoes; the last time this occurred in coastal cities in the United States was in 1905 (New Orleans), but in recent years urban outbreaks have been recognized in Africa. (3) Viruses causing HFRS may infect rats; rats, in turn, have transmitted disease to urban dwellers in Asia and to laboratory personnel working with rat colonies in Europe and Asia. It should be noted that distinction between "urban" and "rural" can be ambiguous in developing countries, particularly if ectoparasite-laden domestic animals are present within large cities.

All the viruses in Table 1 (exception: dengue virus) are infectious by aerosol or fomites. Since most patients are viremic, there is a potential for transmission to patients, medical staff, and particularly laboratory personnel (exception: hantavirus infections, in which, at the time of presentation, viremia is waning and circulating antibody is present).

The age and sex distributions of each disease generally reflect the opportunities for zoonotic exposure. The exception is DHF/DSS, which typically has been a childhood disease in its major focus in Southeast Asia (DHF/DSS will be used to refer to hemorrhagic fever and shock syndrome, the life-threatening complications of dengue fever). DHF/DSS is also unique because it is thought to result most often from infections with a second dengue virus serotype. Although this is the general epidemiologic pattern, dengue virus may cause hemorrhagic fever in adults and in primary infections.

DIFFERENTIAL DIAGNOSIS

Because of the ecologic and geographic determinants of virus circulation, a detailed travel history is essential in making the diagnosis of VHF (see Table 1). Patients with arenaviral or hantaviral infections often recall having seen rodents during the presumed incubation period, but, because the viruses are spread to humans by aerosolized excreta or environmental contamination, actual contact is not necessary. Large mosquito populations are common during Rift Valley fever or flaviviral transmission, but a history of mosquito bite is sufficiently common to be of little assistance, whereas tick bites are of some significance in suspecting Crimean-Congo HF.

VHF should be suspected in any patient presenting with a severe febrile illness and evidence of vascular involvement (subnormal blood pressure, postural hypotension, petechiae, easy bleeding, flushing of face and chest, nondependent edema) who has traveled to an area where the virus is known to occur (see Table 1). Signs and symptoms suggesting additional organ system involvement are common but rarely dominate the picture (headache, photophobia, pharyngitis, cough, nausea or vomiting, diarrhea, constipation, abdominal pain, hyperesthesia, myalgia, dizziness, confusion, tremor). The macular eruption that occurs in most cases of Marburg-Ebola HF should be sought because of its diagnostic importance.

For much of the world, the major differential diagnosis is malaria. It must be borne in mind that parasitemia in patients partially immune to malaria does not prove that symptoms are due to malaria. Typhoid fever and rickettsial and leptospiral diseases are major confounding infections, with nontyphoidal salmonellosis, shigellosis, relapsing fever, fulminant hepatitis, and meningococcemia being some of the other important diagnoses to exclude. Any condition leading to disseminated intravascular coagulation could present in a confusing fashion, as well as diseases such as acute leukemia, lupus erythematosus, idiopathic or thrombotic thrombocytopenic purpura, and hemolytic uremic syndrome.

Because of recent recognition of their worldwide occurrence, additional consideration should be given to infections with Hantaan-related viruses. Classic HFRS (also referred to as Korean hemorrhagic fever or epidemic hemorrhagic fever) has a severe course that progresses sequentially from fever through hemorrhage, shock, renal failure, and polyuria. This clinical form of HFRS is widely distributed in China, the Korean peninsula, and the far eastern USSR, where its reservoir, the striped field mouse (*Apodemus agrarius*), is found. Severe disease also is found in some Balkan states, including Greece, where the yellow-necked field mouse (*Apodemus flavicollis*) is thought to carry a similar virus. However, the Scandinavian and most European virus strains carried by voles (most commonly *Clethrionomys glareolus*) usually produce a milder disease (referred to as nephropathia epidemica) with prominent fever, myalgia, abdominal pain, and oliguria, but without shock or florid hemorrhagic manifestations. The full spectrum of hantaviral infections in humans still is being defined and may include mild illness with fever and myalgia, aseptic meningitis, or hepatic damage.

The clinical laboratory can be very helpful. Thrombocytopenia (exception: Lassa fever) and leukopenia (exceptions: Lassa, Hantaan, and some severe Crimean-Congo HF cases) are the rule. Proteinuria and/or hematuria are common, and their absence virtually rules out Argentine HF, Bolivian HF, and hantaviral infections. A positive tourniquet test has been particularly useful in DSS/DHF, but should be sought in other HF as well.

Definitive diagnosis in an individual case rests on specific virologic diagnosis. Most patients have readily detectable viremia at presentation (exception: hantaviral infections). With the exception of dengue, specialized microbiologic containment is required for safe handling of these viruses. Appropriate precautions should be observed in collection, handling, shipping, and processing of diagnostic samples. Both the Centers for Disease Control (CDC, Atlanta, Georgia) and the US Army Medical Research Institute of Infectious Diseases (USAMRIID, Frederick, Maryland) have diagnostic laboratories functioning at the highest (BSL 4 or P-4) containment level (see below for addresses).

Rapid enzyme immunoassays can detect viral antigens in acute sera from patients with Lassa fever, Argentine HF, Rift Valley fever, Crimean-Congo HF, yellow fever, and specific IgM antibodies in early convalescence. Lassa- and Hantaan-specific IgM often are detectable during the acute illness. Diagnosis by virus cultivation and identification will require 3 to 7 days, or longer.

SPECIFIC THERAPY

Antiviral therapy of proven or probable value exists for several VHF (Table 2). The antiviral drug ribavirin has been shown to reduce mortality from Lassa fever in high-risk patients, and it presumably decreases morbidity in all patients. Lassa fever patients, particularly those with severe disease, should receive 30 mg of ribavirin

TABLE 2 Therapy of Viral Hemorrhagic Fevers

Disease	Indicated	Comments
Lassa fever	Ribavirin	Most effective in first 7 days; convalescent plasma selected for neutralizing antibody may be useful adjunct
Argentine HF	Convalescent plasma	Only effective in first 8 days of illness; ribavirin may also be useful
Bolivian HF	Convalescent plasma	Convalescent plasma effective in preclinical studies; ribavirin may also be useful
Rift Valley fever	Convalescent plasma or ribavirin	Neither of proven value but effective in animal models
Crimean-Congo HF	Ribavirin	Ribavirin effective in preclinical studies; convalescent plasma with neutralizing antibody may be useful or serve as adjunct; IgG available in Bulgaria
HF with renal syndrome	Ribavirin	Useful in first 4 days
Marburg and Ebola HF	—	One survivor received interferon and convalescent plasma; ribavirin ineffective in preclinical testing
Yellow fever	—	Convalescent plasma of possible use
Dengue HF	—	Vigorous fluid replacement live-saving

per kilogram intravenously, followed by 15 mg per kilogram every 6 hours for 4 days, and then 7.5 mg per kilogram every 8 hours for 6 more days. Treatment is most effective if begun within 7 days of onset; lower intravenous doses or oral administration of 2 g followed by 1 g per day for 10 days also may be useful. The only significant adverse effects have been anemia and hyperbilirubinemia, related to a mild hemolysis and reversible block of erythropoiesis. The anemia has not required transfusions or cessation of therapy in African studies. Ribavirin is contraindicated in pregnant women, but, in the case of definite Lassa fever, the predictability of fetal death and the need for uterine evacuation justify its use. Safety in infants and children has not been established. A similar dose of ribavirin begun within 4 days of disease may be effective in HFRS patients. Preclinical ribavirin studies with Argentine and Bolivian HF, Rift Valley fever, and Crimean-Congo HF are promising. The filoviruses are not inhibited by the drug in cell culture and neither dengue- nor yellow fever-infected macaques respond to ribavirin.

Argentine HF responds to therapy with 2 or more units of convalescent plasma containing adequate amounts of neutralizing antibody and given within 8 days of onset.

The life-saving value of appropriate supporting management of DHF/DSS is emphasized by its inclusion in Table 2, even though the treatment is syndrome specific and not virus specific.

SPECIFIC PROPHYLAXIS

The only established virus-specific prophylactic measure for a VHF is yellow fever vaccine, which is mandatory for travelers to endemic areas of Africa and South America. Other vaccines under investigation have some limited utility (Table 3). For circumstances in which risk of infection is judged to be high but transient, reasonable but more speculative approaches are available.

Close personal contacts or medical personnel intensively exposed to blood or secretions from VHF patients (particularly Lassa fever, Crimean-Congo HF, and filoviral diseases) should be monitored for fever and other disease manifestations during a time equal to the established incubation period. In Lassa fever one might administer ribavirin orally (5 mg per kilogram three times per day) for 3 weeks or in Crimean-Congo HF for 10 days. Most subjects will tolerate this drug dose well, but subjects should be under surveillance for breakthrough disease (especially after drug cessation) or adverse drug effects (principally anemia).

SUPPORTIVE THERAPY

Several nonspecific measures apply to all the VHFs. Additional capillary damage and hemostatic impairment should be minimized by prompt hospitalization and gen-

TABLE 3   Prophylaxis of Viral Hemorrhagic Fevers

Disease	Vaccine*	Short-Term, High-Risk Exposure†
Lassa fever	—	Ribavirin
Argentine HF	Live attenuated (phase III, USAMRIID and Argentina)	Convalescent plasma or ribavirin
Bolivian HF	Argentine HF vaccine protects monkeys	Convalescent plasma or ribavirin
Rift Valley fever	Formalin-inactivated (phase II, USAMRIID)	Ribavirin
Crimean-Congo HF	Inactivated (licensed in Bulgaria)	Ribavirin or IgG
HF with renal syndrome	—	Convalescent plasma (infected rodent bite?)
Marburg and Ebola HF	—	—
Yellow fever	Live attenuated (licensed worldwide)	Convalescent plasma
Dengue HF	—	—
Kyasanur Forest disease	Inactivated (phase II, Virus Research Center, Pune, India)	Convalescent plasma

*Vaccines in phase II or III testing are in general indicated for laboratory workers or others at very high risk of infection. Rift Valley fever vaccine should be given to veterinary personnel working with domestic livestock in sub-Saharan Africa.

†Close contacts, exposed medical personnel, or laboratory workers may derive benefit from temporary coverage with ribavirin or convalescent plasma; although neither modality is proven, cell culture and animal studies suggest utility.

Viral Hemorrhagic Fever / **359**

tle handling, preferably in a softly lit room away from regular traffic. Acetylsalicylic acid and other antiplatelet-anticlotting-factor drugs should be avoided. Restlessness, confusion, myalgia, and hyperesthesia frequently are problems and should be managed by reassurance and other supportive measures. Judicious use of oral opiates, diazepam, or chloral hydrate is indicated. Secondary infections are common and should be sought and aggressively treated. Intravenous lines, catheters, and other invasive procedures must be avoided unless clearly indicated in management. Attention should be given to pulmonary toilet, the usual measures to prevent superinfection, and supplemental oxygen. Immunosuppression with steroids or other agents has no empiric and little theoretical basis, except possibly in HFRS. In this disease the onset of the immune response coincides with the onset of symptoms, and uncontrolled observations have suggested that cyclophosphamide therapy may be useful. However, these observations require confirmation before such therapy can be recommended.

The management of bleeding is controversial. Uncontrolled clinical observations support vigorous administration of fresh frozen plasma, clotting factor concentrates, and platelets, as well as early use of heparin for expectant management of disseminated intravascular coagulation. In the absence of definitive evidence, it is recommended that mild bleeding manifestations not be treated at all. More severe hemorrhagic defects should receive appropriate replacement therapy. When definite laboratory evidence of disseminated intravascular coagulation develops, heparin therapy should be employed if appropriate laboratory control is available. Plasma levels of coagulation factors may decrease from lack of synthesis and/or vascular leakage, and viral involvement of bone marrow and liver can complicate interpretation of the usually employed coagulation parameters.

Management of hypotension and shock is difficult. Patients often are modestly dehydrated from heat, fever, anorexia, vomiting, and/or diarrhea. There are covert losses of intravascular volume through hemorrhage and increased vascular permeability. Nevertheless, patients with such problems often respond poorly to fluid infusion and readily develop pulmonary edema, possibly resulting from myocardial impairment and increased pulmonary vascular permeability. Fluid should be given cautiously, and colloid should be used. There is no systematic experience with pharmacologic support of the circulation in patients with the different VHFs. Dopamine is the agent of choice for shock. Alpha-adrenergic agents have not been helpful except when there is need to temporize. Cardiac stimulants, such as digitalis glycosides, could reasonably be applied. High doses of corticosteroids (e.g., 30 mg of methylprednisolone per kilogram) provide another possible therapeutic modality in unrelenting shock.

Treatment for falciparum malaria with a regimen known to be effective for the geographic parasite strain should be given to patients residing in or traveling from malarious areas, unless evaluation by an experienced laboratory excludes malaria. The presence of malarial parasites, particularly in the immune individual, should not preclude the management of a patient for VHF if clinically indicated.

Two hemorrhagic fevers should be clearly separated from the other diseases. Severe consequences of dengue infection are largely due to systemic capillary leakage syndrome and should be managed initially by brisk infusion of crystalloid, followed by albumin or other colloid if there is no response. Severe hantaviral infections present many of the management problems of the other hemorrhagic fevers but will culminate in acute renal failure with subsequent polyuria during recovery. Careful fluid and electrolyte management, and, often, renal dialysis, are necessary for optimal treatment.

ISOLATION AND CONTAINMENT

With the exception of dengue (virus present, but no secondary infection hazard) and hantaviral disease (infectious virus not present in blood or excreta at the time of hospitalization), VHF patients have significant quantities of virus in blood and, perhaps, other excretions. Careful attention to needle disposal and other sources of parenteral exposure is, of course, mandatory. Clinical laboratory personnel are at high risk of exposure and should exercise extreme caution in handling submitted specimens. Certain VHFs (e.g., Crimean-Congo HF) may mimic surgical emergencies, such as bleeding gastric ulcer, leading to secondary infections among personnel of emergency and operating rooms.

Most experience with the various VHFs has been gained in field situations where endoscopy, respirators, arterial lines, routine blood sampling, and extensive laboratory analysis were not available. Under these conditions, mask-gown-glove precautions and other commonly employed barrier nursing procedures have halted transmission in most cases. Experience has shown, however, that these viruses occasionally may disseminate by the airborne route. Well-documented secondary infections among contacts and medical personnel not parenterally exposed have occurred. Thus, caution should be exercised in evaluating and treating the patient with a suspected VHF. Over-reaction of health care providers is inappropriate and detrimental to both patient and staff, but it is prudent to provide isolation as rigorous as is feasible. At a minimum, this should include stringent barrier nursing; mask, gown, glove, and needle precautions; hazard labeling of specimens submitted to the clinical laboratory; restricting access to the patient; and autoclaving or liberally applying hypochlorite or phenolic disinfectants to excreta and other contaminated materials.

No carrier state has ever been observed with any VHF, but excretion of virus in urine or semen may occur in convalescence. Some late-onset complications such as uveitis may be associated with the local presence of infectious virus.

Diagnostic laboratories experienced in dealing with BSL 4/P-4 level pathogens include: United States: US Army Medical Research Institute of Infectious Diseases,

Disease Assessment Division, Fort Detrick, Frederick, Maryland 21701–5011 (telephone 301–663–7193 or evenings 301–663–7373); Centers for Disease Control, Special Pathogens Branch, Atlanta, Georgia 30333 (telephone 404–329–3308); United Kingdom: Center for Applied Microbiology and Research, Special Pathogens Unit, Salisbury, Porton Down, Wiltshire, SP4 0JG, England (telephone 44–0980–610391); South Africa: National Institute for Virology, Private Bag X4, Sandringham, Johannesburg (telephone 27–11–6405031).

INFECTIONS AFFECTING MORE THAN ONE SYSTEM AND CAUSED BY PARASITES OR FUNGI

MALARIA

SUSAN J. JACOBSON, M.D.
DAVID J. WYLER, M.D.

Human malaria is caused by four species of the genus *Plasmodium* (*P. falciparum*, *P. vivax*, *P. malariae*, and *P. ovale*). *P. falciparum* malaria can be fatal, and strains from many parts of the world have developed resistance to certain antimalarial drugs, such as chloroquine. Recognizing malaria and instituting appropriate therapy may be challenging but can be life saving.

LIFE CYCLE

The life cycle of the malaria parasite is important in understanding treatment and prevention. Malaria is transmitted by the bite of infected female anopheline mosquitoes or by inoculation of infected blood (e.g., transfusion malaria or congenital malaria). Mosquitoes inject sporozoites, which enter the liver within minutes of inoculation. In the liver, the parasites multiply as hepatic exoerythrocytic forms (schizonts). After 1 to 2 weeks of development, the hepatic schizonts rupture, releasing thousands of merozoites, which enter the circulation and invade erythrocytes. Some of the exoerythrocytic forms of *P. vivax* and *P. ovale* persist in the liver and remain as latent exoerythrocytic forms (or hypnozoites). These may remain latent in the liver for months or years, resulting in relapses of erythrocytic infection. Once malaria parasites invade the erythrocytes, they never reinvade the liver. Hence, transfusion malaria never results in development of exoerythrocytic forms. There are no latent exoerythrocytic forms in *P. falciparum* or *P. malariae* infections.

Merozoites invade erythrocytes by a complex interaction between specific receptors on merozoites and those on the surface of erythrocytes. Persons whose erythrocytes lack all Duffy blood-group determinants (a common phenotype in most of Africa) are not susceptible to *P. vivax* infection. *P. vivax* and *P. ovale* parasitize young erythrocytes, and *P.* *malariae* infects older erythrocytes, limiting the magnitude of parasitemia. *P. falciparum* can develop in erythrocytes of all ages, and parasitemia can reach very high levels. The magnitude of parasitemia is an important determinant of morbidity and mortality in malaria.

After entering erythrocytes, merozoites of three of the species mature and cause erythrocyte rupture within 48 hours (tertian malaria), while *P. malariae* requires 72 hours (quartan malaria). Maturation involves the development from ring forms through the trophozoite stage to the schizont stage (defined by evidence of nuclear division). Mature schizonts rupture and release many merozoites, which rapidly invade other erythrocytes, continuing the erythrocytic cycle of infection. The sexual cycle begins with some merozoites differentiating into gametocytes. These circulate in the blood and when ingested by an appropriate mosquito can initiate the sporogonic cycle that culminates in the development of sporozoites in about 10 days. At this time, transmission can occur. Only the asexual blood stages cause illness. Gametocytes can persist even after asexual blood stages have been eliminated.

EPIDEMIOLOGY

Malaria transmission occurs in large areas of Central and South America, sub-Saharan Africa, and Indian subcontinent, Southeast Asia, some areas of the Middle East, and Oceania, with an estimated 100 to 200 million cases occurring yearly worldwide. Species distribution varies in different parts of the world: *P. falciparum* predominates in Africa, Haiti, and New Guinea. *P. ovale* occurs primarily in Africa, while *P. vivax* is rarely encountered there. *P. falciparum* and *P. vivax* malaria are both prevalent in Southeast Asia, South America, and Oceania. *P. vivax* predominates on the Indian subcontinent, where infection with *P. falciparum* is infrequent. *P. malariae* distribution is relatively cosmopolitan.

In the United States malaria is generally imported, although occasional small epidemics due to local transmission occur, like that which involved 27 cases of *P. vivax* malaria in San Diego County in 1986. The number of reported cases of malaria in the United States has been stable over the last decade, with approximately 1,000 cases yearly.

Resistance of *P. falciparum* to chloroquine has been reported from all countries with known transmission except the Dominican Republic, Haiti, Central America, the Middle East, and the following countries in West Africa: Chad, Equatorial Guinea, Guinea, Guinea-Bissau, Liberia, Senegal, and Sierra Leone. Resistance to pyrimethamine and sulfonamides (e.g., Fansidar) as well as chloroquine is widespread in Thailand, Burma, and Kampuchea and exists in some areas of Brazil, Kenya, and elsewhere.

DIAGNOSIS

The malarial paroxysm—characterized by high fever, chills, rigor—is the hallmark of acute malaria. Sometimes there is a prodromal period of one to several days. Patients may complain of nonspecific symptoms, such as malaise, headache, myalgia, and fatigue, or have more localized complaints, such as chest pain, abdominal pain, or arthralgias, that may obscure the correct diagnosis. The malarial fever is rarely periodic or regular when it initially occurs in a nonimmune host. Absence of a 48- or 72-hour fever cycle does not exclude a diagnosis of malaria. Prompt diagnosis of malaria by physicians practicing in nonendemic areas requires a high index of suspicion for malaria in travelers in endemic countries. Malaria may occur as early as 9 days following exposure or may present months after the endemic area is left. Chloroquine prophylaxis may delay presenta-

tion of chloroquine-resistant *P. falciparum* malaria. Immune individuals may have relapses (emergence from latent exoerythrocytic stage) or recrudescences (rising wave of intraerythrocytic parasitemia from a persistent low level) years after exposure.

Diagnosis is made by demonstration of the malarial parasites on either thick or thin blood smears that have been stained with Giemsa. Since symptoms may appear a few days before parasites can be detected by blood smear, it is important to continue to obtain blood smears for several days before excluding the diagnosis. Thick smears are primarily used to identify the presence of parasites, and thin smears are used to make species differentiation. The extent of parasitemia should be quantified, either according to percent of parasitized erythrocytes, or—in settings of low-grade parasitemia—by numbers of infected erythrocytes per leukocyte and relating the latter ratio to the leukocyte count.

Clues to *P. falciparum* infection include multiply infected erythrocytes, a high-grade parasitemia (greater than 5 percent), the presence of only ring forms, and the banana-shaped gametocyte (rarely seen). Differentiation of other malaria species is less urgent, because malaria due to the three other species are all initially treated with chloroquine. The choice of therapy for *P. falciparum* infection is more complicated since it depends on the probability that the patient has been infected with a chloroquine-resistant strain and considers the presence of complications.

TABLE 1   Drugs of Choice for Therapy of Malaria

Indication	Drug/Route	Dose	
		Adult	*Pediatric*
Uncomplicated infection with all species except chloroquine-resistant *P. falciparum*	Chloroquine, PO (Aralen)	600 mg base, then 300 mg base in 6 h, then 300 mg base/day × 2 days	10 mg/kg base to maximum of 600 mg, ¹/₂ in 6 h, then qd × 3 days
Uncomplicated infection with *P. falciparum* acquired in areas of chloroquine resistance	Quinine sulfate, PO *plus*	650 mg q8h × 7–10 days	25 mg/kg/day in 3 doses for 10 days
	Pyrimethamine 25 mg/ sulfadoxine 500 mg (Fansidar)	3 tab single dose	2–11 mo: ¹/₄ tab 1–3 yr: ¹/₂ tab 4–8 yr: 1 tab 9–14 yr: 2 tab > 14 yr: 3 tab
	or Doxycyline*	100 mg b.i.d. × 7 days	Tetracyclines are not recommended in children < 8 yr
	or Tetracycline	250 mg q.i.d. × 7 days	
Severe (complicated) *P. falciparum* infection† Patient unable to take PO meds Parasitemia > 5% Presence of organ dysfunction (such as cerebral malaria)	Quinine, IV‡	25 mg/kg/day: ¹/₂ dose in 250–500 ml D5 ¹/₂NS over 4–h infusion. Repeat in 6–8 h if oral therapy cannot be used. Give in same volume over same time, max 1,800 mg/day × 3 days. Adjust fluids for pediatric patients	
	or Quinidine gluconate IV§	15 mg/kg base loading dose in 250 ml NS, infused over 4 h. Subsequent doses 7.5 mg/kg base every 8 h × 7 days either IV or as oral quinidine sulfate or gluconate	
	plus Fansidar or tetracycline	Dose as above	
Prevention of relapses due to *P. vivax* and *P. ovale*	Primaquine, PO#	15 mg base/day × 14 days	0.3 mg base/kg/day × 14 days

* When given in combination with quinine, tetracycline has been shown to be an effective drug in the treatment of *P. falciparum* strains resistant to Fansidar and acquired in Southeast Asia.
† Consider exchange transfusions—see text for further details.
‡ Quinine hydrochloride can be obtained in the U.S. from the Centers for Disease Control, Malaria Branch, Atlanta, GA 30333 (404–488–4046 days; 404–639–2888 nights and weekends). Experts are also available for information regarding alternative regimens.
§ Frequent vital signs and continuous electrocardiographic monitoring should be performed.
# G6PD deficiency should be excluded before administration.

THERAPY

Prompt diagnosis and appropriate therapy are keys to a rapid recovery from malaria. The initial objectives of therapy are rapid reduction of parasitemia and prevention of complications of malaria, such as renal failure or cerebral malaria. The critical factors determining therapy include the clinical status of the patient, the presence of *P. falciparum* malaria parasites, and the potential for drug resistance if the infecting species is *P. falciparum*. Subsequent objectives of therapy may include elimination of dormant hepatic hypnozoites to prevent relapses of *P. vivax* or *P. ovale* malaria.

Drugs used clinically are primarily directed against the asexual parasite within the erythrocyte. These include the 4-aminoquinolines (chloroquine), the cinchona alkaloids (quinine, quinidine), antimetabolities (pyrimethamine, sulfadoxine), and tetracyclines. The 4-aminoquinolines are preferred unless drug resistance is suspected. There are also new drugs, currently not available in the United States, that are effective against chloroquine-resistant malaria. These include mefloquine (an amino alcohol), which is in use in Southeast Asia, is sold in France and Switzerland, and is pending licensing in the United States. Derivatives of a Chinese herbal compound, *quinhaosu*, are currently under study for treatment of multidrug-resistant *P. falciparum* infection.

Drugs of choice for therapy of malaria are indicated in Table 1. Uncomplicated infection with a nonresistant parasite is treated with oral chloroquine. When the patient is infected with *P. falciparum* acquired in areas where chloroquine resistance is a problem and has an uncomplicated infection, oral quinine sulfate should be used in conjunction with another drug. The additional drug can be a combination of pyrimethamine and a sulfonamide (such as Fansidar) in patients not allergic to sulfa drugs. For persons who acquire chloroquine-resistant *P. falciparum* malaria in Southeast Asia, tetracycline or doxycycline should be used with quinine, as Fansidar-resistant strains are widespread in this region. Children less than 8 years old and pregnant women should be administered tetracyclines only for life-threatening infection in which Fansidar resistance is anticipated.

Intravenous quinine or quinidine therapy should be begun in the patient who cannot take medications by mouth or has one or more of the following complications: more than 5 percent parasitized erythrocytes; evidence of organ dysfunction (such as cerebral malaria); or severe anemia. Quinine dihydrochloride (used for intravenous administration) is available in the United States from the Malaria Branch, Centers for Disease Control, Atlanta, Georgia 30333; telephone 404–488-4046 (404–639-2888 nights, weekends). A controlled clinical trial in Thailand showed that intravenous quinidine is as effective (perhaps more so) than quinine. Since intravenous quinidine is available in hospitals in the United States, its immediate use can be life saving. Administration of intravenous quinine or quinidine should be slow and accompanied by continuous cardiac monitoring. The patient can be switched subsequently to quinine administered orally. Pyrimethamine-sulfadoxine (Fansidar) or a tetracycline should be given with quinine once a patient is taking oral medication, as for uncomplicated chloroquine-resistant *P. falciparum* malaria.

For the patient with very high degree of parasitemia (more than 20 percent of erythrocytes infected), exchange transfusions should be considered. There are several anecdotal reports of patients, likely destined to die of malaria with 20 to 70 percent parasitized erythrocytes, recovering without significant sequelae when prompt exchange transfusions were used in conjunction with appropriate intravenous antimalarial therapy. Between 4 and 10 units of whole blood or component therapy (packed erythrocytes and fresh frozen plasma) has been given over a period of up to a day, preceded by venesection. The percent parasitemia is determined frequently (every 4 to 6 hours), and exchange transfusions are usually discontinued once parasitemia is less than 1 to 10 percent.

During the initial treatment of *P. falciparum* malaria, the parasitemia should be determined twice daily for the first 2 or 3 days. For other forms of malaria, a daily determination during the first few days of treatment is adequate. With severe malaria, the clinical status, hemoglobin, platelet count, glucose and electrolyte levels, renal function, and clotting parameters should all be followed.

COMPLICATIONS OF MALARIA

Patients with severe malaria are at risk for hypovolemia, due to salt and water loss from high fever, sweating, and poor fluid intake. Fluid and electrolyte replacement should be carefully undertaken to prevent precipitating noncardiogenic pulmonary edema. Hypoglycemia has been observed as a complication of severe, e.g., cerebral, malaria, often associated with intravenous quinine and particularly in pregnant women. Renal dysfunction occurs through multiple causes: tissue hypoxia, hypovolemia, hemoglobinemia, and disseminated intravascular coagulation (DIC). Correcting the abnormalities and a rapid reduction in parasitemia are the major goals to reducing renal dysfunction.

Hematologic abnormalities—anemia, thrombocytopenia, and rarely DIC—can all occur. If the anemia is severe, transfusions should be administered. Platelet transfusions are not generally necessary, as spontaneous bleeding is rare and the platelet count rapidly returns to normal with appropriate therapy. Heparin should not be used for DIC, although fresh frozen plasma—in conjunction with exchange transfusions—may be appropriate in some settings of DIC.

Cerebral malaria is the most feared complication of malaria. Controlled clinical trials have failed to show any benefit of corticosteroid use in cerebral malaria, which may actually be deleterious; hence, corticosteroids should not be used. With cerebral malaria, as with any coma, maintenance and protection of the airway is critical. If patients survive cerebral malaria, there is usually no major neurologic dysfunction, so supportive care during a malarial coma is important.

RADICAL CURE OF MALARIA

If a patient has had *P. vivax* or *P. ovale* malaria or has had a mixed infection in association with *P. falciparum* malaria, then the patient should receive primaquine therapy to prevent a relapse of *P. vivax* or *P. ovale* at a later time. There is a risk, however, of severe hemolysis if primaquine is given to a person with G6PD deficiency, particularly those of Mediterranean or Oriental background. Hence, G6PD level should be determined prior to the initiation of treatment with primaquine. Occasionally, patients will relapse with *P. vivax* or *P. ovale* malaria despite primaquine therapy and may require repeated therapy.

MALARIA IN PREGNANCY

Malaria during pregnancy poses dangers to the mother and the developing fetus. It can impair fetal growth and increases the risk of spontaneous abortion and stillbirth. Chloroquine therapy during pregnancy is safe, but most of the other antimalarial drugs used to treat chloroquine-resistant malaria are hazardous; hence, all efforts should be exerted to avoid acquiring malaria during pregnancy. Fansidar (pyrimethamine and sulfadoxine), with folinic acid supplementation, should be used in combination with quinine for the pregnant woman with chloroquine-resistant malaria. Relapses of malaria during pregnancy should be treated with the appropriate drugs for the acute episode, with primaquine

administered only postpartum to prevent further relapses. Mefloquine, one of the newer drugs not yet available in the United States, is safe during pregnancy.

PREVENTION

Prevention of malaria in travelers to malarious areas is becoming increasingly difficult. The spread of chloroquine-resistant and multidrug-resistant strains of *P. falciparum* malaria has forced use of drugs in addition to chloroquine. Adverse effects from some of these drugs have limited their safety. New drugs, under development for multidrug resistant malaria, may have a role in prophylaxis, but there are limited studies of efficacy and safety.

All travelers to malaria-endemic areas should be advised to use an appropriate drug regimen and personal protection measures to avoid mosquitoes. The most effective mosquito repellents contain N,N-diethylmetatoluamide (DEET). A pyrethrum-containing flying-insect spray should also be used in living and sleeping areas during evening and nighttime hours. Despite appropriate personal protection measures and use of an appropriate drug prophylaxis, travelers should be advised that they may still contract malaria. They should be instructed to seek prompt medical advise for symptoms of malaria during, or in the months subsequent to, travel to an area endemic for malaria.

There is some controversy concerning the most effective drug regimens for preventing symptoms of malaria, with differing opinions among experts in the field. There are limited studies of efficacy of prophylactic regimens among nonimmune travelers; hence, reliance is frequently placed on studies of suppression of malaria among semiimmune long-term residents in endemic areas. Recommendations for prophylactic regimens may change, depending on the distribution of drug-resistant strains of malaria. The following specific recommendations are accurate as of 1989 and based on the Centers for Disease Control's advice. For updated information consult the *Morbidity and Mortality Weekly Report* or *Health Information for International Travel*. The latter publication, revised annually, is available as DHHS publication no. (CDC)88-8280 from the Superintendent of Documents, U.S. Government Printing Office, Washington, D.C. 20402; telephone 202–783–3238. The Malaria Branch of the Centers for Disease Control has a computerized telephone service. Malaria Information for Travelers, 404–639–1610, which will provide specific advice to travelers to various areas of the world, is suitable for both travelers and their physicians, with frequent updates planned.

Table 2 outlines the drugs used in prophylaxis and the presumptive treatment of malaria. Preferably, malaria chemoprophylaxis should begin 1 to 2 weeks before travel to malarious areas and should continue throughout travel in a malaria endemic area and for 4 weeks after departure from these areas. The exception is doxycycline; because of its short half-life, its use should begin 1 to 2 days prior to entering a malarious area.

For travel to areas where risk of chloroquine-resistant *P. falciparum* malaria has not been reported or is low level or focal, chloroquine alone, once weekly, is recommended. Chloroquine is usually well tolerated. It can be taken with

TABLE 2 Drugs Used in Prophylaxis and Presumptive Treatment of Malaria

Drug	Prophylaxis	
	Adult Dose	*Pediatric Dose*
Chloroquine phosphate (Aralen)	300 mg base (500 mg salt), PO once/wk	5 mg/kg base (8.3 mg/kg salt) PO once/wk, up to maximum adult dose
Hydroxychloroquine sulfate (Plaquenil)	310 mg base (400 mg salt) PO once/wk	5 mg/kg base (6.5 mg/kg salt) PO once/wk, up to maximum adult dose
Doxycycline	100 mg PO once/day	>8 yr: 2 mg/kg PO once/day, up to adult dose
Proguanil (Paludrine)	1 tab (200 mg PO once/day combined with weekly chloroquine	<2 yr: 50 mg/day 2–6 yr: 100 mg/day 7–10 yr: 150 mg/day >10 yr: 200 mg/day
Pyrimethamine-sulfadoxine (Fansidar)	1 tab (25 mg pyrimethamine and 500 mg sulfadoxine) PO once/wk	2–11 mo: 1/8 tab/wk 1–3 yr: 1/4 tab/wk 4–8 yr: 1/2 tab/wk 9–14 yr: 3/4 tab/wk >14 yr: 1 tab/wk
Primaquine	See Table 1	See Table 1
Presumptive Treatment of Malaria for Travelers to Areas of Chloroquine Resistance		
Pyrimethamine-sulfadoxine (Fansidar)	3 tabs (75 mg pyrimethamine and 1,500 mg sulfadoxine) PO as a single dose	2–11 mo: 1/4 tab 1–3 yr: 1/2 tab 4–8 yr: 1 tab 9–14 yr: 2 tabs >14 yr: 3 tabs

food. The related compound hydroxychloroquine may be better tolerated. Occasionally minor adverse effects such as gastrointestinal disturbance, headache, dizziness, blurred vision, and pruritis occur, but these do not generally require discontinuation of the drug. The retinopathy associated with chronic administration of chloroquine in the treatment of rheumatoid arthritis seems not to occur when chloroquine is taken in the doses used for malaria prophylaxis.

For travel to areas where chloroquine-resistant *P. falciparum* malaria is endemic, once-weekly use of chloroquine alone is recommended. In addition, travelers should be given a treatment dose of Fansidar to be carried during travel. They should be instructed to take the Fansidar promptly in the event of a febrile illness during travel when medical care is not promptly available. This presumptive self-treatment of malaria should be understood by a traveler as a temporary measure; prompt medical evaluation is still important. They should continue their weekly chloroquine prophylaxis after presumptive treatment with Fansidar.

Fansidar, taken once weekly in combination with chloroquine, may be considered in certain circumstances involving prolonged exposure in areas with intense transmission of chloroquine-resistant *P. falciparum* malaria. If weekly Fansidar is prescribed, the traveler should be cautioned about the risk of a severe, and possibly fatal, skin reaction. Between 1982 and 1985, there were 24 cases reported (seven fatal) of erythema multiforme, Stevens-Johnson syndrome, and toxic epidermal necrolysis among American travelers using Fansidar. These severe reactions were associated with Fansidar when used as once-weekly prophylaxis. Fansidar also is associated with serum sickness–type reactions, urticaria, and hepatitis. The estimated risk of a fatal, cutaneous reaction among Americans using Fansidar is from 1 in 11,000 to 1 in 25,000 users. If once-weekly Fansidar is prescribed, the traveler should be advised to discontinue it immediately if he or she develops a possible ill effect, especially any skin or mucous membrane irritation, such as itching, redness, rash, mouth or genital lesions, or sore throat. Fansidar should not be given to persons with a history of sulfonamide intolerance or to infants under 2 months of age.

Doxycycline alone, taken daily, is an alternative regimen for the short-term traveler to areas with risk of chloroquine-resistant *P. falciparum* malaria, particularly to areas where chloroquine-resistant and Fansidar-resistant strains are known to occur, such as forested areas of Thailand, Burma, and Kampuchea. It is also appropriate for an individual with a history of sulfonamide intolerance. Doxycycline prophylaxis can begin 1 to 2 days before travel to malarious areas and should be continued daily during travel in malarious areas and for 4 weeks after departure from these areas. Adverse effects of this drug include photosensitivity reactions (usually exaggerated sunburn reaction), and it may be associated with an increased frequency of monilial vaginitis. It is contraindicated in pregnancy and for children under 8 years of age.

Proguanil (Paludrine) is a dihydrofolate reductase inhibitor that is not available commercially in the United States but is widely available elsewhere. Resistance of *P. falciparum* to proguanil is present in some endemic regions such as Southeast Asia, where resistance to Fansidar exists, but the distribution is not well delineated. Travelers using proguanil should take a daily 200-mg dose (adult) in combination with a weekly regimen of chloroquine.

Amodiaquine, a 4-aminoquinoline similar to chloroquine, has been used as an alternative prophylactic drug in areas where chloroquine-resistant *P. falciparum* malaria is endemic. Amodiaquine-associated agranulocytosis has been reported, and hence this drug is NOT recommended for malaria prophylaxis.

Primaquine is used to prevent relapses of *P. vivax* and *P. ovale*. Prophylaxis with primaquine is generally indicated for persons who have had prolonged exposure in malaria-endemic areas, and the dose is as indicated in Table 1. G6PD deficiency should be excluded by appropriate laboratory testing. Primaquine should not be used during pregnancy because the drug may be passed transplacentally to a G6PD deficient fetus and cause life-threatening hemolytic anemia in utero. Chloroquine prophylaxis should be continued weekly through pregnancy and primaquine given after delivery.

Malaria prophylaxis during pregnancy is important to reduce the risk of acute malaria precipitating miscarriage, premature delivery, or stillbirth. Chloroquine or hydroxychloroquine are safe during pregnancy. Fansidar safety during pregnancy has not been completely determined but this drug is recommended to treat chloroquine-resistant *P. falciparum* malaria. Neither doxycycline nor primaquine should be used prophylactically during pregnancy.

Infants and children can contract malaria and should receive prophylaxis. Breast-fed infants do not receive sufficient antimalarial therapy through breast milk and should receive recommended doses of antimalarial agents. Children under the age of 8 years should not receive tetracyclines, and Fansidar is contraindicated in infants younger than 2 months. Chloroquine phosphate is manufactured in the United States only in tablet form and is quite bitter. Pediatric doses should be calculated carefully according to body weight, with pharmacists preparing capsules of calculated pediatric doses. Alternatively, chloroquine in suspension is widely available overseas.

SUGGESTED READING

Centers for Disease Control. Recommendations for the prevention of malaria in travelers. MMWR 1988; 37:277–284.

Chiodini PL, Somerville M, Salam I, et al. Exchange transfusion in severe falciparum malaria. Trans R Soc Trop Med Hyg 1985; 79:865–866.

Lobel HO, Roberts JM, Somaini B, Steffen R. Efficacy of malaria prophylaxis in American and Swiss travelers to Kenya. J Infect Dis 1987; 155:1205–1209.

Phillips RE, Warrell DA, White NJ, et al. Intravenous quinidine for the treatment of severe falciparum malaria. N Engl J Med 1985; 312:1273–1278.

Warhurst DC. Antimalarial drugs: an update. Drugs 1987; 33:50–65.

Wyler DJ. *Plasmodium* species (malaria). In: Mandell GL, Douglas RG Jr, Bennett JE, eds. Principles and practice of infectious diseases. 2nd ed. New York: John Wiley & Sons, 1985:1514.

AMEBIASIS AND GIARDIASIS

JONATHAN I. RAVDIN, M.D.

AMEBIASIS

Entamoeba histolytica is an enteric protozoan that infects 10 percent of the world's population, resulting in 50 to 100 million cases of invasive colitis or liver abscess per year and up to 100,000 deaths. The prevalence is highest in developing countries with poor levels of sanitation; however, modern travel and rates of emigration and the existence of high-risk groups require that physicians throughout the world be familiar with the diverse clinical disease syndromes due to *E. histolytica* and the varied agents used for treatment. The key to diagnosis and treatment of amebiasis is knowledge of the epidemiologic risk factors and clinical manifestations, a rational diagnostic approach, and an understanding of the sites of action of antiamebic drugs.

Epidemiologic Risk Factors

Highly endemic areas include Mexico, India, West and South Africa, and areas of Central and South America. Immigrants from or travelers to these areas are at risk (Table 1); amebic liver abscess occurs within 5 months after leaving an endemic area. An increased incidence of invasive amebiasis in the southwestern United States is solely due to disease in immigrants from Mexico. Institutionalized individuals, especially the mentally retarded, and those living in a communal setting are at particular risk. The oral-anal practices of sexually promiscuous male homosexuals result in a high prevalence of amebic infection. Severe invasive amebiasis can occur in the very young (under age 2 years), pregnant women, malnourished individuals, and those given corticosteroids, the latter often for an incorrect diagnosis of idiopathic inflammatory bowel disease.

Clinical Syndromes and Manifestations

E. histolytica infection has diverse clinical presentations (Table 2). Most common is asymptomatic intestinal luminal infection without evidence of tissue invasion (absence of

TABLE 2   Clinical Syndromes Due to Infection by *Entamoeba histolytica*

Asymptomatic cyst passers (colonization)
Symptomatic cyst passers
Acute rectocolitis
Fulminant colitis
  Toxic megacolon
  Perforation with peritonitis
Chronic nondysenteric colitis
Ameboma
Liver abscess
Peritonitis
Lung abscess, empyema
Pericarditis
Brain abscess
Venereal disease
Cutaneous disease

TABLE 3   Clinical Manifestations of Acute Amebic Colitis

Bloody mucoid diarrhea of 1–4 weeks' duration
Abdominal pain, weight loss
Bloating, tenesmus, cramps
Fever (in only one-third of individuals)
Diffuse abdominal and right upper-quadrant tenderness
Heme-positive stools (in 100%)
Fecal leukocytes variably present

serum antiamebic antibodies, blood in the stool, and mucosal alterations on colonoscopy). Nonspecific symptoms such as bloating, cramps, or decreased appetite have been reported in individuals with noninvasive *E. histolytica* infection; however, the etiologic association of such symptoms is unclear. Amebic colitis (Table 3) has a subacute onset characterized by dysenteric stools; fever occurs in only one-third of individuals. Despite the presence of mucosal ulceration and heme-positive stools, fecal leukocytes may be absent due to the parasite's ability to lyse host neutrophils. Fulminant colitis often results in perforation with peritonitis and has a poor prognosis. Chronic amebic colitis is clinically indistinguishable from idiopathic inflammatory bowel disease presenting with low-grade disease and recurrent episodes of bloody diarrhea. Ameboma is a localized chronic amebic

TABLE 1   Epidemiologic Risk Factors That Apparently Predispose to *Entamoeba histolytica* Infection and Increased Severity of Disease

Prevalence	*Increased Severity*

Lower socioeconomic status in an endemic area including:
  Crowding
  No indoor plumbing
	Children, especially neonates
	Pregnancy and postpartum states
	Corticosteroid use
	Malignancy
	Malnutrition

Immigrants from endemic area	
Institutionalized population; especially mentally retarded	
Communal living	
Promiscuous male homosexuals	

Reprinted with permission from Amebiasis: human infection by *Entamoeba histolytica*. Ravdin JI, ed. New York: John Wiley & Sons, 1988:496.

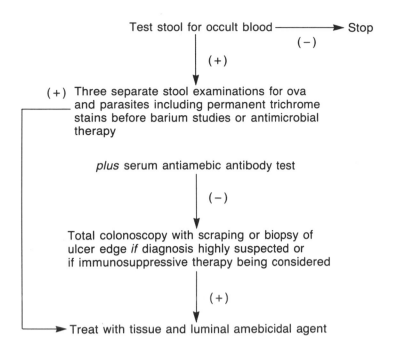

Test stool for occult blood ⟶ Stop

(−)

(+)

(+) Three separate stool examinations for ova and parasites including permanent trichrome stains before barium studies or antimicrobial therapy

plus serum antiamebic antibody test

(−)

Total colonoscopy with scraping or biopsy of ulcer edge *if* diagnosis highly suspected or if immunosuppressive therapy being considered

(+)

Treat with tissue and luminal amebicidal agent

Figure 1   Diagnostic evaluation for acute amebic rectocolitis in a patient with suggestive epidemiology and clinical manifestations.

infection commonly occurring in the cecum or ascending colon that presents as a painful abdominal mass often mistaken on barium enema for a carcinoma.

Amebic liver abscess classically presents with right upper-quadrant pain, fever, and point tenderness over the liver (Table 4). Patients usually present acutely but may exhibit a chronic syndrome in which weight loss and pain predominate. Nonspecific laboratory abnormalities include leukocytosis, elevation of alkaline phosphatase and transaminase, decreased serum albumin and cholesterol, and proteinuria. Elevated bilirubin with jaundice is unusual. Left lobe abscesses are more likely to rupture, with resultant peritonitis or extension to the pericardium, resulting in cardiac tamponade. Pulmonary disease can result from direct extension from a liver abscess or less commonly by hematogeneous spread. Brain abscess is very uncommon; genital infection has been reported in India and can be confused with penile or cervical carcinoma.

Differential Diagnosis and Approach to the Patient

Diagnosis of intestinal amebiasis rests on examination of the stool or mucosal tissue by a skilled microscopist (Fig. 1). Virtually all patients test positive for occult blood; this is a useful, inexpensive screening test. As discussed, the absence or presence of fecal leukocytes is noncontributory. Three separate stool examinations are required to detect 90 percent of infected individuals; interfering substances such as barium, laxatives, antibiotics, and soap enemas should be avoided. Handling of samples and preparation of stained slides are detailed in the Suggested Reading (see below).

Barium x-ray films do not differentiate amebiasis from other types of colonic ulceration. Serum antiamebic antibodies are detected in more than 85 percent of patients with invasive colitis; however, as antiamebic antibodies persist for years in a highly endemic area, these titers may not differentiate acute from remote infection. This is especially true with the indirect hemagglutination assay; gel diffusion, counterimmunoelectrophoresis, or latex agglutination often become negative 6 months after cure of invasive disease and may be useful in differentiating acute from remote infection.

Total colonoscopy with scraping or biopsy of the ulcer edge is definitive. The diagnostic yield is very high and allows for evaluation of patients with ascending colon disease, who often have negative stool examinations. If there is a strong suspicion or a need for immediate diagnosis, colonoscopy should be performed even if the stool examination is negative. Colonoscopy must be performed with care because of the risk of perforation. A tissue diagnosis is especially indicated if corticosteroid therapy is being considered for inflammatory bowel disease. The differential diagnosis

TABLE 4   Clinical Manifestations of Amebic Liver Abscess

Fever
Right upper-quadrant pain
Weight loss
Diarrhea (in 20–40% of individuals)
Exquisite point tenderness over the liver
Hepatomegaly (in <50%)
Elevated white blood cell count, alkaline phosphatase, transaminases, sedimentation rate
Decreased cholesterol and serum albumin levels
Abnormal urinalysis

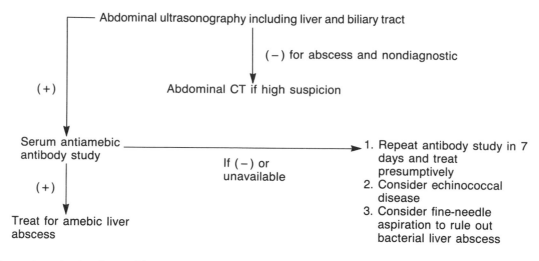

Figure 2 Diagnostic evaluation for amebic liver abscess in a patient with suggestive epidemiology and clinical manifestations.

for acute rectocolitis includes shigellosis, salmonellosis, campylobacteriosis, yersinia infection, invasive *Escherichia coli*, or other less common etiologies of inflammatory diarrhea.

The first step in approaching patients with possible amebic liver abscess (Fig. 2) is to perform an ultrasound examination of the liver and biliary tract. This sensitive nontoxic method detects cavities in the liver or stones and obstruction in the biliary tract. Abdominal computed tomography (CT) may be slightly more sensitive in detecting and delineating a liver abscess but should be reserved for patients with an equivocal nondiagnostic ultrasound examination. Serum antiamebic antibodies are eventually present in 99 percent of patients with amebic liver abscess; however, individuals presenting with fewer than 7 days of symptoms often lack serum antiamebic antibody. In the latter case, a study should be repeated 7 days after presentation.

The differential diagnosis of amebic liver abscess includes pyogenic abscess, echinococcal cyst, and hepatoma. Patients with bacterial abscesses are usually older and have biliary tract disease or abdominal malignancy or have had recent surgery. If the epidemiologic history, clinical profile, and serologic studies are nondiagnostic, a fine-needle aspirate under ultrasound or CT guidance can be performed to rule out bacterial disease. The yield for detection of *E. histolytica* trophozoites is low, especially after initiation of antiamebic therapy. Specific serologic studies must be performed prior to aspiration if there is any clinical suspicion of an echinococcal cyst because of the risk of peritoneal spillage and resultant prophylaxis or seeding.

Therapy and Management

It is uncertain whether noninvasive *E. histolytica* luminal infection requires treatment. Because individuals so infected may develop invasive disease or put others at risk for transmission, I favor eradicating the parasite. Such patients also frequently develop nonspecific gastrointestinal complaints that are difficult to differentiate from the onset of invasive amebiasis. However, I would not routinely screen asymptomatic individuals for amebic infection, nor has mass therapy of institutionalized individuals proved useful.

Agents that successfully eradicate intraluminal infection (Table 5) cannot be relied upon for treatment of deep tissue invasion. For patients with no evidence of invasive amebiasis, diloxanide furoate is the drug of choice. Unfortunately, in the United States this is available only from the Parasite Disease Drug Service of the Centers for Disease Control (CDC), Atlanta, Georgia (telephone 404-329-3670). Intestinal esterases hydrolyze the ester, diloxanide furoate, to the absorbable product, diloxanide. Delayed absorption accounts for high concentrations of diloxanide furoate in the large bowel lumen; adverse effects are uncommon and include flatulence or other mild gastrointestinal complaints. Paromomycin is a highly efficacious nonabsorbable aminoglycoside that is especially advantageous for use in pregnant women or children. Its main adverse effect is increased frequency of stools; in patients with amebic colitis, renal failure or other signs of aminoglycoside toxicity have not been noted. Diiodohydroxyquin is lowest on the list because of the long duration of therapy required, gastrointestinal toxicity, and other less common adverse effects such as fever, headache, generalized furunculosis, and interference with thyroid function tests due to its high iodine content (63 percent).

Metronidazole is the mainstay for treatment of invasive amebiasis. Outside of the United States, an efficacious and less-toxic nitroimidazole, tinidazole, is available and preferred (dose, 2 or 50 mg per kilogram orally once daily for 3 days). Metronidazole distributes throughout the tissues and is metabolized mainly in the liver. Limiting factors for clinical use include its potential carcinogenicity, substantial frequency of gastrointestinal intolerance, disulfiram (Antabuse) effect, and rare neurologic toxicities. The short-course regimens cited (Table 5) may be better tolerated. Urine from patients receiving metronidazole causes genetic changes in bacteria; studies of humans do not reveal a carcinogenic effect, but large-scale, long-term follow-up is lacking. Ten days of

TABLE 5 Therapy for Amebiasis

Presentation, Agent	Adult Dose	Pediatric Dose
Intraluminal infection		
Diloxanide furoate	500 mg orally t.i.d. × 10 days	20 mg/kg/day in 3 divided doses × 10 days
Paromomycin	30 mg/kg/day in 3 divided doses for 10 days	25 mg/kg/day in 3 divided doses × 7 days
Diiodohydroxyquin	650 mg orally t.i.d. × 20 days	30 mg/kg/day in 3 divided doses × 20 days
Invasive colitis		
Metronidazole*	750 mg orally t.i.d. or 500 mg IV q6h × 10 days	35 mg/kg/day in 3 divided doses × 10 days
Metronidazole*	2.4 g PO, single dose	
Tetracycline*†	250 mg orally t.i.d. × 10 days	Adults only
Erythromycin*†	500 mg orally q.i.d. × 10 days	Adults only
Dehydroemetine*	1 mg/kg/day (maximum 90 mg/day) IM in 2 divided doses × 5 days in hospital	Same as in adults, maximum of 60 mg/day
Liver abscess‡		
Metronidazole*†	750 mg PO t.i.d. or 500 mg IV q6h × 10 days	35 mg/kg/day in 3 divided doses × 10 days
Dehydroemetine*†	1 mg/kg/day IM × 5 days in hospital	Same as in adults

* Followed by a drug for luminal infection.
† Chloroquine (base) 600 mg orally per day for 2 days and 300 mg base orally per day for adults and 10 mg base/kg/day for children for 14–21 days is added by some clinicians for severe disease.
‡ Liver abscess needle aspiration only if no response to therapy for 5–7 days or high risk of abscess rupture.

metronidazole will also eliminate intraluminal infection in up to 90 percent of patients; therefore, use of a second agent may not be needed in individuals who complete the whole 10-day course of metronidazole. All patients treated for amebic colitis require careful follow-up stool examinations or colonoscopy to document cure; relapse occurs in 10 percent or more.

In patients who cannot tolerate metronidazoles, tetracycline or erythromycin followed by an intraluminal agent can be used for treatment of colitis, but this therapy will not eradicate amebae in the liver. Chloroquine is active only in the liver and can be added as a third agent; I prefer to avoid its use and carefully follow patients for evidence of hepatic involvement. Dehydroemetine is also available from the Parasite Disease Drug Service of the CDC; emetines have multiple adverse effects including gastrointestinal toxicity in up to 50 percent of patients; neuromuscular complaints including muscle weakness, tenderness, and stiffness; and most importantly, cardiovascular complications such as hypotension, chest pain, electrocardiogram abnormalities (T-wave inversion and prolonged QT interval in 25 to 50 percent), and tachycardia, which may be followed by congestive cardiomyopathy. Patients receiving emetines must be hospitalized and subject to continual monitoring of their cardiac status.

Amebic colitis can be fulminant in pregnant women; metronidazole did not cause untoward effects in one uncontrolled study of 216 pregnant women and should be used for severe amebic disease in this setting. Mild disease can be treated with paromomycin; pregnant women with asymptomatic colonization should be observed or treated with paromomycin. Intestinal perforation during amebic colitis is usually best managed conservatively with antiamebic and antibacterial therapy; attempts at surgical resection should be avoided. Only patients with toxic megacolon require surgery, usually a total colectomy.

Metronidazole alone is adequate initial therapy for amebic liver abscess. Some clinicians add chloroquine or dehydroemetine; however, there are no controlled studies indicating this improves the outcome, and I do not recommend it. Most patients will respond gradually over 3 to 5 days with a decrease in fever, right upper-quadrant pain, and other constitutional complaints. In patients who show no response by 5 to 7 days, aspiration of the abscess may be beneficial. One should also reconsider other diagnostic possibilities. An occasional patient may require open drainage or the addition of a second agent after aspiration, but this is unusual. Therapeutic aspiration of the abscess on presentation is indicated only if the abscess is very large and appears to be at high risk for rupture. Risks of needle aspiration include bacterial suprainfection. Resolution of the abscess cavity is a long-term process, requiring a median of 7 months. Patients should be followed clinically; persistence of a cavity in an asymptomatic individual is not an indication for invasive procedures. Up to one-fifth of patients will have a permanent hepatic cyst.

Avoiding fecal-oral contamination is the only effective means of preventing *E. histolytica* infection. A vaccine is not available; chemoprophylaxis has not been studied nor is it recommended. Boiling is the only certain means of eradicating *E. histolytica* cysts in water. Precautions such as avoidance of uncooked vegetables, salads, fruits that cannot be peeled, and ice cubes are advisable for travelers.

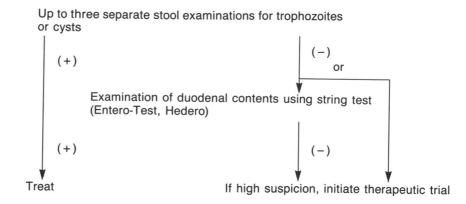

Figure 3 Diagnostic evaluation for giardiasis in a patient with suggestive epidemiology and clinical manifestations.

GIARDIASIS

Giardia lamblia, the most common parasitic cause of diarrhea worldwide, produces appreciable discomfort but not significant mortality. Giardiasis is generally a disease of the very young and presents in nonimmune adults who travel to an endemic area or interface with intense foci of infection in the developed world. The clinical syndrome resulting from *G. lamblia* infection is highly characteristic, easily recognized, and often treated even if the parasite cannot be demonstrated (but one should try). It is unclear whether asymptomatic infection in an endemic area or day care setting merits therapy.

Epidemiologic Risk Factors

At least 23 waterborne outbreaks of giardiasis have been reported; sporadic waterborne acquisition also clearly occurs, with beavers as well as humans implicated. Person-to-person spread in day care centers or among children in the developing world and among sexually promiscuous male homosexuals is also significant. Infection rates in the day care setting can approach 50 percent (Table 6); symptomatic disease occurs in a portion of infected individuals as well as frequent spread of infection to contacts in the home. *Giardia* cysts survive for weeks in surface water, especially at low temperatures. Institutionalized populations are at risk; as mentioned, foreign travel is also important. In addition to a high prevalence in developing countries, areas of the Soviet Union are notorious sites for the acquisition of giardiasis. The majority of infected individuals spontaneously clear the infection and are resistant to rechallenge; however, recent studies of antigenic variation in *G. lamblia* raise the possibility that the parasite can escape from host immune surveillance.

Clinical Manifestations

Up to 70 percent of individuals infected with *G. lamblia* have no manifestations of infection and spontaneously clear the parasite. This is especially so in the very young. Recent studies of experimental infection in volunteers suggest that pathogenicity is strain rather than host specific. After an incubation period of 1 to 2 weeks, infection can manifest as an acute diarrheal syndrome, with watery stools progressing to foul, greasy, malodorous diarrhea (Table 7). Bloating, flatulence, and abdominal cramps are characteristic. Although symptoms may resolve in 3 or 4 days, most patients have persistent complaints for weeks. The stool is heme-negative, and fecal leukocytes are absent. Given appropriate epidemiologic risk factors, the characteristic symptoms and duration of illness are pathognomonic for giardiasis. A minority of these patients have persistent complaints of diarrhea, malaise, headache, and weight loss lasting months (Table 7). Symptoms can be intermittent; lactose intolerance is common and may persist for weeks after therapy.

TABLE 6 Epidemiologic Risk Factors That Apparently Predispose to *Giardia lamblia* Infection and Increased Severity of Disease

Prevalence	Increased Severity
Day care center exposure	Hypogammaglobulinemia
Institutionalization	Common variable type
Foreign travel	X-linked agammaglobulinemia
Ingestion of untreated surface water	? IgA deficiency
	Malnutrition
Promiscuous male homosexual behavior	

TABLE 7 Clinical Manifestations of Giardiasis

Acute diarrhea (days to weeks in duration)
  Diarrhea progresses from watery to greasy and foul-smelling
  Weight loss
  Bloating, flatulence
  Abdominal cramps
  Heme (−), no fecal leukocytes
Chronic diarrhea (>3 weeks in duration)
  Diarrhea: small volume, high frequency, greasy, foul-smelling
  Malaise, lassitude
  Headache
  Diffuse abdominal cramps
  Weight loss

Differential Diagnosis and Approach to the Patient

There are few infectious etiologies that produce the prolonged noninflammatory diarrhea seen in giardiasis. In patients just returned from foreign travel, or others with fewer than 5 days of symptoms, enterotoxigenic *E. coli* or rotavirus is most likely. I begin diagnostic evaluation (Fig. 3) when symptoms persist for more than 5 to 7 days or when the incubation period and risk factors suggest *G. lamblia* infection. Careful examination of three separate stool samples provides a diagnostic yield of up to 90 percent. In a patient with suggestive risk factors and clinical syndrome, if the stool examinations are negative, examination of duodenal contents by a string test may be helpful. Although this is suggested by some studies, in practice one rarely finds a positive string test in a patient with three negative stool examinations. A therapeutic trial, if there are no contraindications, is certainly reasonable and preferable, in my opinion, to performing a duodenal aspirate or biopsy. Patients infected with *G. lamblia* do develop a serum antibody response, but such studies are not yet available for routine clinical use.

Therapy

Many authorities consider quinacrine (Atabrine) the drug of choice for treatment of giardiasis (Table 8). However, given the occasional severe side effect of toxic psychosis as well as other toxicities, including yellow staining of sclerae and skin, gastrointestinal upset, and rarely exfoliative dermatitis, I and many other clinicians prefer to use metronidazole as initial therapy. The toxicities and carcinogenic potential of metronidazole are discussed in the section on amebiasis. Metronidazole, 250 mg orally three times daily for 10 days, has been reported to cure up to 90 percent of individuals, but many adult patients may require the higher dose (750 mg three times daily) for eradication of the parasite. Although metronidazole is better tolerated than quinacrine in children, the U.S. Food and Drug Administration has not officially approved metronidazole for the treatment of giardiasis; its potential risks should be carefully considered before its use. Shorter courses of other nitroimidazoles, such as tinidazole (single dose of 2 g), have been found to be highly efficacious, but these agents are not available in the United States. Furazolidone, a nitrofuran available in a liquid suspension, is useful for treatment of young children, with approximately 80 percent efficacy in the doses described (Table 8). Although it too has gastrointestinal tox-

TABLE 8 Therapy for Giardiasis

Agent	Adult Dose	Pediatric Dose
Metronidazole	750 mg PO t.i.d. × 10 days	15 mg/kg/day PO in 3 divided doses × 7–10 days
Quinacrine	100 mg orally t.i.d. × 7 days	6 mg/kg/day PO in 3 divided doses × 7 days
Furazolidone		8 mg/kg/day PO in 4 divided doses × 10 days
Paromomycin	30 mg/kg/day PO in 3 divided doses × 10 days, especially for pregnant women	Same as adult dose

icity, can turn urine brown, and can cause mild hemolysis in G6PD-deficient individuals, furazolidone is usually better tolerated than quinacrine. Paromomycin is a reasonable alternative agent, especially for use in pregnant patients for whom a nonabsorbable agent is ideal.

Prevention of giardiasis requires avoidance of person-to-person fecal-oral contact and proper handling and treatment of community water supplies. All backcountry surface water should be considered infectious. Boiling water is the most effective means of eradication of cysts; efficacy of added halogens may depend on water temperature and the level of proteinaceous sediment present. Rigorous hand-washing practices in highly endemic foci, such as day care centers, and avoidance of sexual activities that result in fecal-oral contact should be advised.

SUGGESTED READING

Davidson RA. Issues in clinical parasitology: the treatment of giardiasis. Am J Gastroenterol 1984; 79:256–261.

Drugs for parasitic infections. Med Lett Drugs Ther 1986; 28(issue 706): January 31.

Ravdin JI. Intestinal disease caused by *Entamoeba histolytica*. In: Ravdin JI, ed. Amebiasis: human infection by *Entamoeba histolytica*. New York: John Wiley and Sons, 1988:495.

Ravdin JI, Guerrant RL. Current problems in diagnosis and treatment of amebic infections. In: Remington JS, Swartz MN, eds. Current clinical topics in infectious diseases 7. New York: McGraw-Hill, 1980:82.

Reed SL, Braude AI. Extraintestinal disease: clinical syndromes, diagnostic profile, and therapy. In: Ravdin JI, ed. Amebiasis: human infection by *Entamoeba histolytica*. New York: John Wiley and Sons, 1988:511.

TOXOPLASMOSIS

GREGORY A. FILICE, M.D.

Toxoplasma gondii is an ubiquitous protozoan parasite that infects about half of all humans during their lifetimes. Infections in healthy people are usually mild or asympto-

matic. In contrast, primary infection or reactivation of latent infection can be devastating in immunosuppressed people, and treatment is necessary to arrest the process. Women who become infected during pregnancy and who choose not to interrupt the pregnancy should be treated to prevent congenital infection or lessen its severity. Congenitally infected neonates should be treated to prevent progression of the infection and the appearance of sequelae.

Since severe disease is infrequent and often not recognized, there are few systematic studies of therapy. Recommendations are based on clinical experience, anecdotes, and uncontrolled series of treated patients. Clinicians should be prepared to modify their approach in particular clinical circumstances based on the growing knowledge of the pathogenesis *T. gondii* infection. Important facts and principles underlying therapy will be presented in this chapter to allow for rational implementation of the recommendations.

TOXOPLASMA GONDII

T. gondii is a coccidian protozoan parasite of worldwide distribution that infects a wide variety of birds, mammals, and probably reptiles. After an animal ingests an infective form of the parasite, tachyzoites are formed in the intestine and cross the intestinal wall to enter the circulation. They disseminate throughout the body, and after a brief proliferative phase, they give rise to tissue cysts containing up to several hundred, single-celled bradyzoites. Tissue cysts often persist for the life of the host. After the death of the host, the cysts are infectious if ingested along with the tissues by another animal.

Members of the cat family are the definitive hosts for *T. gondii* and support a sexual cycle. The parasite forms oocysts in the intestine that are shed in the feces from 7 to 20 days after acute infection. The oocysts sporulate in the next 2 to 5 days and become infectious. Sporulated oocysts remain infectious for months.

Like other animals, humans become infected by ingesting oocysts or by eating raw or lightly cooked meat. Since oocysts are hardy, it is thought that many infections occur through ingestion of contaminated vegetables or through contact with soil contaminated with cat feces. The prevalence of infection in adults varies throughout the world from 15 to 85 percent. It tends to be higher in the tropics and lower in colder climates, but there are exceptions.

DIAGNOSIS

Serology

Serologic study is the means of diagnosis in most patients suspected of having toxoplasmosis. A discussion of the most helpful serologic tests will enable the reader to understand the present recommendations for therapy.

Tests can be divided into those that measure IgG antibody and those that measure IgM. The Sabin-Feldman dye test (DT) is the standard for measurement of IgG antibodies. Other useful tests for IgG antibodies that usually produce similar results are the agglutination test for IgG antibody (performed with 2-mercaptoethanol to inactivate IgM) and the indirect fluorescent antibody (IFA) test for IgG. Titers rise rapidly after infection, usually before the onset of symptoms and typically to 1,000 or more. High titers persist for months to years and then gradually fall, but IgG antibodies rarely disappear.

There are three useful tests for IgM antibody. The double-sandwich IgM enzyme-linked immunosorbent assay (DS-IgM-ELISA) and IgM immunosorbent assay (IgM-ISA)

are similar. They become positive soon after infection in most infected people and persist for several months to 2 or 3 years. The IgM-IFA test, the original test for IgM antibodies, is less sensitive and remains positive for a shorter time, usually a few months.

The indirect hemagglutination test (IHA) usually becomes positive several weeks after infection and after the IgG tests mentioned above become positive. Since the test is often negative early in infection, it is not useful for screening pregnant women. IHA titers may still rise after other titers have stabilized or are falling.

The behavior of the complement fixation test (CF) depends on the nature of the antigen, and there is no widely accepted standard. With cytoplasmic antigens, the test behaves like the IHA. With cell-membrane antigens, the test behaves more like the DT.

Demonstration of Organisms in Tissues

Tachyzoites in areas of inflammation are indicative of active replication and disease. They are rarely found in the lymph nodes of healthy people with acute lymphadenopathic toxoplasmosis. Cysts can be found in tissues of latently infected people, especially muscle, heart, and brain, but they do not indicate active replication and cannot be taken as evidence of active *T. gondii* infection.

Mouse Inoculation

T. gondii is isolated by inoculation into mice. Material should be triturated if necessary and injected intraperitoneally. If mice sicken or die, peritoneal fluid should be examined for tachyzoites. Unfortunately, many strains are not pathogenic for mice. Such strains are detected by testing serum from the mice for IgG antibody to *T. gondii*.

CLINICAL ILLNESS

Acute Acquired Infection in Immunocompetent People

Most immunocompetent people who become infected with *T. gondii* are asymptomatic. Between 10 and 20 percent have a mild, self-limited illness 1 to 3 weeks after infection, which is usually characterized by fever and lymphadenopathy. Rarely, manifestations of acute acquired toxoplasmosis include encephalitis, myocarditis, hepatitis, pneumonitis, polymyositis, or persistent fevers. The diagnosis is often suggested by the characteristic lymph node histologic findings, characterized by (1) reactive follicular hyperplasia with irregular clusters of epithelioid histiocytes that encroach upon and blur the margins of germinal centers and (2) focal distention of sinuses with monocytoid cells.

The syndrome is not specific, and the diagnosis is usually made by serologic studies. IgG antibody is common in the population, often with relatively high titers. A single positive test for IgG antibody is not sufficient for the diagnosis, although a very high titer ($\geq 16,000$) is suggestive. Usually the titer of IgG antibody has peaked by the time symptoms bring the patient to a physician, and rising titers are seldom documented. IgM antibody should be measured in all patients suspected of having acute toxoplasmosis. A high ($\geq$ 1:2,000) titer of IgG antibody with a positive IgM test in a patient with a compatible clinical syndrome is diagnostic. Exact timing of recent infections can be difficult because IgG titers typically remain 1:2,000 or higher for months to years and the sensitive DS-IgM-ELISA or IgM-ISA tests often remain positive for 2 to 3 years.

Retinochoroiditis

Retinochoroiditis without other manifestations of active disease is usually a late manifestation of congenital infection. In this case it is usually bilateral. Retinochoroiditis occurs in fewer than 1 percent of cases of acute acquired toxoplasmosis, usually only in one eye. Retinochoroiditis is common in infants with generalized congenital toxoplasmosis and in immunocompromised people with reactivated toxoplasmosis.

The diagnosis is suggested by its characteristic ophthalmoscopic appearance. When the process is localized to the eye, serum IgG antibody titers are usually low and may be detectable only in undiluted serum. If antibody is not detected in undiluted serum, eye disease is unlikely to be caused by T. gondii. In patients in whom the retinal appearance is equivocal, the likelihood of the diagnosis is increased if local antibody production can be demonstrated (the ratio of IgG antibody to T. gondii/total IgG in aqueous humor is greater than the ratio of IgG antibody to T. gondii/total IgG in serum.

Toxoplasmosis in Immunosuppressed Patients

People with profound T lymphocyte deficits are unusually susceptible to severe toxoplasmosis, generally from reactivation of latent infection. Common associated conditions include lymphoid malignancies, organ transplantation, and the acquired immunodeficiency syndrome (AIDS). When seronegative organ transplant recipients receive an organ from a seropositive donor, severe toxoplasmosis may occur. Seropositive recipients frequently have increases in antibody to T. gondii during immunosuppressive therapy, but severe toxoplasmosis in these recipients is uncommon.

The most commonly recognized manifestation is encephalitis, which often progresses to necrosis of brain tissue. Computed tomography typically shows low-density masses with ring enhancement and mass effects, but a variety of patterns can occur. Toxoplasmosis of the central nervous system (CNS) should be considered in any AIDS patient with a focal or diffuse CNS lesion. Other common manifestations include pneumonitis, myocarditis, and fever without focal findings. Diagnosis and management are complicated by the fact that these severely immunosuppressed people often have concurrent opportunistic infections.

Recent attention has been focused on disease in AIDS patients. From 15 to 50 percent of adults in the United States are seropositive for T. gondii infection, depending on the region. Approximately 30 percent of seropositive AIDS pa-

tients will develop clinical toxoplasmosis. Nearly all AIDS patients with active toxoplasmosis have IgG antibody; the absence of IgG antibody makes the diagnosis unlikely. However, IgG titers are usually low and stable, and IgM antibody to T. gondii is usually undetectable.

A recent retrospective study indicated that IgG antibody produced locally in CNS toxoplasmosis was secreted into the cerebrospinal fluid (CSF) in sufficient quantitities to help with the diagnosis. In patients with CNS toxoplasmosis, the ratio of specific IgG antibody to total IgG was usually greater in the CSF than in the serum:

$$\frac{CSF\ DT^{-1}}{[CSF\ IgG]} > \frac{serum\ DT^{-1}}{[serum\ IgG]} \ .$$

This was not the case in patients with other CNS diseases. Further prospective experience will be necessary to determine the reliability of the detection of local production of specific IgG.

A definitive diagnosis can be made by obtaining brain tissue for histopathologic study. In cases in which the diagnosis is not apparent from traditional stains, the more sensitive immunochemical staining should be performed. Alternatively, when the clinical presentation is suggestive of T. gondii infection, patients and clinicians may decide to avoid the risk and discomfort associated with brain biopsy and undertake a therapeutic trial directed against T. gondii.

Infection During Pregnancy

The major risk from toxoplasmosis in pregnant women is congenital infection. The risk of transmission to babies born to mothers with primary infection occurring during the first, second, or third trimester is 15, 20, and 60 percent, respectively. In contrast, congenital transmission from mothers who were infected before conception is exceedingly rare; for practical purposes, infants born to women who were seropositive before conception are not at risk for congenital toxoplasmosis.

A major problem is that pregnant women with acute toxoplasmosis, like other healthy adults, are symptomatic only 10 to 20 percent of the time. Screening of women for antibodies to T. gondii should be undertaken before pregnancy and at monthly intervals during pregnancy to detect asymptomatic or mild infections.

For screening, IgG antibody to T. gondii should be measured by DT, agglutination, or IFA. If women are seropositive before pregnancy, further testing is not necessary. If the first test is done after conception, a positive titer should be followed by a test for IgM antibody.

The interpretation of positive serology when the first titer was obtained during pregnancy can be difficult. In the first 6 to 8 weeks after infection, IgG titers are usually unstable; a stable IgG titer in the first 2 months of pregnancy usually signifies infection acquired before pregnancy. After the second month, if the IgG titer is 2,000 or greater or there is IgM antibody, there is a substantial likelihood that infection was acquired during pregnancy.

TABLE 1 Specificity, Sensitivity, and Predictive Value of Nonspecific Tests for Congenital Toxoplasmosis in 746 Pregnancies with Maternal Toxoplasmosis

Test	Specificity (%)	Sensitivity (%)	Predictive value Positive Test (%)	Predictive value Negative Test (%)
Ultrasound findings	99.8	45	95	97
Biologic tests				
White blood cell count	97	38	42	96
Eosinophil count	94	19	17	95
Platelet count	98	28	52	96
Total IgM antibody	97	52	49	97
IgM antibody to *T. gondii*	100	21	100	96
γ-Glutamyl transferase	97	57	52	97
Lactate dehydrogenase	98	17	33	95
Total IgM + white blood cell count	99.8	21	90	96
Total IgM + platelet count	100	21	100	96
γ-Glutamyl transferase + white blood cell count	99.8	26	91	96
γ-Glutamyl transferase + total IgM	99	38	64	96

Adapted from Daffos et al. Prenatal management of 746 pregnancies at risk for congenital toxoplasmosis. N Engl J Med 1988; 318:271–275.

Diagnosis of Fetal Infection

If infection is suspected in a woman during pregnancy, attempts at fetal diagnosis should be made. Between 20 and 28 weeks of gestation, fetal blood should be obtained and tested for the titer of IgM antibodies against *T. gondii* and for concentrations of total IgM antibodies, γ-glutamyl transpeptidase, lactate dehydrogenase, white blood cells, platelets, and eosinophils. A portion should be inoculated into mice for culture. Every 2 weeks ultrasound examinations should be performed to determine the size of the cerebral ventricles and the thickness of the placenta and to seek evidence for fetal ascites, hepatomegaly, or intracranial calcification. The likelihood that congenital infection has occurred should be estimated from these specific and nonspecific indicators (Table 1), and a decision should be made by the woman and her physician. One of three options can be offered: therapy for the mother to arrest fetal infection, termination of the pregnancy, or no treatment.

Congenital Infection

Infection acquired in utero can result in abortion, prematurity, stillbirth, or congenital infection. Only a minority of children with congenital infections are symptomatic at birth. Manifestations include fever, hydrocephalus, microcephalus, hepatosplenomegaly, jaundice, convulsions, chorioretinitis, cerebral calcifications, rash, abnormal CSF (mononuclear pleocytosis and xanthochromia), myocarditis, pneumonitis, deafness, erythroblastosis-like syndrome, thrombocytopenia, lymphocytosis, monocytosis, and nephrotic syndrome. Symptoms are more common at birth in those whose mothers were infected earlier during pregnancy. If those who are asymptomatic are not treated, the majority

will develop neurologic, ocular, or other abnormalities later in life. Treatment appears to reduce the risk of sequelae, and all congenitally infected children should be treated.

In cases of suspected congenital toxoplasmosis, portions of the placenta should be inoculated into mice. Infants should have IgG and IgM titers performed at birth and periodically afterwards. IgM antibody is strongly suggestive of the diagnosis. IgM can be of maternal origin if there has been a leak in the placental barrier, but IgM has a half-life of only 8 days, and the titer in such cases should quickly disappear. If IgM antibody persists or increases in titer, the diagnosis is confirmed. One-fourth of congenitally infected infants will have IgM detectable by IgM-IFA and three-fourths will have IgM detectable by DS-IgM-ELISA. IgG crosses the placenta, and its half-life in the infant is approximately 30 days, which makes early diagnosis difficult. Titers should be followed monthly. If they do not decrease or if they begin to increase, the diagnosis is confirmed. An earlier diagnosis can sometimes be made by calculating "antibody load," the ratio of IgG antibody against *T. gondii* to total IgG. Ordinarily, by the second or third month the ratio falls in uninfected infants with passively acquired maternal antibody. In congenitally infected infants, the ratio levels off and begins to increase as the infant begins to make specific antibody against *T. gondii*.

THERAPEUTIC APPROACH

Chemotherapy

The combination of pyramethamine and sulfadiazine is the standard therapy for toxoplasmosis. The combination has been used extensively in humans, and it is synergistic in experimental infections in mice. Some other agents have activity in vitro or in experimental animals, but they have generally been less active in the laboratory than the combination of pyrimethamine and sulfadiazine. Several new agents are under active investigation, and these recommendations may be superseded over the next few years. When ranges of dosages are recommended, the exact dose should depend on severity of infection and the occurrence of any toxicity.

Pyrimethamine

Pyrimethamine (Daraprim, Chloridin, Malocide), a substituted phenylpyrimidine, inhibits folic acid production in *T. gondii* by interfering with dihydrofolate reductase. It is orally absorbed and has a half-life of 4.5 days in adults. I usually use 1 mg per kilogram per day, up to a maximum of 50 mg for the first 2 days and 25 mg thereafter. Daily doses of 50 mg for prolonged periods have been required in some AIDS patients. After a few weeks of therapy, I give pyrimethamine every 2 or 3 days because of its long half-life. For newborns being treated for congenital infection, I use 0.5 to 1 mg per kilogram per day.

The major toxicity of pyrimethamine is reversible dose-related bone marrow depression. Platelets are most commonly depressed, although leukopenia and anemia also occur. Pyrimethamine can also cause headache, gastrointestinal discomfort, and a bad taste in the mouth. Patients should have complete blood counts performed once or twice a week while taking pyrimethamine. Folinic acid can be absorbed by mammalian cells, but not by *T. gondii*, and it has been suggested that hematologic toxicity may be prevented or treated with folinic acid (citrovorum factor, leucovorin), 5 to 15 mg per day, but there is no good evidence that this is the case in humans.

Large doses of pyrimethamine are teratogenic in animals. Teratogenicity in humans has not been documented, but the drug should be avoided in the first 16 weeks of pregnancy. I recommend its use for documented fetal infection after 20 weeks of gestation (see below) because I believe that the potential benefits outweigh the potential risks in the latter half of pregnancy.

Sulfonamides

Sulfonamides inhibit *T. gondii* by preventing normal use of *p*-aminobenzoic acid in folate metabolism. Sulfadiazine and trisulfapyrimidines (sulfapyrazine, sulfadimidine, and sulfamerazine) are most active; all other sulfonamides are much less active. The half-life of sulfadiazine is 11 hours. I give a loading dose of 75 mg per kilogram (maximum, 4 g) followed by 100 to 150 mg per kilogram per day (maximum, 6 to 8 g per day). For newborns with congenital infection, I use 50 to 100 mg per kilogram per day. The exact dose depends upon the severity of infection and the occurrence of any toxicity.

A wide variety of toxicities have been associated with sulfonamides, including hemolytic anemia, aplastic anemia, agranulocytosis, thrombocytopenia, crystalluria, hepatitis, nephritis, neuritis, anorexia, nausea, vomiting, and reactions due to sensitization. Manifestations of sensitization include rash, arteritis, erythema multiforme, photosensitivity, serum sickness, and drug fever.

Spiramycin

Spiramycin, a macrolide antibiotic, is active against *T. gondii* in experimental animals, and there is clinical, uncontrolled evidence that it is effective in humans. The usual dose is 100 mg per kilogram per day in two to four divided doses.

Because spiramycin is a macrolide, its toxicity resembles that of erythromycin, but it is less toxic than erythromycin. Spiramycin is approved for use in Canada, Mexico, and Europe, but not in the United States. It can be obtained on an investigational basis for treatment of toxoplasmosis by contacting the Division of Antiviral Drug Products, U.S. Food and Drug Administration, Washington, D.C. (telephone, 301–443–0263).

Clindamycin

Clindamycin has activity against *T. gondii* in experimental animals, but its efficacy in humans is unproved. It is concentrated in the choroid, iris, and retina and has been used to treat retinochoroiditis. The usual dose is 15 to 30 mg per kilogram per day in four divided doses (maximum, 2,400 mg per day). Experience with such high doses in children is limited, and the maximal recommended dose for children is 20 mg per kilogram per day.

The most important toxic effect of clindamycin is diarrhea, especially from *Clostridium difficile* colitis. Other untoward effects include rashes, elevations of transaminase levels, granulocytopenia, thrombopenia, and anaphylaxis. Clindamycin has been administered locally through subconjunctival injection, but the toxicity of local therapy appears to outweigh the potential benefits.

Corticosteroids

Corticosteroids have been used to reduce inflammation in toxoplasmosis, especially for sight-threatening ocular disease or encephalitis. There is anecdotal evidence that they are effective in ocular disease, but they should always be used in conjunction with antimicrobial agents against *T. gondii*. I use prednisone, 1 to 2 mg per kilogram per day up to 75 mg per day maximum, or the equivalent. There is no good evidence that corticosteroids are effective for inflammation elsewhere in the body, including the CNS.

Therapy in Specific Clinical Circumstances

Acute Acquired Infection in Immunocompetent People

Most immunocompetent people with acute toxoplasmosis do not require specific therapy. Fevers may require treatment with antipyretics. If symptoms are unusually severe or prolonged, I use pyrimethamine and sulfadiazine. Where spiramycin is available, it may be used as a less-toxic, though probably less-effective, alternative. In the unusual cases when organs other than lymph nodes are clinically involved, I use antimicrobial therapy to prevent significant organ dysfunction.

Retinochoroiditis

Peripheral lesions that do not noticeably affect vision can be observed without the patient's receiving chemotherapy. If lesions progress, affect vision, or threaten important structures (i.e., macula, maculopapillary bundle, or optic nerve), pyrimethamine and sulfadiazine should be administered for 1 month. By 10 days, the borders of retinal lesions should sharpen, and vitreous haze should disappear. Steroids should be used in cases involving the macula, maculopapillary bundle, or optic nerve, always in conjunction with antiparasitic chemotherapy. Clindamycin appears to be an alternative for patients who cannot be treated with pyrimethamine and sulfadiazine.

Disease in Immunosuppressed Patients

Symptomatic toxoplasmosis in patients with severe T cell dysfunction should be treated with pyrimethamine and sulfonamides. The response is often slow and incomplete, and prolonged courses with high doses are often necessary.

Toxoplasmosis is common and particularly difficult to control in AIDS patients, and experiences with AIDS patients are redefining our approach to treatment. AIDS patients frequently become sensitized to sulfonamides and require nonstandard approaches. A few have been treated successfully with clindamycin and pyrimethamine. Others have been treated with 50 mg of pyrimethamine per day alone. The results are anecdotal and difficult to interpret because diagnoses are not always unequivocally established and because the underlying immunosuppression is progressive. At least three groups are studying therapy for toxoplasmosis in persons with AIDS, and further advances should be forthcoming.

Toxoplasmosis relapses in 50 percent or more of AIDS patients after therapy has been discontinued. I maintain AIDS patients on antimicrobial therapy with pyrimethamine and sulfadiazine for life to prevent relapse. I tailor the dose to avoid toxicity and still maintain effective blood levels. Other drugs, alone or in combination, have been used to prevent relapse, but none have emerged as effective substitutes for continual therapy with pyrimethamine and sulfadiazine.

Infection During Pregnancy

If toxoplasmosis is acquired during pregnancy, the parents and physician must decide between termination of the pregnancy and chemotherapy. If chemotherapy is chosen, I use 1 g of spiramycin three times daily, which appears to decrease the risk of fetal infection. Attempts to diagnose fetal infection should be made (see above). If fetal infection occurs and the decision is made to continue with the pregnancy, I prescribe pryimethamine, sulfadiazine, and folinic acid for the rest of the pregnancy.

Congenital Infection

I treat newborns having documented toxoplasmosis with courses of pyrimethamine, sulfadiazine, and folinic acid for 21 days and alternate this with courses of spiramycin for the balance of 2 months (38 to 41 days). If a newborn appears healthy and testing has not yet confirmed or excluded the possibility of congenital toxoplasmosis, I prescribe one course of pryimethamine and sulfadiazine followed by one course of spiramycin.

SUGGESTED READING

Daffos F, Forestier F, Capella-Pavlovsky M, et al. Prenatal management of 746 pregnancies at risk for congenital toxoplasmosis. N Engl J Med 1988; 318:271–275.

Hakes TB, Armstrong D. Toxoplasmosis. Problems in diagnosis and treatment. Cancer 1983; 52:1535–1540.

Luft BJ, Naot Y, Araujo F, Stinson EB, Remington JS. Primary and reactivated toxoplasma infection in patients with cardiac transplants. Clinical spectrum and problems in diagnosis in a defined population. Ann Intern Med 1983; 99:27–31.

McCabe RE, Remington JS. The diagnosis and treatment of toxoplasmosis. Eur J Clin Microbiol 1983; 2:95–104.

Navia BA, Petito CK, Gold JWM, et al. Cerebral toxoplasmosis complicating the acquired immune deficiency syndrome: clinical and neuropathological findings in 27 patients. Ann Neurol 1986; 19:224–238.

Potasman I, Resnick L, Luft BJ, Remington JS. Intrathecal production of antibodies against *Toxoplasma gondii* in patients with toxoplasmic encephalitis and the acquired immunodeficiency syndrome (AIDS). Ann Intern Med 1988; 108:49–51.

Wilson CB, Remington JS, Stagno S, Reynolds DW. Development of adverse sequelae in children born with subclinical congenital *Toxoplasma* infection. Pediatrics 1980; 66:767–774.

NONVENEREAL TREPONEMATOSES

DONALD R. HOPKINS, M.D., M.P.H., D.Sc.(Hon.)

The nonvenereal treponematoses include yaws, endemic syphilis (bejel), and pinta. Pinta is restricted to tropical parts of the Americas, where it is diminishing in incidence and prevalence. Endemic syphilis still occurs in parts of the Middle East and is highly endemic in the Sahel region of West Africa. Yaws is resurgent in West Africa and also still occurs sporadically elsewhere in tropical Africa, Latin America, and Asia.

In diagnosing and treating these infections, one must remember that the nonvenereal treponematoses cannot be distinguished from each other absolutely, nor can they always be distinguished from venereal syphilis. Since venereal syphilis is potentially life threatening in its ability to attack cardiovascular and neurologic organs, and the nonvenereal treponemal syndromes are merely disfiguring (pinta) and/or crippling (endemic syphilis or yaws, both of which attack skin, bones, and cartilage), it is important to evaluate these patients carefully.

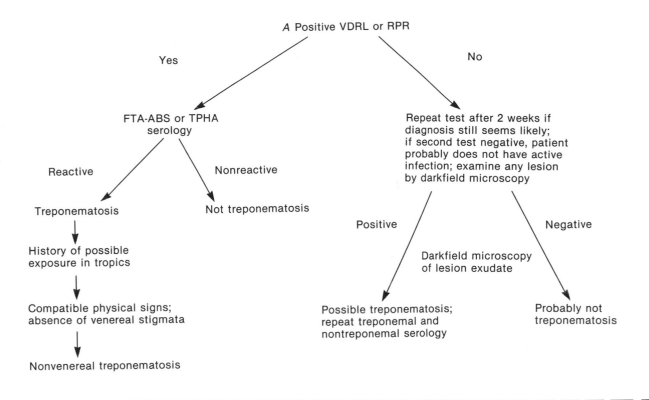

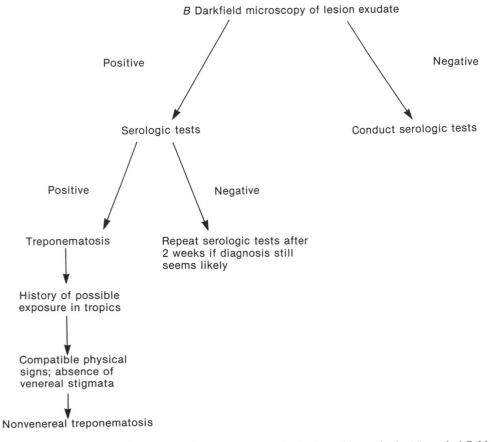

Figure 1 Diagnosis of nonvenereal treponematoses, beginning with serologic (*A*) or darkfield examination (*B*).

DIAGNOSIS

The main basis for diagnosis is to determine whether the patient has a positive nontreponemal test (VDRL, RPR) and a positive treponemal test (FTA-ABS, TPHA). In early stages of the infection (less than 5 years' duration), it should be possible to demonstrate motile treponemes in exudate from primary or secondary lesions under a darkfield microscope. Alternatively, treponemes may be demonstrated in fixed smears of exudate from early lesions by fluorescein-labeled antitreponemal antibody. The most secure diagnosis is based on a positive serologic test (high-titer nontreponemal test and/or reactive treponemal test) plus demonstration of treponemes in exudate from a lesion. In latent stages, and in infections more than 5 years old, the latter will obviously not be possible.

The combination of positive serologic and microscopic tests in the same patient can only confirm that the patient has a treponemal infection, since the venereal and nonvenereal treponemes are physically and antigenically identical (by all current tests), and the serologic reactions in humans also do not differ in any reliable way. In order to determine which of the four syndromes the patient most likely has, one must consider other clues from physical examination and history (Fig. 1).

Typically, yaws manifests first with a large primary lesion on one of the extremities, followed after a few weeks or months by multiple, raised, raspberry-like papillomata. Early lesions of endemic syphilis most commonly appear as patches in and around the mouth, and these are also sometimes followed by a generalized secondary rash, the lesions of which tend to be less exuberant than in yaws. Early yaws and endemic syphilis tend to occur among children younger than 15 years. Early pinta is characterized by slightly elevated, red or bluish circular plaques on the skin. In late stages, both yaws and endemic syphilis may leave a legacy of atrophic superficial scars on the extremities or deep mutilating lesions of the nose or bones. Untreated pinta characteristically results in widespread depigmentation of the skin, although somewhat less widespread depigmentation can also follow yaws or endemic syphilis.

In taking the history, one should seek clues as to the earlier appearance of related signs if the infection is advanced. Whether a patient was born, grew up, or later lived in a known endemic area should be determined and, if so, when and where. The endemic treponematoses were rampant in many tropical countries in the 1940s and 1950s, for example, but were much less prevalent following mass campaigns conducted in many areas in the 1960s. Whether a patient grew up in an urban or rural environment in such a country (as well as the patient's age or sexual maturity) makes a difference in establishing the likelihood of exposure to a venereal or nonvenereal treponematosis. In men, a history of homosexuality increases the likelihood that one is faced with venereal syphilis rather than one of the other treponematoses.

TREATMENT

For patients with an established diagnosis of nonvenereal treponematoses—whether pinta, yaws, or endemic syphilis—an injection of long-acting penicillin G, such as benzathine penicillin G (BPG), is the treatment of choice. Children younger than 10 years old should be given 0.6 million units of BPG. Persons 10 years old and older should be given a total of 1.2 million units of BPG intramuscularly.

Because of the potential confusion with venereal syphilis and the fact that the latter may be life threatening, it is recommended that if, after a careful history and physical examination, there is still some doubt as to whether the treponemal infection in question is venereal or nonvenereal in origin, it may be wisest to treat such patients (pharmacologically, at least) as if they had venereal syphilis. Due to the high transmissibility of yaws and endemic syphilis and the frequency of latent infections, family and other close contacts of confirmed cases should also be treated, prophylactically, at the same time as the index patient.

Little is known about the treatment of endemic treponematoses with antibiotics other than penicillin. A course of oral tetracycline or erythromycin, 0.5 g four times a day for 5 days, is probably adequate therapy in penicillin-allergic adults; children younger than 7 years should not be treated with tetracycline.

TRYPANOSOMIASIS: AFRICAN (SLEEPING SICKNESS) AND AMERICAN (CHAGAS' DISEASE)

JAMES H. MAGUIRE, M.D.

Four different trypanosomes infect human beings. *Trypanosoma brucei rhodesiense* and *Trypanosoma brucei gambiense*, the agents of African sleeping sickness, are transmitted by tsetse flies (*Glossina* species) in sub-Saharan Africa. In warmer regions of the Americas, triatomine or reduviid bugs carry both *Trypanosoma cruzi*, the protozoan responsible for Chagas' disease, and *Trypanosoma rangeli*, a nonpathogenic hemoflagellate that occasionally is mistaken for *T. cruzi*. African and American trypanosomiases differ in their clinical manifestations and require different strategies for diagnosis and treatment.

SLEEPING SICKNESS

African countries report 20,000 cases of sleeping sickness each year. However, many more cases go unreported, and 50 million persons live at risk of becoming infected.

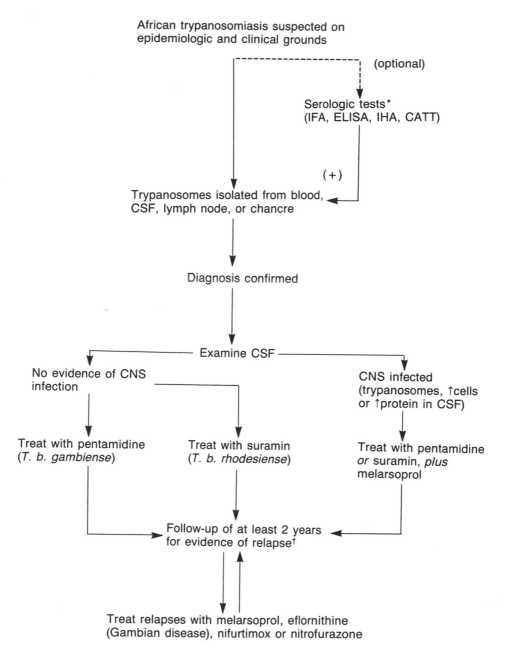

Figure 1 Diagnosis and treatment of African trypanosomiasis. *In the United States, serologic tests available at the Centers for Disease Control, Atlanta, Georgia. †Including examination of CSF at end of treatment, and 3, 6, 12, 18, and 24 months later.

The responsible parasites, *T. b. gambiense* in West and central Africa and the morphologically identical *T. b. rhodesiense* in East Africa, cause a fatal illness if not treated. Infection passes through an early hematolymphatic stage and a late meningoencephalitic stage. Treatment varies according to the stage of infection and the geographic origin of the parasite.

Epidemiologic Clues to Diagnosis

A compatible clinical illness and a history of a painful tsetse bite suggest the diagnosis of African trypanosomia-sis. Tsetse flies inhabit wooded areas along rivers and lakes near human settlements in West Africa and sparsely populated savannahs in East Africa. Except for possible transfusion-induced or congenital infection, transmission occurs only in Africa between the latitudes of 15 degrees north and 15 degrees south.

Several cases of imported infection have been diagnosed in the United States. American citizens most commonly acquired *T. b. rhodesiense* while on safaris in East Africa and became ill shortly after returning home. Infections in African citizens were due to *T. b. gambiense* and became apparent after months to years of residence in the United States.

TABLE 1 Clinical Features of African Trypanosomiasis

Stage	Symptoms and Signs
Chancre	Tender subcutaneous nodule at site of tsetse fly bite lasting several weeks (rare with *T. b. gambiense* infection)
Early (hematolymphatic)	Periodic fever, headache myalgia Lymphadenopathy (especially of posterior cervical nodes in Gambian disease, Winterbottom's sign), splenomegaly Circinate rashes, edema of face and extremities Congestive heart failure, ECG changes Anemia, monocytosis, evidence of disseminated intravascular coagulation, elevated IgM
Late (meningoencephalitic)	Headache, stiff neck, paresthesias Behavioral changes, sleep disturbances, seizures Ataxia, tremor, rigidity, other motor disturbances CSF mononuclear pleocytosis; elevated CSF protein or IgM level Amenorrhea, impotence, other endocrinologic disturbances Coma (with death due to malnutrition or intercurrent infection)

Clinical and Laboratory Diagnosis

Early Stage

Systemic manifestations develop several weeks after the infective bite as trypanosomes spread from the site of inoculation to the bloodstream (Fig. 1, Table 1). Early Rhodesian sleeping sickness runs a rapid course that ends within weeks to months, with invasion of the central nervous system (CNS) or death from myocarditis, secondary infection, or disseminated intravascular coagulation. Symptoms of early Gambian trypanosomiasis, on the other hand, may be mild or absent, and the infection may not be recognized for several years, until CNS invasion occurs.

Definitive diagnosis of African trypanosomiasis requires recovery of parasites from the blood, cerebrospinal fluid (CSF), or aspirates of the chancre or a lymph node. The yield is highest from lymph nodes in Gambian disease, and from the peripheral blood in Rhodesian disease. A wet mount should be examined for motile parasites, and the diagnosis confirmed with a Giemsa or Wright's stained smear. Low levels of parasites often can be detected on thick blood smears, in the buffy coat after centrifugation of blood in a microhematocrit tube, or in centrifuged eluates of blood passed through an anion-exchange column. Because levels of parasitemia fluctuate, examinations should be repeated on multiple occasions, and, if necessary, blood or tissue should be inoculated into laboratory rats or an aspirate of the bone marrow should be examined.

Serologic tests are useful for screening but require parasitologic confirmation. A number of assays detect specific antibodies as early as 2 to 4 weeks after infection. Most African countries employ the card agglutination test for trypanosomiasis (CATT) because it is easily performed in the field on samples of blood obtained by fingerstick.

Late Stage

The CSF should be centrifuged and examined for parasites in all cases of African trypanosomiasis, even in the absence of neurologic signs (see Table 1). The findings of parasites in the CSF, a mononuclear pleocytosis, or an elevated CSF protein level indicate late stage disease.

Treatment

Specific chemotherapy markedly reduces the mortality of African trypanosomiasis (Fig. 1, Table 2). Available drugs are toxic and must be administered parenterally. All patients require prolonged follow-up after treatment for possible relapse.

Early Stage

Suramin and pentamidine usually cure infection during the early stage but are ineffective for late infection because they do not cross the blood-brain barrier. Suramin is the drug of choice for early Rhodesian disease, and pentamidine is preferred for early Gambian disease, except in areas where widespread chemoprophylaxis may have selected for pentamidine-resistant organisms. Suramin may be substituted for pentamidine, but pentamidine should not be used for *T. b. rhodesiense* infection because of possible resistance.

An initial test dose of suramin should be given to exclude hypersensitivity reactions, which cause shock in approximately one person in 20,000 and in persons infected with the filarial worm *Onchocerca vovulus*. Before each injection, urinalysis should be performed, serum creatinine level determined, and treatment delayed if there is evidence of nephrotoxicity. Other adverse effects of suramin include fever, arthralgia, rash, and neuropathy. Pentamidine is given intramuscularly or by slow intravenous infusion over at least 2 hours. It may cause pain or sterile abscesses at the site of intramuscular injection, hypotension, vomiting, hypoglycemia, bone marrow depression, and renal or hepatic damage. Injections may be given every other day if toxicity develops. Patients should remain prone for at least 1 hour after each dose to avoid hypotension.

TABLE 2   Doses of Drugs for Treatment of Trypanosomiasis

Drug	Route	Dose
African trypanosomiasis		
Suramin* (Bayer 205, Antrypol, Germanin, Naganol, etc.)	IV	4 mg/kg (test dose) on day 1; 10 mg/kg on day 3; beginning on day 5, 20 mg/kg (maximum, 1 g)/day every 6 days × 5 doses
Pentamidine isethionate (Pentam) or pentamidine methanesulfonate† (Lomidine)	IV or IM	4 mg/kg (base)/day × 10 days
Melarsoprol* (Mel B, arsobal)	IV	1.5 mg/kg on day 1; 2.0 mg/kg on day 2; 2.2 mg/kg on day 3; 2.5 mg/kg on day 10; 3.0 mg/kg on day 11, and 3.6 mg/kg on days 12, 20, 21, 22
Eflornithine‡ (Difluoromethylornithine, DFMO, Ornidyl)	IV PO	100 mg/kg (IV) q6h × 2 wk, then 75 mg/kg (PO) q6h × 4 wk
American trypanosomiasis		
Nifurtimox* (Bayer 2502, Lampit)	PO	Adults: 10 mg/kg/day in 4 divided doses × 90 days; Age 11–16 yr: 12.5–15 mg/kg/day in 4 divided doses × 90 days Children <11 yr: 15–20 mg/kg/day in 4 divided doses × 90 days
Benznidazole† (Ro7-1051, Rochagan, Radanil)	PO	5 mg/kg/day × 60 days

* Available in the United States from the Parasitic Disease Drug Service, Centers for Disease Control, Atlanta, Georgia.
† Not available in the United States.
‡ Experimental drug available for compassionate treatment only from the manufacturer, Merrell Dow.

Patients should be followed carefully for evidence of relapse, and the CSF should be examined on several occasions for at least 2 years after completion of therapy. Cases of early trypanosomiasis that fail to respond to suramin or pentamidine should be treated with melarsoprol (see below). The effectiveness of eflornithine, an inhibitor of polyamine biosynthesis, for treatment of early stage Gambian trypanosomiasis is currently under evaluation.

Late Stage

At the present time, the drug of choice for treating late stage trypanosomiasis is melarsoprol B, an arsenical compound that penetrates the CNS well. Patients should first receive a short course of suramin (test dose of 4 mg per kilogram followed by a single full dose of 20 mg per kilogram) or pentamidine (two daily doses of 4 mg per kilogram), depending on the geographic origin of the infection. Melarsoprol is then given as outlined in Table 2, or in doses modified according to the severity of the disease (see Suggested Reading, "Epidemiology and Control of African Trypanosomiasis").

Within several days of the first injection of melarsoprol, about 5 percent of persons develop reactive arsenical encephalopathy, a complication that carries a 75 percent mortality. The reaction is probably immune mediated, although corticosteroids do not prevent its occurrence. Treatment consists of discontinuation of melarsoprol and administration of anticonvulsants, mannitol, oxygen, corticosteroids, and epinephrine. Other adverse effects of melarsoprol include exfoliative dermatitis, diarrhea, and jaundice.

Some patients with late Gambian disease fail to respond to melarsoprol. The drug of choice for refractory cases is eflornithine, which appears to be more effective and less toxic than other agents such as tryparsamide, nitrofurazone, and nifurtimox. Eflornithine is well tolerated, but may cause diarrhea or anemia. Its effectiveness as first-line therapy for either early or late Gambian disease has not yet been determined.

Chemoprophylaxis

Prophylactic pentamidine is no longer recommended for persons living in West Africa. The prophylactic dose is not curative and may allow a preexisting *T. b. gambiense* infection to remain undetected until invasion of the CNS occurs. Insect repellents and heavy clothing afford the best protection against tsetse fly bites.

CHAGAS' DISEASE

Trypanosoma cruzi infects more than 10 million persons in the Americas, where it is a major cause of cardiac and gastrointestinal disease. Infection progresses through a brief acute stage and a lifelong chronic stage. Most infected persons show no signs of illness during either stage, yet some persons develop debilitating or life-threatening disease. Strategies for diagnosis and treatment vary according to the stage of infection.

Epidemiologic Clues to Diagnosis

Infection with *T. cruzi* most commonly results from years of residence in a mud-and-stick house in an endemic

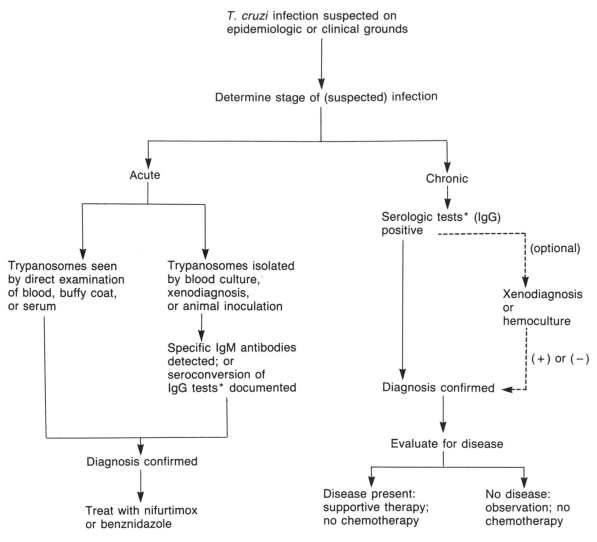

Figure 2 Diagnosis and treatment of Chagas' disease. *Serologic tests available at CDC.

region. Because the reduviid vectors rarely colonize well-built houses, poor persons from rural areas or urban favelas are primarily afflicted. Insect-mediated transmission occurs in all countries of South and Central America and in Mexico, but not in the Caribbean. Transfusion-induced and transplacental infection account for large numbers of cases in these areas as well.

Human infection with *T. cruzi* is rare in the United States. Although infected reduviid bugs and wild mammals inhabit many southern states, only a few autochthonous human infections have been reported. The greatest number of cases are imported cases among immigrants from Central America. The major risk to U.S. citizens seems to be from accidental infection in the laboratory.

Clinical and Laboratory Diagnosis

Acute Stage

Fewer than 10 percent of acute infections come to medical attention because symptoms are absent or mild and flu-like. When present, the typical signs appear 1 to 2 weeks after contact with the vector or up to several months after

transfusion (Fig. 2, Table 3). Five percent of symptomatic acute cases end fatally because of myocarditis or meningoencephalitis.

Acute Chagas' disease is diagnosed most readily by microscopic examination of anticoagulated blood for motile

TABLE 3 Clinical Features of American Trypanosomiasis

Acute Chagas' disease
  Romaña's sign (oculoglandular complex) ⎱ at site of inoculation
  Chagoma (cutaneous nodule) ⎰
  Fever lasting 4 to 8 weeks
  Splenomegaly, hepatomegaly, lymphadenopathy
  Acute myocarditis, meningoencephalitis
  Lymphocytosis with atypical lymphocytes

Chronic Chagas' disease
  ECG abnormalities, especially right bundle branch block
  Congestive heart failure
  Complete atrioventricular block
  Ventricular arrhythmias, sudden cardiac death
  Pulmonary and systemic thromboembolism
  Dysphagia, regurgitation, odynophagia (megaesophagus)
  Constipation, obstipation, volvulus (megacolon)

trypanosomes. Giemsa-stained thick and thin blood smears are less useful because parasites may lyse during processing. When wet mounts are negative, the buffy coat or the sediment of centrifuged serum often reveals trypanosomes. Occasionally, parasites can be isolated only by cultivation of blood on NNN or other special medium, animal inoculation, or xenodiagnosis. In the latter procedure, laboratory-raised, uninfected reduviid bugs feed on the patient or a sample of the patient's blood and are examined for trypanosomes 3 to 4 weeks later. Demonstration of parasitemia by blood culture, animal inoculation, or xenodiagnosis does not distinguish acute from chronic infection, however, and serologic testing may be necessary to make the distinction. Serum IgM antibodies to *T. cruzi*, detected by the indirect fluorescent antibody test (IFAT) or enzyme-linked immunosorbent assay (ELISA), indicate acute infection, as does seroconversion of tests for specific IgG.

Chronic Stage

Chronic infection is suspected in asymptomatic persons who have been exposed to the parasite or in symptomatic persons who show the characteristic signs (see Table 3). Serologic tests are superior to parasitologic tests for confirmation, since parasitemia during this stage is subpatent. Available assays for detecting IgG antibodies to *T. cruzi* include the highly sensitive and specific complement fixation (Machado-Guerreiro), IFAT, ELISA, and indirect hemagglutination tests. Rare false-positive reactions occur in persons infected with *Leishmania donovani*, *Leishmania braziliensis*, or *T. rangeli* and can be avoided by use of purified glycoprotein antigens. Hemoculture or xenodiagnosis confirm the diagnosis of chronic infection in up to 70 percent of cases but are seldom necessary.

All persons with chronic *T. cruzi* infection should undergo a periodic history and physical examination, electrocardiogram (ECG), and radiograph of the chest. More sensitive studies such as echocardiograms or gastrointestinal radiographs should be reserved for persons with positive findings. While the majority of infected persons remain disease free for life, in certain geographic areas, 30 to 40 percent of persons develop cardiac or gastrointestinal complications after an asymptomatic interval of years to decades. The ECG helps determine prognosis: adults with a normal tracing have a normal life expectancy, while those with right bundle branch block are seven times more likely to die prematurely from cardiac disease.

Treatment

Persons with acute or congenital Chagas' disease should always receive chemotherapy (see Fig. 2, Table 2). Persons with chronic infections should not be treated because of the limited effectiveness and toxicity of the available drugs, nifurtimox and benznidazole.

Acute Stage

Both drugs clear parasitemia, shorten the duration of illness, and reduce the immediate mortality of acute Chagas' disease. Cure of infection is certain only when serologic tests and xenodiagnoses remain negative for several years.

Rates of cure are low in Brazil, but higher in Argentina and Chile, perhaps because of regional variation of parasites' susceptibility to chemotherapy. Whether treatment of the acute stage prevents the complications of the chronic stage is not yet known.

Because of its availability, nifurtimox is the drug of choice for acute Chagas' disease in the United States. Both it and the alternative, benznidazole, are administered orally and are better tolerated by children than by adults. Adverse effects are frequent, and few patients are able to complete the long course of therapy. Both drugs produce reversible neuropathies, rashes, and gastrointestinal and psychic disturbances. Many patients develop profound anorexia and weight loss while taking nifurtimox.

Chronic Stage

Treatment during the chronic stage temporarily suppresses parasitemia but rarely produces parasitologic cure and does not prevent or ameliorate disease. Chronic infection is best not treated, except in the setting of a controlled trial, as has been advocated for infections of less than 2 years' duration.

The complications of chronic Chagas' disease are managed supportively. The response of congestive heart failure to diuretics and vasodilators is often short lived, and heart transplantation should be considered in selected cases. Permanent pacemakers prolong survival of persons with complete heart block and a normal-sized heart. Antiarrhythmic agents such as amiodarone control symptomatic ventricular arrhythmias, but their ability to prevent sudden cardiac death has not been studied. Repeated mechanical dilatation alleviates the symptoms of mild Chagas' megaesophagus, and surgery can offer a lasting solution for advanced megaesophagus or megacolon.

Chemoprophylaxis and Prevention of Transmission by Blood Transfusion

No effective vaccine or chemoprophylaxis for preventing infection with *T. cruzi* exists. Travelers to endemic areas should not sleep out of doors or in poorly constructed dwellings that may harbor reduviid bugs.

The Centers for Disease Control does not recommend treatment of persons exposed to the parasite during a laboratory accident until infection is documented by serologic tests or isolation of the parasite. However, consideration should be given to presumptive treatment when there has been unequivocal inoculation of the highly infective trypomastigote forms.

Careful serologic screening of blood donors virtually eliminates transfusion-induced Chagas' disease. In endemic areas where accurate serology is not available, gentian violet should be added to blood prior to transfusion to kill trypanosomes.

TRYPANOSOMA RANGELI INFECTION

Reduviid bugs transmit *T. rangeli* in many parts of Central America and northern South America where *T. cruzi* is endemic. The laboratory must take care to distinguish these two parasites when examining blood smears, hemocultures, or bugs used for xenodiagnosis. *T. rangeli* infection may cause falsely positive serologic tests for *T. cruzi* infection if purified antigens are not used. Persons infected with the nonpathogenic *T. rangeli* do not require treatment.

SUGGESTED READING

Gutteridge WE. Trypanosomiasis. Existing chemotherapy and its limitation. Br Med Bull 1985; 41:162–168.

Marr JJ, Docampo R. Chemotherapy for Chagas' disease: a perspective of current therapy and considerations for future research. Rev Infect Dis 1986; 8:884–903.
Stolf NAG, Higushi L, Bocchi E, et al. Heart transplantation in patients with Chagas' disease cardiomyopathy. J Heart Transplant 1987; 6:307–312.
Taelman H, Schechter PJ, Marcelis L, et al. Difluoromethylornithine, an effective new treatment of Gambian trypanosomiasis. Am J Med 1987; 82:607–614.
WHO Expert Committee. Epidemiology and control of African trypanosomiasis. Geneva: World Health Organization, Tech Rep Ser No 739, 1986.

LEISHMANIASIS

RICHARD D. PEARSON, M.D., F.A.C.P.
THOMAS R. NAVIN, M.D.
ANASTACIO DE Q. SOUSA, M.D.
THOMAS G. EVANS, M.D.

Leishmania species produce a spectrum of disease referred to collectively as leishmaniasis. It is estimated that several hundred thousand to as many as a million people are affected worldwide. The clinical manifestations vary depending on the infecting *Leishmania* species (Table 1) and the host's immune responses. Most cases fit into one of three clinical syndromes: cutaneous, mucosal, or visceral leishmaniasis. The manifestations of cutaneous leishmaniasis range from single, localized ulcers to diffuse, nonulcerative involvement of the skin. In mucosal leishmaniasis an initial skin lesion(s) is followed months to years later by involvement of mucosal areas of the nose, oral pharynx, or rarely the larynx. In visceral leishmaniasis there is generalized involvement of the reticuloendothelial system with hepatosplenomegaly, fever, and wasting.

The *Leishmania* live within the gut of their arthropod vectors—sandflies of the genera *Phlebotomus* in the Old World and *Lutzomyia* and *Psychodopygus* in the Americas—as extracellular, flagellated promastigotes. They are inoculated into susceptible human or animal hosts when sandflies attempt to take a blood meal. Promastigotes gain access to mononuclear phagocytes in the skin and convert within them to the intracellular amastigote form. Amastigotes are 2 to 5 μm in diameter, round or oval in shape, and lack an exteriorized flagellum. They appear somewhat larger in touch preparations than in biopsies. Wright or Giemsa staining reveals an eccentrically placed nucleus and a characteristic, bar-shaped, intensely stained kinetoplast. In most areas leishmaniasis is a zoonosis. The animal reservoirs vary with *Leishmania* species and geographic location. For example, *Leishmania major* is found in rodents in the Middle East, whereas domestic dogs and wild foxes are the presumed

reservoirs of *Leishmania chagasi* in South America. In the case of *Leishmania donovani* in India, there is no apparent animal reservoir; infection is spread among humans by anthropophilic sandflies.

The diagnosis of leishmaniasis in a suspected case is confirmed by identification of leishmanial amastigotes in tissue or isolation of promastigotes in culture using NNN (Novy-McNeal-Nicolle) medium, Schneider's insect medium with fetal calf serum, or one of several alternatives. The taxonomy of *Leishmania* is still in a state of flux. Although slight differences exist, the morphology of amastigotes and promastigotes cannot be used to differentiate among *Leishmania* species. Speciation is usually based on isoenzyme analysis or on species-specific monoclonal antibody, restriction endonuclease, or kDNA hybridization probes. Pentavalent antimonial compounds have been the mainstay of treatment of leishmaniasis for decades. Their pharmacology and use in the major clinical syndromes are detailed in the sections to follow. A number of alternative drugs and forms of local therapy have also been proposed. The pyrazolopyrimidines (of which allopurinol is the prototype) and ketoconazole are the most promising, but clinical experience is still insufficient to warrant their use except in controlled trials or unusual situations.

PHARMACOLOGY OF PENTAVALENT ANTIMONIAL DRUGS

Two pentavalent antimonial compounds are available for the treatment of leishmaniasis. Stibogluconate sodium (Pentostam) has been widely used in India, Africa, the Mediterranean littoral, and the Middle East. Meglumine antimonate (Glucantime) has been used in Latin America and in countries formerly under French influence. Neither is licensed in the United States, but stibogluconate sodium is available for investigational use through the Drug Service of the Centers for Disease Control (telephone, 404-639-3670). Physicians requesting the drug must register as clinical investigators with the CDC Drug Service. Permission to use stibogluconate sodium at dosages or durations in excess of the CDC recommendations must be obtained from the federal Food and Drug Administration.

Stibogluconate sodium contains 100 mg of pentavalent antimony (SbV) per milliliter. It is supplied in 100-ml bottles. Meglumine antimonate contains SbV, 85 mg per mil-

Use of trade names is for identification only and does not imply endorsement by the U.S. Public Health Service or by the U.S. Department of Health and Human Services.

TABLE 1 Clinical Manifestations of Leishmanial Infection

Clinical Syndromes	Leishmanial Species	Location
Visceral leishmaniasis (kala-azar)		
General involvement of the reticuloendothelial system (spleen, bone marrow, liver etc.)	L. donovani donovani	Indian subcontinent, China
	L. d. infantum	Middle East, Mediterranean littoral, Balkans, western Asiatic area, northwestern Iberia, China, subsaharan Africa
	L. d. chagasi	Latin America
Post-kala-azar dermal leishmaniasis	L. d. donovani	Indian subcontinent
	L. d. species	Kenya, possibly Ethiopia and Somalia
Old World cutaneous leishmaniasis		
Single or limited number of skin lesions	L. major	Middle East, central Asia, Africa, Indian subcontinent
	L. tropica	Mediterranean littoral, Middle East, west Asiatic area, Indian subcontinent
	L. aethiopica	Ethiopian highlands, Kenya
Diffuse cutaneous leishmaniasis	L. aethiopica	Ethiopian highlands, Kenya
New World cutaneous leishmaniasis		
Single or limited number of skin lesions	L. mexicana mexicana (chiclero ulcer)	Mexico, Central America Texas (?)
	L. m. amazonensis	Amazon basin and neighboring areas, Brazil, Panama, Venezuela, Trinidad
	L. m. pifanoi	Venezuela
	L. m. garnhami	Venezuela
	L. m. venezuelensis	Venezuela
	L. m. species undetermined	Dominican Republic
	L. braziliensis braziliensis	Brazil, Peru, Ecuador, Bolivia, Paraguay, Argentina
	L. b. guyanensis (pian) bois, bush yaws	Guyana, Surinam, northern Amazon Basin
	L. b. peruvian (uta)	Peru, western Andes, Argentinian highlands
	L. b. panamensis	Panama and adjacent areas
Diffuse cutaneous leishmaniasis	L. m. amazonensis	Amazon basin and neighboring areas
	L. m. pifanoi	Venezuela
	L. m. mexicana	Mexico, Central America (rare)
	L. m. species	Dominican Republic
Mucosal leishmaniasis	L. b. braziliensis (Espundia)	Multiple areas in South America
	L. b. panamensis (rare)	Panama and adjacent areas

The taxonomy of *Leishmania* species is still in a state of flux. Three species complexes have been traditionally identified: *L. donovani* complex, *L. mexicana* complex, and *L. braziliensis* complex, each having multiple subspecies as indicated above. Lainson and Shaw, who have been leaders in the classification of *Leishmania*, have recently proposed that the various subspecies be reclassified as distinct species, e.g., *L. donovani chagasi* as *L. chagasi* (Lainson R, Shaw JJ. Evolution, classification and geographic distribution. In: Peters W, Killick-Kendrick R, eds. The leishmaniases in biology and medicine. Vol 1. London: Academic Press, 1987;2–103).

liliter, and is available in 5-ml vials. These drugs are prescribed on the basis of SbV content. The two compounds are thought to be equivalent in terms of efficacy and toxicity, but comparative clinical studies are lacking and the bioavailability may vary with manufacturer. Stibogluconate has been the most widely studied internationally and is the only one available in the United States. It can be administered intramuscularly, but newer regimens call for larger doses and the drug is usually given intravenously, either as undiluted solution (injected over a 5-minute period) or diluted in 50 ml of 5 percent dextrose-in-water or saline and administered over 20 minutes. Stibogluconate is rapidly cleared through the kidney. The blood SbV concentration as a function of time is best described by a three-compartment pharmacokinetic model, with a very short initial distribution phase followed by biexponential elimination. The mean half-lives for the elimination phases have been reported to be 1.7 and 33 hours after intravenous administration and 2 and 76 hours after the drug is given intramuscularly. It has been suggested that the slow, terminal, elimination phase may be due to in vivo conversion of SbV to trivalent Sb, which could be responsible for the toxicity associated with long-term, high-dose therapy. SbV is thought to be concentrated in cells of the reticuloendothelial system, where it probably affects parasite metabolism.

SbV is relatively well tolerated, even in children less than 2 years of age. The most common adverse effects include abdominal pain, nausea, vomiting, malaise, headache, elevated hepatic transaminase levels, nephrotoxicity, weakness, myalgias, arthralgias, fever, skin rash, cough, and pneumonia, but these seldom prevent completion of the treatment course. Dose-related changes in the electrocardiogram are observed; the most frequent are T-wave inversion and prolonged QT interval. Rarer but more serious adverse effects include atrial and ventricular arrhythmias and rarely anaphylaxis. Sudden death has occurred in patients given high doses of SbV (30 mg per kilogram per day) for visceral leishmaniasis. The use of SbV is contraindicated or should be used only with great care in patients with myocarditis, hepatitis, and nephritis. Most of the data on adverse effects caused by stibogluconate have been gathered from young patients, usually children. Whether these findings can be applied to older patients is not known. Until such data are available, it is probably wise to lower the dose or shorten the treatment for patients over 60 years of age. The safety of SbV in pregnancy has not been evaluated, and it should be avoided in that setting if possible.

TREATMENT OF VISCERAL LEISHMANIASIS

Visceral leishmaniasis is almost always caused by *L. donovani* in the Old World or *L. donovani chagasi* in the Americas, but *Leishmania mexicana* and *Leishmania tropica* have been isolated from a few patients with the syndrome. The disease is most common in children in Latin America and the Mediterranean littoral. In East Africa and India, adolescents and adults are also involved. On the average, one or two persons, usually travelers, are treated for visceral leishmaniasis in the United States each year. Sporadic cases have also been reported among northern Europeans who vacation in Mediterranean countries, including Italy, Spain, or Greece. Immunocompromised persons, particularly those with AIDS or taking corticosteroids, are at increased risk of developing progressive disease. Several cases of visceral leishmaniasis have been reported in renal transplant recipients many years after they moved from endemic areas.

Persons with visceral leishmaniasis generally present with fever, weight loss, massive splenomegaly, hepatomegaly, and occasionally with lymphadenopathy. There is associated anemia, leukopenia, eosinopenia, thrombocytopenia, hypoalbuminemia, hypergammaglobulinemia, and often bleeding tendencies. The course is usually subacute, but a few persons have a precipitous onset that can be confused with malaria. Some patients have chronic, fluctuating, oligosymptomatic disease. Asymptomatic, self-resolving infections are also common. Classic visceral leishmaniasis is usually not difficult to diagnose in an endemic area, but there is often a delay in making the diagnosis in patients presenting in the United States. Visceral leishmaniasis should be considered in the differential diagnosis of fever of undetermined origin among travelers or immigrants from endemic areas.

Persons with visceral leishmaniasis have high titers of antileishmanial antibodies as measured by ELISA, indirect immunofluorescence, or other assays. The diagnosis is confirmed by identification of amastigotes in bone marrow aspirates, liver biopsies, peripheral blood mononuclear cells, splenic aspirates, or other tissue. Both *L. donovani* and *L. d. chagasi* grow as promastigotes in NNN, Schneider's insect, or other media. Splenic aspiration was found in studies in East Africa to be the most sensitive diagnostic method, but many clinicians do not use this approach because of concern for life-threatening hemorrhage. Bone marrow aspirate is the next-most-sensitive approach, but it is positive in only 60 percent of cases. The Montenegro skin test, in which promastigote antigen is inoculated into the skin, is characteristically negative. Patients with progressive visceral leishmaniasis demonstrate no *Leishmania* antigen-specific T cell responsiveness. In many cases, a diagnosis of visceral leishmaniasis is based on the clinical presentation, history of exposure in an endemic area, positive serology, and exclusion of other febrile diseases associated with hepatosplenomegaly, such as malaria, typhoid fever, tuberculosis, schistosomiasis with concurrent salmonellosis, and myeloproliferative disorders.

Stibogluconate (or meglumine antimonate) 20 mg SbV per kilogram per day (with a maximal daily dose of 850 mg) for 20 days is the treatment of choice for visceral leishmaniasis. The limitation to a maximal daily dose is based on concerns about potential cardiac toxicity, but therapy can be extended for more than 30 days without serious side effects. The efficacy of treatment can be affected by geographic differences among infecting *Leishmania*, the health status and immune responsiveness of the host, the extent of disease at the time therapy is initiated, and the amount and possibly the type of SbV. In studies from different geographic areas, the initial response rate of visceral leishmaniasis to SbV has exceeded 90 percent. Primary unresponsiveness, defined as no clinical or parasitologic improvement during the first course of pentavalent antimony, varies from 2 to 8 percent. Few of the *L. donovani* isolates from such persons have been resistant to pentavalent antimony in vitro. Visceral leishmaniasis in East Africa tends to be less responsive than disease acquired in other areas, and the relapse rate after apparently successful therapy in Kenya has ranged from 5 to 36 percent. The relapse rate in other regions is less than 10 percent. Interrupted or incomplete therapy increases the risk of relapse.

Persons who relapse often respond to a second or third course of pentavalent antimony. There is no consensus on the optimal therapy for patients with multiple relapses or primary unresponsiveness. Higher doses of SbV can be given for longer periods of time. The combination of allopurinol plus stibogluconate sodium has been effective in treating some patients who failed with stibogluconate sodium alone. Alternative drugs include pentamidine isethionate, a diamidine that can be given intramuscularly or slowly intravenously at a dose of 2 to 4 mg per kilogram per day three times a week for up to 15 doses. Adverse effects are frequent and include hypotension (if the drug is given too rapidly), headache, nausea, vomiting, abdominal discomfort, generalized or localized urticarial eruptions, and life-threatening hypoglycemia. The latter is due to pancreatic β-cell damage and insulin release. It may be followed later by hyperglycemia and in some cases insulin-dependent diabetes mellitus. Sterile abscesses are common at the site of intramuscular injections; thrombophlebitis may follow intravenous administration. Amphotericin B, 0.5 mg per kilogram given daily or 1.0 mg per kilogram every other day for up to 8 weeks, has also been used successfully. Field studies of related pyrazolopyrimidines are underway, but the clinical experience is still insufficient to determine how they compare with SbV.

Visceral leishmaniasis is often associated with secondary viral or bacterial infections and severe wasting. Bacterial complications, including pneumonia and tuberculosis, must be treated with appropriate antibiotics. Children with visceral leishmaniasis should be isolated from those with measles and other contagious diseases. Dietary and vitamin supplementation are important in wasted patients.

TREATMENT OF CUTANEOUS AND MUCOSAL LEISHMANIASIS

Cutaneous leishmaniasis due to *L. mexicana* subspecies or *L. braziliensis* subspecies is endemic in Latin America from the Yucatan Peninsula of Mexico in the north to the northern parts of Chile, Uruguay, and Argentina in the south. Occasional cases occur in central and northern Mexico. Cutaneous leishmaniasis in the Western Hemisphere is endemic in many low-lying tropical forests. Epidemics have occurred in Brazil as forests are cleared for roads or farms. In the Old World, cutaneous leishmaniasis due to *L. major* and *L. tropica* is found in countries surrounding the Mediterranean Sea as well as in the Middle East, Afghanistan, and the southern USSR. *Leishmania major* infection is often acquired in rural areas by settlers or soldiers. It has been a major problem among troops operating in desert regions. *L. tropica* on the other hand is commonly transmitted in urban areas. In East Africa cutaneous leishmaniasis due to *Leishmania aethiopica* occurs in countries bordering on the southern edge of the Sahara Desert. Cases of autochthonous cutaneous leishmaniasis occur, but rarely, in Texas, and each year approximately 25 cases of cutaneous leishmaniasis are reported in the United States among travelers returning from endemic areas.

The manifestations of cutaneous leishmaniasis vary with the infecting *Leishmania* species and the host. The typical lesion begins as a papule at the site where promastigotes are injected. The papule enlarges slowly and eventually ulcerates. Less commonly, verrucous lesions may develop. Cutaneous ulcers may be single or multiple, large or small, painful or painless. They usually heal after several months

to more than a year, leaving atrophic scars. In mucosal disease due to *L. braziliensis*, an initial cutaneous lesion heals only to be followed months to years later by metastatic involvement of mucosal areas of the nose, mouth, lips, or oral pharynx. In diffuse cutaneous leishmaniasis, an unusual anergic variant caused by *L. mexicana* or *L. aethiopica*, the initial papule does not ulcerate and amastigotes spread throughout the skin, causing nodular or papular lesions. Another unusual variant is leishmaniasis recidiva, which is encountered in Iran, Iraq, and adjacent areas. It is a chronic condition, persisting for many years, in which lesions expand slowly while healing at the center. Finally, post-kala-azar dermal leishmaniasis is a macular or papular eruption that follows treatment of visceral leishmaniasis in India and Africa. In Africa, cutaneous lesions tend to resolve spontaneously after several months, but in India they can persist for years.

Consensus is lacking on the optimal way to diagnose cutaneous leishmaniasis. The following approach is used in Guatemala. The skin surrounding a suspected cutaneous lesion is anesthetized, any scab is removed, and the surrounding hair is shaved. The lesion is scrubbed well with a surgical brush and soap. It is rinsed thoroughly with sterile saline, and as a final step, the area is scrubbed with alcohol. Aspirates of the lesion are obtained using syringes filled with 0.1 ml of sterile saline that contains no bacteriostatic agent. The needle of the syringe is directed tangentially to the ulceration. The goal is to avoid bacteria and fungi that colonize the ulcer and to sample tissue as close to the margin of the ulcer as possible. While suction is applied, the needle is rotated as it is advanced in the skin to obtain a core of tissue from just below the epidermis. Suction is maintained as the needle is withdrawn. The aspirated material is inoculated into a sterile tube containing culture medium and/or into the hind footpad of a hamster or BALB/c mouse. A punch biopsy is then taken with a disposable 3-, 4-, or 5-mm punch. The punch is positioned so that most of the biopsy contains nonulcerated tissue. One-third of the biopsy is used for pathology, one-third is cultured for fungi, and the rest is macerated in a sterile tissue grinder. One aliquot is then cultured for leishmania; another is injected into the footpad of a hamster or a BALB/c mouse. Impression smears are prepared by scraping the edge of the ulcerated area with a scalpel. The best smears are made by obtaining as little blood as possible and preparing a thin smear. The diagnosis is confirmed by identifying amastigotes in touch preparations or biopsy material or by isolating promastigotes in culture.

Treatment of Cutaneous Leishmaniasis Acquired in Areas Without Mucosal Disease

There is some latitude in the treatment of patients who contract cutaneous disease in areas where mucosal leishmaniasis is unknown or very rare (Europe, the Middle East, Asia, Africa, Mexico, and Guatemala). This includes areas with cutaneous disease caused by *L. tropica, L. major, L. mexicana,* or *Leishmania peruviana.* Some authorities suggest that cutaneous ulcers due to these species can be left untreated, since most lesions will eventually heal spontaneously. Placebo-controlled trials of SbV are lacking. In our experience, therapy with SbV is usually advisable unless the lesion has begun to heal spontaneously. As initial therapy, stibogluconate, 20 mg of SbV per kilogram (maximum of 850 mg) daily for 10 days, is recommended. Ulcers often continue to heal after one course of therapy, and patients should be observed for several weeks after the end of therapy before a decision is made to administer more SbV. If additional drug is indicated, a total of 30 days of therapy can be given without producing serious toxicity. Secondary bacterial and fungal infections should be managed with local care and antibiotics as necessary.

A number of alternative therapeutic approaches have been used. There have been reports of cure after injection of SbV directly into lesions. Various forms of cryotherapy or local hyperthermic therapy alone or in conjunction with systemic drugs have been used. Several antibiotic and antifungal agents have also been studied. The preliminary results have been promising with oral ketoconazole, oral allopurinol, and topical paromomycin with methylbenzethonium chloride, but clinical experience is still insufficient to warrant their general use. Oral metronidazole, rifampin, and clofazimine have also been used to treat cutaneous leishmaniasis. In most instances these drugs have not been studied in a placebo-controlled manner.

In some situations, therapy with SbV is known to be less effective. Specifically, *L. aethiopica* infection is less responsive to SbV than are other *Leishmania* species. High doses of stibogluconate, 20 mg per kilogram twice daily for 30 days, have been effective in some patients, but the potential for cardiac toxicity increases at these doses. Pentamidine isethionate, 2 to 4 mg once or twice a week up to 15 doses, has been used successfully in some patients, but pentamidine has potentially serious adverse effects, as reviewed earlier.

Diffuse cutaneous leishmaniasis, an anergic variant usually due to *L. aethiopica* or *L. mexicana*, also responds poorly to pentavalent antimony and other drugs. Even when there is an initial response, relapses are common. Several persons with diffuse cutaneous leishmaniasis acquired in the Dominican Republic have been successfully treated with heat applied to affected areas. Leishmaniasis recidiva tends to progress despite systemic SbV therapy. Finally, post-kala-azar dermal leishmaniasis in India responds poorly to SbV, although some cases have been successfully treated.

Treatment of Cutaneous Lesions Acquired in Areas With Mucosal Disease Due to *L. braziliensis* Subspecies.

For patients who present with cutaneous leishmanial lesions in areas of Latin America where mucosal leishmaniasis is endemic, stibogluconate, 20 mg per kilogram (maximal daily dose 850 mg) for at least 20 days, is recommended to reduce the likelihood of late mucosal disease. An increased rate of relapse with *L. b. braziliensis* has been associated with inadequate dosage or interruption of therapy. Identification of the infecting *Leishmania* species is particularly helpful in areas where *L. braziliensis* subspecies coexist with

other *Leishmania* species, since in most areas only in infection with *L. braziliensis* subspecies is curative therapy necessary to prevent the development of mucosal disease.

Treatment of Mucosal Lesions

The most important complication of *L. b. braziliensis* infection is the development of mucosal lesions, which appear months to years after the primary lesion(s) has healed. Amastigotes are usually scant in mucosal lesions and difficult to find in histologic sections. *L. b. braziliensis* grows poorly in culture and slowly in animals. Consequently, a putative diagnosis is often made on the basis of the clinical findings, the presence of antileishmanial antibodies, a positive skin test with leishmanial antigen, and the exclusion of other diagnoses, including paracoccidioidomycosis, syphilis, tertiary yaws, histoplasmosis, sarcoidosis, midline granuloma, and basal cell carcinoma. The initial recommended dose of stibogluconate for mucosal leishmaniasis is 20 mg per kilogram (maximum of 850 mg daily) for a minimum of 4 weeks. Persons who respond slowly or relapse should receive the same dose for at least twice the duration. Those who fail can be given either pentamidine isethionate, 2 to 4 mg per kilogram daily once or twice weekly for up to 15 doses, or amphotericin B, 0.5 daily or 1.0 mg per kilogram every other day for up to 8 weeks—a total dose of approximately 2 g. Some have advocated the addition of steroids in patients who develop pronounced inflammation at the site of mucosal lesions during therapy. Jarisch-Herxheimer-like reactions with fever and erythema of cutaneous lesions have been noted in a small percentage of persons; they are of particular concern in the rare patient with laryngeal involvement.

There are no rigid criteria with which to document cure in mucosal leishmaniasis. The relapse rate at 1 year is as high as 50 percent in some areas of Brazil. Improved forms of chemotherapy are clearly needed. Plastic surgery is often necessary to ameliorate the sequelae of mucosal leishmaniasis but should not be performed earlier than 1 year after chemotherapy since relapse of infection can result in graft rejection.

Prophylaxis

Spontaneous resolution of cutaneous leishmaniasis due to *L. major* is associated with acquisition of protective immunity against the infecting strain. People have been successfully immunized in Israel and the USSR with live *L. major* promastigotes inoculated at inconspicuous sites on the body. Although this approach has been successful, it has been discontinued because some of the resulting lesions heal slowly, others become secondarily infected, and even after healing, live parasites may persist at the site of inoculation. A killed promastigote vaccine formulated with five *Leishmania* strains has been developed in Brazil. Preliminary studies suggest that it provides partial protection against cutaneous disease. Intensive efforts are now ongoing to identify specific leishmanial antigens that can elicit protective T cell responses in order to develop a defined, component vaccine. Until an effective vaccine is available, vector control with insect repellents containing *N,N*-diethyl-*m*-toluamide (deet) and fine-mesh sandfly nets are recommended for travelers.

SUGGESTED READING

Anabwani GM, Dimiti G, Ngira JA, Bryceson ADM. Comparison of two dosage schedules of sodium stibogluconate in the treatment of visceral leishmaniasis in Kenya. Lancet 1983; 1:210–212.

Berman JD. Chemotherapy for leishmaniasis: biochemical mechanisms, clinical efficacy, and future strategies. Rev Infect Dis 1988; 10:560–586.
Centers for Disease Control. Information material for physicians —Pentostam (sodium antimony gluconate): HHS, PHS, CDC protocol. Atlanta: CDC.
Chulay JD, Fleckenstein L, Smith DH. Pharmacokinetics of antimony during treatment of visceral leishmaniasis with sodium stibogluconate or meglumine antimoniate. Trans R Soc Trop Med Hyg 1988; 82:69–72.
Pearson RD, Sousa AQ. *Leishmania* species: visceral (kala-azar) cutaneous and mucosal leishmaniasis. In: Mandell GL, Douglas RG Jr, Bennett JE, eds. Principles and practice of infectious diseases. 3rd ed. New York: John Wiley, 1989 (in press).
Report of a WHO Expert Committee. The leishmaniases. Geneva: WHO Tech Rep Ser no. 710, 1984.

SCHISTOSOMIASIS

JOSEPH A. COOK, M.D.

In the past 10 years, chemotherapy for schistosomiasis has undergone a dramatic change: the cure is no longer worse than the disease. Only a decade ago, it was still possible (and necessary) to administer dangerous intravenous antimonials, obtained through the Centers for Disease Control. Now, however, two safe oral drugs are available, both approved by the U.S. Food and Drug Administration.

INFECTION

Schistosomiasis results from infection with one of the three common (or two rare) human schistosomes, the only trematode with separate sexes that infects humans. The extent of the disease is determined by the number of invading larval stages (cercariae). These cercariae penetrate the skin during contact with fresh water containing the appropriate, infected snail intermediate host. Because schistosomes, like most helminths, do not multiply within the human host, the intensity of infection depends on the number of cercariae that penetrate and develop into adult worms. In areas where schistosomiasis is endemic, relatively few persons sustain a heavy infection; most have a light infection. This means that severe disease is confined to 10 percent or less of those infected. The majority have mild or no symptoms and, perhaps, no pathology from the infection whatsoever. In fact, in endemic areas schistosomiasis remains largely asymptomatic until the late chronic stages of severe disease. In the case of *Schistosoma mansoni* and *Schistosoma japonicum* infection, liver fibrosis occurs; with *Schistosoma haematobium* infection, chronic obstructive uropathy results. The development of severe chronic disease from schistosomes depends primarily on the duration and intensity of infection. The actual pathology is caused by the body's reaction to those eggs that are not passed in feces or urine but, rather, remain in tissues. Individuals with greater numbers of worm pairs over longer periods of time sustain damage. In isolated cases the focality of infection, that is, the location of adult worm pairs,

can play a role; in the case of *S. haematobium*, a few worm pairs strategically placed near the ureteral orifices may cause obstructive uropathy even in the absence of severe infection. Likewise, the infrequent cases of transverse myelitis are thought to be the result of ectopic location of adult worm pairs. Because it is not possible to determine the longevity of any particular infection and because it is clear that children treated early in their infections respond better to therapy than adults, early diagnosis and treatment is desirable. Also, because the drugs now available have few adverse effects, there is a compelling case to be made for treating any person found to be excreting eggs from one of the schistosome species.

DIAGNOSIS

Signs of infection with schistosomiasis are not immediately obvious. Patients who have grown up in an endemic area, acquiring their worms at a relatively slow rate, are likely to manifest fewer symptoms than those expatriates who are suddenly exposed to large numbers of infectious cercariae at one time. In these cases the individual may evince such acute symptoms as fever, cough, diarrhea, arthralgias, and anorexia, accompanied by leukocytosis with eosinophilia. Eosinophilia, in general, suggests the presence of helminthic infection and, together with a history of exposure to fresh water in geographic areas where schistosomes are found, dictates a search for schistosome eggs in the urine or feces. *S. mansoni* infection is found in Africa, the Middle East, Venezuela and Brazil in South America, and some of the Caribbean islands; *S. japonicum* occurs in China, the Philippines, and Southeast Asia; the urinary schistosome, *S. haematobium*, is found in Africa and the Middle East.

Definitive diagnosis is made by finding the characteristic eggs in the patient's feces or urine. Two simple methods for detection are the Kato fecal smear for *S. mansoni* and *S. japonicum* and the nucleopore filtration method for urinary schistosomiasis. Because both tests are also quantitative, providing information on the intensity of infection, both indicate the likelihood that disease is present or will develop. Although a number of immunologic techniques that demonstrate the presence of antibodies to schistosomes exist, they are not reliable in detecting active infection.

TREATMENT

The drug of choice is praziquantel (Biltricide). The detailed mechanism of praziquantel action remains undefined, although it is thought to be associated with increased entry of calcium ions and other cations into the parasite cells, resulting in a tetanic contraction. Effects are greater on male schistosome worms than on females. The drug is rapidly and efficiently absorbed (80 to 100 percent), and peak plasma levels are achieved in 1 to 3 hours after ingestion. Serum half-life is 1 to 1½ hours; in contrast, drug metabolites have a half-life of 4 to 6 hours. More than 80 percent of the drug is eliminated as metabolic products in the urine over 4 days. The treatment regimen for *S. mansoni* and *S. haematobium* infection is a single dose of 40 mg per kilogram of body weight. For *S. japonicum* infection, 20 mg per kilogram is given three times in 1 day at approximately 3- to 4-hour intervals for a total of 60 mg per kilogram. The pediatric dose is the same. Side effects of praziquantel are transient and generally dose related. Abdominal pain, by far the most common side effect, is infrequently severe and is associated with vomiting and diarrhea. Patients with impaired liver function sustain higher peak plasma concentrations, increased bioavailability of the drug, and some increase in side effects. However, for reasons that remain unclear, abdominal pain and bloody diarrhea after ingestion of praziquantel occur more frequently in patients with the most intense infections, without respect to plasma concentration. Even the most severe adverse effects, however, have not required hospitalization and generally cease within 24 hours. Cure rates reach approximately 85 percent; equally important, in those not cured there is a greater than 95 percent reduction in the egg excretion and, hence, a parallel reduction in the likelihood of disease.

Two second-line drugs are also available. Oxamniquine (Vansil) is effective only against *S. mansoni* and is administered in a single dose (20 mg per kilogram for children and 15 mg per kilogram for adults) against the South American and Caribbean strains of *S. mansoni*. Higher doses of oxamniquine are required for strains from other geographic regions, making it a less useful drug in these cases. Dizziness is the primary side effect of oxamniquine; also, it must be given with caution to any person with a history of seizure disorders as seizures have been a reported side effect, though rare.

The other second-line drug, metrifonate, is effective only in *S. haematobium* infections. It has the disadvantage of requiring three doses (7.5 mg per kilogram of body weight) at 2-week intervals in order to give results comparable to praziquantel. Although it is easily obtained elsewhere, it is not available in the United States. There are virtually no side effects ascribed to metrifonate. However, it is a cholinesterase inhibitor, and the potential for cholinergic clinical adverse effects in humans exists, especially if metrifonate is given at the time of exposure to other cholinesterase-inhibiting compounds.

SUGGESTED READING

Mahmoud AAF, ed. Clinical tropical medicine and communicable diseases. Vol II, no 2. London: Bailliere Tindall, 1987.

Nash TE, Cheever AW, Ottesen EA, Cook JA. Schistosome infection in humans: perspectives and recent findings. Ann Intern Med 1982; 97:740–754.

Watt GF, White NJ, Padre L, et al. Praziquantel pharmacokinetics and side effects in *Schistosoma japonicum*–infected patients with liver disease. J Infect Dis 1988; 157:530–535.

SUPERFICIAL FUNGAL INFECTION

SERGIO RABINOVICH, M.D.

The usual superficial fungal infections are the dermatophytoses that are almost always limited to the skin, hair, and nails. Three distinct species cause these common infections: *Microsporum*, *Trichophyton*, and *Epidermophyton*. Two other common fungal agents, *Malassezia furfur*, the cause of tinea versicolor, and *Candida albicans*, complete the basic mycology. *Candida* is unique among these agents because it often involves the mucosa and may involve every organ in the body.

Conveniently, superficial fungal infections are classified by the area of the body involved and are frequently called tineas. The ones that need to be remembered are capitis (scalp and hair), barbae (beard area), cruris (groin), and pedia (feet and occasionally hands). In addition, onychomycosis (nails) and tinea versicolor complete the necessary glossary.

As in any other infection the first issue is having the correct diagnosis; most of the time this is simple. In fact, the patient will know that he has athletes' foot or jock itch. Unfortunately, this is not always the case. Experienced dermatologists are required who have the proper means for diagnosis. The diagnostic reagents include simple 10 percent or 20 percent potassium hydroxide to be added to the sample obtained, staining solution such as a mixture of Quick ink with potassium hydroxide or Gram stain, and the ability to culture the organism for identification. In addition a Wood's lamp is required. Cultures are not necessary if the diagnosis is obvious and if it can be predicted that the treatment is going to be successful. Cultures are necessary in a small proportion of patients when the diagnosis is in doubt and examinations of skin scrapings are not helpful.

Seeing or growing the organism does not always assure the diagnosis. The fungus might be a commensal or might be only part of the problem. The other part might be a coexisting bacterial infection or the presence of contact dermatitis to previous remedies or other external agents. Heat, moisture, and tissue maceration enhance the growth and persistence of superficial fungal infections. This is true at least in the predisposed host. The reasons why some people are not infected with superficial fungi in spite of lack of preventive measures is not known. For the infected person, local treatments, if they can be effectively applied, are most useful. For example, for athletes' foot, in addition to the chosen antifungal agent, drying the feet well, keeping them ventilated, and wearing sandals will make an important difference, especially in severe cases.

ATHLETES' FOOT (TINEA PEDIS)

This is a common infection; transmission occurs in public showers, and lack of drying the feet predisposes to infection. The reasons why some people do not become infected in spite of being exposed are not known. Bacterial superinfections that use the cracks in the skin must be kept in mind and treated. Occasionally, cellulitis involving feet and the lower legs occurs, mainly with group A or β-hemolytic streptococci or staphylococcus and requires treatment with systemic antibiotics. Dicloxacillin 250 mg PO four times daily is a useful regimen for these gram-positive infections. The fungal infection must be treated for several weeks to prevent recurrence.

INFECTIONS OF SCALP AND HAIR (TINEA CAPITIS)

Dermatophytes of the genera *Microsporum* and *Trichophyton* are the causative agents. In the United States *Microsporum audouinii* was once very common. Today *Trichophyton tonsurans* is the most common cause of tinea

capitis and its presence is often difficult to prove. The hair infected with tinea tonsurans does not exhibit the characteristic yellow-green fluorescence seen in hair infected with *M. audouinii* and *Microsporum canis*. The diagnosis is suspected based on the appearance of the lesion with areas of alopecia and the presence of "black dots." As the infected hairs break just below the folliculus orifice, these follicles or "black dots" are apparent and are the best source of material to be examined with potassium hydroxide (KOH) and culture. These infections occur almost exclusively in the prepuberal period and often in groups of children. Treatment is with microcrystalline griseofulvin, 10 mg per kilogram taken with food; if there is no improvement in 4 to 6 weeks, higher doses are needed until all clinical evidence of disease is not apparent, but not less than 6 to 8 weeks. Ultramicrosized griseofulvin, which is more expensive, can be used in similar doses if microcrystalline fails, but proof of its advantage is lacking. Selenium sulfide shampoo or lotion is an important added therapeutic measure. The patient should use the shampoo daily, and as improvement begins, space the shampoo to twice a week.

INFECTIONS OF THE FACE (TINEA BARBAE, BARBER'S ITCH)

This type of infection affects the bearded area of the face and neck. It is caused by *Trichophyton* and *Microsporum*. The infection is often superficial and mimics ringworm of other parts of the body. It is associated with temporary loss of hair in the involved areas. Sometimes it involves deeper areas of the skin, with follicular pustules or nodules mimicking severe acne. It also can mimic bacterial folliculitis in what is called the sycosiform type. Topical treatments are not successful by themselves. Systemic treatments with griseofulvin for 6 to 8 weeks is required. Alternatively, ketoconazole or other oral imidazoles are used.

TABLE 1 Treatment of Superficial Fungal Infections

Agent	Tinea Capitis	Tinea Cruris	Tinea Pedis	Tinea Corporis	Tinea Barbae	Tinea Versicolor	Candida	Onychomycosis
Undecylenic acid	−	+	+	+	−	−	−	−
Tolnaftate	−	+	+	+	+	−	−	−
Nystatin	−	−	−	−	−	−	+	−
Clotrimazole	−	+	+	+	+	+	+	−
Miconazole	−	+	+	+	+	+	+	−
Ketoconazole cream	−	+	+	+	−	+	+	−
Econazole	−	+	+	+	+	+	+	−
Cicloprixolamine	−	+	+	+	+	+	+	−
Amphotericin B, topical	−	−	−	−		−	+	−
Other	Systemic therapy	Use cotton underwear	Treat bacterial infection, sandals			Selenium; repeat in 1 wk Ketoconazole 400 mg qd for 3 days	Systemic therapy in immunosuppressed patient	None very good; systemic and removal of nails

INFECTIONS OF THE BODY (TINEA CORPORIS)

This form excludes infections of the hair, face, feet, hands, groin, and nails. Produced by *Trichophyton* and *Epidermophyton*, these infections are often worse in persons with uncontrolled leukemia, lymphomas, or diabetes mellitus.

Several forms have special names; circinate is the common variety; kerion is a term to describe severe inflammatory reactions with edema, vesicle formation, and occasionally pustulation. The inflammatory reaction is able to control the infection and makes it self-limited. Majocchi granuloma involves the hair follicles, more often in the lower extremities, and requires systemic therapy similar to that for tinea barbae.

GROIN INFECTIONS (TINEA CRURIS)

These infections are more common in males than in females, and the lesion often has an inflammatory margin. It is produced by *Trichophyton* and *Epidermophyton*. *Candida* does involve the inguinal area but usually involves a wider area and has distinct satelliting.

Tolnaftate is quite effective. Small amounts of the cream suffice, but it must be used for at least 3 weeks, and the infection has a high rate of recurrence. If *Candida* is involved or there is no certainty of the nature of the offending fungus, 2 percent miconazole or any imidazole, also in small amounts, should be used.

TINEA VERSICOLOR

This infection manifests as asymptomatic hypopigmented lesions of 2 to 5 mm covered with a fine scale. It is caused by the yeast *Malassezia furfur*. The hypopigmented areas become more noticeable with sun exposure, as the surrounding skin becomes darker and the lesions remain the same.

The treatment is 1 percent selenium sulfide in a shampoo base over the entire body. Ketoconazole 400 mg daily for 3 days clears the lesions. Long-term cures are likely.

MUCOCUTANEOUS CANDIDIASIS

Candida species involve the skin in a variety of ways. It is the one fungus that in addition to involving the skin and nails affects the mucosa, including the areas between mucosa and skin, such as perianal, perioral, and vaginal introitus, and indeed may produce systemic infections that may involve any organ in the body, with serious consequences.

Candida albicans is the most common pathogen, but any of a long list of *Candida* species may be present: *C. parapsilosis, C. tropicalis, C. krusei, C. guillermondi, C. glabrata* (previously known as *torulosis glabrata*), and others.

The presence of *Candida*, demonstrated by culture, does not necessarily signify infection. Candida can be grown frequently from the mouth of a healthy person with dentures. Yet in hospitalized or chronically ill patients, candidal dermatitis, with its characteristic satelliting lesions, is common. The inguinal, perianal, and axillary areas and areas under the breast are often involved. Topical treatment with effective anticandidal agents, such as miconazole nitrate, is quite effective.

Occasionally, systemic treatment with ketoconazole is needed. In immunosuppressed patients systemic treatment is almost always necessary. In patients with human immunodeficiency virus infection, candidal infection of the mouth is common, sometimes as the initial manifestation and commonly as one of the problems late in the disease. Topical treatment can be tried but most of the time is not sufficient. Ketoconazole, 200 mg daily, usually suppresses the infection but may have to be taken indefinitely. Amphotericin B is almost never necessary in superficial infections but is quite effective when used for the treatment of deep infections and the patient has a concurrent superficial infection.

In other immunosuppressed states, candidal as well as other superficial fungal infections are more common than in the immunocompetent person. Candidal vaginitis is probably more frequent in pregnant women and may be more common in women taking contraceptive hormones. Persistent topical treatment suffices most of the time. Seldom is it necessary to discontinue hormonal therapy in favor of other contraceptives.

In the newborn and in children in diapers, *Candida* may be the causative organism of diaper rash. In buccal candidiasis of the infant, the nipple of the mother needs to be treated. The physician must keep in mind that the presence of candidal superficial infection needs to be treated, but some thought should be given to the possible presence of an immunodeficiency state, including malnutrition. The use of antibiotics for reasons not totally understood but probably related to decrease of the normal flora of mucosal areas predisposes to candidal infection.

SUGGESTED READING

Moschellz SL, Hurley HJ. Dermatology. 2nd ed. Philadelphia: WB Saunders, 1985.

Rook A, Wilkinson DS, Ebling FJG, et al. Textbook of dermatology. 4th ed. Boston: Blackwell Scientific Publications, 1986.

NOSOCOMIAL INFECTIONS

URINARY CATHETER–ASSOCIATED INFECTION

JOHN P. BURKE, M.D.
DAVID C. CLASSEN, M.D.

The urinary catheter is an ancient device that continues to have an indispensable role in medical care. It is employed in a wide variety of clinical circumstances to permit drainage of the anatomically or functionally obstructed urinary tract, to control drainage in incontinent patients, or to obtain precise measurement of urinary output. The most important clinical distinctions in the use of urinary catheters relate to the duration of use: brief in-and-out catheterization, short periods of indwelling catheterization (1 to 7 days) in postoperative patients, intermediate durations (7 to 30 days) in critically ill medical patients, and long-term (>30 days) catheterization in patients who are incontinent or have incorrectable obstruction of the bladder outlet.

The use of a urinary catheter always entails some risk of both infective and noninfective complications; the former includes the risk of death from gram-negative rod bacteremia and perhaps from other as yet undefined mechanisms. The sequelae of catheter-induced infections include acute and chronic pyelonephritis; perinephric, vesical, and urethral abscesses; bladder and renal stones; renal failure; polyposis and squamous metaplasia; and carcinoma of the bladder, suppurative epididymitis, and urethral strictures. In addition, patients with catheter-associated infections harbor a formidable reservoir of antibiotic-resistant pathogens that may be responsible for cross-infection in health care institutions.

Bacteriuria, i.e., literally the presence of bacteria in urine, is a necessary antecedent of these infectious complications. The normal urinary tract above the distal urethra is free of bacteria and able to clear rapidly small numbers of organisms that may be introduced through urethral trauma or instrumentation. The indwelling urinary catheter breaches this normal mucosal defense mechanism, not only by providing a continuing means of entry for bacteria, but also by serving as a foreign body that promotes infection through a number of additional mechanisms: (1) bacterial adherence to uroepithelial cells may be transiently increased; (2) biofilm production by bacteria adherent to the catheter itself may protect the bacterial colonies from systemic antibiotics as well as from host defenses; and (3) indwelling catheters with retention balloons incompletely empty the bladder, thereby compromising the physical removal of bacteria.

The usual organisms responsible for catheter-associated bacteriuria are gram-negative bacilli and enterococci derived from the fecal flora. Anaerobic bacteria, however, are rarely found. *Candida* and staphylococcal species may account for as many as one-third of the cases. A single infecting species is usual, but serial infections are common; most patients with long-term catheters have polymicrobial bacteriuria with spontaneous turnover of individual species.

There are only two pathways by which microorganisms commonly enter the catheterized urinary tract: through the catheter lumen or through the potential space between the urethral mucosa and the outside surface of the catheter. Candiduria and bacteriuria due to *Staphylococcus aureus* may result from bloodstream infection, but gram-negative rods virtually never infect the urinary tract by the hematogenous route.

Bacteriuria associated with indwelling catheterization may have diverse origins. For example, asymptomatic bacteriuria may precede placement of the catheter, or bacteriuria may arise from organisms pushed into the bladder during transurethral catheter insertion. Bacteriuria may also be acquired through ascent of organisms that are allowed to contaminate the inside of the drainage bag (from improper emptying) or the catheter tubing (from nonsterile disconnection of the catheter drainage tube junction). Finally, bacteria colonizing the perineum and the meatal surface may also migrate to the bladder in the pericatheter space, a pathway that appears to account for 70 percent or more of acquired bacteriurias during short and intermediate durations of catheterization.

Organisms, especially *Pseudomonas* and *Serratia* species, that enter through the intraluminal route are commonly acquired from transient carriage of gram-negative bacilli on the hands of personnel or on collection containers (exogenous infection) and may be transmitted by cross-infection. Organisms that enter through the pericatheter space are generally part of the patient's normal fecal and perineal flora (endogenous infection), although these organisms may become a part of the perineal and meatal flora as a consequence of hospitalization or as a result of cross-infection.

DIAGNOSIS

The diagnosis of catheter-associated bacteriuria in a patient with a standard Foley catheter with a retention balloon depends upon quantitative culture of urine obtained by aseptic needle aspiration from the distal catheter or through a sampling port on the drainage tube. The catheter should not be disconnected from the drainage tube in order to collect a specimen because contamination of the closed system may result.

For occasional sampling, one can avoid the need for clamping the tubing to collect urine by aspirating directly through the catheter itself distal to the channel for inflating the balloon using a 22- or 25-gauge needle. The site should be cleansed with an alcohol wipe before needle puncture, and aseptic precautions should be observed; disposable gloves should be worn and care taken to avoid needle-stick injury.

Despite the concern that continuous drainage through an indwelling catheter may not permit retention of urine in the bladder long enough for bacterial growth to yield high colony counts, especially for organisms with fastidious growth requirements, small numbers of bacteria introduced into the system do generally multiply rapidly and exceed 100,000 or more colonies per milliliter in a day or two in patients not receiving systemic antibiotics. The criterion selected to define bacteriuria depends largely on the purpose to be served. Lower colony counts are commonly selected as a breakpoint in clinical trials of catheter care in order to provide greater sensitivity for detection. Theoretically, any number of bacteria obtained by aspiration should be considered significant. In clinical practice and especially in long-term catheterized patients, the criterion of 100,000 or more colony-forming units (cfu) is quite satisfactory.

Caution in interpreting colony counts is necessary, however, because some rapid tests for bacteriuria are insensitive to low colony counts, and bacteremia does occasionally occur in those with colony counts of less than 100,000 per milliliter. Moreover, colony counts of urine from long-term catheters may not accurately reflect the density of bladder bacteriuria, and some suggest that in these patients the catheter should be changed before a specimen is obtained for culture.

No reliable criteria exist to distinguish bladder colonization from infection. Most patients with catheter-associated bacteriuria also have pyuria and remain asymptomatic. A long-term catheterization patient almost always has pyuria and bacteriuria. Culture of the tip of the Foley catheter has no role in the diagnosis of infection.

PREVENTION OF INFECTION

Although urinary tract infection is an inevitable consequence of long-term catheterization, bacteriuria can be successfully avoided in the majority of patients with short periods of catheterization by the correct use of techniques for closed sterile urinary drainage. In those with intermediate durations, bacteriuria can be successfully postponed. While the benefits of delaying the onset of bacteriuria have not been well defined, complicated infections and urosepsis may be less common and bacteriuria may be better tolerated once the acute stage of the underlying illness has resolved. The prompt removal of catheters that are no longer necessary may result in true prevention. Moreover, cross-infection with antibiotic-resistant organisms can be successfully prevented regardless of the duration of catheterization and is a worthwhile clinical goal.

Nearly all of the commercially available systems for urinary drainage are closed, i.e., the drainage tube is fused to a vented collection bag so that the urine is not exposed to air, and the distal end of the tube is not exposed to the reservoir of urine in the bag. The introduction and widespread use of closed sterile drainage was a major advance and has undoubtedly prevented thousands of deaths from gram-negative bacteremia in the past 25 years. Closed drainage systems represent a passive infection control measure that requires little effort by personnel. However, closed systems must be opened, for example, when urine is emptied from the bag or when the catheter is disconnected from the system for irrigation or by accident.

Unfortunately, the principles of closed drainage are not well understood by all health care workers, and errors in the care of closed systems are commonplace. Improper handling can introduce bacteria that can ascend to the bladder, especially when backflow of urine occurs if the bag is raised above the bladder or placed beside the patient being transported, for example, to the radiology department. Regular and continuing in-service education of personnel, emphasizing the principles of closed drainage, is obviously necessary but appears to hold little promise for major reductions in the rate of catheter-associated bacteriuria, in part because the majority of infections appear to result from the pericatheter pathway. Periodic culture studies as recommended by Kunin (see Suggested Reading) may help individual institutions identify excessive rates of bacteriuria and improper catheter care.

Efforts to block the periurethral pathway of infection by the frequent application of topical antimicrobial agents to the meatal surface have not been cost effective, and the use of povidone-iodine preparations was associated with an increased incidence of bacteriuria in one controlled study.

At present, removal of crusts and debris from the external surface of the catheter, especially around the meatal insertion site, with plain soap and a washcloth during daily bathing is generally recommended and may help to reduce urethral irritation.

Disconnections of the catheter drainage tube can be discouraged by the application of taped seals to the junction, and contamination of the drainage bag can be prevented by the use of disposable gloves for handling the outflow spigot. Other adjuncts to closed drainage have generally been unsuccessful or have had questionable cost benefits.

Modifications of closed drainage have included coating or impregnation of the catheter with proprietary compounds to inhibit bacterial adherence or growth. One such coating using silver oxide has shown promising results in a randomized controlled trial in selected patients; it is currently being evaluated in more broadly representative hospitalized patients. The instillation of antibacterial substances into the drainage bag remains controversial but may have some efficacy in settings where contamination of bags is frequent.

This latter approach may become more practical as longer-acting agents are developed so that frequent instillations are not needed. In addition, disinfection of the drainage bag urine could eliminate a reservoir for potential cross-infection.

Urinary drainage equipment is marketed in an aggressively competitive environment in which infection control properties are stressed, usually without supporting clinical evidence of efficacy. Currently the selection of such equipment should be based on factors other than extravagant and unsupported claims for prevention of infection; cost and acceptability to nursing personnel should be the decisive factors.

There seems to be no justification for the use of expensive silicone-coated catheters for patients with brief or intermediate durations of catheterization, although they may be associated with less encrustation, blockage, urethritis, and discomfort with longer-term use. No set interval should be adopted for changing the catheter; in general, patients with long-term catheters will require changing at monthly intervals, but broad individual variation occurs and the "catheter life" of each patient should be determined by examining the removed catheter for encrustations and blocked flow.

The smallest suitable catheter diameter should be selected, and larger catheters are usually needed only for postoperative urologic patients who are passing blood clots. The balloon volume should also be small (5 to 10 ml) since forcible removal of catheters with 30-ml balloons can occur with greater resulting urethral trauma.

In 1983 the Centers for Disease Control (Atlanta) published guidelines for the prevention of catheter-associated infections that represented a consensus of experts and that remain relevant today. Particularly noteworthy is the admonition to catheterize only when necessary and then using correct aseptic technique and closed drainage. Alternatives to indwelling catheterization such as condom catheters, incontinence clothing, or intermittent catheterization should be utilized when possible. At times, the risk of indwelling catheterization may be judged to be more acceptable than the nursing problems associated with incontinence, especially when tissue maceration and decubitus ulcers are present.

The use of suprapubic catheter placement has become prevalent in postoperative gynecologic procedures and appears to be associated with a lower risk of bacteriuria, improved patient comfort, and more rapid restoration of normal voiding mechanisms. Techniques have also been developed for the "nonoperative" placement of small-bore suprapubic catheters without retention balloons. However, further evaluation of the safety, efficacy, and benefits of this approach is needed.

The use of systemic antimicrobial agents to prevent catheter-associated bacteriuria has generally been condemned because of the benign nature of most of these infections and because of the cost, adverse effects, and selection of resistant organisms associated with antibiotic use. A reduced incidence of bacteriuria during the first 4 days of catheterization has been found in patients receiving systemic antibiotics. However, their use for this purpose cannot be recommended except possibly in certain high-risk or immunocompromised patients in whom a short duration of catheterization is anticipated. Suitably controlled studies to define the optimal agents, regimens, and, if present, cost benefits are currently needed. At present, no prophylactic antimicrobial regimen has been found to prevent infection in long-term catheterized patients. Methenamine preparations are not effective in the prevention or treatment of bacteriuria in catheterized patients but may have a role in reducing encrustations and blockage of catheters (by a mechanism unrelated to its antibacterial property), thereby lengthening the interval between required catheter changes in selected patients.

TREATMENT

In the past, investigators have directed less attention to the management than to the prevention of catheter-associated bacteriuria. Consequently, there is a dearth of well-controlled trials to serve as a basis for specific recommendations, in contrast to the many therapeutic trials in other urinary tract infection syndromes. Nonetheless, there is a consensus that catheter-associated bacteriuria should not be treated with systemic antimicrobial agents as long as the patient remains catheterized and asymptomatic.

The basis for this view is that treatment is effective only in making the urine culture-negative while the antibiotic is being given but not in eliminating bacterial colonies adherent to the catheter and protected by the bacterial glycocalyx from exposure to the antibiotic. Relapse of bacteriuria following treatment usually occurs. Replacement of the catheter and drainage bag with a new sterile system within 24 to 48 hours after therapy has begun is a potentially useful strategy that has been incompletely evaluated.

Bacteremia may occur at any time during indwelling catheterization and not only at times of catheter insertion or change. Moreover, fever in a patient with an indwelling catheter should not be attributed to bacteriuria unless other potential causes have been evaluated. Blood and urine specimens should be obtained for culture (a single blood culture should suffice in most instances), and the patient should be empirically treated for bacteremia, usually with either an aminoglycoside or an expanded-spectrum β-lactam antibiotic (see the chapter *Gram-Negative Rod Bacteremia*).

In the nonneutropenic patient who is not in septic shock, there is no adequate justification for the use of combination antimicrobic regimens. However, microscopic examination of a Gram-stained urine specimen can be helpful in selecting empiric therapy, for example, by suggesting the presence of enterococci and the use of ampicillin, either alone or in combination with gentamicin.

A common clinical problem is colonization by yeast, especially in patients receiving systemic antimicrobics. Most often, these patients do not develop invasive disease, and the "infection" clears with removal of the catheter. However, in selected patients, continuous irrigation with amphotericin B (50 mg per liter of sterile water per day) through a triple-lumen catheter for 5 days has been associated with resolution of candiduria and is preferable to systemic antifungal treatment.

Daily monitoring of urine cultures from patients with short or intermediate durations of catheterization has not proved to be a useful strategy to permit the treatment of bacteriuria and, thereby, the prevention of bacteremia. Nonetheless, it seems reasonable to culture the urine at the time of catheter insertion and again immediately before its removal in order to identify asymptomatic infections that require follow-up. In most patients bacteriuria will spontaneously clear after the catheter is removed, but the physician's goal should be to see that the now-noncatheterized urinary tract is left sterile and not to rely on a normal urinalysis or the absence of symptoms for this assurance. A follow-up urine culture 1 to 2 weeks after catheter removal will help to identify persistently bacteriuric patients who are candidates for treatment.

A further indication for urine culture in an asymptomatic catheterized patient occurs when a urologic operation or a surgical procedure involving the placement of prosthetic material or an organ transplant is planned. Systemic antimicrobial treatment selected on the basis of culture and susceptibility data may help to reduce the risk of bacteremia originating from the urinary tract in these patients.

Cultures of urine from asymptomatic long-term catheterized patients may, on the other hand, invite unnecessary antibiotic treatment and lead to antibiotic-resistant infections, adverse effects from the drugs used, and increased costs.

The complications of bacteriuria in long-term catheterized patients are often associated with obstruction and/or stones. Intermittent irrigation, either with normal saline or with antimicrobial solutions, such as 0.25 percent acetic acid, has not proved useful in preventing obstructions or in eradicating established bacteriuria.

Patients with long-term catheters who become febrile ($\geq$ 38.9 °C) should be managed as above for possible bacteremia and should also be evaluated for catheter obstruction and local periurethral infection. Patients with recurrent high fevers, bacteremia, or increasing renal dysfunction should be evaluated for urinary tract stones. For such patients, operative intervention may be required.

SUGGESTED READING

Kunin CM. Care of the urinary catheter. In: Detection, prevention and management of urinary tract infections. 4th ed. Philadelphia: Lea & Febiger, 1987:245.
Slade N, Gillespie WA. The urinary tract and the catheter. Infection and other problems. New York: John Wiley & Sons, 1985.
Warren JW. Catheter-associated urinary tract infections. Infect Dis Clin North Am 1987; 1:823–854.

INTRAVASCULAR CATHETER– ASSOCIATED INFECTION

CYRUS C. HOPKINS, M.D.

Infection associated with intravascular catheters can involve several different parts of the system: the entry site of the catheter into the skin, the subcutaneous tissue between the skin entry site and the vessel, the intravascular portion of the catheter, or the intraluminal fluid within the catheter, tubing, bottle or bag, or pressure transducers.

Infection at each of these sites has its own likely organisms and may appear with different clinical presentations. The skin entry site is probably the most common site of entry of the organism. Clinically significant infection at this site may present as a purulent cellulitis centered around the entry site. Colonization of this site and extension through the subcutaneum to the intravascular catheter segment can occur without signs of infection. In the case of a "tunneled" catheter with a long subcutaneous segment, tunnel infection alone may occur, in which case a red streak of apparent cellulitis is often visible. Infection may involve the intravascular segment alone, either serving as a focus of origin or as a nidus for adherence of organisms hematogenously disseminated to it from another source. Finally, some species will grow readily within the fluid itself, which provides logarithmic growth, yielding a high inoculum of organisms (usually gram-negative bacilli) or a source of endotoxin.

DIAGNOSIS

Appropriate treatment rests on clinical suspicion, for most primary clinical diagnoses of catheter-associated infections are diagnoses of exclusion, except for the few catheter entry-site or tunnel infections, which are clinically manifest at the site. Fevers—or septic signs occurring in hospital in a patient with intravascular catheters—should always raise the question of a catheter-associated infection but are statistically far more likely to be caused by infections at other common sites of nosocomial infection, such as the catheterized urinary tract, the surgical wound, or the lower respiratory tract. Initial evaluation, then, rests on a complete history, focusing on recent in-hospital events, and physical and laboratory examination of the most commonly infected sites. During this initial evaluation, the catheter site should be examined and inquiries made into the duration of use of any indwelling catheter; the frequency of change of fluids, tranducers, and tubings; and any recent manipulation of the catheter.

TREATMENT

The general principle of therapy involves: (1) search for the organism by blood culture, Gram stain, and culture of drainage (if any) and, in some instances, culture of the intravenous fluids; (2) in general, removal of the catheter; (3) then, but before waiting for culture results, initiation of broad-spectrum antibiotics, especially covering for *Staphylococcus aureus* unless otherwise guided by the results of the above; and finally, (4) simplification of the antibiotics when culture results become available.

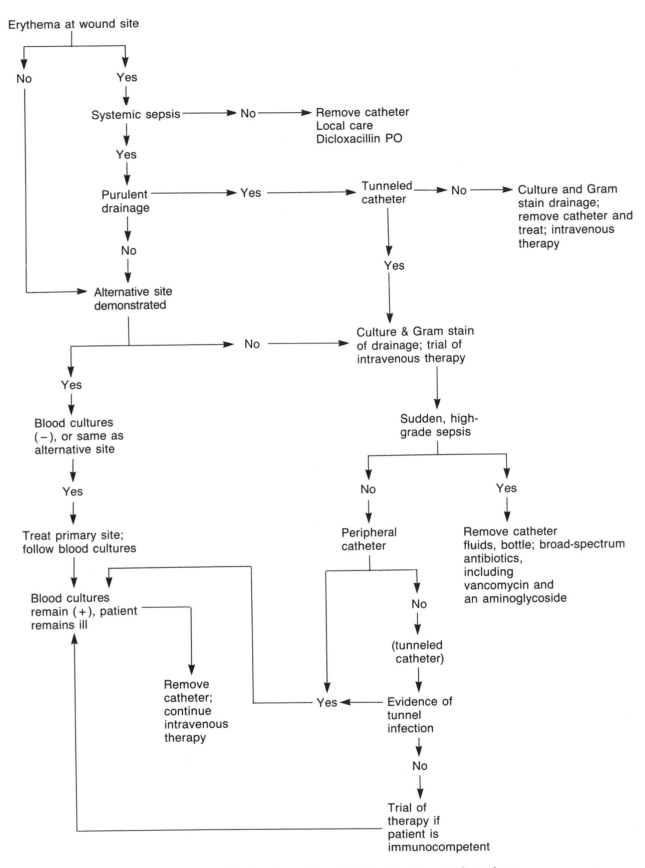

Figure 1 Possible infection in a patient with indwelling intravascular catheter.

If erythema and purulence are found, the catheter is removed whenever possible. Peripheral or non-tunneled catheters should always be removed, and purulent drainage should be Gram stained and cultured. Occasionally, a trial of therapy can be successful for tunneled, hard-to-replace catheters (Hickman, Broviac). Blood cultures should also be obtained before treatment is begun (Fig. 1).

If only local signs of erythema and tenderness are found without any signs of systemic sepsis, a non-tunneled catheter should be removed, and a short course of oral antibiotics, such as dicloxacillin, 500 mg orally four times a day, can be used.

If no local signs of catheter-related infection are found, the search for other unrelated sites should continue. Physical examination, chest roentgenogram, urinalysis, and inspection of wound sites should be performed to exclude other sites. Blood cultures should be obtained. If another focus is found, Gram stain and culture of material reflecting this site should be performed and treatment of this focus begun.

If blood cultures are positive for the same organism found in another infected site (urine, wound, sputum), and if the clinical course is favorable with appropriately directed therapy, the catheter need not be removed, unless the bacteremia-causing organisms are staphylococci (either coagulase-positive or coagulase-negative). If so, the catheter should then be removed and cultured. If not, the underlying infection should be treated and the catheter and catheter changes handled in a routine manner and then reevaluated. Catheters removed for documented sepsis should not be changed over a guidewire, as infection of the new catheter remains a risk.

If the catheter remains in place, treatment should generally begin with vancomycin, until *Staphylococcus epidermidis,* or even methicillin-resistant *S. aureus* (MRSA) has been excluded by culture results.

If the initial evaluation reveals signs of severe sepsis of sudden onset, such as septic shock, the intravenous fluid should be immediately suspected. In that case, all intravascular lines, tubing, and fluid sources should be removed and saved intact for culture and identification. Treatment must include both vancomycin (in case of MRSA) and an aminoglycoside, since there is little margin for error.

Antibiotic Selection

Always begin with antistaphylococcal therapy (nafcillin 1 g intravenously every 4 hours or cefazolin 1 g intravenously every 8 hours), then revise or add aminoglycosides (gentamicin, 1.5 mg per kg per dose) if gram-negative rods are found on Gram stain or culture of drainage of blood. If MRSA is known to be present in the institution, or if the catheter must be retained, treatment is better begun with vancomycin (2 g per day, for an adult with normal renal function). If yeasts are found in blood cultures, amphotericin B is the drug of choice.

Duration

The duration of therapy is not well defined. Prolonged *Staphylococcus aureus* bacteremia requires 4 weeks of intravenous therapy with a penicillinase-resistant semisynthetic penicillin (oxacillin, nafcillin), a first-generation cephalosporin (cefazolin), or vancomycin. If the infection has been detected promptly and the offending catheter is immediately removed, and if no hardware is present, many experts recommend only 2 weeks of therapy, assuming that the patient responds promptly (bacteremia with a removable focus). In this era of increasing use of home delivery of intravenous antibiotics, I use this shorter course only infrequently. Coagulase-negative staphylococci will require 4 weeks of treatment only if other indwelling hardware is present (e.g., prosthetic cardiac valves). Gram-negative bacteremia usually requires up to 3 weeks of therapy, depending on the response of the patient. Management of fungal sepsis is also unclear: fundoscopic examination should be performed initially and later in the course. If the fundi show no evidence of candidal infection, 500 mg (total dose) of amphotericin B will suffice for an immunocompetent patient, but there are no good data to guide us on this at this time.

Failure of Treatment

Failure to respond to appropriate therapy requires reevaluation of several clinical issues, especially the certainty of the diagnosis, the exclusion of other sites, and whether secondary endocarditis or septic phlebitis is likely. Reexamination of the site is critical; persistent pain and induration over the involved vein and signs of impaired venous drainage (especially for central catheters) prompt consideration of septic phlebitis. "Milking" the involved vein toward the insertion will occasionally produce purulent drainage. Persistent purulence, induration, and lack of response necessitate surgical involvement.

SPECIAL PROBLEMS

Hyperalimentation solutions provide a source (presumably because they provide a special growth medium) for organisms not often associated with septicemia, such as *Candida albicans* or similar yeasts, or, especially in infants, *Malassezia furfur.* In both cases, initial conventional blood cultures may be negative. The catheter should be removed and blood cultures performed with special techniques, such as lysis-centrifugation, which may have a higher yield. Comparing colony counts on specimens obtained through the catheter versus peripheral specimens may allow some prediction of whether the catheter is the source. If fungal infection is a possibility, Gram stain of the catheter may be helpful, since it may be positive even though blood cultures are negative.

Hickman, Broviac, and other central tunneled catheters become infected much less frequently than do peripheral catheters or other centrally inserted catheters. There is increasing evidence that treatment of an intravascular site, or even of the entry site alone, may often be successfully completed even if the catheter is left in place. Infections along the track of the tunneled catheter, however, particularly if caused by gram-negative bacilli, are unlikely to respond, and the catheter will have to be removed. Bacteremia in children with a Hickman catheter in place will often be cured without removing the catheter. There are inadequate data to guide us in adults.

Immunocompromised patients may develop catheter-associated sepsis with a wide variety of organisms. Positive blood cultures, or even fever of unclear origin in a catheterized patient, should be followed by removal of the catheter. New skin lesions, especially at the entry site, but even peripherally, should be biopsied.

SUGGESTED READING

Allo MD, Miller J, Townsend T, et al. Primary cutaneous aspergillosis associated with Hickman intravenous catheters. N Engl J Med 1987; 317:1105–1108.

Benezra D, Kiehn TE, Gold JWM, et al. Prospective study of infections in indwelling central venous catheters using quantitative blood cultures. Am J Med 1988; 85:495–498.

Bernhardt LL, Antopol SC, Simberkoff MS, et al. Association of teichoic acid antibody with metastatic sequelae of catheter-associated Staphylococcus aureus bacteremia. A failure of the two-week antibiotic treatment. Am J Med 1979; 66:355–357.

Pettigrew RA, Lang SDR, Haydock DA, et al. Catheter-related sepsis in patients on intravenous nutrition: a prospective study of quantitative catheter cultures and guidewire changes for suspected sepsis. Br J Surg 1985; 72:52–55.

Raucher HS, Hyatt AC, Barzilai A, et al. Quantitative blood cultures in the evaluation of septicemia in children with Broviac catheters. J Pediatr 1984; 104:29–33.

Walsh TJ, Bustamante CI, Vlahov D, et al. Candidal suppurative peripheral thrombophlebitis: recognition, prevention, and management. Infect Control 1986; 7:16–32.

POSTOPERATIVE WOUND INFECTION

JOHN E. McGOWAN Jr., M.D.

THE PROBLEM

Wound infections following operation are a frequent and important cause of surgical morbidity and mortality. The Centers for Disease Control reported surgical wound infections in 0.47 percent of all hospital discharges in 1984 from hospitals participating in their National Nosocomial Infections Survey (NNIS). The infection rate markedly increases when pus or a perforated viscus is found at operation. In "clean" surgery (no infection encountered, no hollow muscular organ opened, no break in aseptic technique during the procedure) the rate of infection is 1 to 2 percent, while after "contaminated" procedures (those with acute inflammation without pus, gross spillage from a hollow viscus, a major break in aseptic technique during the operation, or acute trauma of less than 4 hours), rates of approximately 15 percent are encountered.

The presence of a wound infection has economic as well as patient consequences. The average hospital stay increases by about 10 days when a postoperative patient acquires a wound infection. Thus, making sure that optimal therapy is given at the time that the wound infection is discovered can be cost-effective as well as salutary for the patient.

DIAGNOSIS

Most infections occur between the fourth and 10th day after surgery, but this latent period varies markedly with the site and type of operation, the use of perioperative prophylaxis (discussed in a separate chapter), the infecting organism(s), and whether the infection is superficial or deep to the incision site.

The usual definition of infection depends on the presence of a purulent exudate at the site. Most postoperative wound infections are uncomplicated, involving only the skin and subcutaneous tissues. Infrequently, they progress to involve the fascia and muscle. Local pain at the site of the incision, tenderness, redness, swelling, and increased warmth are the usual initial manifestations of infection. At this stage, it may be difficult to determine whether an infection exists, as no exudate may be present. Deep wound infections also are difficult to detect; often the persistence of patient infirmity, development of fever, positive blood culture, or laboratory studies suggesting continued inflammation (e.g., abnormally high levels of C-reactive protein, leukocytosis) permit recognition, or trigger the studies (e.g., ultrasonography, computed tomography, nuclear scanning, aspiration or biopsy, surgical exploration) needed for diagnosis. Development of a mass or dehiscence can occasionally be the clues to the existence of infection.

TREATMENT

Once one has decided that the patient's clinical manifestations represent infection and not other potential causes of postoperative fever, and after appropriate specimens have been obtained for culture and other laboratory studies, therapy is instituted. Appropriate treatment depends on the sites involved.

Nonantimicrobial Management—The Key to Success

Local (superficial) postoperative wound infections are those involving the incisional site, without spread to adjacent areas. Stitch abscess or mild inflammation at the site of a stitch, while technically a local wound infection, usually is of such little clinical import that it is often not considered local postoperative wound infection. The cardinal elements of treatment for a local postoperative wound infection are drainage of pus and local wound care, including debridement when necessary.

Complicated wound infections are those from which spread beyond the initial incision site is suspected. Possible problems may include abscess formation or other tissue in-

TABLE 1 Recommendations for Initial Empiric Therapy for Postoperative Wound Infection, Based on Gram-Stain Evaluation of Exudate

Gram-Stain Findings	Likely Pathogens	Antimicrobial Drug Regimen* Local Infection	Antimicrobial Drug Regimen* Complicated Infection
Gram-positive cocci in chains	Enterococci (group A *Streptococcus*†)	A C	B C
Gram-positive cocci in clusters	*Staphylococcus aureus* (coagulase-negative *Staphylococcus*†)	D None	E F
Gram-positive bacilli	Clostridia	C	C
Gram-negative bacilli	Depends on site of surgery	G	See Table 2
Fungi	*Candida*	None	Only if severe immunocompromise (see text)

Note. This table presents usual guidelines for situations in which therapy must be started before information about organism identification and susceptibility can be obtained from culture. Certain diagnostic and epidemiologic factors may make it necessary to modify the recommendations given here (see text). In all cases, these initial recommendations should be modified when definitive microbiologic information becomes available.

* Drugs and administration:
Regimen A: ampicillin 1 g IV q4h (alternative: no therapy).
Regimen B: penicillin G 2 million units IV q4h plus gentamicin 2 mg/kg IV given slowly over 1 hour once, then 1.5 mg/kg IV given slowly over 1 hour q8h (assuming normal renal function). If high-level resistance to gentamicin is frequent among enterococci at the institution, or if the patient is allergic to penicillin, give vancomycin (regimen F) instead.
Regimen C: penicillin G 1 million units IV q4h (alternative, clindamycin 900 mg IV q8h).
Regimen D: dicloxacillin 250 mg PO q.i.d. (alternative, cephalexin 500 mg PO q.i.d. or cefadroxil 750 mg PO b.i.d. or cephradine 500 mg PO q.i.d.).
Regimen E: nafcillin 2 g IV q4h (alternative, cefazolin 1 g IV q8h, but if methicillin-resistant organisms prevalent in hospital, use regimen F instead of either of these).
Regimen F: vancomycin 500 mg IV q6h (alternative, none).
Regimen G: cefazolin 1 g IV q8h.
† Certain clinical or epidemiologic features may make this organism likely enough that empiric therapy is warranted (see text).

vasion deep to the incision, involvement of tissues adjacent to the incision, or spread by bloodstream or lymphatics to distant sites. A critical component of care for these complicated infections is obtaining effective drainage of loculated pus, accompanied by debridement of dead tissue when necessary. On occasion, surgical reexploration will be required to provide these remedies; aspiration through the skin has been effective in some situations.

Antimicrobial Management

Antimicrobial agents are an adjunctive measure for therapy of local infection at the incision site. In complicated infections, antimicrobial therapy is as essential as local wound care and drainage of pus from both incision and deeper sites. In both local and complicated infections, the correct therapy depends on the likely microorganisms causing the infection.

First Choice: Therapy Based on Examination of Exudate

The best way to choose therapy is to obtain exudate from the wound (and other sites, if present) and examine a Gram-stained smear of the pus. On the basis of the appearance of the Gram stain, one can establish a likely etiology and choose therapy tailored more specifically to these organisms. Table 1 shows the organisms most likely to be involved in postoperative wound infection, in the order of their occurrence in the NNIS survey. For most of these organism groups, usual drugs and regimens employed are indicated in the table. When gram-negative bacilli are seen on smear,

the likely organisms depend on the type of operation, so initial therapy is chosen on this basis (Table 2). When yeast are seen on the smear, the likelihood is high that *Candida* (most likely *Candida albicans*) is present; however, amphotericin B, the treatment of choice, is so toxic that therapy usually is withheld pending further documentation of disseminated candidal infection. However, such delay may be unwise if the patient has severely compromised host defenses.

Second Choice: Antimicrobial Therapy Based on Type of Operation

In some circumstances it will not be possible to obtain material from the wound to assess likely organisms, or the material obtained may not provide helpful information. In these cases one must make an empiric choice of antimicrobial agents on the basis of the type of operation performed. The organisms involved are most likely to be those present or adjacent to the sites opened during surgery or those introduced by trauma.

Infecting organisms vary greatly according to the site of the procedure. In "clean" operations, in which sites of endogenous flora have not been entered, *Staphylococcus aureus* is the most likely cause of infection. By contrast, operations involving areas with endogenous flora are likely to have multiple organisms at the site of postoperative infection.

Table 2 presents usual guidelines for therapy for postoperative wound infections based on the operative procedure. These guidelines are drawn from consideration of the likely pathogens in each case.

**TABLE 2   Recommendations for Initial Empiric Therapy for Postoperative Wound Infection,
Based on Type of Surgery Performed**

Gastrointestinal surgery
  Likely pathogens: enteric gram-negative aerobic bacilli, especially *Escherichia coli*, *Proteus mirabilis*, *Klebsiella*; anaerobes, especially
    Bacteroides species resistant to β-lactams; enterococci; group A *Streptococcus* or *Clostridium* (if infection appears in first 24–48 hours
    after surgery)
  Therapy for local infection: regimen A
  Therapy for complicated infection: regimen B or regimen C
  Therapy for onset in first 24–48 hours after surgery: regimen D
Obstetric and gynecologic surgery
  Likely pathogens: gram-negative aerobic bacilli, especially *E. coli, P. mirabilis, Klebsiella;* anaerobes, especially *Bacteroides* species
    resistant to β-lactams; group B *Streptococcus*; group A *Streptococcus* or *Clostridium* (if infection appears in first 24–48 hours after surgery)
  Therapy for local infection: regimen A
  Therapy for complicated infection: regimen B or regimen C
Urologic surgery
  Likely pathogens: Enterobacteriaceae, especially *E. coli, P. mirabilis, Klebsiella*; enterococci;
  Therapy for local infection: regimen E
  Therapy for complicated infection: regimen F
Burn surgery
  Likely pathogens: *Staphylococcus aureus; Pseudomonas aeruginosa*; group A *Streptococcus* (if infection appears in first 24–48 hours after
    surgery)
  Therapy for local infection: no systemic therapy—only topical antibiotics
  Therapy for complicated infection: regimen G
  Therapy for onset in first 24–48 hours after surgery: regimen D
Head and neck surgery
  Likely pathogens: *S. aureus;* oral streptococci; oral anaerobes (including *Bacteroides* species NOT usually resistant to β-lactams)
  Therapy for local infection: regimen M
  Therapy for complicated infection: regimen I
Other surgical procedures
  Likely pathogens: *S. aureus*; coagulase-negative staphylococci; gram-negative aerobic bacilli, especially *E. coli, P. mirabilis, Klebsiella*
    (group A *Streptococcus* or *Clostridium* if infection appears in first 24–48 hours after surgery)
  Therapy for local infection: regimen I
  Therapy for complicated infection: regimen J
  Therapy for onset in first 24–48 hours after surgery: regimen D

Note. This table presents usual guidelines for situations in which therapy must be started before microbiologic information can be obtained from culture or
gram-stain of exudate. Certain diagnostic and epidemiologic factors may make it necessary to modify the recommendations given here (see text). In all cases,
these initial recommendations should be modified when more definitive microbiologic information becomes available.
* Drugs and administration:
  Regimen A: cefoxitin 1 g IV q6h (alternatives: cefotetan, 1 g IV q12h; ceftizoxime 1 g q12h).
  Regimen B: cefoxitin 2 g IV q6h *plus* gentamicin 2 mg/kg IV give slowly over 1 hour once, then 1.5 mg/kg IV give slowly over 1 hour q8h (assuming normal
    renal function). If gentamicin resistance is frequent at institution, give instead amikacin 7.5 mg/kg IV slowly over 1 hour q12h (alternative: clindamycin 900
    mg IV q8h *plus* gentamicin administered as above).
  Regimen C: metronidazole 500 mg IV q8h (assuming normal hepatic insufficiency) *plus* gentamicin 1.5 mg/kg IV given slowly over 1 hour q8h (assuming normal
    renal function). Give metronidazole PO instead of IV as soon as patient tolerates full liquids.
  Regimen D: penicillin G 1 million units IV q4h (alternative: clindamycin 900 mg IV q8h).
  Regimen E: trimethoprim-sulfamethoxazole, one double-strength tablet orally b.i.d. (alternative: ampicillin 1 g IV q4h).
  Regimen F: ampicillin 2 g IV q4h *plus* gentamicin 2 mg/kg IV given slowly over 1 hour once, then 1.5 mg/kg IV given slowly over 1 hour q8h (assuming normal
    renal function). If gentamicin resistance is frequent at institution, give instead amikacin 7.5 mg/kg IV slowly over 1 hour q12h.
  Regimen G: ticarcillin 3 g IV q4h *plus* gentamicin 2 mg/kg IV given slowly over 1 hour once, then 1.5 mg/kg IV give slowly over 1 hour q8h (assuming normal
    renal function). If gentamicin resistance is frequent at institution, give instead amikacin 7.5 mg/kg IV slowly over 1 hour q12h.
  Regimen H: penicillin G 1 million units IV q4h.
  Regimen I: cefazolin 1 g IV q8h.
  Regimen J: cefazolin 2 g IV q8h *plus* gentamicin 2 mg/kg IV given slowly over 1 hour once, then 1.5 mg/kg IV given slowly over 1 hour q8h (assuming normal
    renal function). If gentamicin resistance is frequent at institution, give instead amikacin 7.5 mg/kg IV slowly over 1 hour q12h.

Many other drugs have effective spectra of activity against most of the organisms listed in Tables 1 and 2. However, the use of some is better reserved for situations in which follow-up microbiologic information shows that the organism is resistant to the first-line drug choices listed in the tables. In addition, a number of drugs with pertinent microbiologic spectra (e.g., clavulanic acid and sulbactam combinations, aztreonam, ciprofloxacin) had been approved for general clinical use only recently when this chapter was written. These are deferred from the tables until more information is available about their relative benefit and risk.

The recommendations in Table 2 must be considered as a starting point for the treatment decision. They must be used in light of further diagnostic and epidemiologic fac-tors, which may make it necessary to modify the recommendations given in Table 2. Some of these modifying factors and their impact on the choice of therapy are considered here.

How Long After Operation Did the Infection Occur? The shorter the period, the greater the likelihood that organisms with increased virulence are involved. For example, infection during the first 24 to 48 hours after surgery is likely to be caused by streptococci (usually group A) or clostridia (often those associated with gas gangrene). The clinical presentation of these infections is often as distinct as their time course; the patient becomes rapidly ill and the infection quickly spreads away from the incision site, advancing through many different tissue areas at a fearsome pace. Here, aggressive surgical debridement of the infected and dying tissue is crucial to survival, as is parenteral administration of drugs that will affect both of the likely pathogens. High doses of penicillin G (4 million units intravenously every 4 hours) are appropriate as support for the major step, surgical debridement.

What Perioperative Antimicrobial Prophylaxis (If Any) Was Given? The spectrum of activity of the prophylactic antimicrobial agent may have major impact on the infecting organisms. For example, increasing use of the broad-spectrum β-lactam drugs is thought to be a major factor in the increasing prevalence of enterococci as nosocomial pathogens.

How Long Was the Patient in the Hospital Before Operation? A long preoperative hospitalization increases the chances that the patient has become colonized with nosocomial organisms, which might be more resistant to antibiotics than usual flora acquired in the community.

How Good Are the Patient's Host Defenses? Host defenses ordinarily handle invading microorganisms without problem. In some patients, however, these defenses can be inhibited by the patient's underlying diseases or their therapy (e.g., diabetes mellitus, malnutrition, use of immunosuppressive drugs) or by the presence of a foreign body prosthesis. In such cases, the cause of infection may include less virulent microorganisms than would otherwise be the case. For example, the presence of a hip prosthesis or vascular shunt would increase the likelihood that relatively less virulent organisms like coagulase-negative staphylococci or diphtheroids were involved in the infection.

What Unusual Patterns of Susceptibility Exist in This Hospital? Resistance patterns of nosocomial pathogens vary markedly from place to place, even within the same city. Uncommon patterns of resistance within a given hospital must be taken into account. For example, infections due to *S. aureus* usually can be treated with methicillin or one of several cephalosporins. In a hospital where methicillin-resistant strains of *S. aureus* are common, vancomycin must be the drug of choice whenever this organism is strongly suspected.

What Special Patient Circumstances Influence Drug Choice? Drug allergies, pregnancy, other medications which might interact with the chosen antimicrobial agent— these and similar factors can change the usual guidelines appreciably.

FOLLOW-UP—ASSESSING VALIDITY OF THERAPY CHOICE

In all cases, the initial choice for therapy should be modified when microbiologic information from the various specimens becomes available. Recovery of organisms from wound culture can be especially helpful in evaluating the therapy chosen, either because the organism has a predictable susceptibility pattern or because susceptibility now can be tested. However, two situations must be considered further in evaluating results of wound culture.

First, false-negative wound culture is a possibility. A postoperative wound infection is defined by the presence of purulent exudate at the site of the wound, whether or not a culture of this drainage is positive. There are many factors which can lead to a negative culture result that does not reflect the true etiology of the infection. Some of these are therapy with antimicrobial agents prior to the time that the specimen is taken (especially agents for operative prophylaxis), the presence of pathogens that are not easily grown in culture, and improper specimen collection, transport, or laboratory analysis. For example, anaerobic bacteria cannot usually be recovered from swab or superficial cultures, and most laboratories will not process such specimens for recovery of anaerobes.

In many of these cases in which culture is unsuccessful, the Gram stain of the original exudate will provide important clues to the etiology of the infection, and guide completion of therapy.

Second, false-positive wound culture, i.e., the presence of usual skin flora in exudate cultures, may mislead the prescriber about cause of the infection. Particularly problematic is recovery of coagulase-negative staphylococci from the site of an infection. Coagulase-negative staphylococci can be pathogens in surgical wound infection, especially when prosthetic devices have been implanted or the patient has severely compromised host defenses. In all other cases, isolation of this group of organisms must be regarded with suspicion and treatment given only when the organism is repeatedly recovered in the presence of ongoing infection.

Recovery of possibly pathogenic organisms from culture may represent colonization of the site rather than a true infection, especially when the patient has received perioperative antimicrobial agents and time has elapsed since the procedure. This problem is particularly likely to arise when cultures have been taken from surface or other areas in which endogenous flora are present. Determining whether these organisms should prompt therapy requires consideration of the patient's clinical course.

DURATION OF THERAPY

How quickly the infection resolves determines the duration of therapy. In the usual course of local infection, therapy with parenteral agents should not be needed beyond 2 or 3 days. For complicated infection that resolves uneventfully, intravenous treatment is continued until the patient has been afebrile for 1 to 2 days; then oral therapy is continued for 1 week after the apparent resolution of the process.

SUGGESTED READING

Eiseman B, Stahlgren L, eds. Cost-effective surgical management. Philadelphia: WB Saunders, 1987.

Lubin MF, Walker HK, Smith RB, eds. Medical management of the surgical patient. 2nd ed. Boston: Butterworths, 1988.

Pollock A, Evans M. Surgical infections. Baltimore: Williams and Wilkins, 1987.

SYSTEMIC PROPHYLACTIC ANTIBIOTICS IN SURGERY

JAN V. HIRSCHMANN, M.D.

GENERAL PRINCIPLES

Prophylactic antibiotics can reduce the frequency and the enormous costs of postoperative wound infections in many surgical procedures, but maximal benefit occurs only when certain principles govern their use. For an operation to warrant antimicrobial prophylaxis, the adverse consequences of infection must exceed the costs of the antibiotics used. These costs include not only the price of the drug and its administration, but also those arising from toxic and allergic reactions to the agents, the development of antibiotic-resistant infections, and the effect of widespread antimicrobial use on hospital flora and subsequent nosocomial infections.

To justify the routine administration of prophylatic antibiotics, the surgical procedure must have frequent or extraordinarily severe postoperative infections. Because the risk of wound infections varies considerably according to the type of procedure, operations have been classified into four groups: clean, clean-contaminated, contaminated, and dirty.

Clean procedures constitute about 75 percent of all operations and have an expected wound infection rate of less than 5 percent, in most centers less than 2 percent. By definition, these wounds are nontraumatic, with no break in sterile technique, and no entry into the respiratory, alimentary, or genitourinary tracts. Postoperative wound infections are not only infrequent, but also usually minor, requiring local measures for treatment and no prolonged hospitalization or antimicrobial therapy. The costs of antimicrobial prophylaxis in clean procedures exceed the costs of infectious complications, with one major exception—the insertion of prosthetic devices, such as artificial joints or cardiac valves. The wound infection rate in these operations is higher because, in the presence of these foreign bodies, infection occurs with lower numbers of organisms than usual and with bacteria like *Staphyloccocus epidermidis* that are ordinarily not pathogens. Furthermore, the consequences of infected prostheses are severe: hospitalization is lengthy, antimicrobial therapy is prolonged, and removal of the prosthesis is usually necessary.

Clean-contaminated procedures, constituting 15 percent of all operations, have an expected wound infection rate of 10 percent but in certain procedures it approaches 40 percent. These operations involve entry into the alimentary or respiratory tract, the vagina, or uninfected urinary or biliary tracts. For those procedures where transection occurs across a mucosal surface that normally harbors a teeming population of bacteria, such as the upper airway or the large bowel, the wound infection rate is very high, and prophylaxis is clearly justified.

Contaminated cases, about 5 percent of operative procedures, have a wound infection rate of about 20 percent. Such cases involve fresh trauma, a major break in sterile technique, gross spillage from the gastrointestinal tract, or acute, nonpurulent inflammation.

Dirty operations have a wound infection rate of 30 to 40 percent and involve traumatic wounds with retained, devitalized tissue, foreign bodies, fecal contamination, or delayed treatment. Also included are operations for acute bacterial infections, perforated viscera, or transection of clean tissue to drain pus. Because inflammaton, infection, or severe bacterial contamination are already present at the time of surgery in contaminated or dirty operations, antimicrobial agents function as treatment rather than prophylaxis, and different principles of antibiotic administration apply. Thus, prophylaxis deals with clean and clean-contaminated cases only.

The major discoveries from both experimental and clinical investigations relate to the timing and duration of drug administration. To be effective, prophylactic antibiotics must be present in adequate concentration in the wound tissue concurrent with or only shortly after contamination occurs. Antimicrobial agents begun after this brief "decisive period" fail to prevent wound infections. The practical conclusion is that the prophylactic antibiotic must be given shortly before or during the operation, not afterwards. Postoperative doses alone are ineffective. A second principle is that postoperative doses following preoperative or intraoperative antibiotics are unnecessary. Effective tissue levels of the agent must persist for the duration of contamination, but this contamination ceases at the time of wound closure. Accordingly, for most procedures a single dose of an agent given just before surgery provides adequate coverage. Only for prolonged operations is a second (intraoperative) dose appropriate, and then only if the prophylactic antimicrobial agent has a short half-life.

A third major principle is that the antibiotic chosen for prophylaxis should be active against the major pathogens likely to be encountered in a specific operation. The agent need not be effective against all possible contaminating organisms, but must be able to reduce the number below the level required to cause infection.

Cephalosporins have been especially popular prophylactic agents because of their wide spectrum of activity, infrequent adverse effects, and extensive promotion by drug companies. Most trials have investigated cephalosporins rather than other agents for these reasons. Their efficacy and safety have been impressive. For most surgical procedures, a first-generation cephalosporin is the drug of choice. Because cefazolin has some special advantages, it has emerged as the preferred agent. Unlike cephalothin, it can be given intramuscularly and has the additional benefit of high serum levels and a long half-life. Because cefazolin and other first-generation cephalosporins are inactive against *Bacteroides fragilis,* cefoxitin or cefotetan—second-generation cephalosporins effective against this organism—should be used in colorectal surgery and appendectomies, in which *B. fragilis* is a frequent cause of postoperative infections. Cefotetan has the advantage of a very long half-life, ensuring that a single preoperative dose will suffice, even for protracted operations. For other procedures, however, second-generation cephalosporins have no advantage and are more expensive than cefazolin. Third-generation cephalosporins such as ceftriaxone, ceftazidime, and cefotaxime are inappropriate agents for prophylaxis. They are much more costly, and their

TABLE 1 Systemic Prophylactic Antibiotics in Surgery

Procedure	Recommended Antibiotic	Preoperative Adult Dosage*
Gastroduodenal surgery (high-risk patients only)	Cefazolin	1 g IM or IV
Biliary tract surgery (high-risk patients only)	Cefazolin	1 g IM or IV
Appendectomy	Cefoxitin or cefotetan	1 g IV
Colorectal surgery	Oral: erythromycin and neomycin	1 g each at 1 PM, 2 PM, and 11 PM the day before surgery
	Parenteral: cefoxitin or cefotetan	1 g IV
Open heart surgery	Cefazolin or	1 g IV q4h throughout procedure
	Cefonicid (for prolonged procedure)	1 g IV before surgery
Pacemaker implantation	Cefazolin	1 g IM or IV
Pulmonary resection	Cefazolin	1 g IM or IV
Peripheral vascular surgery (abdominal aortic graft, lower extremity graft through groin incision, amputation for ischemic lower extremity, hemodialysis graft)	Cefazolin	1 g IM or IV
Vaginal or abdominal hysterectomy	Cefazolin	1 g IM or IV
Cesarean section (high-risk patients only)	Cefazolin	1 g IV after cord clamping
Head and neck surgery (incision through oral or pharyngeal mucosa)	Cefazolin	1 g IM or IV
Joint replacement or internal fixation of proximal femoral fracture	Cefazolin	1 g IM or IV

* Single dose except where noted otherwise.

activity against unusual gram-negative bacilli confers no advantage since these organisms are extremely uncommon causes of wound infections following clean and clean-contaminated surgery. Indeed, comparative trials have confirmed that they are not superior to the first- and second-generation cephalosporins for prophylaxis in elective surgery.

PROPHYLAXIS IN SPECIFIC SURGICAL PROCEDURES

Abdominal Surgery

Gastroduodenal

Ordinarily, the stomach and duodenum have a relatively sparse flora of aerobic organisms because the low pH from gastric acidity and the vigorous intestinal motility discourage bacterial growth. With impairment of either of these protective mechanisms, aerobic bacteria, including gram-negative bacilli, flourish, and the wound infection rate, ordinarily negligible in gastroduodenal surgery, rises substantially. The indications for prophylactic antibiotics, therefore, are obstruction; hemorrhage, where blood buffers the acid; gastric ulcer and malignancy, where both acidity and motility decrease; and chronic use of H_2 blockers, such as cimetidine, which markedly reduce acid secretion.

Biliary Tract

The wound infection rate following biliary tract surgery is low unless the bile is infected. Situations in which bile cultures are likely to be positive include common duct obstruction, previous biliary tract surgery, patient age greater than 70 years, and acute cholecystitis. Patients in these circumstances should receive antimicrobial prophylaxis against the likely organisms, usually *Escherichia coli, Klebsiella* species, and various streptococci.

Appendectomy

Agents effective against *B. fragilis* and especially *E. coli* reduce the frequency of wound infections following appendectomy. For patients with a normal or inflamed appendix, a single preoperative or intraoperative dose of cefoxitin or cefotetan suffices; patients with appendiceal perforation or abscess require postoperative antibiotics to eradicate the established infection.

Colorectal

Postoperative wound sepsis is very common following colorectal surgery, even with preceding mechanical bowel preparations using liquid diet, cathartics, and enemas. The commonest infecting organisms are *E. coli* and *B. fragilis.* Oral or parenteral agents active against these bacteria markedly reduce infectious complications. Some regimens have employed nonabsorbable oral agents to reduce the concentration of intraluminal bacteria below that necessary to cause infection when minor spillage of bowel contents occurs; other programs have used parenteral agents to provide effective tissue levels to prevent infection when such contamination develops. The distinction between these two approaches is partly fallacious: oral agents are absorbed in sufficient quantity to yield measurable tissue levels, and parenteral agents, even if given immediately before surgery, reduce the concentration of intraluminal intestinal bacteria.

Oral programs have included an agent effective against coliforms—usually an aminoglycoside such as neomycin or kanamycin—and one active against *B. fragilis* such as erythromycin or metronidazole. Oral doxycycline alone is effective against both types of organisms. Alternatively, a parenteral regimen using cefoxitin, cefotetan, doxycycline, or a combination of an aminoglycoside and clindamycin or metronidazole has also been effective. Whether a combination of oral and parenteral agents together is superior to either alone remains unsettled. A reasonable approach for elective colorectal surgery is a combination of oral erythromycin and neomycin supplemented with a single preoperative dose of cefoxitin or cefotetan. For emergency surgery, bowel obstruction, or other circumstances where the oral route is not feasible, cefoxitin or cefotetan should be used alone in a single dose.

Cardiothoracic Surgery

Valvular

The serious consequences of prosthetic valve endocarditis justify the use of a prophylactic agent effective against the usual causes of this infection: *Staphylococcus aureus, S. epidermidis,* and, less commonly, coliforms. The most important elements in preventing endocarditis and other postoperative infections is to have effective serum levels sustained throughout the operation. Cefazolin given every 4 hours during the procedure is an excellent choice, but cefonicid, with its very long serum half-life, may have a special advantage in protracted cases where a single, preoperative dose would provide satisfactory serum and tissue levels.

Coronary Artery Bypass

Unless there is a concomitant valvular surgery, endocarditis is a rare complication. Sternal wound infections, with the serious potential of sternal osteomyelitis, however, seem to be frequent, and several studies have shown a significant reduction with the use of prophylactic antibiotics. *S. aureus* is the commonest pathogen, but, especially with contaminated or inadequate topical antiseptic preparation of the chest, other organisms can be responsible.

Pacemaker Implantation

Skin flora, usually *S. aureus* or *S. epidermidis,* causes pacemaker pocket infections. Prophylactic antibiotics have reduced their incidence significantly in some studies, but others suggest that they are unnecessary in centers where the infection rate is low.

Noncardiac Thoracic Surgery

Several trials of prophylaxis in noncardiac thoracic surgery have reached conflicting conclusions about its benefit. It is not clear what factors predispose to postoperative infectious complications. A reasonable approach may be to give a first-generation cephalosporin for major lung resection, but its efficacy remains unsettled.

Peripheral Vascular Surgery

Vascular grafts of the abdominal aorta or of the lower extremities through a groin incision have fewer complicating infections with prophylactic antibiotics than without. *S. aureus* is the major pathogen. Surgery of the brachiocephalic vessels requires no prophylaxis, since the incidence of the postoperative infections is very low. Prophylactic antibiotics do, however, reduce the frequency of infections following implantation of vascular grafts for hemodialysis access and after lower extremity amputations for ischemia.

Obstetrical and Gynecologic Surgery

Vaginal Hysterectomy

Prophylactic antibiotics reduce the incidence of febrile morbidity defined as temperatures greater than 38°C on two separate occasions at least 6 hours apart—excluding the first 24 hours following surgery. Studies have employed this criterion because the determination of the presence of a wound infection is so difficult following vaginal hysterectomy. Although there are numerous possible causes of this postoperative fever, infectious complications—urinary tract infections, pelvic cellulitis, vaginal cuff infections, and infected hematoma or abscess—apparently account for most cases. Several antimicrobial agents have been effective in reducing febrile morbidity, but a first-generation cephalosporin enjoys the widest use. The bacteriology of the pelvic infections is predominantly aerobic and anaerobic gram-positive organisms, nonfragilis *Bacteroides* species, and coliforms.

Abdominal Hysterectomy

The preponderance of studies illustrates the value of prophylactic antibiotics in abdominal hysterectomy, although the incidence of febrile morbidity is usually less than in vaginal hysterectomies. The infecting flora appears to be the same.

Cesarean Section

With ruptured membranes at the commencement of labor, the risk of postoperative infection, predominantly endometritis, increases. In these circumstances prophylactic antibiotics significantly reduce infectious complications. To avoid administering antibiotics to the baby, the agent may be given after cord clamping without any diminution in efficacy.

Head and Neck Surgery

Because the saliva contains an abundant flora of aerobic and anaerobic organisms, infections following neck incision through the oral or pharyngeal mucosa are common and usually polymicrobial. The usual bacteria found include streptococci, staphylococci, *Klebsiella* species, anaerobic gram-positive cocci, and nonfragilis *Bacteroides* species. A cephalosporin significantly reduces these infectious complications.

Orthopedic Surgery

Joint Replacement

Skin flora, such as *S. aureus* and *S. epidermidis,* diphtheroids, and *Propionibacterium acnes,* causes the preponderance of infections complicating total joint replacement. Although studies have examined only total hip replacement where prophylactic antistaphylococcal agents significantly reduce deep infections, implantation of any artificial joint seems to warrant antimicrobial prophylaxis.

Hip (Proximal Femoral) Fractures

Proximal femoral fractures repaired by nails, plates, or other orthopedic hardware have a low incidence of postoperative wound infection (5 to 8 percent), but the frequency of these serious infections is significantly reduced by prophylactic antistaphylococcal agents.

Genitourinary Surgery

Prostatectomy

In patients with sterile preoperative urine, the incidence of postoperative bacteriuria following prostatectomy is about 25 percent. Although prophylactic antibiotics can reduce this to less than 5 percent, they do not diminish the frequency of postoperative fever and gram-negative bacillary sepsis. Since postoperative bacteriuria is often asymptomatic and self-limited, prophylactic antibiotics do not seem to be indicated.

Neurosurgery

Several studies have failed to demonstrate any benefit for prophylactic antibiotics in the insertion of ventricular shunts for hydrocephalus. For cranial procedures the information is conflicting, but with spinal surgery the frequency of postoperative infection is too low to justify prophylaxis.

SUGGESTED READING

Antimicrobial prophylaxis in surgery. Med Lett 1987; 29:91–94.

DiPiro JT, Bowden TA, Hooks VA. Prophylactic parenteral cephalosporins in surgery. Are the newer agents better? JAMA 1984; 252:3277–3279.

DiPiro JT, Cheung RPF, Bowden TA, Mansberger JA. Single-dose systemic antibiotic prophylaxis of surgical wound infection. Am J Surg 1986; 152:552–559.

Hirschmann JV, Inui TS. Antimicrobial prophylaxis: a critique of recent trials. Rev Infect Dis 1980: 2:1–23.

INDEX